Peptide and Protein Engineering for Biotechnological and Therapeutic Applications

Peptide and Protein Engineering for Biotechnological and Therapeutic Applications

Pierre Rousselot-Pailley
Aix Marseille Université, France

Olga Iranzo
Aix Marseille Université, France

World Scientific

NEW JERSEY • LONDON • SINGAPORE • BEIJING • SHANGHAI • HONG KONG • TAIPEI • CHENNAI • TOKYO

Published by

World Scientific Publishing Co. Pte. Ltd.
5 Toh Tuck Link, Singapore 596224
USA office: 27 Warren Street, Suite 401-402, Hackensack, NJ 07601
UK office: 57 Shelton Street, Covent Garden, London WC2H 9HE

Library of Congress Cataloging-in-Publication Data
Names: Rousselot-Pailley, Pierre, editor. | Iranzo, Olga, editor.
Title: Peptide and protein engineering for biotechnological and therapeutic applications / [edited by] Pierre Rousselot-Pailley, Olga Iranzo, Aix Marseille Université, France.
Description: New Jersey : World Scientific, [2023] | Includes bibliographical references and index.
Identifiers: LCCN 2022037229 | ISBN 9789811261657 (hardcover) | ISBN 9789811261664 (ebook for institutions) | ISBN 9789811261671 (ebook for individuals)
Subjects: MESH: Protein Engineering--methods | Proteins--therapeutic use | Peptides--therapeutic use | Biotechnology--methods | Biomimetic Materials--therapeutic use
Classification: LCC RS431.P75 | NLM QU 55.95 | DDC 615.1/9--dc23/eng/20220902
LC record available at https://lccn.loc.gov/2022037229

British Library Cataloguing-in-Publication Data
A catalogue record for this book is available from the British Library.

For any available supplementary material, please visit
https://www.worldscientific.com/worldscibooks/10.1142/13005#t=suppl

Desk Editors: Aanand Jayaraman/Yugarani

Typeset by Stallion Press
Email: enquiries@stallionpress.com

https://doi.org/10.1142/9789811261664_fmatter

Preface

Peptides and proteins are crucial biomolecules in life. The manifold functions they carry out range from molecular recognition and signaling to catalysis and immune response. However, the native systems are limited to a reduced toolbox of chemical functionalities as well as tridimensional structures. Scientists quickly realize that widening these toolboxes could indeed pave the way to engineer peptides and proteins with enhanced properties with respect to their native counterparts and/or with structures and functions unprecedented in Nature. This is a great scientific challenge but advances in the chemical and biological synthesis of these biomolecules, in computational tools, in molecular biology and in high-throughput screening are making possible this realm. Additionally, this challenge is fostered by the need to develop tailor-made systems that can outperform Nature and thus fulfill tasks that are required to solve current societal challenges in health, energy and environment.

With the aim of giving an overview of the last developments in the field of peptide and protein engineering, we started writing this book in the second semester of 2018. At the time when the invitations were sent, positive and encouraging replies were obtained from all the authors. However, when the deadline for submission of the contributions was fast approaching, COVID-19 pandemic arrived. This unprecedented worldwide situation affected the schedule of this book to the point that we considered giving up the book project due to several cancellations. This has clearly been a challenging time for all and we are immensely grateful to all who have contributed and finally have made possible the publication of this book.

The book *Peptide and Protein Engineering for Biotechnological and Therapeutic applications* comprises a collection of chapters that cover different chemical and biological approaches to either redesign or create peptides and proteins with desired properties. It starts with the contribution of Surajit *et al.* describing the importance of the configuration of the amide bond and how the *cis* conformation is crucial for the structure and biological function of peptides and proteins. Different families of conformationally constrained building blocks known to stabilize exclusively the *cis* amide bond when incorporated into peptides are nicely described. These units either induce or themselves mimic *β*-turns, important elements of peptide/protein secondary structure. The book continues with two chapters focused on antimicrobial peptides (AMPs) and derivatives. Namely, Maresca *et al.* describe the use of peptides and peptidomimetics as a promising alternative to the conventional antibiotics treatment for Helicobacter pylori infection. Native AMPs obtained from diverse sources (e.g., amphibians, fungi, insects, immune mammal cells) are first presented and subsequently, different families of peptidomimetics are described (e.g., *β*-peptides, peptoids, oligoacyllysines). The chapter by Lafond *et al.* gives a nice overview of antimicrobial Ribosomally synthesized and Post-translationally modified Peptides (RiPPs). After briefly describing each class of RiPPs, the chapter focuses on the sactipeptides and ranthipeptides families. In the following chapter, Novelli and Granja nicely provide an insight into the theoretical and experimental efforts made for the design and synthesis of self-assembling cyclic peptide nanotubes (SCPNs) with special attention on their dynamic behavior. Additionally, they reviewed recent advances in developing multi-responsive hybrid self-assemblies and bioactive materials with applications in biology, chemistry, and materials science. The contribution by Satriano *et al.* gives an overview of the classification and properties of protein and peptide-based nanomaterials used in the field of nanomedicine. Excitingly this review highlights the opportunities for the use of these hybrid peptide/protein nanomaterials as effective scaffolds for tissue engineering, biosensors, drug delivery and theranostic systems.

Next, Delsuc *et al.* describe the different protein- and peptide-based strategies developed so far to engineer mimics of glutathione peroxidase (GPx), an important enzyme that plays an essential role in the redox homeostasis by controlling the levels of hydroperoxides. The review emphasizes the need to develop new GPx mimics with enhanced stability and efficacy in tissues and cells. The following chapter by Vázquez *et al.*

gives an overview of artificial metallopeptides designed to selectively recognize different DNA secondary structures (i.e., regular B-DNA, three-way junctions, G-quadruplex). Although challenging, these designed systems search for a synergistic action of both units, the peptide and metal complex, in recognizing their DNA target. Additionally, achieving (intra)cellular targeting and internalization are highlighted as added-value features that will foster the development of these systems beyond the merely academic setting. The chapter by Odaert *et al.* deals with the use of high-field 3D NMR spectroscopy for the determination of the tridimensional structure of the Extracellular Domain of the Death Receptor 5 (DR5-ED). Death Receptors selectively drive cancer cells to apoptosis upon binding to the Tumor necrosis factor-a-Related Apoptosis-Inducing Ligand (TRAIL). The data reported will enable binding experiments with TRAIL peptidomimetics. In the following chapter, using CALB (lipase B of *Candida antarctica*) and TAP (thioesterase of *Escherichia coli*) enzymes as models, Pleiss and Carvalho report on the importance of modeling by unbiased molecular dynamics simulations the binding free energy profiles of enzymes at different substrate concentrations. The described methodology is a valuable predictive tool for enzyme engineering and bioprocess design since can allow the identification and removal of kinetic bottlenecks.

Three more chapters are finally presented which are dedicated to the development of artificial metalloenzymes. Lombardi *et al.* provide a review covering recent advances in the design of peptide-based artificial metalloenzymes. The chapter highlights the advantages of using peptides as scaffolds to host and fine-tune different metal-ion binding sites, namely hemes and metalloporphyrins as well as mononuclear and dinuclear metal sites, and how these systems successfully carry out natural enzymatic as well as abiotic transformations. Next, Onoda and Hayashi report on biohybrid catalysts developed in their group by incorporating various transition metal complexes into the β-barrel nitrobindin protein. The chapter concludes by describing an affinity purification system based on a maltose-binding protein-tag that has allowed the development of a reliable platform for high-throughput screening and thus, for the directed evolution of their biohybrid catalysts. Finally, the contribution by Mahy *et al.* focuses on recent strategies that have allowed the production of artificial metalloenzymes capable of catalyzing abiotic reactions in living cells, among them olefin metathesis, polymerization of phenylacetylene, allylic deallylations, nitrene and carbene transfer reactions and Diels–Alder reactions. A wide range of applications in the fields of green chemistry, biotechnology, health, and environment are foreseen for these systems in near future.

The chapters summarized above span from simple building blocks production and peptidic scaffolds of different sizes and structures to more complex systems including enzymes and artificial metalloenzymes. Different strategies that combine both chemical and biological tools have been developed to access the desired properties and thus attain the sought functionalities. This is an expanding field that will afford functional biomolecules and hybrid systems capable of addressing key societal challenges of our times in relevant areas such as health, environment and energy.

Pierre Rousselot-Pailley and *Olga Iranzo*

https://doi.org/10.1142/9789811261664_fmatter

Contents

https://doi.org/10.1142/9789811261664_0001

Chapter 1

Cis-Amide Stabilizing Proline Analogs: Synthesis and Applications

Isita Banerjee, Indranil Duttagupta, Abhishek Gupta, and Surajit Sinha*

School of Applied and Interdisciplinary Sciences, Indian Association for the Cultivation of Science, Jadavpur, Kolkata, India

**ocss5@iacs.res.in*

1. Introduction

Redesigning natural peptide sequence in order to achieve desired structure and function has immensely helped in developing a new class of therapeutic peptides with enhanced bioactivity and stability. These modifications are often imparted by the introduction of tailor-made non-proteinogenic amino acids for desired properties and function. Recent advances in the synthesis of artificial amino acids have enormously boosted the research in this field [1].

Introduction of cyclic amino acids with limited conformational space is an effective approach for structural modification of peptides and proteins. The cyclic nature of the unique amino acid proline places major constrains on the ϕ, ψ, and ω dihedral angles of the polypeptide backbone and introduces a complete 180° turn in the direction of the peptide chain, defined as the β-turn. One special type of VI-β turn is observed in the case of proline with a *cis* amide bond. Consequently, the inclusion of a proline or a modified proline residue in the sequence of a peptide or protein is expected to result in unique conformational properties.

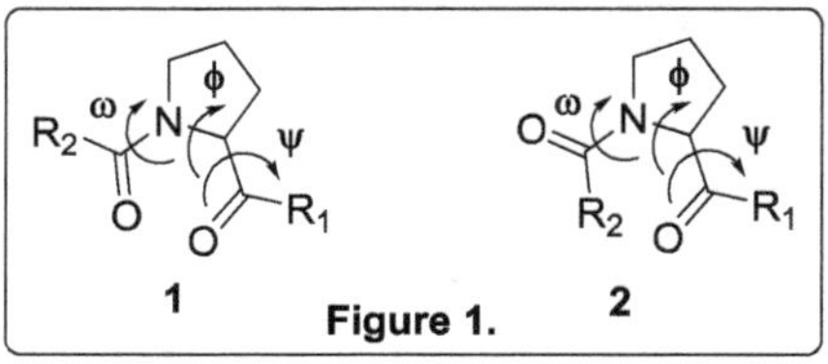

Figure 1.

In peptides, amide bonds are mostly found in their thermodynamically more stable *trans* conformation (**1**, Figure 1: *Trans* and *Cis* conformations of amide bonds preceding proline), [2] although, the thermodynamically less stable *cis* conformation (**2**, Figure 1) is also observed in proteins (~0.03–0.05% of non-proline *cis* amide bonds), [3] primarily due to the steric demands of the preceding or succeeding amino acids in the sequence [4]. On the other hand, the amide bond preceding the proline has a higher propensity of *cis* conformation (~10%). As a result, conformationally constrained amino acids are a crucial target for backbone modification in order to stabilize the *cis* conformer in proteins and peptides.

Over the years, numerous groups have reported *cis*-inducing artificial amino acids most of which are covalent modifications of the proline motif [5,6] These classes of molecules may bear a resemblance in ring size or structure and at the same time contain heteroatoms or alkyl groups embedded in order to impart the requisite steric or thermodynamic demand for a *cis* stabilized structure.

2. Importance of *cis* Peptide Bonds

The configuration of the amide bond in a peptide is central to the nature of the secondary structure that the protein backbone can adopt. *Cis/trans* isomerization of these bonds is known to play a crucial role in protein folding, transmembrane active transport, splicing, and cell signaling [7]. Although rare in occurrence, *cis* peptide bonds are crucial in a variety of biological processes mostly because of their presence near the active sites of enzymes such as in β-lactamase (Glu166–Ile167), dihydrofolate reductase (Gly98–Gly99), carboxypeptidase (Ser197–Tyr198 and Arg272–Asp273), and *N*-carbamoylsarcosine amidohydrolase (Ala172–Thr173) [8]. Similarly, in the case of Ribonuclease A, residues 103 to 124 form a β-sheet structure with a type VI-β-bend containing a *cis* peptide bond at Asn^{113}–Pro^{114} [9]. Naturally, the *trans-cis* isomerization of proline-containing amide is catalyzed by the peptidyl prolyl isomerases (PPIases). This process sometimes acts as a timer to help control the amplitude and duration of a cellular process [10,11]. Additionally, recent research has demonstrated the importance of *cis* proline in the proper functioning of numerous proteins responsible for routine biological activities [12–14].

3. *Cis*-Inducing Amino Acids

The development of building blocks that ensure a *cis* conformation when incorporated into a peptide structure has not only helped in addressing countless questions regarding the structure and functioning of proteins but also has facilitated the development of therapeutic peptides with enhanced stability and bioactivity. Accordingly, the conformational properties of a wide number of synthetic proline derivatives have been reported. These compounds were obtained by: (a) incorporating a substituent at the α-carbon [15–17]; (b) replacing α-carbon by "nitrogen" [18] in the pyrrolidine ring, [19,20]; (c) altering the chemical nature of the pyrrolidine ring either by changing the ring size, [21] or replacing a carbon atom by a heteroatom, [22,23]; and (d) incorporating an intracyclic double bond [24]. However, in these cases, only 15–20% *cis* amide bond is observed. Bulkier substitution like methyl (Me) either at the α-carbon or 3- or 4-position did not improve the conformational changes.

3.1. *Proline analogs*

Herein, we discuss the proline analogs which are known to stabilize the *cis* amide bond exclusively.

3.1.1. *Pseudoprolines*

Pseudoprolines (ψ-Pro) (**3**, Figure 2: Pseudoprolines) are synthetic proline analogs originally developed to assist in structure-disruption and solubilization in solid-phase peptide synthesis [25–27]. Synthetically, these are readily accessed by cyclocondensation of the amino acids with a side chain thiol or hydroxyl functionality (cysteine, threonine, or serine) with aldehydes or ketones [28]. Extensive conformational investigations concerning the ψ-Pro preceding peptide bond led to the development of 2,2-dimethylated thiazolidine class

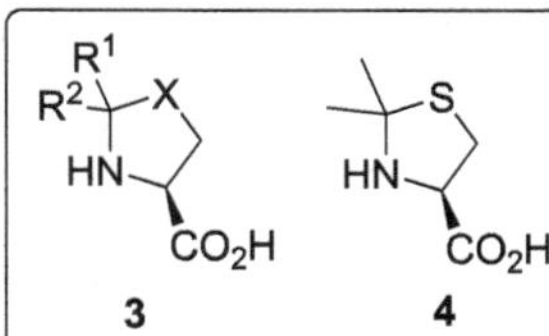

Figure 2.

of compounds which, unlike other pseudoprolines, could induce up to 100% *cis* conformation in the preceding peptide bond in model di- and tripeptides [29,30]. The 2,2-Dimethyl-1,3-thiazolidine-4-carboxylic acid (**4**) was synthesized by the condensation of cysteine with acetone (Scheme 1(a)) [31]. Being sterically demanding, this pseudoproline analog is not directly introduced in the sequence as a single unit but rather as a dipeptide unit [25–27] (**5**) to achieve the desired conformational effect (Scheme 1(b)).

The efficacy of thiazolidine-based pseudoproline in inducing *cis* conformation in peptides has been unambiguously proved [32] and exploited in order to design bioactive peptides and aid in the formation of macrocyclic peptides [33]. Mutter *et al.* reported the 2,2-dimethylated thiazolidine derivative of V3 loop of HIV-1 with the sequence cyclo(-Arg-His-Ile-Gly-Xaa-Gly-Arg-Ala-Phe-Cys-Tyr-) which exclusively adopted a *cis* conformation [34]. Schiller *et al.* reported the ψ-Pro analogs of Morphiceptin and Endomorphin-2 with excellent μ-opioid agonistic activity in the nanomolar range. The studies validated the importance of cisoid conformation around the Tyr-Pro amide for the opioid activity of these Morphiceptin analogs [35]. ψ-Pro analogs have also been successfully used as a turn-inducing element for solution-phase head-to-tail cyclization reactions of side chain-protected linear peptides [36–42].

3.1.2. *5,5-Dimethylproline*

Scheraga *et al.* [43] reported that the substituted proline, 5,5-dimethylproline (dmP, **6**, Figure 3: 5,5-dimethyl proline (dmP)), has the ability to

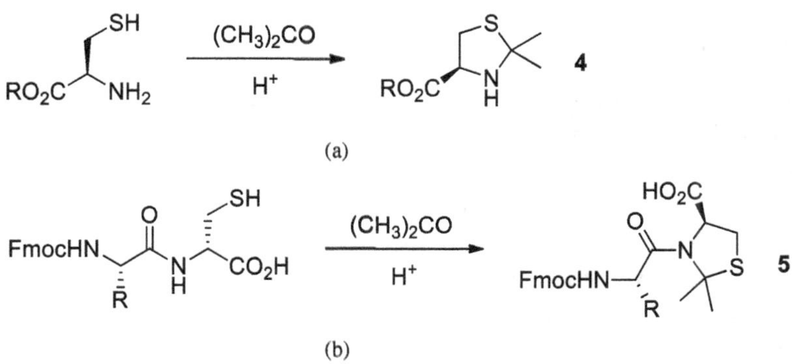

Scheme 1. Synthesis of (a) 2,2-dimethyl-1,3-thiazolidine-4-carboxylic acid 4 and (b) dipeptide analogs of ψ-Pro.

impart *cis* conformation when incorporated into the synthetic protein bovine pancreatic ribonuclease A (RNase A). Moore *et al.* [44] first reported the convenient synthesis of dmP using commercially available 5,5-dimethylpyrroline-l-oxide. Treatment of compound **7** with KCN in the presence of hydrochloric acid afforded **8** which was immediately reduced to racemic **6** by catalytic hydrogenation (Scheme 2). Following the sequence of residues in RNase A, this group reported the synthesis of the tripeptides Ac-Tyr-dmP-Asn (YdmPN) and Ac-Asn-dmP-Tyr (NdmPY). NMR study revealed that these analogs solely exist in *cis* conformation. This conformational preference arises from the steric interactions of two methyl groups at the δ-carbon atom of dmP with the preceding residue.

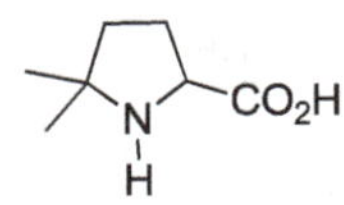

6, Figure 3.

3.2. *Aromatic amino acids*

3.2.1. *1,5-disubstituted tetrazole*

The tetrazole ring system as an alternate means of mimicking the *cis* configuration of a peptide bond was initially conceptualized by Marshall *et al.* [45] The synthesis of such 1,5-disubstituted tetrazole ($\psi[CN_4]$) (**9**, Figure 4: 1,5-disubstituted tetrazoles) and their use as *cis* peptide bond mimic were first described by R. L. Johnson *et al.* [46] Starting from a dipeptide (**10**) the corresponding imidoyl chloride (**11**) was generated which was then converted to the corresponding $\psi[CN_4]$ (**12**) using hydrazoic acid with some degree of racemization (Scheme 3).

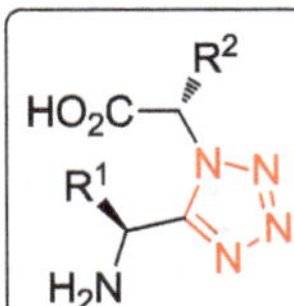

9, Figure 4.

The resulting tetrazole system (**12**) was reported to readily undergo racemization at the α-carbon of C-terminal when treated with base, hence

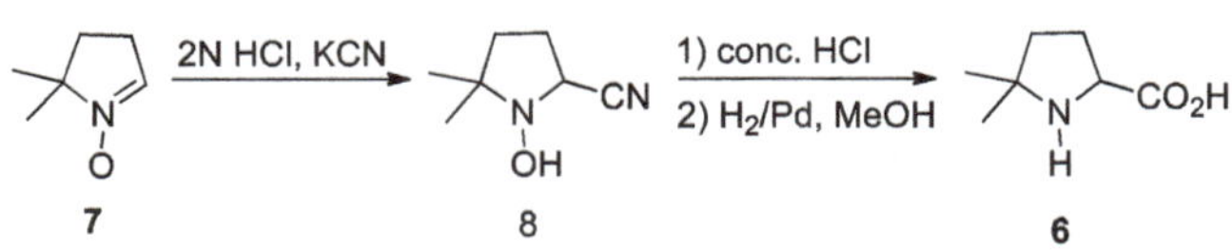

Scheme 2. Synthesis of 5,5- dimethlyproline 6.

their synthetic utility in peptide synthesis remained limited until Marshall *et al.* [47] developed the synthetic protocol to generate the ψ[CN_4] (**13**) with substantial diastereo purity and its incorporation into larger peptides using mixed anhydride protocol (Scheme 4).

The ability of the 1,5-disubstituted tetrazole-based peptide bond mimic to adopt a cisoid conformation was confirmed by comparing the biological activity of naturally occurring peptides with a known *cis* amide bond to that of the ψ[CN_4] containing analog [45,46,48–50] and using X-ray crystallography [51].

3.2.2. *N-methyl-α-benzyl-o-aminomethylphenylacetic acid* (14)

G. Van Binst *et al.* reported a *cis* peptide bond mimic derived from 2-aminomethylphenylacetic acid. The synthesis consisted in the *N* and *C*-methylation of 2-(Boc-aminomethyl)phenylacetic acid (**15**) in order to prevent the *δ*-turn stabilizing H-bond formation, and subsequent introduction of a phenyl side chain at the *α*-position of the carboxyl group by alkylation (Scheme 5) [52].

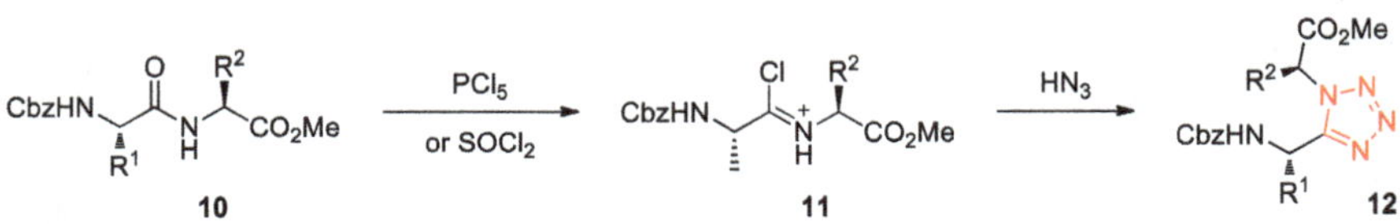

Scheme 3. Synthesis of tetrazole dipeptides.

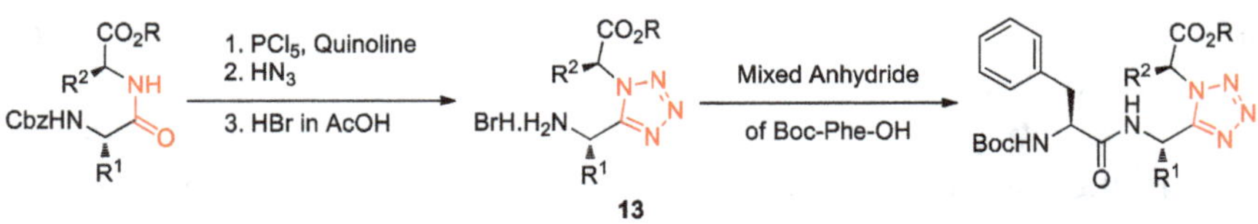

Scheme 4. Synthesis and peptide coupling with ψ[CN_4].

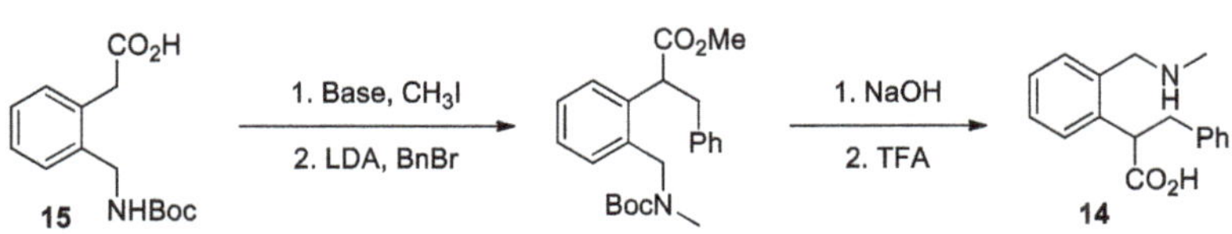

Scheme 5. Synthesis of *N*-methyl-*α* -benzyl-o-aminomethylphenylacetic acid 14.

The group synthesized cyclic somatostatin analogs using their *cis* peptide bond mimic, which were structurally similar to synthetic somatostatin analog (SMS 201–995) [53]. Comparable bioactivity of both SMS 201–995 and its *N*-Me-*α*-Bzl-*o*-AMPA (**14**)-containing analog confirmed its capacity as an effective dipeptide mimic for a *cis* peptide bond.

3.2.3. *1,2-disubstituted pyrroles*

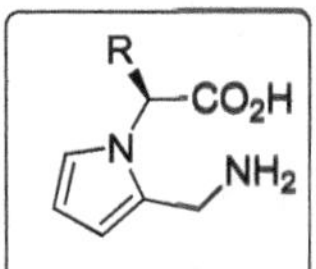

16, Figure 5.

Building on the concept of 1,5-disubstituted tetrazole (ψ[CN_4]) (**12**) and following a similar design, Jamieson *et al.* reported the synthesis of 1,2-disubstituted pyrrole (ψ[C_4N]) type dipeptide surrogates as *cis* amide mimics (**16**, Figure 5: 1,2 Disubstituted pyrrole containing amino acid) [54]. Starting from 2,5-dimethoxytetrahydrofuran, the synthesis of Gly-X (ψ[C_4N]) (**16**) was completed in four steps for amino acids containing a side chain. The condensation of 1,4-dimethoxytetrahydrofuran with amino acid methyl ester hydrochloride yielded the 1-substituted pyrrole (**17**). Formylation of **17** followed by ester hydrolysis and reductive amination generated the (ψ[C_4N]) **16** (Scheme 6). The glycine analog was synthesized from pyrrole-2-carboxaldehyde by alkylation with bromoacetic acid.

3.3. *Lactam-based cis inducer*

3.3.1. *(L,L)-3-amino-Z-piperidone-6-carboxylic acid* (18)

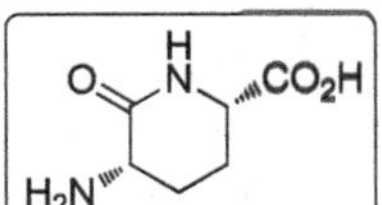

L,L-Acp, 18, Figure 6.

D.S. Kemp *et al.* reported the lactam-based *β*-turn inducer L,L-3-amino-*Z*-piperidone-6-carboxylic acid (L,L-Acp, **18**, Figure 6: (L,L)-3-amino-Z-piperidone-6-carboxylic acid) [55]. The group reported its stereoselective synthesis starting from *N*-carbobenzoxy-*O*-*tert*-butyl-L-serine. The oxidation of the side chain hydroxyl (to yield **19**) followed by dicyclohexylcarbodiimide-mediated coupling with *L*-homoserine lactone yielded the dipeptide (**20**), which on *N*-carbobenzoxy deprotection underwent *in situ* lactamization to yield the corresponding diketopiperazine (**21**). The side chain alcohol of

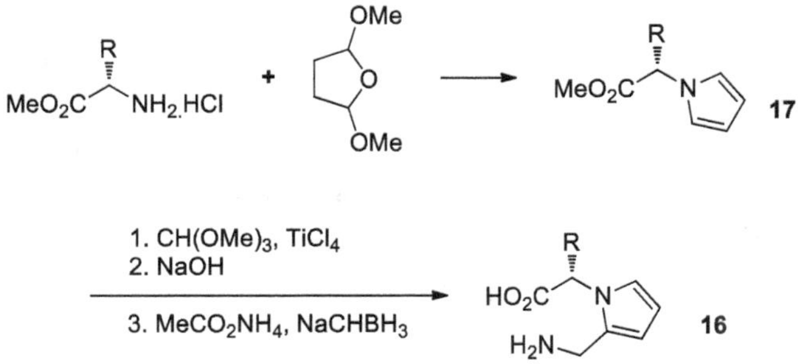

Scheme 6. Synthesis of ψ[C$_4$N] 16.

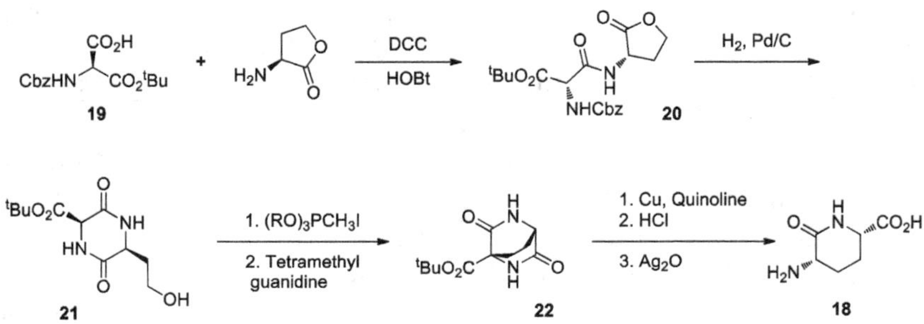

Scheme 7. Synthesis of L,L-Acp 18.

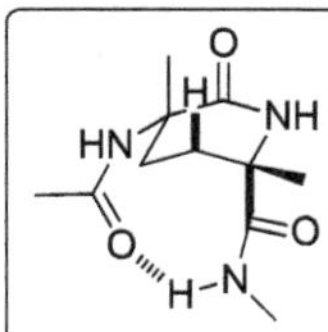

22, Figure 7.

diketopiperazine on iodination followed by an S_N2 reaction with the enolate generated from the 1,3-dicarbonyl system yielded the bicyclic diketopiperazine (**22**). Copper-mediated decarboxylation followed by lactam hydrolysis generated the desired L,L-Acp (**18**) with acceptable diastereo purity (Scheme 7).

In a preceding publication, [56] the group rationalized the *β*-turn-inducing capacity of L,L-Acp using simple amides, dipeptides and tripeptides. The chair conformation (**22**, Figure 7: Chair conformation of piperidone ring of Acp residue enforces the *Cis* amide confirmation.) of the piperidone of the Acp residue, with H^b and H^d in axial and equatorial positions, respectively, enforces a turn conformation on peptides containing the Acp residues.

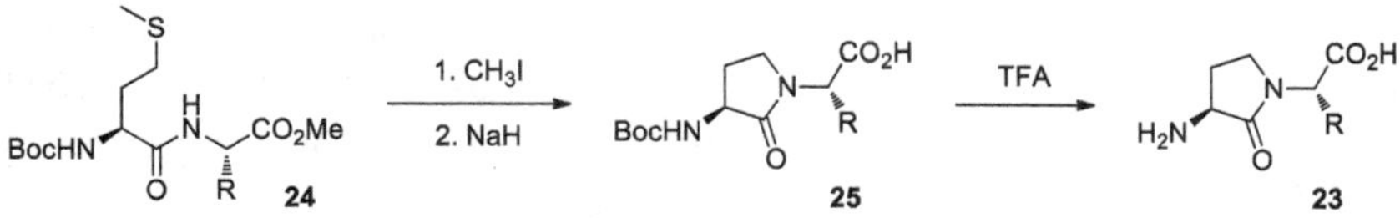

Scheme 8. Synthesis of γ-lactam 23.

3.3.2. *γ-lactams*

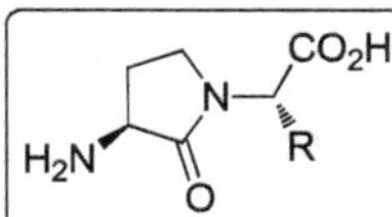

23, Figure 8.

Freidinger *et al.* reported a five-membered lactam-based β-turn mimic (**23**, Figure 8: γ-lactam based amino acids) [57]. Computational analysis assisted in the design and hinted towards the ability of this dipeptide mimic to stabilize a backbone conformation similar to an ideal type II β-turn. The γ-lactam was synthesized from the S-methylated protected dipeptide (**24**) in two steps. The protected dipeptide (**24**) was converted to a sulfonium salt using methyl iodide followed by a stereospecific cyclization to the lactam (**25**) using sodium hydride. *N*-Boc deprotection yielded the γ-lactam (23, Scheme 8). The β-turn mimic could be introduced into peptide sequence using standard peptide coupling protocols.

Freidinger *et al.* [58,59] and other groups [60,61] synthesized several analogs of bioactive peptides using their β-turn mimic, which were similar to the original bioactive peptides both structurally and in terms of bioactivity confirming its capacity as an effective mimic for a *cis* peptide bond. The same group later reported the synthesis of other similar δ and ε lactams using a very similar protocol [62].

3.3.3. *Bicyclic lactams*

3.3.3.1. 2(*S*)-2,3,4,4a,7,7a-hexahydro-6-oxo-5*H*-pyrano [2,3-b]-pyrrole (26)

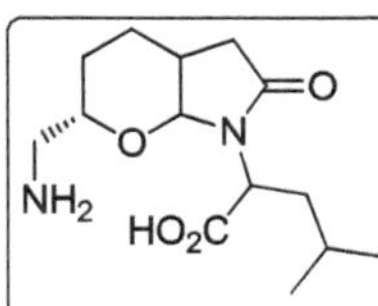

26, Figure 9

B. L. Currie *et al.* first conceptualized and reported this class of β-turn mimic. Based on conformational calculations on projected dihedral angles of enkephalin and its analog, 2(*S*)-2,3,4,4a,7,7a-hexahydro-6-oxo-5*H*-pyrano [2,3-b]-pyrrole (**26**, Figure 9:

Bicyclic lactam amino acid, 2(*S*)-2,3,4,4a,7,7a-hexahydro-6-oxo-5*H*-pyrano [2,3-b]-pyrrole) was chosen as the most suitable mimic [63]. Synthesis of **26** from the pthalimido compound (**27**) was reported by the same group in a succeeding publication. The pthalimido compound (**27**) upon Rhodium (II)-catalyzed cyclopropanation with diazoethyl-acetate gave the cyclopropane ester (**28**). Acid hydrolysis of (**28**) generated the lactone (**29**) which was then converted to the corresponding bicyclic lactam (**30**) using methanolic ammonia. *N*-alkylation of **30** with 2-bromo-4-methylpentanoate produced the protected *β*-turn mimic **31** (Scheme 9) [64]. The same group published later a better protocol for accessing the mimic in better yields [65]. An extensive study of the *β*-turn-inducing capacity in enkephalin analogs was also performed using NMR spectroscopy and molecular modelling studies [66].

3.3.3.2. (3S, 6S, 9R)-2-oxo-3-amino-7-thia-l-azabicyclo[4.3.0] nonane-9-carboxylic acid (32)

Nagai *et al.* reported a similar bicyclic lactam-based *β*-turn mimic which bore resemblance to that of the mimic reported by B. L. Currie [63]. Molecular modelling studies revealed that the proposed compound **32** Figure 10: Bicyclic lactam-based dipeptide having a thiazolidine ring) has almost superimposable conformation with that of D-Ala-L-Pro residues in [D-Ala[4,4']]-gramicidin S (GS), which is known to be type II' *β*-turn [67,68]. Encouraged by these results, the group proceeded to synthesize the protected **32**, Figure 10: Bicyclic lactam-based

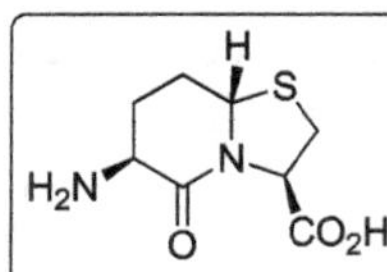

32, Figure 10

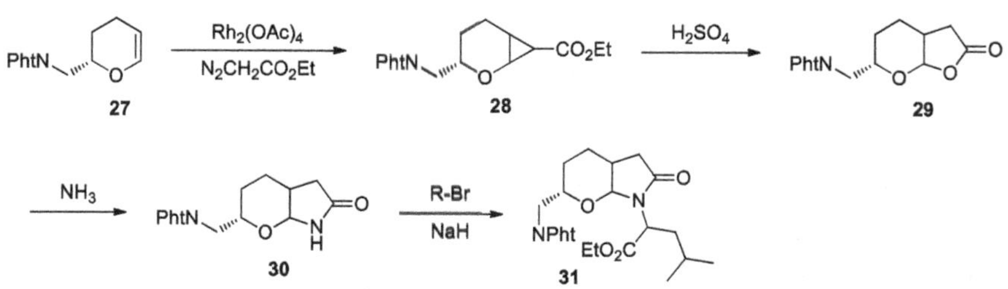

Scheme 9. Synthesis of protected 2(S)-2,3,4,4a,7,7a-hexahydro-6-oxo-5H-pyrano-[2,3-b]-pyrrole, 31.

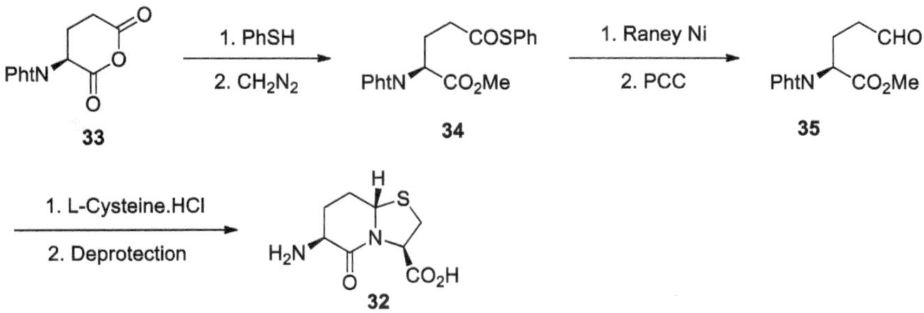

Scheme 10. Synthesis of β-turn mimic 32.

dipeptide having a thiazolidine ring) The anhydride of N-phthalyl-L-glutamic anhydride (**33**) was opened with thiophenol in the presence of dicyclohexylamine followed by esterification with diazomethane to yield (**34**). The compound **34** was then converted to the aldehyde **35** using Raney-nickel, followed by oxidation with pyridinium chlorochromate (PCC). The reaction of the aldehyde **35** with L-cysteine hydrochloride in aqueous ethanol containing sodium acetate followed by heating generated thiazolidine compound **32** (Scheme 10).

In order to confirm the ability of the bicyclic dipeptide skeleton to adopt a β-turn, the group synthesized the lactam analog of Dnp-Gly-D-Ala-L-Pro-Gly-pNA, a peptide known to predominantly adopt a type II' β-turn [69]. The CD spectrum of both peptides in MeOH resembled closely indicating a type II' β-turn in both cases. Later investigations further elaborated on the ability of the bicyclic dipeptide skeleton (**32**) to impart a β-turn into peptides [70–72]. W. D. Lubell *et al.* [73] and J. E. Baldwin *et al.* [74] later reported the synthesis of structurally similar analogs.

3.3.3.3. (6R, 8a R)-6-amino-5-oxohexahydroindolizine-8a (1H)-carboxylic acid (36)

J. P. Germanas *et al.* and J. A. Robinson *et al.* almost simultaneously reported the synthesis of a bicyclic lactam-based β-turn mimic **36** (Figure 11: (6R, 8a R)-6-amino-5-oxohexahydroindolizine-8a (1H)-carboxylic acid) utilizing two different methodologies. Both synthetic methods utilized amine and carboxylate protected (R)-allylproline as

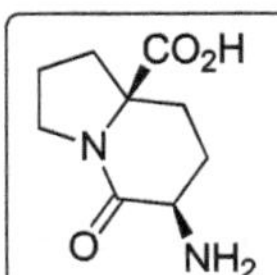

36, Figure 11.

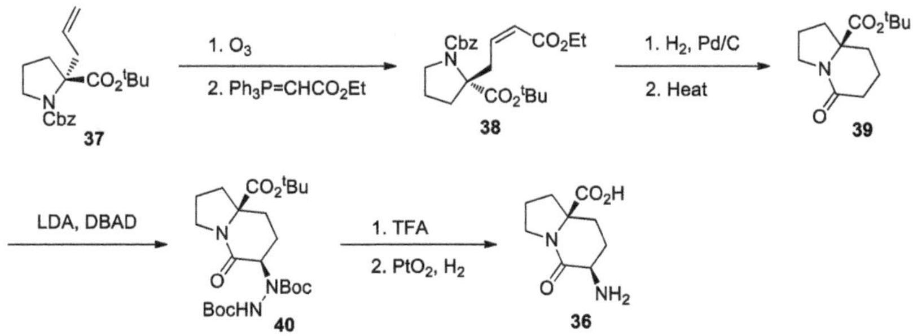

Scheme 11. Synthesis of β-turn mimic 36.

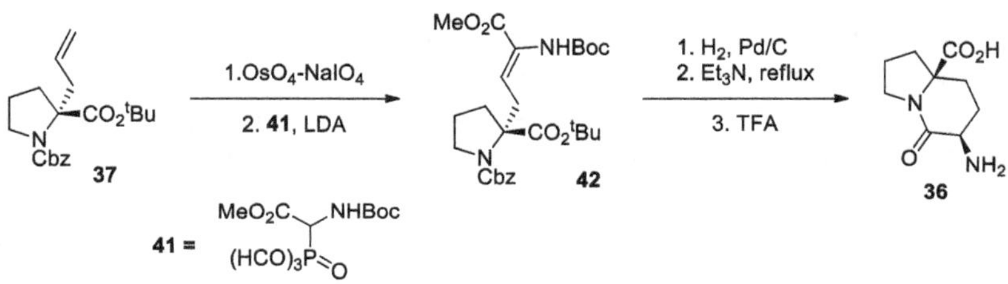

Scheme 12. Synthesis of β-turn mimic 36.

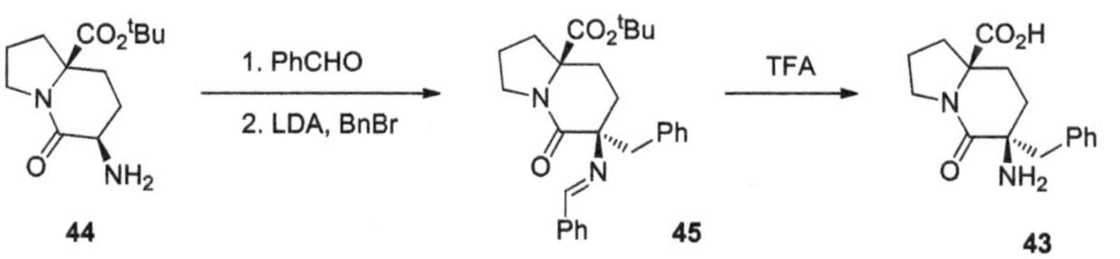

Scheme 13. Synthesis of β-turn mimic 43.

the starting material. J. A. Robinson *et al.* used ozone for the oxidative cleavage of the double bond of **37** followed by a Wittig reaction that yielded the α,β unsaturated ester **38,** which on hydrogenolysis and heating in toluene produced the bicyclic lactam **36**. Lithium enolate of the lactam **39** on treatment with di-*tert*-butyl-azodicarboxylate (DBAD) generated the azo-lactam intermediate **40**. Compound **40** on *tert* butyl deprotection followed by Platinum dioxide (PtO_2)-mediated reductive deamination generated the target β-turn mimic **36** (Scheme 11) [75].

J. P. Germanas *et al.* subjected the protected (R)-allylproline **37** to osmium tetroxide-metaperiodate-mediated oxidative cleavage. The resulting aldehyde was subjected to a Horner–Wadsworth–Emmons reaction with phosphonate **41** to yield the *α,β* unsaturated ester **42**. The compound **42** on hydrogenolysis followed by lactamization in refluxing triethyl amine and subsequent deprotection generated the target *β*-turn mimic **36** (Scheme 12) [76,77].

J. A. Robinson *et al.* reported later a better version of his previously described *β*-turn mimic **36** by introducing an additional benzyl group adjacent to the amine functionality (**43**) [75]. Introduction of the benzylic functionality utilizing enolate chemistry (Scheme 13) helped in better rigidity of the imparted *β*-turn, which was proved by comparing the bioactivity of the *β*-turn mimic-containing somatostatin analog to that of the authentic peptide [78].

3.4. *Azo-containing β-turn mimics*

3.4.1. *2-((1R,9R)-9-((R)-amino(phenyl)methyl)-6,10-dioxo-1,4,7,8,9,10-hexahydro-6H-pyridazino[1,2-a][1,2]diazepin-1-yl) acetic acid (46)*

Kahn *et al.* [79,80] introduced **46** (Figure 12: 2-((1R,9R)-9-((R)-amino(phenyl)methyl)-6,10-dioxo-1,4,7,8,9,10-hexahydro-6H-pyridazino[1,2-a][1,2]diazepin-1-yl) acetic acid) as a *β*-turn mimic and accomplished the synthesis using an intramolecular hetero Diels-Alder reaction as a key step.

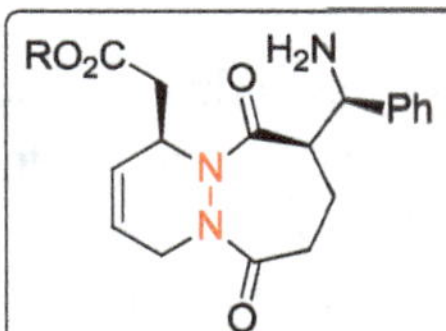

46, Figure 12.

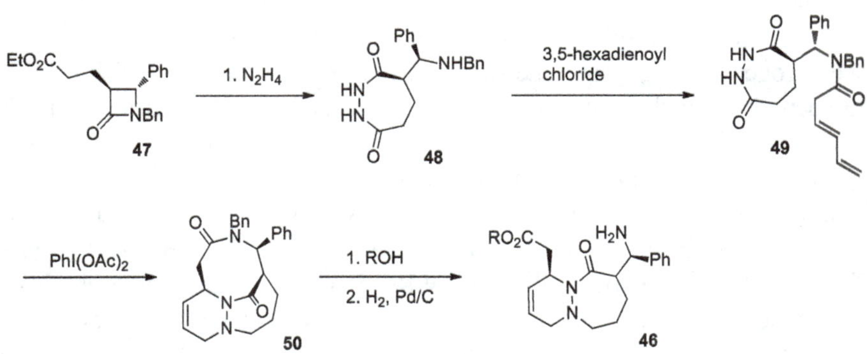

Scheme 14. Synthesis of *β*-turn mimic 46.

The structure of the mimic **46** comprised an aza-bridged 6-7 fused bicyclic di-lactam system that resembled the previously discussed bicyclic lactams (Section 3.3) to some extent. The benzyl-protected trans β-lactam **47** on treatment with hydrazine in refluxing methanol yielded the 7-membered diacylhydrazide **48,** which on acylation with 3,5-hexadienoylchloride provided the intermediate **49**. Compound **49** on *N-N* bond oxidation with iodosobenzene diacetate generated the requisite dienophile that undergoes an extremely facile intramolecular hetero Diels–Alder reaction to yield the tricyclic compound **50**. Compound **50** yielded the β-turn mimic **46** on methanolysis or by treating with amino acid methyl ester (Scheme 14).

The same group later reported the synthesis of peptide analogs of the β-turn mimic **46** using solid phase methodology [81] to design β-turn-containing inhibitors of thrombin [82–84].

3.4.2. *3-Pyrazolidine carboxylic acid* (*Delta-azaproline*) (51)

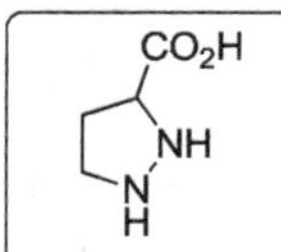

51, Figure 13.

Recently, Sinha *et al.* and Jamart-Grégoire *et al.* reported the synthesis and use of δ-azaproline **51** (Figure 13: 3-Pyrazolidine carboxylic acid (δ-azaproline) as a β-turn enforcer when incorporated into peptides. Being structurally closest to proline (compared to other proline mimetics), it has the potential for wider applications in the field of peptide research. Sinha *et al.* [85,86] subjected diethyl allylmalonate to electrophilic amination to yield the azo-containing diethyl allylmalonate **52**. The compound **52** on decarboxylation followed by diazomethane-mediated esterification yielded the advanced precursor **53**. Osmium tetroxide-metaperiodate-mediated oxidative cleavage of **53** yielded the aldehyde **54,** which upon reductive cyclization and deprotection generated the δ-azaproline (Scheme 15(a)). The difference in reactivity of the two nitrogen of the δ-azaproline was utilized to incorporate the proline mimic into peptides in both the δ-protected and deprotected forms (Scheme 15(b)).

Jamart-Grégoire *et al.* [87] synthesized δ-azaproline **51** from (*R*)-α-hydroxy-γ-butyrolactone by using Mitsunobu reaction as the key step. Namely, the hydroxy group in (*R*)-α-hydroxy-γ-butyrolactone was replaced by N-benzyloxycarbonylamino-phthalimide to yield **57**. Phthalimide deprotection followed by Boc protection and lactone hydrolysis generated the precursor **58**. This precursor on esterification followed by cyclization using another Mitsunobu reaction yielded the protected δ-aza- proline **59**. The protecting groups in **59** were removed to yield the δ-azaproline **51** (Scheme 16).

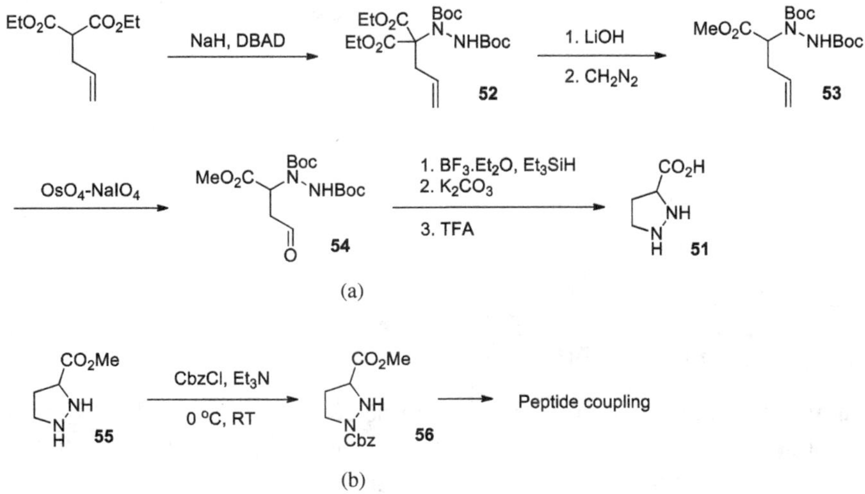

Scheme 15. (a) Synthesis of the δ-aza-proline 51; (b) Reactivity difference of hydrazino nitrogens of the δ-azaproline.

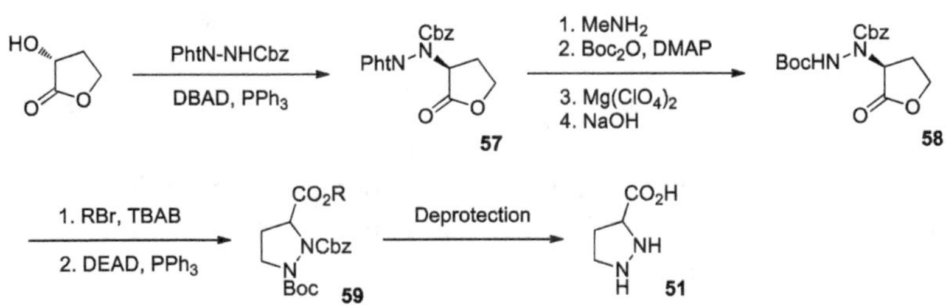

Scheme 16. Synthesis of δ-azaproline 51.

Sinha *et al.* [88] used the δ-azaproline to control the structure of both linear and cyclic peptides, which allowed them to exclusively switch between the *cis* and *trans* conformations around the AA-Xaa-AA bonds using the δ nitrogen protecting group as the chemical tool. The δ-azaproline adopted the *cis* conformation in simple amides, dipeptides and tripeptides whereas its δ-nitrogen protected forms adopted a *trans*-conformation. In the case of longer linear or cyclic peptides, the δ-azaproline adopted a *trans* conformation whereas the δ-nitrogen protected forms adopted the *cis* conformation. The δ-azaproline was also reported to be able to control the structure of rigid cyclic peptides. Similar observations were also reported by Jamart-Grégoire *et al.* [89].

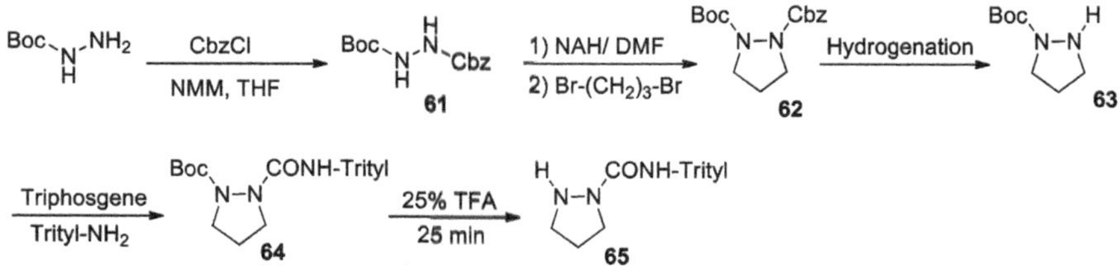

Scheme 17. Synthesis of protected α-azaproline 65.

3.4.3. *α-Azaproline* (60)

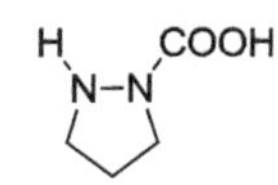

60, Figure 14.

Another approach to stabilize the *cis* amide conformer of the peptide bond is replacement of the α-carbon of azaproline by a N atom (Figure 14: 1-Pyrazolidine carboxylic acid (α-Azaproline) which imparts a VI-β turn in the peptide sequence. The synthesis of these azapeptides was first introduced by Goldschmidt and Wick [90] and further developed in solution phase and solid phase by Andre *et al.* [91] using triphosgene chemistry. Encouraged by these results, Marshall *et al.* [18] synthesized the protected azaproline **65**. The Boc-hydrazine was acylated with carbobenzoxychloride to afford compound **61,** which on subsequent alkylation generated compound **62**. Compound **62** on Cbz deprotection followed by triphosgene and tritylamine-mediated amidation provided compound **64**. Further Boc deprotection generated the protected azaproline **65**. In order to confirm the conformational preference of azaproline, the group performed NMR experiments on the biologically relevant thyrotropin-releasing hormone (TRH) containing azaproline analogs. The substitution of azaproline for Pro in the TRH analogs with *cis* amide constraints produced a significant loss in binding affinity for TRH receptor as compared to that of TRH itself.

4. Concluding Remarks

β-Turns in peptides and proteins are a crucial factor for their activity, function and degradation. Although rare in nature, the high evolutionary conservation of these turns hints towards its significance in the protein function. Advances in peptide research have challenged researchers to synthesize customized molecules with desirable electronic or structural properties to mimic these turns. Conformationally constrained amino acids that either induce or themselves mimic a β-turn are changing the landscape of peptide research by answering a fundamental question on peptide secondary structure and folding. Designing degradation-resistant peptide-based inhibitors is another field where these molecules are contributing immensely.

Acknowledgments

S.S. thanks the Indo-French Centre for the Promotion of Advanced Research (CEFIPRA) for financial support [IFC/A/5105-2/2014/1060].

List of abbreviations

Standard 3 letter codes for amino acids have been used throughout the chapter

Boc	tert-Butyloxycarbonyl
CD spectrum	Circular dichroism (CD) spectroscopy
NMR	Nuclear Magnetic Resonance Spectroscopy
ψ-Pro	Pseudoproline
RNase	Ribonuclease
Xaa	Conformationally constrained amino acid

References

1. Liu, J., Han, J., Izawa, K., Sato, T., White, S., Meanwell, N. A. and Soloshonok, V. A. (2020) Cyclic Tailor-Made Amino Acids in the Design of Modern Pharmaceuticals. *Eur. J. Med. Chem.* 208, pp. 112736–112810.
2. Ramachandran, G. N. and Sasisekharan, V. (1968) Conformation of Polypeptides and Proteins. *Advan. Prot. Chem.* 23, pp. 283–437.
3. Stewart, D. E., Sarkar, A. and Wampler, J. E. (1990) Occurrence and Role of *cis* Peptide Bonds in Protein Structures. *J. Mol. Biol.* 214, pp. 253–260.
4. Jabs, A., Weiss, M. S. and Hilgenfeld, R. (1999) Non-Proline *Cis* Peptide Bonds in Proteins. *J. Mol. Biol.* 286, pp. 291–304.
5. Ganguly, H. K. and Basu, G. (2020) Conformational Landscape of Substituted Prolines. *Biophys. Rev.* 12, pp. 25–39.
6. Pandey, A. K., Naduthambi, D., Thomas, K. M. and Zondlo, N. J. (2013) Proline Editing: A General and Practical Approach to the Synthesis of

Functionally and Structurally Diverse Peptides. Analysis of Steric versus Stereoelectronic Effects of 4-Substituted Prolines on Conformation within Peptides. *J. Am. Chem. Soc.* 135, pp. 4333–4363.

7. Dugave, C. and Demange, L. (2003) *Cis-Trans* Isomerization of Organic Molecules and Biomolecules: Implications and Applications. *Chem. Rev.* 103, pp. 2475–2532.
8. Pal, D. and Chakrabarti, P. (1999) *Cis* Peptide Bonds in Proteins: Residues Involved, Their Conformations, Interactions and Locations. *J. Mol. Biol.* 294, pp. 271–288.
9. Montelione, G. T., Arnold, E., Meinwald, Y. C, Stimson, E. R., Denton, J. B., Huang, S-G., Clardy, J. A. and Scheraga, A. (1984) Chain-Folding Initiation Structures in Ribonuclease A: Conformational Analysis of *trans*-Ac-Asn-Pro-Tyr-NHMe and *trans*-Ac-Tyr-Pro-Asn-NHMe in Water and in the Solid State. *J. Am. Chem. Soc.* 106, pp. 7946–7958.
10. Lu, K. P., Finn, G., Lee, T. H. and Nicholson, L. K. (2007) Prolyl *cis-trans* Isomerization as a Molecular Timer. *Nat. Chem. Biol.* 3, pp. 619–629.
11. Eckert, B., Martin, A., Balbach, J. and Schmid, F. X. (2005) Prolyl Isomerization as a Molecular Timer in Phage Infection. *Nat. Struct. Mol. Biol.* 12, pp. 619–623.
12. Lummis, S. C. R., Beene, D. L., Lee, L. W., Lester, H. A., Broadhurst, R. W. and Dougherty, D. A. (2005) *Cis-trans* Isomerization at a Proline Opens the Pore of a Neurotransmitter-Gated Ion Channel. *Nature.* 438, pp. 248–252.
13. Sarkar, P., Saleh, T., Tzeng, S. R., Birge, R. B. and Kalodimos, C. G. (2011) Structural Basis for Regulation of the Crk Signaling Protein by a Proline Switch. *Nat. Chem. Biol.* 7, pp. 51–57.
14. Vogel, M., Bukau, B. and Mayer, M. P. (2006) Allosteric Regulation of Hsp70 Chaperones by a Proline Switch. *Mol. Cell.* 21, pp. 359–367.
15. Flores-Ortega, A., Jimenez, A. I., Cativiela, C., Nussinov, R., Aleman, C. & Casanovas, J. (2008) Conformational Preferences of α-Substituted Proline Analogs. *J. Org. Chem.* 73, pp. 3418–3427.
16. Judith, L., Anderson, F., Gilardi, R., Karle, I. L., Frey, M. H., Opella, S. J., Gierasch, L. M., Goodman, M., Madison, V. and Delaney, N. G. (1983) Crystal Structures, Molecular Conformations, Infrared Spectra, and ^{13}C NMR Spectra of Methylproline Peptides in the Solid State. *J. Am. Chem. Soc.*105, pp. 6609–6614.
17. Delaney, N. G. and Madison, V. (1982) Novel Conformational Distributions of Methylproline Peptides *J. Am. Chem. Soc.* 104, pp. 6635–6641.
18. Zhang, W.-J., Berglund, A., Kao, J. L.-F., Couty, J.-P., Gershengorn, M. C. and Marshall, G. R. (2003) Impact of Azaproline on Amide *Cis-Trans* Isomerism: Conformational Analyses and NMR Studies of Model Peptides Including TRH Analogs. *J. Am. Chem. Soc.* 125, pp. 1221–1235.

19. Song, K. I. and Kang, Y. K. (2005) Puckering Transition of 4-Substituted Proline Residues. *J. Phys. Chem. B.* 109, pp. 16982–16987.
20. Flores-Ortega, A., Casanovas, J., Nussinov, R. & Alema, C. (2008) Conformational Preferences of β- and γ-Aminated Proline Analogs. *J. Phys. Chem. B.* 112, pp. 14045–14055.
21. Jhon, J. S. and Kang, Y. K. (2007) Conformational Preferences of Proline Analogs with Different Ring Size. *J. Phys. Chem. B.* 111, pp. 3496–3507.
22. Kang, Y. K. and Park, H. S. (2007) Conformational Preferences of Pseudoproline Residues. *J. Phys. Chem. B.* 111, pp. 12551–12562.
23. Kang, Y. K. and Byun, B. J. (2007) Conformational Preferences and *cis-trans* Isomerization of Azaproline Residue. *J. Phys. Chem. B.* 111, pp. 5377–5385.
24. Flores-Ortega, A., Casanovas, J., Zanuy, D., Nussinov, R. and Alema, C. (2007) Conformations of Proline Analogs Having Double Bonds in the Ring. *J. Phys. Chem. B.* 111, pp. 5475–5482.
25. Mutter, M., Nefzi, A., Sato, T., Sun, X., Wahl, F. and Wöhr, T. (1995) Pseudo-Prolines (psi Pro) for accessing "Inaccessible" Peptides. *Pept. Res.* 8, pp. 145–153.
26. Wöhr, T., Wahl, F., Nefzi, A., Rohwedder, B., Sato, T., Sun, X. and Mutter M. (1996) Pseudo-Prolines as a Solubilizing, Structure-Disrupting Protection Technique in Peptide Synthesis. *J. Am. Chem. Soc.* 118, pp. 9218–9227.
27. Wöhr, T. and Mutter, M. (1995) Pseudo-Prolines in Peptide Synthesis: Direct Insertion of Serine and Threonine Derived Oxazolidines in Dipeptides. *Tetrahedron Lett.* 36, pp. 3847–3848.
28. Haack, T. and Mutter, M. (1992) Serine Derived Oxazolidines as Secondary Structure Disrupting, Solubilizing Building Blocks in Peptide Synthesis. *Tetrahedron Lett.* 33, pp. 1589–1592.
29. Keller, M., Sager, C., Dumy, P., Schutkowski, M., Fischer, G. S. and Mutter, M. (1998). Enhancing the Proline Effect: Pseudo-Prolines for Tailoring *Cis/Trans* Isomerization. *J. Am. Chem. Soc.* 120, pp. 2714–2720.
30. Dumy, P., Keller, M., Ryan, D. E., Rohwedder, B., Wöhr, T. and Mutter, M. (1997) Pseudo-Prolines as a Molecular Hinge: Reversible Induction of *cis* Amide Bonds into Peptide Backbones. *J. Am. Chem. Soc.* 119, pp. 918–925.
31. Woodward, G. E. and Schroeder, E. F. (1937) The Reaction of Cysteine with Acetone. A Note on the Titration of Cysteine by the Acetone-Hydrochloric Acid Method of Linderstrom-Lang. *J. Am. Chem. Soc.* 59, pp. 1690–1694.
32. Kantharaju, R. S., Raghavender, U. S., Aravinda, S., Shamala, N. and Balaram, P. (2009) Conformations of Heterochiral and Homochiral Proline-Pseudoproline Segments in Peptides: Context dependent *Cis–Trans* Peptide Bond Isomerization. *Bioploymers*. 92, pp. 405–416.
33. Postma, T. M. and Albericio, F. (2014) Cysteine Pseudoprolines for Thiol Protection and Peptide Macrocyclization Enhancement in Fmoc-Based Solid-Phase Peptide Synthesis. *Org. Lett.* 16, pp. 1772–1775.

34. Wittelsberger, A., Keller, M., Scarpellino, L., Patiny, L., Acha-Orbea, H. and Mutter, M. (2000) Pseudoprolines: Targeting a *cis* Conformation in a Mimetic of the gp120 V3 Loop of HIV-1. *Angew. Chem. Int. Ed. Engl.* 39, pp. 1111–1115.
35. Keller, M., Boissard, C., Patiny, L., Chung, N. N., Lemieux, C., Mutter, M. and Schiller P. W. (2001) Pseudoproline-Containing Analogs of Morphiceptin and Endomorphin-2: Evidence for a *Cis* Tyr-Pro Amide Bond in the Bioactive Conformation. *J. Med. Chem.* 44, pp. 3896–3903.
36. Rückle, T., de Lavallaz, P., Keller, M., Dumy, P. and Mutter, M. (1999) Pseudo-Prolines in Cyclic Peptides : Conformational Stabilisation of Cyclo [Pro-Thr($\psi^{Me,Me}$pro)-Pro]. *Tetrahedron.* 55, pp. 11281–11288.
37. Sayyadi, N., Skropeta, D. and Jolliffe, K. A. (2005) N,O-Isopropylidenated Threonines as Tools for Peptide Cyclization: Application to the Synthesis of Mahafacyclin B. *Org Lett.* 7, pp. 5497–5499.
38. Fairweather, K. A., Sayyadi, N., Luck, I. J., Clegg, J. K. and Jolliffe, K. A. (2010). Synthesis of All-L Cyclic Tetrapeptides Using Pseudoprolines as Removable Turn Inducers. *Org. Lett.* 12, pp. 3136–3139.
39. Skropeta, D., Jolliffe, K. A. and Turner, P. (2004) Pseudoprolines as Removable Turn Inducers: Tools for the Cyclization of Small Peptides. *J. Org. Chem.* 69, pp. 8804–8809.
40. Sayyadi, N., Taleski, D., Leesch, S., & Jolliffe, K. A. (2014) Investigating the Scope of Pseudoproline Assisted Peptide Cyclization. *Tetrahedron.* 70, pp. 7700–7706.
41. Fairweather, K. A, Sayyadi, N., Roussakis, C. and Jolliffe K. A. (2010) Synthesis of the cyclic Heptapeptide Axinellin A. *Tetrahedron.* 66, pp. 935–939.
42. Schmiedeberg, N. and Kessler, H. (2002) Reversible Backbone Protection Enables Combinatorial Solid-Phase Ring-Closing Metathesis Reaction (RCM) in Peptides. *Org. Lett.* 4, pp. 59–62.
43. An, S. S. A., Lester, C. C, Peng, J. L., Li, .Y-J., Rothwarf, D. M., Welker, E., Thannhauser, T. W., Zhang, L. S., Tam, J. P. and Scheraga, H. A. (1999) Retention of the *Cis* Proline Conformation in Tripeptide Fragments of Bovine Pancreatic Ribonuclease A Containing a Non-natural Proline Analogue, 5,5-Dimethylproline. *J. Am. Chem. Soc.* 121, pp. 11558–11566.
44. Magaard, V. W., Sanchez, R. M., Bean, J. W. and Moore M. L. (1993) A Convenient Synthesis of the, Conformationally Constrained Amino Acid 5,5-dimethylproline. *Tetrahedron Lett.* 34, pp. 381–384.
45. Marshall, G. R., Humblet, C., Van Opdenbosch, N. and Zabrocki, J. (1981) Peptides: Synthesis-Structure-Function: *Proc. 7th American Peptide Symposium*, Rich, D. H., Gross, E., Eds. Pierce Chemical Company: Rockford, IL, p 669.
46. Yu, K. L. and Johnson, R. L. (1987) Synthesis and Chemical Properties of Tetrazole Peptide Analogs. *J. Org. Chem.* 52, pp. 2051–2059.

47. Zabrocki, J., Dunbar, Jr J. B., Marshall, K. W., Toth, M. V. and Marshall, G. R. (1992) Conformational Mimicry: Synthesis and Incorporation of 1,5-Disubstituted Tetrazole Dipeptide Analogs into Peptides with Preservation of Chiral Integrity: Bradykinin. *J. Org. Chem.* 57, pp. 202–209.
48. Valle, G., Crisma, M., Yu, K.-L., Toniolo, C., Mishra, R. K. and Johnson, R. L.(1988) Synthesis and X-ray Diffraction Analysis of the Tetrazole Peptide Analog Pro-LeuΨ[CN_4]Gly-NH_2. *Coll. Czech. Chem. Commun.* 53, pp. 2863–2876.
49. Lebl, M., Slaninova, J., and Johnson R. L. (1990) Analogs of oxytocin containing a pseudopeptide Leu-Gly bond of *cis* and *trans* configuration. *Int. J. Pept. Protein Res.* 33, pp. 16–21.
50. Garofalo, A., Tarnus, C., Remy, J. M., Leppik, R., Piriou, F., Harris, B. and Pelton, J. T. (1990) In Peptides: Chemistry, Structure and Biology: Rivier, J., and Marshall, G. R., Eds: ESCOM Leiden, pp. 833–834.
51. Zabrocki, J., Smith, G. D., Dunbar, Jr. J. B., Iijima, H. and Marshall, G. R. (1988) Conformational Mimicry. 1. 1,5-Disubstituted Tetrazole Ring as a Surrogate for the *Cis* Amide Bond. *J. Am. Chem. Soc.* 110, pp. 5875–5880.
52. Elseviers, M., Van Der Auwera, L., Pepermans, H., Tourwe, D. and Van Binst, G. (1988) Evidence For Tee Bioactive Conformation in a Cyclic Hexapeptide Analog of Somatostatin Containing a *Cis*-Peptide Bond Mimic. *Biochem. Biophys. Res. Commun.* 154, pp. 515–521.
53. Bauer, W., Briner, U., Doepfner, W., Haller, R., Huguenin, R., Marbach, P., Petcher, T. J. and Pless, J. (1982) SMS 201–995: A Very Potent and Selective Octapeptide Analog of Somatostatin with Prolonged Action, *Life Sci.* 31, pp. 1133–1140.
54. Abell, A. D., Hoult, D. A. and Jamieson, E. J. (1992) Synthesis of 1,2-Disubstituted Pyrroles: A *Cis* Peptide Bond Surrogate. *Tetrahedron Lett.* 33, pp. 5831–5832.
55. Kemp, D. S. and Sun, E. T. (1982) Amino Acid Derivatives That Stabilize Secondary Structures of Polypeptides: Synthesis of LL-3-Amino-Z-Piperidone-6-Carboxylic Acid (LL-Acp), a Novel Beta-Turn-Forming Amino Acid. *Tetrahedron Lett.* 23, pp. 3759–3760.
56. Kemp, D. S. and McNamara, P. (1982) Amino Acid Derivatives That Stabilize Secondary Structures of Polypeptides II. The Most Stable Conformation of Peptides Containing 3-Amino-2-Piperidone-6-Carboxylic Acid (Acp). *Tetrahedron Lett.* 23, pp. 3761–3764.
57. Freidinger, R. M., Veber, D. F., Perlow, D. S., Brooks, J. R. and Saperstein, R. (1980) Bioactive Conformation of Luteinizing Hormone Releasing Hormone: Evidence from a Conformationally Constrained Analog. *Science.* 210, pp. 656–658.
58. Freidinger, R. M. (1981) Computer Graphics and Chemical Synthesis in the Study of Conformation of Biologically Active Peptides. In *Peptides: Synthesis-Structure-Function.*, Rich, D. H. and Gross, E., eds., pp. 673–683. Pierce Chemical Company, Rockford.

59. Freidinger, R. M., Brady, S. F., Paleveda, W. J., Perlow, D. S., Colton, C. D., Whitter, W. L., Saperstein, R., Brady, E. J., Cascieri, M. A. and Veber, D. F. (1987) Synthesis of New Peptides Based on Models of Receptor-Bound Conformation. In *Clinical Pharmacology in Psychiatry.* Dahl, S. G. and Gram, L. F., ed., pp. 12–19. Springer-Verlag: Berlin.
60. Douglas, A. J., Mulholland, G., Walker, B., Guthrie, D. J. S., Elmore, D. T. and Murphy, R. F. (1988) The Preparation of a C-Terminal Gastrin Peptide Containing a Synthetic β-Bend Mimic. *Biochem. Soc. Trans.* 16, pp. 175–176.
61. Peggion, E., Foffani, M. T., Wunsch, E., Moroder, L., Borin, G., Goodman, M. and Mammi, S. (1985) Conformational Properties of Gastrin Fragments of Increasing Chain Length. *Biopolymers*. 24, pp. 647–666.
62. Freidinger, R. M., Perlow, D. S. and Veber, D. F. (1982) Protected Lactam-Bridged Dipeptides for Use as Conformational Constraints in Peptides. *J. Org. Chem.* 47, pp. 104–109.
63. Krstenansky, J. L., Bsrsnowski, R. L., and Currie, B. L. (1982) A New Approach to Conformationally Restricted Peptide Analogs: Rigid β-Bends. 1. Enkephalin as an Example. *Biochem. Biophys. Res. Commun.* 109, pp. 1368–1374.
64. Krstenansky J. L., Rosario-Chow, M. D. and Currie, B. L. (1992) The Synthesis of Syn-and Anti-2(*S*)-phthalimido-methyl-2,3,4,4a,7,7a-hexahydro-6oxo-5H-pyrano-[2,3-b]Pyrroles as Rigid β-Bend Peptide-Mimetics. *J. Heterocyclic. Chem.* 29, pp. 707–711.
65. Rosario-Chow, M. D., Ungwitayatom, J. and Currie, B. L. (1991) Manganic Acetate Mediated Transformation of Enol-Ethers into Gamma-Lactones. *Tetrahedron Lett.* 32, pp. 1011–1014.
66. Krstenansky, J. L., Lin, Z. L., Ungwitayatom, J., Lee, Y. H., Rosario-Chow, M. D., Sheu, W. S., Johnson, M. E. and Currie, B. L. (1993) Design and Synthesis of a Bicyclic Non-Peptide β-Bend Mimetic of Enkephalin. *Tetrahedron.* 49, pp. 3489–3500.
67. Kawai, M. and Nagai, U. (1978) Comparison of Conformation and Antimicrobial Activity of Synthetic Analogs of Gramicidin S: Stereochemical Consideration of the Role of D-Phenylalanine in the Antibiotic. *Biopolymers.* 17, pp. 1549–1565.
68. Shiba, T. (1977) Peptide Chemistry*: Proceedings of the 15th Symposium on Peptide Chemistry,* Osaka, November 4–5, 1977.
69. Higashijima, T., Sato, K. and Nagai, U. (1983) Studies on the β-Turn of Peptides. VI. Nuclear Magnetic Resonance Study on the Conformations of N-(2,4-Dinitrophenyl)tetrapeptide p-Nitroanilides Related to the β-Turn Part of Gramicidin S. *Bull. Chem. Soc. Jpn.* 56, pp. 3323–3328.
70. Sato, K. and Nagai U. (1986) Synthesis and Antibiotic Activity of a Gramicidin S Analog Containing Bicyclic β-Turn Dipeptides. *J. Chem. Soc. Perkin. Trans.* 1, pp. 1231–1234.

71. Bach, II A. C., Markwalder, J. A. and Ripka, W. C. (1991) Synthesis and NMR Conformational Analysis of a β-Turn Mimic Incorporated into Gramicidin S. *Int. J. Peptide Protein Res*. 38, pp. 314–323.
72. Nagai, U., Sato, K., Nakamura, R. and Kato, R. (1993) Bicyclic Tuned Dipeptide (BTS) as a β-Turn Mimetics: Its Design, Synthesis and Incorporation into Bioactive Peptides. *Tetrahedron*. 49, pp. 3577–3592.
73. Lombart, H. G. and Lubell W. D. (1994) Synthesis of Enantiopure α,ω-Diamino Dicarboxylates and Azabicycloalkane Amino Acids by Claisen Condensation of α-[N-(Phenylfluorenyl)amino] Dicarboxylates. *J. Org. Chem*. 59, pp. 6147–6149.
74. Baldwin, J. E., Hulme, C., Schofield, C. J. and Edwards, A. J. (1993) Synthesis of Potential β-Turn Bicyclic Dipeptide Mimetics. *J. Chem. Soc. Chem. Commun*. 11, pp. 935–936.
75. Gramberg, D. and Robinson, J. A. (1994) Design and Synthesis of a *cis*-Gly-Pro, Type-VI Turn, Dipeptide Mimetic and its Use in Fmoc-Solid Phase Peptide Synthesis. *Tetrahedron Lett*. 35, pp. 861–864.
76. Dumas, J. P. and Germanas, J. P. (1994) Design, Syntheses and Evaluation of a Novel Bicyclic Lactam as a Gly-Pro Type VI Beta-Turn Mimic. *Tetrahedron Lett*. 35, pp. 1493–1496.
77. Kim, K., Dumas, J. P. and Germanas, J. P. (1996) Novel Bicyclic Lactams as XaaPro Type VI β Turn Mimics: Design, Synthesis, and Evaluation. *J. Org. Chem*. 61, pp. 3138–3144.
78. Gramberg, D., Weber, C., Beeli, R., Inglis, J., Bruns, C. & Robinson J. A. (1995) Synthesis of a Type-VI β-Turn Peptide Mimetic and Its Incorporation into a High-Affinity Somatostatin Receptor Ligand. *Helv. Chim. Acta*. 78, pp. 1588–1606.
79. Kahn, M., Wilke, S., Chen, B. and Fujita, K. (1988) Nonpeptide Mimetics of β-Turns: A Facile Oxidative Intramolecular Cycloaddition of an Azodicarbonyl System. *J. Am. Chem. Soc*. 110, pp. 1638–1639.
80. Kahn, M., Wilke, S., Chen, B. and Fujita, K. (1988) The Design and Synthesis of Mimetics of Peptide β-Turns. *J. Mol. Recognit*. 1, pp. 75–79.
81. Kahn, M. and Bertenshaw, S. (1989) The Incorporation of β-Turn Prosthetic Units into Merrifield Solid Phase Peptide Synthesis. *Tetrahedron Lett*. 30, pp. 2317–2320.
82. Wu, T. P., Yee, V., Tulinksy, A., and Chmsciel, R. A., Nakanishi, H., Shen, R., Priebe, C. and Kahn, M. (1993) The Structure of a Designed Peptidomimetic Inhibitor Complex of α-thrombin. *Protein Eng*. 6, pp. 471–478.
83. Mathews, II. and Tulinsky, A. (1995) Structure-Based Design of Protease Inhibitors: Active-Site Mimetic Inhibition of Thrombin. *Acta Cryst*. D51, pp. 550–559.
84. Nakanishi, H., Chrusciel, R. A., Shen, R., Bertenshaw, S., Johnson, M. E., Rydel, T. J., Tulinsky, A. and Kahn, M. (1992) Peptide Mimetics of the Thrombin-Bound Structure of Fibrinopeptide A. *Proc. Natl. Acad. Sci*. 89, pp. 1705–1709.

85. Duttagupta, I., Goswami, K. and Sinha, S. (2012) Synthesis of Cyclic α-Hydrazino Acids. *Tetrahedron*. 68, pp. 8347–8357.
86. Duttagupta, I., Goswami, K., Chatla, P. and Sinha, S. (2014) Improved Synthesis of Cyclic α-Hydrazino Acids of Five- to Nine-Membered Rings and Optical Resolution of 5,6,7-Membered Ring Hydrazino Acids. *Synth. Commun*. 44, pp. 2510–2519.
87. Voss, E., Arrault, A., Bodigue, J. and Jamart-Gregoire, B. (2009) Efficient Synthesis of Enantiomerically Pure (*S*)-δ-Azaproline Starting from (*R*)-α-hydroxy-γ-butyrolactone via the Mitsunobu Reaction. *Tetrahedron*. 20, pp. 1809–1812.
88. Duttagupta, I., Misra, D., Bhunya, S., Paul, A. and Sinha, S. (2015) *Cis-Trans* Conformational Analysis of δ-Azaproline in Peptides. *J. Org. Chem.* 80, pp. 10585−10604.
89. Humbert-Voss, E., Arrault, A. and Jamart-Gregoire B. (2014) Synthesis and Conformational Behavior of Pseudopeptides Containing δ-azaproline. A Cis Conformational Preference for Xaa_1-δ-azaPro Bond. *Tetrahedron*. 70, pp. 363–370.
90. Goldschmidt, S. and Wick, M. (1952) Uber Peptid-Synthesen I. *Justus Liebigs Ann. D Chem.* 575, pp. 217–231.
91. Andre, F., Marraud, M., Tsouloufis, T., Tzartos, S. J. and Boussard, G. (1997) Triphosgene: An Efficient Carbonylating Agent for Liquid and Solid-Phase Aza-Peptide Synthesis. Application to the Synthesis of Two Aza-Analogs of the AChR MIR decapeptide. *J. Pept. Sci*. 3, pp. S429–441.

https://doi.org/10.1142/9789811261664_0002

Chapter 2

Antimicrobial Peptides and Peptidomimetics as Treatment Option for *Helicobacter pylori* Infection

Hamza Olleik[*,†,¶], Josette Perrier[*], Akram Hijazi[‡], Elias Baydoun[§], and Marc Maresca[*,||]

[*]*Aix Marseille Univ, CNRS, Centrale Marseille, iSm2, Marseille, France*
[†]*Sorbonne Université, Université de Technologie de Compiègne, CNRS Enzyme and Cell Engineering Laboratory, France*
[‡]*Doctoral School of Science and Technology, Research Platform for Environmental Science (PRASE), Lebanese University, Lebanon*
[§]*Department of Biology, American University of Beirut, Lebanon*

[¶]*hamza.olleik@live.com*
[||]*m.maresca@univ-amu.fr*

1. General View Regarding Infection by *H. pylori*, Its Consequences and Its Actual Treatment with Conventional Antibiotics

Helicobacter pylori is a Gram-negative microaerophilic bacterium of helical bacillus form, causing gastric ulcer and cancer [1–8]. JR Warren and BJ Marshall (Nobel Prize of physiology and medicine 2005) discovered it in the early 1980s [1,9]. This bacterium colonizes exclusively the gastric mucosa of humans and some primates [10,11]. The mechanism of transmission from person to person is still not fully understood but the oral-oral and oral-fecal routes are more likely the modes of transmission, the infection being acquired mainly during the first two decades of life [12].

H. pylori infection is one of the most common infections worldwide with around 55% of humans being infected. Its prevalence, the measurement of all individuals affected at a particular time, is greater in developing countries (around 80–90%) than in the developed ones (around 20–30%). In Europe for example, in 2018, the prevalence was 23.5% in the Czech Republic, 28.9% in Germany, and 42.9% in Denmark. In France, the prevalence was shown to be 46.9% in a meta-analysis published in 2017 [13]. In other developed countries, China, the USA, and Australia have a prevalence of 34.4%, 25.3%, and 21.5%, respectively [14]. In the Middle East, the prevalence is much higher with 72.8% in Iran and 75.7% in Afghanistan. Similarly, in Africa, the percentages were high. In Ghana, 71.1% of the tested patients were positive. Algeria had a decrease in the prevalence from 80% to 57% since 1980 [14]. Overall, a gradual reduction in the rate of infection has been observed resulting in a decreased prevalence of infection that remains however greater in underprivileged areas [13,14].

Regarding the physiological consequences of *H. pylori* infection, the imbalance between aggression factors (acid and peptic secretions) and defense factors (inflammation, mucus and prostaglandins) induced by *H. pylori* infection is the main cause of gastric or duodenal ulcer [15,16]. *H. pylori* infection also results in chronic gastritis. It is a histological anomaly related to the inflammatory reaction at the level of the mucosa, most often asymptomatic, and whose spontaneous healing is rare. Over time, signs of atrophy appear that are associated with gastric cancer [17,18].

H. pylori is flagellated with about 4–7 flagella which give its high motility property [7]. Furthermore, it is microaerophilic, which means that it requires oxygen but at lower concentrations than those found in the atmosphere [19]. It uses hydrogen and hydrogenase as energy sources. It also uses other enzymes such as urease, oxidase, and catalase (Figure 1) [20]. Although *H. pylori* lives in the stomach, it is not affected by its acidic pH. Several mechanisms protect this bacterium from being destroyed by acidity. First, urease transforms urea into ammonia and carbon dioxide. Ammonia partially neutralizes gastric acidity [16]. *H. pylori* takes advantage of its flagella and its spiral shape where it drills the layer of mucus in the stomach and adheres to epithelial cells through its adhesins [21]. Furthermore, *H. pylori* has the ability to form coccoid and

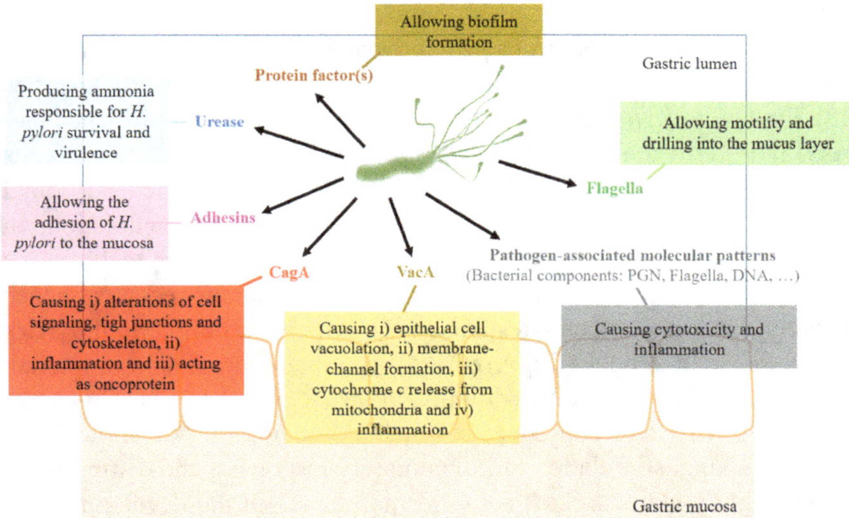

Fig. 1. Survival and virulence factors involved in *H. pylori*'s pathogenicity (inspired from [34]). The survival and the virulence of *H. pylori* are associated with various factors as explained in the main text.

bacterial biofilms as a defensive mechanism. This can also participate in the transmission of infection [22,23].

H. pylori has a lot of other characteristics that help it adapt to the gastric environment, one of which is its enormous genetic diversity by frequent mutations [24]. Lots of studies were conducted to better understand the effect of this genetic diversity on *H. pylori*'s virulence and pathology. For example, nickel is a metal cofactor of urease and thus plays a role in *H. pylori* survival and gastric colonization. Nickel transport is controlled by two different genes (*nixA* and *niuBDE*). They were acquired from the last common ancestor of the gastric *Helicobacter* species by horizontal gene transfer and function independently from each other. The gene *niuBDE* is not only responsible for the transport of nickel, but also for the transport of cobalt and bismuth, a metal used in *H. pylori* therapy (see in what follows). Other examples for genetic diversity between strains are the alcohol/aldehyde-producing enzymes that are important for acid resistance and production of toxic aldehydes. Difference of expression was seen in different areas worldwide which was highest in the African lineages. One more example is the genes encoding for membrane proteins. *H. pylori* from American populations has three genes encoding for outer membrane proteins (*alpB, hofC*, and *frpB4*) evidencing that different genes' sequences frequently have distinct evolutionary histories [25]. Finally, *H. pylori* produces proteins that are part of its virulence factors (Figure 1). Vacuolating Cytotoxin (VacA) is a polypeptide that exerts some detrimental effect on the epithelial cells, altering the endosomal maturation, which consequently leads to epithelial cell vacuolation. In addition, VacA induces membrane-channel formation, cytochrome c release from mitochondria, and binding to cell membrane receptors hence activating proinflammatory response [16]. Another example is the cytotoxin-associated gene A (CagA). CagA is an oncoprotein able to interact with numerous host proteins within the gastric epithelial cells. This interaction leads to major consequences such as perturbation of intracellular actin trafficking, stimulation of inflammatory responses, and disruption of cellular tight junctions. Such activities participate in the development of gastric cancer [26]. CagA is thus associated with gastrointestinal adenocarcinoma, myeloid leukemia, and B cell lymphoma. It also increases gastric inflammation via NFκB signaling and causes IL-8 secretion [27].

All the virulence factors of *H. pylori* described in Figure 1 are responsible for its physiological consequences and its pathogenicity. They cause dyspepsia, gastroesophageal reflux disease, gastric inflammation, ulcers and cancer [4–6]. For example, uncharacterized secreted protein(s) play a role in biofilm formation and increased resistance of *H. pylori* to physical or chemical insults and to antibiotics [23]. Using urease, *H. pylori* transforms urea to ammonia that is toxic to epithelia cells. Ammonia, with the help of other proteases and toxins produced by *H. pylori,* causes gastric ulcer [28]. *H. pylori* also causes chronic gastritis, an inflammation which in turn increases the risk of ulcers [20]. In addition, *H. pylori* is the leading cause of gastric cancer [4–6] (ranked by the World Cancer Research Fund International as the fourth most commonly occurring cancer in men and the seventh most commonly occurring cancer in women, with over 1 million new cases in 2018) [29]. It is also classified as carcinogenic to humans by the International Agency for Research on Cancers and the WHO. Different mechanisms are proposed for causing cancer. CagA acts as an oncoprotein once injected into gastric cells [26]. In addition, the production of free radicals during chronic gastric inflammation caused by pathogen-associated molecular patterns (PAMPs), VacA and CagA [30–32] increases the risk of mutation to epithelial cells. Regarding PAMPs of *H. pylori* involved in inflammation, it has to be noted that although

H. pylori, as other Gram-negative bacteria, harbors lipopolysaccharide (LPS) on its membrane, the LPS of *H. pylori* does not have the ability to induce inflammation [33], meaning that other PAMPs are involved (such as peptidoglycan, flagella, and DNA).

In addition to its health impact, *H. pylori* has also a major economic impact in both direct and indirect ways. For example, just for the United States, the annual cost is estimated to be $6 billion other than hospitalization and decrease in work productivity cost [35,36]. Furthermore, additional burden is due to the indirect costs of *H. pylori* which are the costs of maintenance treatment of peptic ulcer disease, mainly caused by the infection. This cost could be decreased to half by the eradication of the infection instead of maintenance with antacids medications [37].

Different approaches have been considered to treat *H. pylori* [38–40]. Although vaccines are still under investigation to prevent its transmission without real success [17,41,42], until now, the only way to treat patients already infected by *H. pylori* is the use of conventional antibiotics. Unfortunately, similar to what is observed with other bacterial pathogens, *H. pylori* became resistant to many conventional antibiotics (see in what follows).

Hence, the first line of treatment is normally a triple therapy. It consists of a proton pump inhibitor in addition to two different antibiotics for ten days. Depending on the antibiotic resistance of the infecting strain, the choice of the antibiotic combination differs. Normally, it is a combination of two of clarithromycin, amoxicillin, metronidazole, and/or fluoroquinolone.

The second option for the treatment of *H. pylori* is the quadruple therapy which is the addition of a bismuth salt to the triple therapy. Bismuth salt exerts a direct bactericidal effect on *H. pylori* in a number of ways: by forming complexes in the bacterial wall and in the periplasmic space. Bismuth also aids ulcer healing by increasing the production of mucosal protective factors such as prostaglandin, epidermal growth factor, and bicarbonate secretion [39,43,44].

There are other "off label" approaches for the treatment of *H. pylori* used by clinicians, some of which are culture-guided treatment, addition of probiotics, sequential vs. hybrid therapy, and some plant extracts [38,45–48]. All these approaches showed opposing results within studies, that is why they do not have clear recommendations.

As mentioned, even though combinations of two or three antibiotics are used with a treatment duration of 10–14 days, treatment failure rates are worrying. As observed with its prevalence differing from one country to another, the resistance of *H. pylori* to antibiotics and treatment failure rates differs too. For example, quinolone resistance rates have grown sharply in many countries. It has been found to be 11% in Europe, 10% in Brazil and 28% in South Korea [49]. High primary resistance rates to clarithromycin (20≥40%) and fluoroquinolones (20≥33%) have been reported mostly in the developed countries [50]. In France, the failure rates were up to 44% in the use of the first-line therapy [51]. Similar results were seen in the developing countries. For example, in Syria, a study showed insufficient responses to both clarithromycin and levofloxacin-based triple therapies with eradication rates as low as 35.1% and 29.7% [52].

Accordingly, in 2017, WHO published a list of antibiotic-resistant "priority pathogens" — a catalog of 12 families of bacteria that pose the greatest threat to human health. Due to its increasing resistance, *H. pylori* was classified in the high-risk group (priority group 2) just after methicillin-resistant *Staphylococcus aureus* (MRSA) [53].

To better solve the problem of treatment failure, it is important to understand the reason of *H. pylori* resistance to conventional antibiotics (Table 1).

Resistance mechanisms in *H. pylori* classically involve mutations in different enzymes, membrane proteins or in ribosome-associated proteins and also an increase in the expression of efflux pumps.

Nowadays, although conventional antibiotics were and are the primary treatment option and the gold standard for the treatment of *H. pylori* [39], resistance and treatment failure are very high even with triple and quadruple therapies [49]. Thus, conventional antibiotics, although efficient for decades, are now failing at totally eradicating *H. pylori*. In addition, due to their low-to-no selectivity, the use of cocktail antibiotics for a long period (10–14 days) to treat *H. pylori* leads to various side effects, including microbiota dysbiosis at the level of epithelia (intestine, vagina, airways and skin). Since normal flora are responsible for the "barrier effect" limiting the colonization of epithelia by pathogenic bacteria and fungi, the dysbiosis caused by conventional antibiotics used to eradicate *H. pylori* ironically can increase the risk of infection by other pathogens. As an example, the intestinal dysbiosis caused by conventional antibiotics used to eradicate *H. pylori*, in addition to provoking moderate-to-severe diarrhea, has been also reported to increase the risk of secondary fatal clostridial infection [54,55].

Table 1. Mechanisms of resistance of *H. pylori.*

Antibiotic	Mechanism of Action	Mechanism of Resistance
Amoxicillin	Beta-lactamase antibiotic which inhibits cell wall	• Point mutations in the penicillin-binding proteins gene • Beta-lactamase in *H. pylori* • Efflux pump
Clarithromycin	Macrolide group which inhibits bacterial protein synthesis	• 23S ribosomal RNA A2143G, A2142G, and A2142C mutations are the most frequent cause • A2115G, G2141A, G2172T, T2182C, T2190C, C2195T, A2223G, G2224A, G2245T, G2254T, T2289C, and C2611A mutations • Efflux pumps (Phe-Arg-β-naphthylamide for example) • Outer membrane proteins alterations
Levofloxacin	Fluoroquinolone drug which interacts with DNA gyrase (encoded by *gyrA* and *gyrB*)	• Point mutations in the quinolone resistance-determining regions of *gyrA* or *gyrB*
Metronidazole	Synthetic nitroimidazole which induces nitro and superoxide radicals leading to the destruction of the DNA helical structure	• Mutations of rdxA, a gene that encodes an oxygen-insensitive NADPH nitroreductase • Inactivation of frxA (encoding the NADPH flavin oxidoreductase) and fdxB (encoding the ferredoxin-like protein) • Efflux pump (RND pumps for example)
Tetracycline	Macrolide antibiotic which inhibits protein synthesis	• Point mutations in tet-1 in 16S • Triple-base-pair 16S rDNA AGA (926–928) mutations • Efflux pump

For the above reasons, researchers are trying to find alternatives to conventional antibiotics [38]. Among them, antimicrobial peptides and their chemical mimics (peptidomimetics) gave promising results as detailed in what follows.

2. Antimicrobial Peptides as a Treatment Strategy Against *H. pylori*

Antimicrobial peptides (AMPs) are part of the innate immune response of all living organisms [56]. They are potent, broad-spectrum antibiotics that are expected to be novel therapeutic agents [57,58]. Experiments have shown that antimicrobial peptides can kill Gram-negative and -positive bacteria (including those resistant to conventional antibiotics), mycobacteria (including *Mycobacterium tuberculosis*), viruses, fungi, and even cancer cells [59–62].

AMPs can have multiple activities at the same time, including antibacterial, anti-fungal, anti-viral, anti-parasitic and anti-cancer activities [59–62]. Also, AMPs appear to be bactericidal rather than bacteriostatic [63]. In addition to directly killing bacteria and unlike conventional antibiotics, some AMPs also have immunoregulatory functions that can be involved in the clearance of infections [64], including the ability to alter host gene expression [65], as a chemokine-like or chemokine-inducing agent [66], and to inhibit inflammation including LPS-mediated one [67]. AMPs can also promote wound healing, modulate dendritic cell responses, and regulate innate and adaptive immune responses [68,69].

AMPs are small proteins, typically between 12 and 50 amino acid residues [70]. Although some AMPs are anionic due to the presence of negatively charged residues (aspartic or glutamic acid), most of the described AMPs are cationic with one or more positively charged residues provided by arginine, lysine, or histidine [71,72]. They also generally contain more than 50% of hydrophobic amino acid residues making them amphiphilic (both polar/hydrophilic and apolar/hydrophobic) [73]. AMPs are classified in many different ways, one of which is into anionic vs. cationic peptides [74], but the most used one is according to the secondary structure. This includes alpha helix, beta sheet attributed to the presence of disulfide bond(s), loop type structure due to the presence of a simple disulfide bond in the peptide chain, and those who have an extended structure [75]. Other classifications are according to origin (mammal, amphibians, insects, plants, virus, and bacteria) [76] or synthesis pathway (ribosomal synthesis vs. non-ribosomal synthesis). Whereas ribosomal peptides are produced like other peptides and proteins by ribosomes, non-ribosomal peptides are synthesized by non-ribosomal peptide synthetases (which are specific for one type of peptides) independent of the messenger RNA. This procedure can be used by the microorganism to cyclize, branch, or connect repeats [77].

The mechanisms of action of AMPs are very diverse. There are two types of AMPs according to their mechanism of action, the permeabilizing peptides that permeabilize the bacterial membrane and the non-permeabilizing peptides acting through their interaction with targets located inside the bacteria such as nucleic acids, synthesis machineries, proteins and/or enzymes [72].

The permeabilizing peptides (most common type) are characterized mainly by their cationic charge, associated with their amphipathic characteristic (presenting hydrophobic fractions and polar fractions that are hydrophilic) explaining their interaction with the bacterial membrane formed mainly of anionic phospholipids and their ability to permeabilize it [72]. Different types of mechanisms have been described to explain the membrane permeabilization caused by the AMPs:

(i) *The barrel mechanism*: After being introduced into the interior of the membrane and having reached a sufficient concentration, the peptides are placed perpendicular to the membrane creating hydrophilic pores that cause the loss of osmotic equilibrium and of the membrane potential of the bacteria.
(ii) *The carpet mechanism*: The peptides are associated with the extracellular face of the membrane, creating a carpet, and weakening the bacterial membrane, eventually leading to cell death due to loss of cytoplasm.
(iii) *The micellar aggregate mechanism (toroidal)*: When a high concentration of peptides is reached, they are reoriented forming channels and cell death occurs due to loss of cytoplasmic content. This model resembles the Barrel-stave model, but here, AMPs are always in contact with phospholipid head groups of the membrane [75].

The reason for the innocuity of AMPs against human cells is that they neither insert nor cause damage to the membrane of eukaryotic cells since these cells are rich in neutral phospholipids and cholesterol which are substances that inhibit the incorporation of AMPs and the formation of pores in the membranes. Indeed, the membrane of eukaryotic cells is positive, unlike the extracellular bacterial membrane, therefore the positive charge of the AMPs allows them to penetrate only bacterial cells [78]. Also, the presence of negatively charged lipids into the membrane of cancer cells may explain their sensitivity to AMPs compared to normal cells [79].

A lot of factors can affect the activity, toxicity, and mechanism of action of AMPs such as length, sequence, helicity, charge, or hydrophobicity. It is not well understood how or which mechanism each type of peptide forms, though different studies gave various hypotheses regarding their structure/activity relationship (SAR). Lengthwise, for example, at least 22 amino acids are needed to transverse the lipid bilayers. Also, increasing or decreasing the charge of a peptide can change both activity and toxicity dramatically [80].

The main advantage of AMPs over conventional antibiotics is their lower (or null) ability to select resistant strains. WHO defines antimicrobial resistance as the ability of a microorganism (like bacteria, viruses, and some parasites) to stop an antimicrobial (such as antibiotics, antivirals and antimalarials) from working against it. As a result, standard treatments become ineffective, the infection persists and may spread to others [81]. The resistance of bacteria, including *H. pylori*, to common medicines, has become a threat to global health and a serious problem, which has led to increased transmission and, as a consequence, increased mortality rate [82].

Due to their particular mechanism of action (MOA) relying on their fast insertion into the bacterial membrane leading to its permeabilization, AMPs are (i) active against bacteria already resistant to classical antibiotic targeting intracellular enzyme and (ii) nearly impossible to cause resistance [83,84]. Indeed, resistances to AMPs are rare although some cases have been observed due to (i) bacterial cell envelope modification, (ii) AMPs degradation, sequestration and/or expelling, (iii) release of membrane vesicles, (iv) formation of biofilm or (v) capsulation [85,86].

H. pylori causes a bacterial infection involving biofilm formation and leads to gastric inflammation, ulcer, and cancer. For those reasons, the antibacterial, anti-biofilm, anti-inflammatory, wound-healing and anticancer activities of AMPs [77] make them an attractive strategy, the same drug being able to treat all aspects of this pathology.

Finally, contrarily to conventional antibiotics that display low-to-no selectivity against a particular bacterial strain, some AMPs and their mimics have been proved to be more specific (see in what follows) limiting the risk of side effects such as dysbiosis as observed with classical antibiotics.

Since the 1990s, AMPs started to be recognized as a potential treatment for *H. pylori*. Neshani *et al.* were the first in 2018 to review literature data regarding AMPs and *H. pylori* [87]. From that date, only three more studies described AMPs active on *H. pylori*, i.e. the amphibian temporin SHa and its derivatives [88], the fungal cyclodepsipeptides (enniatins and beauvericin) [89] and four uncharacterized AMPs from the insect black soldier fly (BSF; *Hermetia illucens* Linnaeus) [90].

Among the AMPs described as active on *H. pylori*, four are from amphibians: pexiganan (magainin 2's derivative), PGLa-AM1, odorranain-HP and temporin Sha.

- Pexiganan (H-GIGKFLKKAKKFGKAFVKILKK-NH2) is an alpha-helical cationic peptide of 22 amino acids derivative of magainin 2 isolated originally from *Xenopus laevis*. It was the first to be described in the literature, in 1997, as active against *H. pylori* [91]. Results were promising with good activity although hemolytic side effects were observed. Peptide was improved over years, and in 2015, the evaluation of its nanoparticle form gave good activity (minimal inhibitory activity (MIC) of 4 μg/ml), good stability, rapid bacteriolytic effect (99.99% killing after 20 min of contact) and importantly, a confirmed *in vivo* efficiency [92]. The alpha-helical structure of pexiganan allows it to cause membrane permeabilization through toroidal pores [93]. Regarding additional activities of pexiganan, although no tests were performed in the particular case of *H. pylori*, magainin 2 and/or pexiganan are known to have anti-biofilm [94] anti-inflammatory [95,96], anti-cancer [97] and wound-healing [98–100] effects, reinforcing the interest for this peptide as a treatment option in *H. pylori* infection.
- PGLa-AM1 (H-GMASKAGSVLGKVAKVALKAAL-NH2) is an alpha-helical cationic peptide of 22 amino acids isolated from octaploid frog *Xenopus amieti*. It was found active against *H. pylori* with an MIC value of 1 μg/ml with fast bacteriolytic action (in 15 to 30 minutes) and a confirmed *in vivo* efficiency. Its mechanism of action is still not characterized [101]. Although it is known to stimulate insulin and glucagon release, no data are available regarding anti-biofilm, anti-cancer, or wound-healing activities. Importantly, PGLa-AM1 displays a selective activity against *H. pylori* over other tested bacterial strains with MIC against *H. pylori* being 50 to 100 times lower compared to MIC against other tested bacteria. This makes it very attractive as an alternative to conventional antibiotics causing dysbiosis due to their poor selectivity [54,55].

- Odorranain-HP (H-GLLRASSVWGRKYYVDLAGCAKA-OH) is a cationic 23 amino acids peptide isolated from the skin secretions of diskless-fingered odorous frog *(Odorrana grahami)*. It gave an MIC value on *H. pylori* of 20 μg/ml. No other data regarding its structure, activity and/or mechanism of action are available making it hard to evaluate its potential use as *H. pylori* treatment [102].
- Temporins, particularly temporin SHa and its derivatives, are the last to date amphibian AMPs described as active against *H. pylori* [88]. They are alpha-helical amphipathic cationic peptides of 8–17 amino acids with a *C*-terminal amidation isolated from the European red frog *Rana temporaria*. The activity against *H. pylori* and innocuity against human gastric cells of the various types of temporins described so far were tested and results are presented in Table 2 (personal unpublished data).

The comparison of the therapeutic index (IC_{50} obtained from toxicity analysis divided by the MIC obtained on *H. pylori*) of the different forms of temporins allowed to identify temporin SHa as the best candidate (more active and safer one).

In addition to natural temporin SHa (H-FLSGIVGMLGKLF-NH2), analogs obtained by Gly to Ala substitutions were then tested [88]. Temporin SHa and its derivatives gave MIC values on *H. pylori* (including clinical strains resistant to conventional antibiotics) as low as 3.12 μM (corresponding to 4.3 μg/ml) and an IC_{50} on the viability of human gastric cells of 1558 μM (corresponding to 2147 μg/ml) resulting in a therapeutic index of 499. The safety of temporin SHa and its derivatives was further confirmed *ex vivo* using explants of the human stomach. Time-kill assay showed that temporin SHa and its derivatives had a strong bacteriolytic action, killing 90–99% of bacteria after 20 min of incubation in accordance with the demonstrated membranolytic activity of these peptides. Although the presence of stomach mucus did not inhibit their anti-*H. pylori* effect, temporin SHa was found sensitive to proteolysis by pepsin, whereas some of its derivatives were found partially pepsin-resistant. In addition to its anti-*H. pylori* activity, temporins, including temporin Sha, are also known to possess anti-biofilm [103] antimicrobial peptides (AMPs anti-inflammatory [104], anti-cancer [105] and wound-healing [106] activities. Unfortunately, *in vivo* efficiency against *H. pylori* was not tested, the therapeutic potential of temporin SHa and its derivatives is still to be confirmed.

Table 2. Sequence, anti-*H. pylori* activity and innocuity of the different isoforms of temporins. Anti-*H. pylori* activity and innocuity of temporins on human gastric cells were measured as described in Olleik *et al* [88]. MIC and IC_{50} are expressed in μM and the therapeutic index was calculated by dividing IC_{50} by MIC values.

Temporin	**Sequence**	**MIC *H. pylori* (μM)**	**IC_{50} gastric cells (μM)**	**Therapeutic Index**
SHa	H-FLSGIVGMLGKLF-NH2	3.12	1558	499.3
K_3-SHa	H-FLKGIVGMLGKLF-NH2	3.12	477.2	152.9
L	H-FVQWFSKFLGRIL-NH2	3.12	191.7	61.4
SHb	H-FLPIVTNLLSGLL-NH2	>100	2146	–
SHc	H-FLSHIAGFLSNLF-NH2	>100	>1000	–
SHd	H-FLPAALAGIGGILGKLF-NH2	50	589.8	11.7
SHe	H-FLPALAGIAGLLGKIF-NH2	50	186.5	3.7
SHf	H-FFFLSRIF-NH2	>100	>1000	–
1DRa	H-HFLGTLVNLAKKIL-NH2	3.12	96.5	30.9
1Va	H-FLSSIGKILGNLL-NH2	25	483.8	19.3

The second source of AMPs shown to be active against *H. pylori* are peptides produced by immune cells of mammals: the cathelicidins and defensins families. The idea to test these peptides against *H. pylori* came from the fact that (i) they are known to be active against other bacteria, (ii) their expressions are altered during *H. pylori*'s infection, and (iii) mouse knockout for these AMPs shows stronger colonization by *H. pylori* [87].

- Cathelicidins are alpha-helical cationic peptides produced mainly by immune cells. Both the human cathelicidin LL-37 (H-LLGDFFRKSKE-KIGKEFKRIVQRIKDFLRNLVPRTES-OH) and the mouse cathelicidin CRAMP (H-GLLRKGGEKIGEKLKK IGQKIKNFFQKLVPQPEQ-OH) have been described active against *H. pylori* [107,108]. In addition to having anti-*H. pylori* activity due to pore formation, cathelicidins are also able to destroy biofilm, regulate immunity, stimulate wound-healing, inhibit inflammation, including the one caused by *H. pylori*, showing also anticancer activity [87,109].
- Cbf-K_{16} (H-KFFRKLKKSVKKRAKKFFKKPRVIGVSIPF-OH), a variant of a cathelicidin-like antimicrobial peptide found in the venom

of the snake *Bungarus fasciatus*, was reported to be active on *H. pylori* including drug-resistant bacteria at 16 μg/ml. Antimicrobial activity was then confirmed *in vivo* in a mouse gastritis model, with a decrease in bacterial counts of 3.9-$\log_{10}$ units in stomach tissues and a decrease in the secretion of inflammatory cytokine IL-8. Mechanistic studies revealed that Cbf-K_{16} acts through membrane disruption, DNA-binding and modulation of gene expression [110].

- Defensins are β-sheeted cationic AMPs expressed by immune and epithelial cells of animals and by higher plants as well. To date, two defensins have been reported as active on *H. pylori*: the human neutrophil peptide 1 (HNP-1) and SolyC, a synthetic cationic AMP derived from tomato defensin. The activity of HNP-1 (H-ACYCRIPACIAGE-RRYGTCIYQGRLWAFCC-OH) requires the presence of three intramolecular disulfide bonds. Chemically synthesized or bacterially expressed none-bridged HNP-1 is inactive. The use of a *Pichia pastoris* expression system was thus necessary to produce the active HNP-1. *In vitro* and *in vivo* data confirmed that HNP-1 is active against *H. pylori*, including resistant strains (MIC 8 μg/ml). In addition, HNP-1 did not cause selection of resistant strain after repeated exposure, in contrast to the conventional antibiotics clarithromycin and metronidazole [111]. HNP-1 also possesses anti-cancer [112], anti-biofilm [113], anti-inflammatory [114] and wound-healing [115] activities. SolyC (H-FSGGNCRGFRRRCFCTK-NH2) is a synthetic cationic AMP derived from tomato defensin. It is active against *H. pylori* including resistant strains with an MIC and bactericidal action at 10–15 μg/ml. SolyC also possesses anti-inflammatory activity [116,117]. Other activities on biofilm, cancer, or wound-healing of SolyC were not described so far.

Two families of AMPs from fish were also described as active on *H. pylori*: the piscidins and epinecidin-1.

- Tilapia piscidins form another group of host defense peptides described as active against *H. pylori*. They are alpha-helical cationic antimicrobial peptides. Testing of the different members of this family showed that Tilapia piscidin 3 (TP3) (H-FIHHIIGGLFSVGKHIHSLIHGH-OH) and Tilapia piscidin 4 (TP4) (H-FIHHIIGGLFSAGKAIHRLIRRRRR-OH) were more active with MIC values ranging from 8 to 12 and 1.5-3 μg/ml, respectively. Activity was maintained on clinical strains resistant to conventional antibiotics. In addition, piscidins are also known to possess anti-biofilm [118], anti-inflammatory [119], anti-cancer [120,121], and wound-healing [122] activities. Importantly, the anti-*H. pylori* activity of piscidins was confirmed *in vivo* using the mouse model [123].

- Epinecidin-1 (H-GFIFHIIKGLFHAGKMIHGLV-OH) is an alpha-helical cationic peptide isolated from the fish *Epinephelus coioides*. Epi-1 is active against various bacteria, including *H. pylori* with an MIC value of 8–12 μg/ml. It has a bactericidal action with 99% killing after 1 hour related to pore formation and membrane lysis [124]. It is active on clinical strains resistant to conventional antibiotics. Not tested for other AMPs active on *H. pylori*, Epi-1 has, in addition to its direct effect on *H. pylori*, a synergistic effect with the conventional antibiotics classically used to treat the infection (amoxicillin, clarithromycin, and metronidazole). Epi-1 also possesses anti-cancer [125,126] and wound-healing [127] activities. *In vivo* assay on the mouse model of infection of *H. pylori* confirmed the efficiency of Epi-1 [124].

Some AMPs produced by probiotic bacteria and called bacteriocins were also described as active against *H. pylori*. This includes nisin A, lacticins, leucocin, pediocins and bulgaricin [128]. Although not all these AMPs are well characterized, their activity against *H. pylori* is very interesting as it allows the design of treatment based not only on purified AMPs but also based on the use of live bacteria able to colonize the stomach (as lactic bacteria are tolerant to acidic media) and, in addition, to produce locally these AMPs to compete with *H. pylori* for the binding to the gastric mucosa.

- Among the most studied, nisin A is a polycyclic lantibiotic peptide produced by *Lactococcus lactis* used as food preservative for decades. It possesses an MIC on *H. pylori* ranging from 0.39 to 25 μg/ml depending on the reference strain tested.
- Pediocin BA28 is a bacteriocin, not fully characterized in terms of sequence and mechanism of action, produced by probiotic *Pediococcus acidilactici* BA28. It shows activity against *H. pylori* with complete killing at 500 μg/ml [129]. Another pediocin, pediocin L50, was also demonstrated to be active against *H. pylori* [130].
- Bulgaricin BB18 (H-KIYRGNVGHCGKSTVDWGTAIGNGNN-AASFL-OH), a bacteriocin produced by *Lactobacillus delbrueckii*

subsp. *bulgaricus*, was found active against *H. pylori* in diffusion assay but without further characterization [131].

- Similarly, another study described two other bacteriocins of 4.5 and 6.5 kDa isolated from *Enterococcus faecalis* BK61 and *Lactobacillus brevis* BK11 active against *H. pylori* but no further characterization was performed [132].

Few insects' AMPs have been described as active on *H. pylori.*

- The most known insect AMPs active on *H. pylori* is bicarinalin. It is an alpha-helical cationic peptide of 20 amino acids (H-KIKIPWGK-VKDFLVGGMKAV-NH2) isolated from the venom of the ant *Tetramorium bicarinatum.* It was found active against reference strain and clinical strains of *H. pylori* resistant to conventional antibiotics with MIC values ranging from 2.2 to 8.6 μg/ml. It exerts its activity through membrane leakage and inhibits the adhesion of *H. pylori* to human gastric cells [133,134]. It also has anti-biofilm activity [135].
- The insect black soldier fly (BSF; *Hermetia illucens* Linnaeus) was shown to produce four AMPs, still to be characterized, having anti-*H. pylori* properties [90].

Finally, the fungal cyclodepsipeptides (enniatins and beauvericins) corresponding to non-ribosomal AMPs were tested and found active against *H. pylori* [89]. These fungal AMPs were found only active on Gram-positive bacteria and not on Gram-negative ones, except *H. pylori* and *V. alginolyticus*. Although it could be found surprising that an antibiotic selective of Gram-positive bacteria is also specifically active on *H. pylori* (and *V. alginolyticus*), this phenomenon was also observed with other antibacterial compounds derived from the plant molecules, berberine and aurones [136,137]. This suggests that *H. pylori* and *V. alginolyticus,* although belonging to Gram-negative, behave like Gram-positive ones in terms of susceptibility to certain antibiotics, potentially in relation to particularity in their membrane composition and/or LPS.

Overall, AMPs found active on *H. pylori* are very diverse in terms of length, spatial structure, and charge (from slightly charged to strongly cationic). It seems thus surprising that among the thousands of known AMPs, only few of them were described as active on *H. pylori*. One explanation may be that a lot of AMPs were tested and found not or poorly active on *H. pylori*. Indeed, polymyxin B (PMB), a cyclic AMP active against numerous bacteria, is inactive on *H. pylori* due to LPS and membrane modifications [138]. Another explanation, more likely, may be that *H. pylori* was not considered as a priority target until recently and so a lot of already characterized AMPs found active on other priority bacteria (such as *S. aureus*, *A. baumannii* or *P. aeruginosa*) were not tested on *H. pylori*. The fact that the WHO recently classified *H. pylori* as a member of the high priority group makes it reasonable to predict that more and more AMPs will be tested and found active on *H. pylori* in the near future.

3. Antimicrobial Peptidomimetics as Treatment Strategy Against *H. pylori*

Natural AMPs have two major limitations: (i) their sensitivity to proteases present in the intestinal lumen, blood, and cells and (ii) their production cost and time. Indeed, the purification of a native peptide from a biological matrix takes months to years with potentially a low yield. For chemically produced peptides, although it decreases over years, buying 1 g of linear peptide still costs between 500 and 1,000 euros and takes 2–3 weeks, even more for AMPs with disulfure bridges, with 1 g at 10,000 to 30,000 euros and 4–8 weeks of production. Although the first limitation (i.e. the protease sensitivity) can be addressed easily by cyclization or by incorporation of non-natural amino acids and/or *D*-amino acids, it increases further the cost and production time. For that reason, peptidomimetics have been designed. Peptidomimetics are chemically synthesized bioinspired molecules mimicking AMPs. A large number of strategies have been used to produce the very diverse library of peptidomimetics that are described in the literature [139]. The term peptidomimetic describes any sequence designed to mimic a peptide structure and/or function(s), but in which the backbone is not based on α-amino acid residues alone like in natural peptides. Peptidomimetics correspond thus to alternative AMPs, the natural peptide serving as starting template/pharmacophores in terms of length, backbone, side chains, hydrophobicity, charge and amphipathicity that are further subject to optimization using rational design. The resulting peptide mimics (or peptidomimetics) to maintain some or all the activities of the natural AMPs used as model (i.e. antibacterial, selectivity profiles, antibiofilm, anti-inflammatory, anti-cancer and/or wound-healing properties) with an improved bioavailability, stability, lower cost and time of production/purification compared to natural AMPs extracted from biological samples. Although others exist, the main peptidomimetics studied are *N*-alkylated glycines (peptoids), *β*-peptoids (*N*-alkylated *β*-alanine oligomers), *β*-peptides, *α*-peptide/*β*-peptoids, *α*/*γ* *N*-acylated *N*-aminoethy lpeptides (AA peptides) and oligoacyllysines (OAKs). Although the antibacterial activity of such peptidomimetics has been proved using different bacterial strains, to date, only two types of peptidomimetics have been described as active on *H. pylori*.

In 2009, a total of five oligoacyllysines (OAKs) sequences were screened against *H. pylori* allowing to identify $C_{(12)}K\text{-}2\beta_{(12)}$ as the more active one [140]. C12K-KlK-KlK with $\beta_{(12)}$ representing lysylaminododecanoyl-lysyl subunits, C12, dodecanoic acid; K, lysine. and l, aminododecanoic acid. $C_{(12)}K\text{-}2\beta_{(12)}$ was found active *in vitro* against *H. pylori* with an MIC of 6.5 to 26 μM (corresponding to 8–32 μg/ml) depending on the strain tested. $C_{(12)}K\text{-}2\beta_{(12)}$ was furthermore found bactericidal and able to totally kill *H. pylori in vitro* in 6–8 hours. As expected, $C_{(12)}K\text{-}2\beta_{(12)}$ was found to be very stable and not affected by pH or temperature (although the sensitivity to pepsin was not tested). Later, in 2012, the same group characterized further this peptidomimetic in terms of mechanism of action and *in vivo* efficiency [141]. The authors demonstrated that $C_{(12)}K\text{-}2\beta_{(12)}$ rapidly permeabilizes the bacterial membrane and creates pores that cause bacterial cell lysis. In addition, they found that once it has crossed the bacterial membranes, $C_{(12)}K\text{-}2\beta_{(12)}$ binds to bacterial DNA, RNA, and proteins, inhibiting enzymatic activities and macromolecule synthesis. The selectivity against *H. pylori* as well as additional activities (anti-biofilm, anti-inflammatory, anti-cancer, wound-healing) of $C_{(12)}K\text{-}2\beta_{(12)}$ were not tested/described. Importantly, the fact that the *in vivo* assay performed on *H. pylori*-infected gerbils confirmed the efficiency of this OAK peptides strongly suggests its potential value as therapeutic treatment of *H. pylori* infection.

In 2017, a second family of peptidomimetic was described as active on *H. pylori* [142]. It corresponds to a class of pH-sensitive, helix–coil conformation transitional antimicrobial polypeptides (HCT-AMPs) (PGA) m-r-(PHLG-MHH)n, bearing randomly distributed negatively charged glutamic acid and positively charged poly(*γ*-6-N-(methyldihexylammonium) hexyl-*L*-glutamate)(PHLG-MHH) residues. The design of these peptidomimetics allows them to change their conformation depending on the pH. At physiological pH when they adopt a random coiled conformation, these peptidomimetics did not show any bactericidal activity against *H. pylori* or *E. coli* nor toxicity against human cells. However, under acidic conditions, similar to the one of the stomach, they transformed to a helical structure active against *H. pylori* (active dose as low as 1–2 μM) including clinical strains resistant to conventional antibiotics by causing membrane permeabilization. This nice strategy makes HCT-AMPs selective of *H. pylori*. Indeed, the pH-dependent structural change of HCT-AMPs revealing their activity only at acidic pH will make them active on *H. pylori* only when they are present in the stomach. Once they leave the stomach, they will reach the neutral pH of the intestine and not be active against commensal colonic flora. The efficiency of HCT-AMPs against *H. pylori* activity was further confirmed *in vivo* in a mouse model with killing efficacy comparable to the triple therapy approach based on conventional antibiotics. In addition, HCT-AMPs did not cause any signs of toxicity against the intestinal tissues and cells. Importantly, whereas the conventional antibiotics used in the triple therapy caused an important dysbiosis and the death of 86% of the commensal bacteria, HCT-AMPs did not cause any dysbiosis, confirming *in vivo* their selectivity against *H. pylori*. It will be interesting to evaluate if HCT-AMPs possess some additional activities of the AMPs such as anti-biofilm, anti-inflammatory, anti-cancer and/or wound-healing effects.

4. Conclusion

In conclusion, it appears that AMPs and antimicrobial peptidomimetics represent an alternative to conventional antibiotics in the eradication of *H. pylori*'s infection. Indeed, due to their mechanism of action relying mostly on membrane alteration and/or permeabilization, AMPs and peptidomimetics are active on clinical strains of *H. pylori* already resistant to conventional antibiotics. In addition, and contrarily to conventional antibiotics, they have also been found to be less prompt at selecting strains resistant to them.

Furthermore, since the actual treatment of *H. pylori*'s infection by conventional antibiotics requires the use of cocktails of molecules for a long period, it is associated with side effects, including dysbiosis that can have severe and even lethal consequences. The selectivity of the natural AMP PGLa-AM1 or the pH-sensitive peptidomimetics HCT-AMPs against *H. pylori* makes them thus a better and safer option.

Finally, as *H. pylori* infection involves the formation of biofilms and the induction of inflammation, ulcer, and cancer, the additional activities of AMPs and peptidomimetics (i.e. anti-biofilm, anti-inflammatory, anti-cancer and/or wound-healing activities) make them more efficient, all symptoms and consequences of *H. pylori*'s infection being treated with the same drug.

Without a doubt, it can be predicted that future works will confirm the high potential of AMPs and peptidomimetics in the eradication of *H. pylori*'s infection.

References

1. Dunn, B. E., Cohen, H. and Blaser, M. J. (1997) Helicobacter pylori. *Clin. Microbiol. Rev.* 10, pp. 720–741.
2. Mobley, H. L. T., Mendz, G. L. and Hazell, S. L. (2001) Overview. In *Helicobacter pylori: Physiology and Genetics*; Mobley, H. L., Mendz, G. L., Hazell, S. L., eds. ASM Press: Washington, DC.
3. Vandenplas, Y. (200) *Helicobacter pylori* Infection. *World J. Gastroenterol.* 6, pp. 20–31, doi:10.3748/wjg.v6.i1.20.
4. Duarte, H. O., Gomes, J., Machado, J. C. and Reis, C. A. (2018) Gastric Cancer: Basic Aspects. *Helicobacter.* 23, pp. e12523, doi:10.1111/hel.12523.
5. Jonaitis, L., Pellicano, R. and Kupcinskas, L. (2018) *Helicobacter pylori* and Nonmalignant Upper Gastrointestinal Diseases. *Helicobacter* 23, pp. e12522, doi:10.1111/hel.12522.
6. Venerito, M., Vasapolli, R. and Rokkas, T. (2018) Malfertheiner, P. Gastric Cancer: Epidemiology, Prevention, and Therapy. *Helicobacter.* 23, pp. e12518, doi:10.1111/hel.12518.
7. O'Rourke, J. and Bode, G. (2001) Morphology and Ultrastructure. In *Helicobacter pylori: Physiology and Genetics.* Mobley, H. L., Mendz, G. L. and Hazell, S. L., eds. ASM Press: Washington, DC.
8. Waskito, L. A., Salama, N. R. and Yamaoka, Y. (2018) Pathogenesis of *Helicobacter pylori* Infection. *Helicobacter.* 23, pp. e12516, doi:10.1111/hel.12516.
9. Watts, G. (2005) Nobel Prize is Awarded to Doctors Who Discovered *H pylori. BMJ.* 331, pp. 795.
10. Allen, A., Newton, J., Oliver, L., Jordan, N., Strugala, V., Pearson, J. P. and Dettmar, P. W. (1997) Mucus and *H. pylori. J. Physiol. Pharmacol. Off. J. Pol. Physiol. Soc.* 48, pp. 297–305.
11. Solnick, J. V., Chang, K., Canfield, D. R. and Parsonnet, J. (2003) Natural Acquisition of *Helicobacter pylori* Infection in Newborn Rhesus Macaques. *J. Clin. Microbiol.* 41, pp. 5511–5516, doi:10.1128/JCM.41.12.5511-5516.2003.

12. Brown, L. M. (2000) *Helicobacter pylori*: Epidemiology and Routes of Transmission. *Epidemiol. Rev.* 22, pp. 283–297, doi:10.1093/oxfordjournals.epirev.a018040.
13. Hooi, J. K. Y., Lai, W. Y., Ng, W. K., Suen, M. M. Y., Underwood, F. E., Tanyingoh, D., Malfertheiner, P., Graham, D. Y., Wong, V. W. S., Wu, J. C. Y., *et al.* (2017) Global Prevalence of *Helicobacter pylori* Infection: Systematic Review and Meta-Analysis. *Gastroenterology*. 153, pp. 420–429, doi:10.1053/j.gastro.2017.04.022.
14. Sjomina, O., Pavlova, J., Niv, Y. and Leja, M. (2018) Epidemiology of *Helicobacter pylori* Infection. *Helicobacter.* 23, pp. e12514, doi:10.1111/hel.12514.
15. Narayanan, M., Reddy, K. M. and Marsicano, E. (2018) Peptic Ulcer Disease and *Helicobacter pylori* Infection. *Mo. Med.* 115, pp. 219–224.
16. Roesler, B. M., Rabelo-Gonçalves, E. M. A. and Zeitune, J. M. R. (2014) Virulence Factors of *Helicobacter pylori*: A Review. *Clin. Med. Insights Gastroenterol.* 7, pp. 9–17, doi:10.4137/CGast.S13760.
17. Blosse, A., Lehours, P., Wilson, K. T. and Gobert, A. P. (2018) Helicobacter: Inflammation, Immunology, and Vaccines. *Helicobacter*. 23, pp. e12517, doi:10.1111/hel.12517.
18. Graham, D. Y., Malaty, H. M., Evans, D. G., Evans, D. J., Klein, P. D. and Adam, E. (1991) Epidemiology of *Helicobacter pylori* in an Asymptomatic Population in the United States: Effect of Age, Race, and Socioeconomic Status. *Gastroenterology.* 100, pp. 1495–1501, doi:10.5555/uri:pii:001650859190644Z.
19. Percival, S. L. and Williams, D. W. (2014) Chapter Seven — Helicobacter pylori. In *Microbiology of Waterborne Diseases (Second Edition)*; Percival, S. L., Yates, M. V., Williams, D. W., Chalmers, R. M. and Gray, N. F., eds. Academic Press: London, pp. 119–154.
20. Nilius, M. and Malfertheiner, P. (1996) *Helicobacter pylori* Enzymes. *Aliment. Pharmacol. Ther.* 10 Suppl 1, pp. 65–71.
21. Gu, H. (2017) Role of Flagella in the Pathogenesis of *Helicobacter pylori. Curr. Microbiol.* 74, pp. 863–869, doi:10.1007/s00284-017-1256-4.
22. Yonezawa, H., Osaki, T. and Kamiya, S. (2015) Biofilm Formation by *Helicobacter pylori* and Its Involvement for Antibiotic Resistance. *BioMed Res. Int.* 2015, doi:10.1155/2015/914791.
23. Hathroubi, S., Zerebinski, J., Clarke, A. and Ottemann, K. M. (2020) *Helicobacter pylori* Biofilm Confers Antibiotic Tolerance in Part via A Protein-Dependent Mechanism. *Antibiotics*. 9, pp. 355, doi:10.3390/antibiotics9060355.
24. Linz, B., Windsor, H. M., McGraw, J. J., Hansen, L. M., Gajewski, J. P., Tomsho, L. P., Hake, C. M., Solnick, J. V., Schuster, S. C. and Marshall, B. J. (2014) A Mutation Burst During the Acute Phase of *Helicobacter pylori*

Infection in Humans and Rhesus Macaques. *Nat. Commun.* 5, pp. 4165, doi:10.1038/ncomms5165.

25. Thorell, K., Lehours, P. and Vale, F. F. (2017) Genomics of *Helicobacter pylori. Helicobacter.* 22, pp. e12409, doi:10.1111/hel.12409.
26. Chen, S.-Y., Zhang, R.-G. and Duan, G.-C. (2016) Pathogenic Mechanisms of the Oncoprotein CagA in *H. pylori*-Induced Gastric Cancer (Review). *Oncol. Rep.* 36, pp. 3087–3094, doi:10.3892/or.2016.5145.
27. Chang, W.-L., Yeh, Y.-C. and Sheu, B.-S. (2018) The Impacts of *H. pylori* Virulence Factors on the Development of Gastroduodenal Diseases. *J. Biomed. Sci.* 25, doi:10.1186/s12929-018-0466-9.
28. Tsujii, M., Kawano, S., Tsuji, S., Fusamoto, H., Kamada, T. and Sato, N. (1992) Mechanism of Gastric Mucosal Damage Induced by Ammonia. *Gastroenterology*. 102, pp. 1881–1888, doi:10.1016/0016-5085(92)90309-M.
29. Bray, F., Ferlay, J., Soerjomataram, I., Siegel, R. L., Torre, L. A. and Jemal, A. (2018) Global Cancer Statistics 2018: GLOBOCAN Estimates of Incidence and Mortality Worldwide for 36 Cancers in 185 Countries. *CA. Cancer J. Clin.* 68, pp. 394–424, doi:10.3322/caac.21492.
30. Piao, J.-Y., Lee, H. G., Kim, S.-J., Kim, D.-H., Han, H., Ngo, H.-K.-C., Park, S.-A., Woo, J.-H., Lee, J.-S., Na, H.-K. *et al.* (2016) *Helicobacter pylori* Activates IL-6-STAT3 Signaling in Human Gastric Cancer Cells: Potential Roles for Reactive Oxygen Species. *Helicobacter* 21, pp. 405–416, doi:10.1111/hel.12298.
31. Servetas, S. L., Bridge, D. R. and Merrell, D. S. (2016) Molecular Mechanisms of Gastric Cancer Initiation and Progression by *Helicobacter pylori*: *Curr. Opin. Infect. Dis.* 29, pp. 304–310, doi:10.1097/QCO.0000000000000248.
32. Thalmaier, U. (2002) Role of Tumor Necrosis Factor Alpha in *Helicobacter pylori* Gastritis in Tumor Necrosis Factor Receptor 1-Deficient Mice. *Infect. Immun.* 70, pp. 3149–3155, doi:10.1128/IAI.70.6.3149-3155.2002.
33. Matsuyama, N., Kirikae, T., Kirikae, F., Hashimoto, M., Amano, K.-I., Hayashi, S., Hirai, Y., Kubota, T. and Nakano, M. (2001) Non-standard Biological Activities of Lipopolysaccharide from *Helicobacter pylori. J. Med. Microbiol.* 50, pp. 865–869, doi:10.1099/0022-1317-50-10-865.
34. Morales-Guerrero, E. S., Mucito-Varela, E., Ruben, G., Lopez-Vidal, Y. and Castillo-Rojas, G. (2013) The Role of CagA Protein Signaling in Gastric Carcinogenesis — CagA Signaling in Gastric Carcinogenesis. In *Current Topics in Gastritis – 2012.* Mozsik, G., ed. InTech.
35. Sonnenberg, A. and Everhart, J. E. (1997) Health Impact of Peptic Ulcer in the United States. *Am. J. Gastroenterol.* 92, pp. 614–620.
36. Testerman, T. L. and Morris, J. (2014) Beyond the Stomach: An Updated View of *Helicobacter pylori* Pathogenesis, Diagnosis, and Treatment. *World J. Gastroenterol.* 20, pp. 12781–12808, doi:10.3748/wjg.v20.i36.12781.

37. Taylor, J. L., Zagari, M., Murphy, K. and Freston, J. W. (1997) Pharmacoeconomic Comparison of Treatments for the Eradication of *Helicobacter pylori*. *Arch. Intern. Med.* 157, pp. 87–97, doi:10.1001/archinte.1997.00440220091012.
38. Ayala, G. (2014) Exploring Alternative Treatments for *Helicobacter pylori* Infection. *World J. Gastroenterol.* 20, pp. 1450, doi:10.3748/wjg.v20.i6.1450.
39. Chey, W. D., Leontiadis, G. I., Howden, C. W. and Moss, S. F. (2017) ACG Clinical Guideline: Treatment of *Helicobacter pylori* Infection. *Am. J. Gastroenterol.* 112, pp. 212, doi:10.1038/ajg.2016.563.
40. O'Morain, N. R., Dore, M. P., O'Connor, A. J. P., Gisbert, J. P. and O'Morain, C. A. (2018) Treatment of *Helicobacter pylori* Infection in 2018. *Helicobacter*. 23, pp. e12519, doi:10.1111/hel.12519.
41. Malfertheiner, P., Selgrad, M., Wex, T., Romi, B., Borgogni, E., Spensieri, F., Zedda, L., Ruggiero, P., Pancotto, L., Censini, S. *et al.* (2018) Efficacy, Immunogenicity, and Safety of a Parenteral Vaccine Against *Helicobacter pylori* in Healthy Volunteers Challenged with a Cag-Positive Strain: A Randomised, Placebo-Controlled Phase 1/2 Study. *Lancet Gastroenterol. Hepatol.* 3, pp. 698–707, doi:10.1016/S2468-1253(18)30125-0.
42. Stubljar, D., Jukic, T. and Ihan, A. (2018) How Far are we From Vaccination Against *Helicobacter pylori* Infection? *Expert Rev. Vaccines*. 17, pp. 935–945, doi:10.1080/14760584.2018.1526680.
43. Alkim, H., Koksal, A. R., Boga, S., Sen, I. and Alkim, C. (2017) Role of Bismuth in the Eradication of *Helicobacter pylori*. *Am. J. Ther.* 24, pp. e751, doi:10.1097/MJT.0000000000000389.
44. Konturek, S. J., Stachura, J., Radecki, T., Drozdowicz, D. and Brzozowski, T. (1987) Cytoprotective and Ulcer Healing Properties of Prostaglandin E2, Colloidal Bismuth and Sucralfate in Rats. *Digestion*. 38, pp. 103–113, doi:10.1159/000199579.
45. Goderska, K., Agudo Pena, S. and Alarcon, T. (2018) *Helicobacter pylori* Treatment: Antibiotics or Probiotics. *Appl. Microbiol. Biotechnol.* 102, pp. 1–7, doi:10.1007/s00253-017-8535-7.
46. Cogo, L. L., Monteiro, C. L. B., Miguel, M. D., Miguel, O. G., Cunico, M. M., Ribeiro, M. L., de Camargo, E. R., Kussen, G. M. B., Nogueira, K. da S. and Costa, L. M. D. (2010) Anti-*Helicobacter pylori* Activity of Plant Extracts Traditionally used for the Treatment of Gastrointestinal Disorders. *Braz. J. Microbiol.* 41, pp. 304–309, doi:10.1590/S1517-83822010000200007.
47. Cammarota, G., Ianiro, G., Bibbò, S., Di Rienzo, T. A., Masucci, L., Sanguinetti, M. and Gasbarrini, A. (2014) Culture-Guided Treatment Approach for *Helicobacter pylori* Infection: Review of the Literature. *World J. Gastroenterol. WJG*. 20, pp. 5205–5211, doi:10.3748/wjg.v20.i18.5205.

48. Ashokkumar, S., Agrawal, S., Mandal, J., Sureshkumar, S., Sreenath, G. S. and Kate, V. (2017) Hybrid Therapy versus Sequential Therapy for Eradication of *Helicobacter pylori*: A Randomized Controlled Trial. *J. Pharmacol. Pharmacother.* 8, pp. 62–67, doi:10.4103/jpp.JPP_24_17.
49. Savoldi, A., Carrara, E., Graham, D. Y., Conti, M. and Tacconelli, E. (2018) Prevalence of Antibiotic Resistance in *Helicobacter pylori*: A Systematic Review and Meta-analysis in World Health Organization Regions. *Gastroenterology*. 155, pp. 1372–1382.e17, doi:10.1053/j.gastro.2018.07.007.
50. Mitov, I. and Vladimirov, B. (2011) *Helicobacter Pylori*; Horizon Scientific Press.
51. Dupas, J.-L. (2003) First Line Therapy for *Helicobacter pylori* Eradication in France. *Gastroenterol. Clin. Biol.* 27, pp. 467–472.
52. Cheha, K. M., Dib, S. O. A. and Alhalabi, M. M. (2018) Pilot Study: Comparing Efficacy of 14-Day Triple Therapy Clarithromycin versus Levofloxacin on Eradication of *Helicobacter pylori* Infection in Syrian Population Single-Center Experience. *Avicenna J. Med.* 8, pp. 14–17, doi:10.4103/ajm.AJM_70_17.
53. World Health Organization (WHO) publishes list of bacteria for which new antibiotics are urgently needed Available online: https://www.who.int/news-room/detail/27-02-2017-who-publishes-list-of-bacteria-for-which-new-antibiotics-are-urgently-needed (accessed on Jul 21, 2019).
54. Trifan, A., Girleanu, I., Cojocariu, C., Sfarti, C., Singeap, A. M., Dorobat, C., Grigore, L. and Stanciu, C. (2013) Pseudomembranous Colitis Associated with a Triple Therapy for *Helicobacter pylori* Eradication. *World J. Gastroenterol.* 19, pp. 7476–7479, doi:10.3748/wjg.v19.i42.7476.
55. Nei, T., Hagiwara, J., Takiguchi, T., Yokobori, S., Shiei, K., Yokota, H., Senoh, M. and Kato, H. (2020) Fatal fulminant Clostridioides Difficile Colitis Caused by Helicobacter pylori Eradication Therapy; A Case Report. *J. Infect. Chemother.* 26, pp. 305–308, doi:10.1016/j.jiac.2019.10.021.
56. Sørensen, O. E., Borregaard, N. and Cole, A. M. (2008) Antimicrobial peptides in innate immune responses. *Contrib. Microbiol.* 15, pp. 61–77, doi:10.1159/000136315.
57. Hancock, R. E. W. and Falla, T. J. (1996) Antimicrobial Peptides: Broad-Spectrum Antibiotics from Nature. *Clin. Microbiol. Infect.* 1, pp. 226–229, doi:10.1016/S1198-743X(15)60279-8.
58. Kang, H.-K., Kim, C., Seo, C. H. and Park, Y. (2017) The Therapeutic Applications of Antimicrobial Peptides (AMPs): A Patent Review. *J. Microbiol. Seoul Korea.* 55, pp. 1–12, doi:10.1007/s12275-017-6452-1.
59. Chen, Q., Cheng, P., Ma, C., Xi, X., Wang, L., Zhou, M., Bian, H. and Chen, T. (2018) Evaluating the Bioactivity of a Novel Broad-Spectrum Antimicrobial Peptide Brevinin-1GHa from the Frog Skin Secretion of *Hylarana guentheri* and Its Analogues. *Toxins.* 10, doi:10.3390/toxins10100413.

60. Hsieh, I.-N. and Hartshorn, K. L. (2016) The Role of Antimicrobial Peptides in Influenza Virus Infection and Their Potential as Antiviral and Immunomodulatory Therapy. *Pharmaceuticals*. 9, doi:10.3390/ph9030053.
61. Jin, G. and Weinberg, A. (2019) Human Antimicrobial Peptides and Cancer. *Semin. Cell Dev. Biol.* 88, pp. 156–162, doi:10.1016/j.semcdb.2018.04.006.
62. Portell-Buj, E., Vergara, A., Alejo, I., López-Gavín, A., Monté, M. R., San Nicolás, L., González-Martín, J. and Tudó, G. (2019) *In vitro* Activity of 12 Antimicrobial Peptides Against Mycobacterium Tuberculosis and Mycobacterium Avium Clinical Isolates. *J. Med. Microbiol.* 68, pp. 211–215, doi:10.1099/jmm.0.000912.
63. Dosler, S. (2017) Antimicrobial Peptides: Coming to the End of Antibiotic Era, The Most Promising Agents. *Istanb. J. Pharm.* 47, pp. 72–76, doi:10.5152/IstanbulJPharm.2017.0012.
64. Nijnik, A. and Hancock, R. (2009) Host Defence Peptides: Antimicrobial and Immunomodulatory Activity and Potential Applications for Tackling Antibiotic-Resistant Infections. *Emerg. Health Threats J.* 2, doi:10.3134/ehtj.09.001.
65. Lai, Y. and Gallo, R. L. (2009) AMPed Up Immunity: How Antimicrobial Peptides Have Multiple Roles in Immune Defense. *Trends Immunol.* 30, pp. 131–141, doi:10.1016/j.it.2008.12.003.
66. Hieshima, K., Ohtani, H., Shibano, M., Izawa, D., Nakayama, T., Kawasaki, Y., Shiba, F., Shiota, M., Katou, F., Saito, T. *et al.* (2003) CCL28 Has Dual Roles in Mucosal Immunity as a Chemokine with Broad-Spectrum Antimicrobial Activity. *J. Immunol.* 170, pp. 1452–1461, doi:10.4049/jimmunol.170.3.1452.
67. Sun, Y. and Shang, D. (2015) Inhibitory Effects of Antimicrobial Peptides on Lipopolysaccharide-Induced Inflammation. *Mediators Inflamm.* 2015, doi:10.1155/2015/167572.
68. Diamond, G., Beckloff, N., Weinberg, A. and Kisich, K. O. (2009) The Roles of Antimicrobial Peptides in Innate Host Defense. *Curr. Pharm. Des.* 15, pp. 2377–2392.
69. Mangoni, M. L., McDermott, A. M. and Zasloff, M. (2016) Antimicrobial Peptides and Wound Healing: Biological and Therapeutic Considerations. *Exp. Dermatol.* 25, pp. 167–173, doi:10.1111/exd.12929.
70. Wu, Q., Patočka, J. and Kuča, K. (2018) Insect Antimicrobial Peptides, a Mini Review. *Toxins* 10, doi:10.3390/toxins10110461.
71. Jenssen, H., Hamill, P. and Hancock, R. E. W. (2006) Peptide Antimicrobial Agents. *Clin. Microbiol. Rev.* 19, pp. 491–511, doi:10.1128/CMR.00056-05.
72. Kumar, P., Kizhakkedathu, J. N. and Straus, S. K. (2018) Antimicrobial Peptides: Diversity, Mechanism of Action and Strategies to Improve the Activity and Biocompatibility In Vivo. *Biomolecules*. 8, 4, doi:10.3390/biom8010004.
73. Le, C.-F., Yusof, M. Y. M., Hassan, H. and Sekaran, S. D. (2015) In Vitro Properties of Designed Antimicrobial Peptides that Exhibit Potent

Antipneumococcal Activity and Produces Synergism in Combination with Penicillin. *Sci. Rep.* 2015, *5*, 9761, doi:10.1038/srep09761.
74. Laverty, G., Gorman, S. P. and Gilmore, B. F. (2011) The Potential of Antimicrobial Peptides as Biocides. *Int. J. Mol. Sci.* 12, pp. 6566–6596, doi:10.3390/ijms12106566.
75. Bahar, A. A. and Ren, D. (2013) Antimicrobial Peptides. *Pharmaceuticals.* 6, pp. 1543–1575, doi:10.3390/ph6121543.
76. Hancock, R. E. W. and Chapple, D. S. (1999) Peptide Antibiotics. *Antimicrob. Agents Chemother.* 43, pp. 1317–1323, doi:10.1128/AAC.43.6.1317.
77. Mahlapuu, M., Håkansson, J., Ringstad, L. and Björn, C. (2016) Antimicrobial Peptides: An Emerging Category of Therapeutic Agents. *Front. Cell. Infect. Microbiol.* 6, doi:10.3389/fcimb.2016.00194.
78. Malanovic, N. and Lohner, K. (2016) Antimicrobial Peptides Targeting Gram-Positive Bacteria. *Pharmaceuticals.* 9, doi:10.3390/ph9030059.
79. Deslouches, B. and Di, Y. P. (2017) Antimicrobial Peptides with Selective Antitumor Mechanisms: Prospect for Anticancer Applications. *Oncotarget.* 8, pp. 46635–46651, doi:10.18632/oncotarget.16743.
80. Huang, Y., Huang, J. and Chen, Y. (2010) Alpha-Helical Cationic Antimicrobial Peptides: Relationships of Structure and Function. *Protein Cell.* 1, pp. 143–152, doi:10.1007/s13238-010-0004-3.
81. WHO Antimicrobial resistance Available online: http://www.who.int/antimicrobial-resistance/en/ (accessed on Aug 19, 2019).
82. Reardon, S. (2014) WHO Warns Against "Post-Antibiotic" Era. *Nat. News*, doi:10.1038/nature.2014.15135.
83. Benkhaled, B. T., Hadiouch, S. and Olleik, H. Elaboration of Antimicrobial Polymeric Materials by Dispersion of Well-Defined Amphiphilic Methacrylic SG1-Based Copolymers. *Polym. Chem.* 7, pp. 36–43, doi:10.1039/C5PY01483B.
84. Fjell, C. D., Hiss, J. A., Hancock, R. E. W. and Schneider, G. (2012) Designing Antimicrobial Peptides: Form Follows Function. *Nat. Rev. Drug Discov.* 11, pp. 37–51, doi:10.1038/nrd3591.
85. Abdi, M., Mirkalantari, S. and Amirmozafari, N. (2019) Bacterial Resistance to Antimicrobial Peptides. *J. Pept. Sci.* 25, e3210, doi:10.1002/psc.3210.
86. Murray, B. O., Dawson, R. A., Alsharaf, L. M. and Anne Winter, J. (2020) Protective Effects of *Helicobacter pylori* Membrane Vesicles Against Stress and Antimicrobial Agents. *Microbiology*, doi:10.1099/mic.0.000934.
87. Neshani, A., Zare, H., Eidgahi, M. R. A., Chichaklu, A. H., Movaqar, A. and Ghazvini, K. (2019) Review of Antimicrobial Peptides with Anti-*Helicobacter pylori* Activity. *Helicobacter.* 24, pp. e12555, doi:10.1111/hel.12555.
88. Olleik, H., Baydoun, E., Perrier, J., Hijazi, A., Raymond, J., Manzoni, M., Dupuis, L., Pauleau, G., Goudard, Y., Villéon, B. de L. *et al.* (2019)

Temporin-SHa and Its Analogs as Potential Candidates for the Treatment of Helicobacter pylori. *Biomolecules*. 9, 598, doi:10.3390/biom9100598.

89. Olleik, H., Nicoletti, C., Lafond, M., Courvoisier-Dezord, E., Xue, P., Hijazi, A., Baydoun, E., Perrier, J. and Maresca, M. (2019) Comparative Structure–Activity Analysis of the Antimicrobial Activity, Cytotoxicity, and Mechanism of Action of the Fungal Cyclohexadepsipeptides Enniatins and Beauvericin. *Toxins*. 11, pp. 514, doi:10.3390/toxins11090514.
90. Alvarez, D., Wilkinson, K. A., Treilhou, M., Téné, N., Castillo, D. and Sauvain, M. (2019) Prospecting Peptides Isolated From Black Soldier Fly (Diptera: Stratiomyidae) With Antimicrobial Activity Against *Helicobacter pylori* (Campylobacterales: Helicobacteraceae). *J. Insect Sci.* 19, doi:10.1093/jisesa/iez120.
91. Iwahori, A., Hirota, Y., Sampe, R., Miyano, S., Takahashi, N., Sasatsu, M., Kondo, I. and Numao, N. (1997) On the Antibacterial Activity of Normal and Reversed Magainin 2 Analogs Against *Helicobacter pylori*. *Biol. Pharm. Bull.* 20, pp. 805–808, doi:10.1248/bpb.20.805.
92. Zhang, X.-L., Jiang, A.-M., Ma, Z.-Y., Li, X.-B., Xiong, Y.-Y., Dou, J.-F. and Wang, J.-F. (2015) The Synthetic Antimicrobial Peptide Pexiganan and Its Nanoparticles (PNPs) Exhibit the Anti-*Helicobacter pylori* Activity *in vitro* and *in vivo*. *Molecules*. 20, pp. 3972–3985, doi:10.3390/molecules20033972.
93. Ramamoorthy, A., Thennarasu, S., Lee, D.-K., Tan, A. and Maloy, L. (2006) Solid-State NMR Investigation of the Membrane-Disrupting Mechanism of Antimicrobial Peptides MSI-78 and MSI-594 Derived from Magainin 2 and Melittin. *Biophys. J.* 91, pp. 206–216, doi:10.1529/biophysj.105.073890.
94. Ostrowska, K., Kamysz, W., Dawgul, M. and Różalski, A. (2014) Synthetic Amphibian Peptides and Short Amino-Acids Derivatives Against Planktonic Cells and Mature Biofilm of Providencia Stuartii Clinical Strains. *Pol. J. Microbiol.* 63, pp. 423–431.
95. Giacometti, A., Ghiselli, R., Cirioni, O., Mocchegiani, F., D'Amato, G., Orlando, F., Sisti, V., Kamysz, W., Silvestri, C., Naldoski, P. *et al.* (2004) Therapeutic Efficacy of the Magainin Analogue MSI-78 in Different Intra-Abdominal Sepsis Rat Models. *J. Antimicrob. Chemother.* 54, pp. 654–660, doi:10.1093/jac/dkh390.
96. Nan, Y. H., Jeon, Y. J., Park, I.-S. and Shin, S. Y. (2008) Antimicrobial Peptide P18 Inhibits Inflammatory Responses by LPS- But not by IFN-γ-Stimulated Macrophages. *Biotechnol. Lett.* 30, pp. 1183–1187, doi:10.1007/s10529-008-9682-9.
97. Yang, D., Zou, R., Zhu, Y., Liu, B., Yao, D., Jiang, J., Wu, J. and Tian, H. (2014) Magainin II Modified Polydiacetylene Micelles for Cancer Therapy. *Nanoscale*. 6, pp. 14772–14783, doi:10.1039/C4NR04405C.

98. Rishi, P., Vashist, T., Sharma, A., Kaur, A., Kaur, A., Kaur, N., Kaur, I. P. and Tewari, R. (2018) Efficacy of Designer K11 Antimicrobial Peptide (A Hybrid of Melittin, Cecropin A1 and Magainin 2) Against Acinetobacter Baumannii-Infected Wounds. *Pathog. Dis.* 76, doi:10.1093/femspd/fty072.
99. Lipsky, B. A., Holroyd, K. J. and Zasloff, M. (2008) Topical versus Systemic Antimicrobial Therapy for Treating Mildly Infected Diabetic Foot Ulcers: A Randomized, Controlled, Double-Blinded, Multicenter Trial of Pexiganan Cream. *Clin. Infect. Dis.* 47, pp. 1537–1545, doi:10.1086/593185.
100. Gopinath, D., Kumar, M. S., Selvaraj, D. and Jayakumar, R. (2005) Pexiganan-Incorporated Collagen Matrices for Infected Wound-Healing Processes in Rat. *J. Biomed. Mater. Res. A.* 73A, pp. 320–331, doi:10.1002/jbm.a.30303.
101. Zhang, X., Jiang, A., Wang, G., Yu, H., Qi, B., Xiong, Y., Zhou, G., Qin, M., Dou, J. and Wang, J. (2017) Fusion Expression of the PGLa-AM1 With Native Structure and Evaluation of its Anti-*Helicobacter Pylori* Activity. *Appl. Microbiol. Biotechnol.* 101, pp. 5667–5675, doi:10.1007/s00253-017-8302-9.
102. Chen, L., Li, Y., Li, J., Xu, X., Lai, R. and Zou, Q. (2007) An Antimicrobial Peptide with Antimicrobial Activity Against *Helicobacter pylori*. *Peptides.* 28, pp. 1527–1531, doi:10.1016/j.peptides.2007.07.007.
103. Oger, P.-C., Piesse, C., Ladram, A. and Humblot, V. (2019) Engineering of Antimicrobial Surfaces by Using Temporin Analogs to Tune the Biocidal/antiadhesive Effect. *Molecules.* 24, 814, doi:10.3390/molecules24040814.
104. Capparelli, R., Romanelli, A., Iannaccone, M., Nocerino, N., Ripa, R., Pensato, S., Pedone, C. and Iannelli, D. (2009) Synergistic Antibacterial and Anti-Inflammatory Activity of Temporin A and Modified Temporin B In Vivo. *PLOS ONE.* 4, pp. e7191, doi:10.1371/journal.pone.0007191.
105. Shaheen, F., Nadeem-ul-Haque, M., Ahmed, A., Simjee, S. U., Ganesan, A., Jabeen, A., Shah, Z. A. and Choudhary, M. I. (2018) Synthesis of Breast Cancer Targeting Conjugate of Temporin-SHa Analog and its Effect on Pro- and Anti-Apoptotic Protein Expression in MCF-7 Cells. *Peptides.* 106, pp. 68–82, doi:10.1016/j.peptides.2018.07.002.
106. Simonetti, O., Cirioni, O., Goteri, G., Ghiselli, R., Kamysz, W., Kamysz, E., Silvestri, C., Orlando, F., Barucca, C., Scalise, A. *et al.* (2008) Temporin A is Effective in MRSA-Infected Wounds Through Bactericidal Activity and Acceleration of Wound Repair in a Murine Model. *Peptides.* 29, pp. 520–528, doi:10.1016/j.peptides.2007.12.011.
107. Zhang, L., Yu, J., Wong, C. C. M., Ling, T. K. W., Li, Z. J., Chan, K. M., Ren, S. X., Shen, J., Chan, R. L. Y., Lee, C. C. *et al.* (2013) Cathelicidin Protects Against *Helicobacter pylori* Colonization and the Associated Gastritis in Mice. *Gene Ther.* 20, pp. 751–760, doi:10.1038/gt.2012.92.
108. Zhang, L., Wu, W. K. K., Gallo, R. L., Fang, E. F., Hu, W., Ling, T. K. W., Shen, J., Chan, R. L. Y., Lu, L., Luo, X. M., *et al.* (2016) Critical Role of Antimicrobial Peptide Cathelicidin for Controlling *Helicobacter pylori*

Survival and Infection. *J. Immunol. Baltim. Md 1950.* 196, pp. 1799–1809, doi:10.4049/jimmunol.1500021.

109. Kuroda, K., Okumura, K., Isogai, H. and Isogai, E. (2015) The Human Cathelicidin Antimicrobial Peptide LL-37 and Mimics are Potential Anticancer Drugs. *Front. Oncol.* 5, doi:10.3389/fonc.2015.00144.
110. Jiang, M., Ma, L., Huang, Y., Wu, H., Dou, J. and Zhou, C. (2020) Antimicrobial Activities of Peptide Cbf-K16 Against Drug-Resistant *Helicobacter pylori* Infection In Vitro and In Vivo. *Microb. Pathog.* 138, pp. 103847, doi:10.1016/j.micpath.2019.103847.
111. Zhang, X., Jiang, A., Qi, B., Yu, H., Xiong, Y., Zhou, G., Qin, M., Dou, J. and Wang, J. (2018) Secretion Expression of Human Neutrophil Peptide 1 (HNP1) in Pichia Pastoris and Its Functional Analysis Against Antibiotic-Resistant *Helicobacter pylori*. *Appl. Microbiol. Biotechnol.* 102, pp. 4817–4827, doi:10.1007/s00253-018-8982-9.
112. Ferdowsi, S., Pourfathollah, A. A., Amiri, F., Rafiee, M. H. and Aghaei, A. (2019) Evaluation of Anticancer Activity of α-Defensins Purified from Neutrophils Trapped in Leukoreduction Filters. *Life Sci.* 224, pp. 249–254, doi:10.1016/j.lfs.2019.03.072.
113. Moazzezy, N., Karam, M. R. A., Rafati, S., Bouzari, S. and Oloomi, M. (2020) Inhibition and Eradication Activity of Truncated α-Defensin Analogs Against Multidrug Resistant Uropathogenic *Escherichia coli* Biofilm. *PLOS ONE.* 15, e0235892, doi:10.1371/journal.pone.0235892.
114. Brook, M., Tomlinson, G. H., Miles, K., Smith, R. W. P., Rossi, A. G., Hiemstra, P. S., Wout, E. F. A. van't; Dean, J. L. E., Gray, N. K., Lu, W. *et al.* (2016) Neutrophil-Derived Alpha Defensins Control Inflammation by Inhibiting Macrophage mRNA Translation. *Proc. Natl. Acad. Sci.* 113, pp. 4350–4355, doi:10.1073/pnas.1601831113.
115. Li, J., Raghunath, M., Tan, D., Lareu, R. R., Chen, Z. and Beuerman, R. W. (2006) Defensins HNP1 and HBD2 Stimulation of Wound-Associated Responses in Human Conjunctival Fibroblasts. *Invest. Ophthalmol. Vis. Sci.* 47, pp. 3811–3819, doi:10.1167/iovs.05-1360.
116. Avitabile, C., Capparelli, R., Rigano, M. M., Fulgione, A., Barone, A., Pedone, C. and Romanelli, A. (2013) Antimicrobial Peptides from Plants: Stabilization of the γ Core of a Tomato Defensin by Intramolecular Disulfide Bond. *J. Pept. Sci.* 19, pp. 240–245, doi:10.1002/psc.2479.
117. Rigano, M. M., Romanelli, A., Fulgione, A., Nocerino, N., D'Agostino, N., Avitabile, C., Frusciante, L., Barone, A., Capuano, F. and Capparelli, R. (2012) A Novel Synthetic Peptide from A Tomato Defensin Exhibits Antibacterial Activities Against *Helicobacter pylori*. *J. Pept. Sci.* 18, pp. 755–762, doi:10.1002/psc.2462.
118. Libardo, M. D. J., Bahar, A. A., Ma, B., Fu, R., McCormick, L. E., Zhao, J., McCallum, S. A., Nussinov, R., Ren, D., Angeles-Boza, A. M., *et al.*

(2017) Nuclease Activity Gives An Edge to Host-Defense Peptide Piscidin 3 Over Piscidin 1, Rendering It More Effective Against Persisters and Biofilms. *FEBS J.* 284, pp. 3662–3683, doi:10.1111/febs.14263.

119. Kumar, A., Mahajan, M., Awasthi, B., Tandon, A., Harioudh, M. K., Shree, S., Singh, P., Shukla, P. K., Ramachandran, R., Mitra, K. *et al.* (2017) Piscidin-1-Analogs with Double *L*- and *D*-lysine Residues Exhibited Different Conformations in Lipopolysaccharide but Comparable Anti-Endotoxin Activities. *Sci. Rep.* 7, pp. 39925, doi:10.1038/srep39925.

120. Su, B.-C., Pan, C.-Y. and Chen, J.-Y. (2019) Antimicrobial Peptide TP4 Induces ROS-Mediated Necrosis by Triggering Mitochondrial Dysfunction in Wild-Type and Mutant p53 Glioblastoma Cells. *Cancers.* 11, pp. 171, doi:10.3390/cancers11020171.

121. Ting, C.-H., Liu, Y.-C., Lyu, P.-C. and Chen, J.-Y. (2018) Nile Tilapia Derived Antimicrobial Peptide TP4 Exerts Antineoplastic Activity Through Microtubule Disruption. *Mar. Drugs.* 16, pp. 462, doi:10.3390/md16120462.

122. Huang, H.-N., Chan, Y.-L., Wu, C.-J. and Chen, J.-Y. (2015) Tilapia Piscidin 4 (TP4) Stimulates Cell Proliferation and Wound Closure in MRSA-Infected Wounds in Mice. *Mar. Drugs.* 13, pp. 2813–2833, doi:10.3390/md13052813.

123. Narayana, J. L., Huang, H.-N., Wu, C.-J., and Chen, J.-Y. (2015) Efficacy of the Antimicrobial Peptide TP4 Against *Helicobacter pylori* Infection: In Vitro Membrane Perturbation via Micellization and *in vivo* Suppression of Host Immune Responses in a Mouse Model. *Oncotarget.* 6, pp. 12936–12954.

124. Narayana, J. L., Huang, H.-N., Wu, C.-J. and Chen, J.-Y. (2015) Epinecidin-1 Antimicrobial Activity: *In vitro* Membrane Lysis and *in vivo* Efficacy Against *Helicobacter pylori* Infection in a Mouse Model. *Biomaterials.* 61, pp. 41–51, doi:10.1016/j.biomaterials.2015.05.014.

125. Lin, W.-J., Chien, Y.-L., Pan, C.-Y., Lin, T.-L., Chen, J.-Y., Chiu, S.-J. and Hui, C.-F. (2009) Epinecidin-1, An Antimicrobial Peptide from Fish (*Epinephelus coioides*) Which has an Antitumor Effect like Lytic Peptides in Human Fibrosarcoma Cells. *Peptides.* 30, pp. 283–290, doi:10.1016/j.peptides.2008.10.007.

126. Chen, J.-Y., Lin, W.-J., Wu, J.-L., Her, G. M. and Hui, C.-F. (2009) Epinecidin-1 Peptide Induces Apoptosis Which Enhances Antitumor Effects in Human Leukemia U937 Cells. *Peptides.* 30, pp. 2365–2373, doi:10.1016/j.peptides.2009.08.019.

127. Huang, H.-N., Rajanbabu, V., Pan, C.-Y., Chan, Y.-L., Wu, C.-J. and Chen, J.-Y. (2013) Use of the Antimicrobial Peptide Epinecidin-1 to Protect Against MRSA Infection in Mice with Skin Injuries. *Biomaterials.* 34, pp. 10319–10327, doi:10.1016/j.biomaterials.2013.09.037.

128. Kim, T. S., Hur, J. W., Yu, M. A., Cheigh, C. I., Kim, K. N., Hwang, J. K. and Pyun, Y. R. (2003) Antagonism of *Helicobacter pylori* by Bacteriocins

of Lactic Acid Bacteria. *J. Food Prot.* 66, pp. 3–12, doi:10.4315/0362-028X-66.1.3.

129. Kaur, B., Garg, N., Sachdev, A. and Kumar, B. (2014) Effect of the Oral Intake of Probiotic Pediococcus Acidilactici BA28 on *Helicobacter pylori* Causing Peptic Ulcer in C57BL/6 Mice Models. *Appl. Biochem. Biotechnol.* 172, pp. 973–983, doi:10.1007/s12010-013-0585-4.
130. Chelliah, R., Saravanakumar, K., Daliri, E. B.-M., Kim, J.-H., Lee, J.-K., Jo, H., Kim, S.-H., Ramakrishnan, S. R., Madar, I. H., Wei, S. *et al.* (2020) Unveiling the Potentials of Bacteriocin (Pediocin L50) from Pediococcus Acidilactici with Antagonist Spectrum in a Caenorhabditis Elegans Model. *Int. J. Biol. Macromol.* 143, pp. 555–572, doi:10.1016/j.ijbiomac.2019.10.196.
131. Simova, E. D., Beshkova, D. B. and Dimitrov, Z. P. (2009) Characterization and Antimicrobial Spectrum of Bacteriocins Produced by Lactic Acid Bacteria Isolated from Traditional Bulgarian Dairy Products. *J. Appl. Microbiol.* 106, pp. 692–701, doi:10.1111/j.1365-2672.2008.04052.x.
132. Lim, E. S. (2015) Purification and Characterization of Two Bacteriocins from Lactobacillus brevis BK11 and Enterococcus faecalis BK61 Showing Anti-Helicobacter pylori Activity. *J. Korean Soc. Appl. Biol. Chem.* 58, pp. 703–714, doi:10.1007/s13765-015-0094-y.
133. Guzman, J., Téné, N., Touchard, A., Castillo, D., Belkhelfa, H., Haddioui-Hbabi, L., Treilhou, M. and Sauvain, M. (2017) Anti-*Helicobacter pylori* Properties of the Ant-Venom Peptide Bicarinalin. *Toxins.* 10, doi:10.3390/toxins10010021.
134. Téné, N., Bonnafé, E., Berger, F., Rifflet, A., Guilhaudis, L., Ségalas-Milazzo, I., Pipy, B., Coste, A., Leprince, J. and Treilhou, M. (2016) Biochemical and Biophysical Combined Study of Bicarinalin, An Ant Venom Antimicrobial Peptide. *Peptides.* 79, pp. 103–113, doi:10.1016/j.peptides.2016.04.001.
135. Eales, M. G., Ferrari, E., Goddard, A. D., Lancaster, L., Sanderson, P. and Miller, C. (2018) Mechanistic and Phenotypic Studies of Bicarinalin, BP100 and Colistin Action on *Acinetobacter baumannii*. *Res. Microbiol.* 169, pp. 296–302, doi:10.1016/j.resmic.2018.04.005.
136. Olleik, H., Yahiaoui, S., Roulier, B., Courvoisier-Dezord, E., Perrier, J., Pérès, B., Hijazi, A., Baydoun, E., Raymond, J., Boumendjel, A., *et al.* (2019) Aurone Derivatives as Promising Antibacterial Agents Against Resistant Gram-Positive Pathogens. *Eur. J. Med. Chem.* 165, pp. 133–141, doi:10.1016/j.ejmech.2019.01.022.
137. Olleik, H., Yacoub, T., Hoffer, L., Gnansounou, S. M., Benhaiem-Henry, K., Nicoletti, C., Mekhalfi, M., Pique, V., Perrier, J., Hijazi, A. *et al.* (2020) Synthesis and Evaluation of the Antibacterial Activities of 13-Substituted Berberine Derivatives. *Antibiotics.* 9, 381, doi:10.3390/antibiotics9070381.
138. Tran, A. X., Whittimore, J. D., Wyrick, P. B., McGrath, S. C., Cotter, R. J. and Trent, M. S. (2006) The Lipid A 1-Phosphatase of *Helicobacter pylori*

Is Required for Resistance to the Antimicrobial Peptide Polymyxin. *J. Bacteriol.* 188, pp. 4531–4541, doi:10.1128/JB.00146-06.

139. Molchanova, N., Hansen, P. R. and Franzyk, H. (2017) Advances in Development of Antimicrobial Peptidomimetics as Potential Drugs. *Molecules*. 22, pp. 1430, doi:10.3390/molecules22091430.
140. Makobongo, M. O., Kovachi, T., Gancz, H., Mor, A. and Merrell, D. S. (2009) *In Vitro* Antibacterial Activity of Acyl-Lysyl Oligomers against Helicobacter pylori. *Antimicrob. Agents Chemother.* 53, pp. 4231–4239, doi:10.1128/AAC.00510-09.
141. Makobongo, M. O., Gancz, H., Carpenter, B. M., McDaniel, D. P. and Merrell, D. S. (2012) The Oligo-Acyl Lysyl Antimicrobial Peptide C12K-2*β*12 Exhibits a Dual Mechanism of Action and Demonstrates Strong *In Vivo* Efficacy against Helicobacter pylori. *Antimicrob. Agents Chemother.* 56, pp. 378–390, doi:10.1128/AAC.00689-11.
142. Xiong, M., Bao, Y., Xu, X., Wang, H., Han, Z., Wang, Z., Liu, Y., Huang, S., Song, Z., Chen, J. *et al.* (2017) Selective Killing of Helicobacter pylori with pH-Responsive Helix–Coil Conformation Transitionable Antimicrobial Polypeptides. *Proc. Natl. Acad. Sci.* 114, pp. 12675–12680, doi:10.1073/pnas.1710408114.

https://doi.org/10.1142/9789811261664_0003

Chapter 3

Antimicrobial Ribosomally Synthesized and Post-Translationally Modified Peptides as a Source of Alternatives to Antibiotics: A Focus on the Sactipeptides and Ranthipeptides Subclasses

Clarisse Roblin*, Pierre Rousselot-Pailley*, Victor Duarte†, Josette Perrier*, and Mickael Lafond*,‡

**Aix Marseille Univ, CNRS, Centrale Marseille, iSm2, Marseille, France, ADISSEO France SAS, Centre d'Expertise et de Recherche en Nutrition, Commentry, France*
†University Grenoble Alpes, CEA, IRIG, CBM, Grenoble, France

‡mickael.lafond@univ-amu.fr

1. Introduction

One of the major concerns in Public Health nowadays is antibiotic resistant bacteria. It has been estimated that millions of people will perish from infections caused by multi-drug resistant (MDR) bacteria in the decades to come [1]. The history of antibiotic therapy has shown that whenever a new class of antibiotics has been introduced into the clinic, very quickly, resistant bacterial populations have emerged. This phenomenon based either on an intrinsic or acquired resistance mechanism gives the bacteria a survival advantage, leading overall to the emergence of an increasing number of resistant bacteria and their spread [2]. In addition, only two new classes of antibiotics have been discovered since the 1960s [3]. Therefore, it is essential and urgent to find new antibiotics. Several alternatives to antibiotic treatment such as phage therapy, immunotherapy, or microbiota transplantation are investigated to overcome the antibiotic resistance crisis [4]. Notably, one of these alternatives is the use of antimicrobial peptides i.e. peptides able to inhibit the growth of microorganisms or to kill them. In particular, **Ri**bosomally synthesized and **P**ost-translationally modified **P**eptides (RiPPs) compose a class of highly diverse peptides with promising therapeutic applications including the treatment of infectious diseases caused by bacteria (i.e. antibacterial activity) or other microorganisms such as fungi, viruses, and parasites (i.e. antimicrobial activity).

2. Definition and Generalities

RiPPs are peptides defined by a size limit of 10 kDa that are ribosomally translated in a mRNA-dependent manner and undergo various post-translational modifications (PTMs). They are produced by organisms from the three domains of Life (archaea, prokaryotes and eukaryotes) and exert multiple types of biological activities including antibacterial and antimicrobial activities but also insecticidal, nematoxic and anti-cancer effects among others. The PTMs carried by RiPPs and the structure of RiPPs are highly diverse and determine their classification that will be presented below. However, all RiPPs share a common biosynthesis pathway [5,6]. This pathway starts with the transcription and translation of a structural gene in a precursor peptide composed of 20–110 amino acid residues. The precursor peptide is composed of at least two distinct domains named leader peptide and core peptide. The core peptide defines the region that is subjected to PTMs whereas the leader peptide defines a region that is cleaved by proteolysis subsequently to the core peptide modification. In most RiPPs, the leader peptide is located at the *N*-terminus of the core peptide, but it can also be located at the *C*-terminus as in the case of bottromycins [5]. While most PTMs occur when the leader peptide is still attached to the core peptide, some modifications that require the free *N*-terminus of the core peptide can happen after the excision of the leader peptide. Such examples are found in the cyanobactin and lanthipeptide subclasses whose RiPPs might undergo head-to-tail cyclization or

N-terminus alterations, respectively [7]. Additionally, some RiPPs have a recognition sequence at the *C*-terminus that is required for cleavage and cyclization of the peptide such as amatoxins, phallotoxins, borosins or orbitides [6]. In some cases, like cyanobactins, recognition sequences can be present at both *N*- and *C*-termini [8]. In RiPPs produced by eukaryotes, such as cyclotides or conopeptides [6], a signal domain can be also found at the *N*-terminus that directs the precursor peptide to a specific cellular compartment where modifications of the core peptide occur. The fully mature and active RiPP corresponds to the modified core peptide excised from all the other domains, i.e. signal, recognition and leader (Figure 1).

The genes involved in the production and maturation of RiPPs are in most cases regrouped in genetic clusters. The number of genes composing these genetic clusters greatly varies but at least two Open Reading Frames (ORFs) are found for all RiPPs: the structural sequence and a sequence encoding a modification enzyme (also called maturation enzyme) [9] Multiple sequences encoding precursor peptides can be found instead of a single copy. Likewise, multiple maturation enzymes, whether with similar activity or not, can be encoded in RiPP biosynthesis genetic clusters (BGC). In some examples, the genes involved in RiPP biosynthesis are

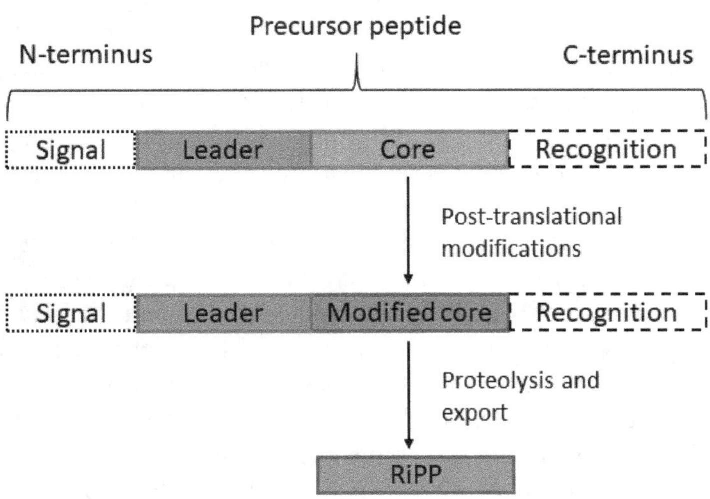

Fig. 1. Common modular organization and maturation pathway of RiPPs. Solid lines indicate sequences found in all RiPPs whereas dashed lines represent optional sequences. In some cases, the leader is found at the C-terminus of the core peptide rather than at the *N*-terminus.

not clustered but rather distant in the genome. For example, in the genome of *Bacillus anthracis*, the sequence encoding the precursor peptide of heterocycloanthracin is located 1.27 Mbases upstream of two clustered ORFs encoding distinct enzymes both involved in PTM formation: a cyclodehydratase and a dehydrogenase [10]. Another example is found in the genome of the cyanobacterium *Prochlorococcus*. A gene encoding a modification enzyme typical of the subclass lanthipeptide is clustered with seven sequences encoding putative peptide precursors. However, 22 other similar structural sequences are found elsewhere in the bacterial genome [11]. Additionally, genes involved in the regulation of production, in proteolysis and export as well as in the cell immunity to its own RiPP are also commonly found in the RiPP BGC [12].

3. Roles of the Leader Peptide

3.1. *Involvement in the maturation process*

The leader peptides among RiPPs greatly vary in length as well as in amino acid composition. Several roles have been proposed for the leader peptide. First, the removal of the leader sequence in most RiPPs prevents or highly diminishes the incorporation of PTMs on the core peptide [7]. Therefore, it has been hypothesized that the leader peptide acts as a recognition sequence for the maturation enzymes or as an activator of these enzymes. This hypothesis was corroborated by the successful modification and export of non-natural peptides expressed as fusions with the leader peptide of the extensively studied lanthipeptide nisin in its natural producer strain *Lactococcus lactis* [13]. Many RiPPs with high variability in the core peptide exhibit the same PTMs. As it is unlikely that the enzyme could have such substrate tolerance, it has been proposed that the enzymes could recognize conserved motifs in the leader peptide of different RiPPs and exert their catalytic activities on the core peptide [14]. In fact, some classes of RiPPs, such as lanthipeptides, exhibit conserved leader sequences but variable core sequences [15]. In particular, in the case of prochlorosins cited earlier, the 29 putative peptide precursors share more than 90% of similarity in their leader sequence whereas no conserved motifs have been found in the core sequences. The single lanthipeptide modification enzyme is able to process the different precursors by incorporating the same type of PTMs, but at different positions resulting from the core sequence variability [11,15,16]. Moreover, a binding motif of the maturation enzyme to the leader peptide has been identified in some RiPPs such as for class I lanthipeptides. Their leader sequences almost all contain a Phe-Asp/Asn-Leu-Asn/Asp motif. Mutation of this motif in NisA — the precursor of nisin — prevented binding to the dehydratase NisB which is the first enzyme catalyzing the two-step modification of this lanthipeptide, suggesting that this motif is essential for substrate recognition [17]. Co-crystallization of NisA with NisB provided more information on their interaction: the leader domain of NisA binds to NisB as an anti-parallel β-strand at a position ensuring that the core peptide is in contact with the catalytic site of NisB. The Phe-Asp/Asn-Leu-Asn/Asp conserved motif of the NisA leader peptide is involved in hydrophobic interactions with NisB [18] (Figure 2(a)). Additional crystallization studies on other coupled precursor peptides and maturation enzymes, such as the cyanobactin heterocyclase LynD with an artificial precursor PatE' as well as the adenyltransferase MccB with MccA, the precursor of microcin C7, showed that the binding of the leader peptide to the enzyme involves similar interactions and structures [19,20] (Figures 2(b) and 2(c)). Specifically, the domain of the enzymes involved in leader peptide binding corresponds to a winged helix-turn-helix. It was then proposed that RiPP maturation enzymes harbor a specific RiPP precursor peptide Recognition Element (RRE). Analyses of known RREs revealed structural similarity with the small protein PqqD that is also involved in the multi-enzymes maturation of a RiPP — the pyrroloquinoline quinone (PQQ) — as a chaperone [21] (Figure 2(d)).

In silico analyses based on the structure of PqqD revealed that at least half of the prokaryotic subclasses of RiPPs are modified by enzymes containing an RRE [22]. Interaction of the leader peptide and the maturation enzyme through a PqqD-like RRE were confirmed in five other subclasses of RiPPs: lasso peptides, linear azoline-containing peptides, thiopeptides, sactipeptides [22–25] **(see details in Section 1.5.4.)** and recently for the CteA ranthipeptide [26] (**see details in Section 1.6.3.**). For example, it was shown that the precursor of therbactin from the lasso peptides subclass binds to a PqqD-like RRE through hydrophobic interactions of a Tyr-X-X-Phe-X-Leu-X-X-X-Gly leader peptide motif that is essential and sufficient for the recognition by the maturation enzyme. Therefore, recognition of the leader peptide by the maturation enzyme is mediated through steric complementarity, rather than sequence specificity [27]. Noteworthy, many RRE domains were identified in the family of radical-S-adenosylmethionine (SAM) enzymes involved in the maturation of several subclasses of RiPPs including bottromycin, proteusin, sactipeptide, and

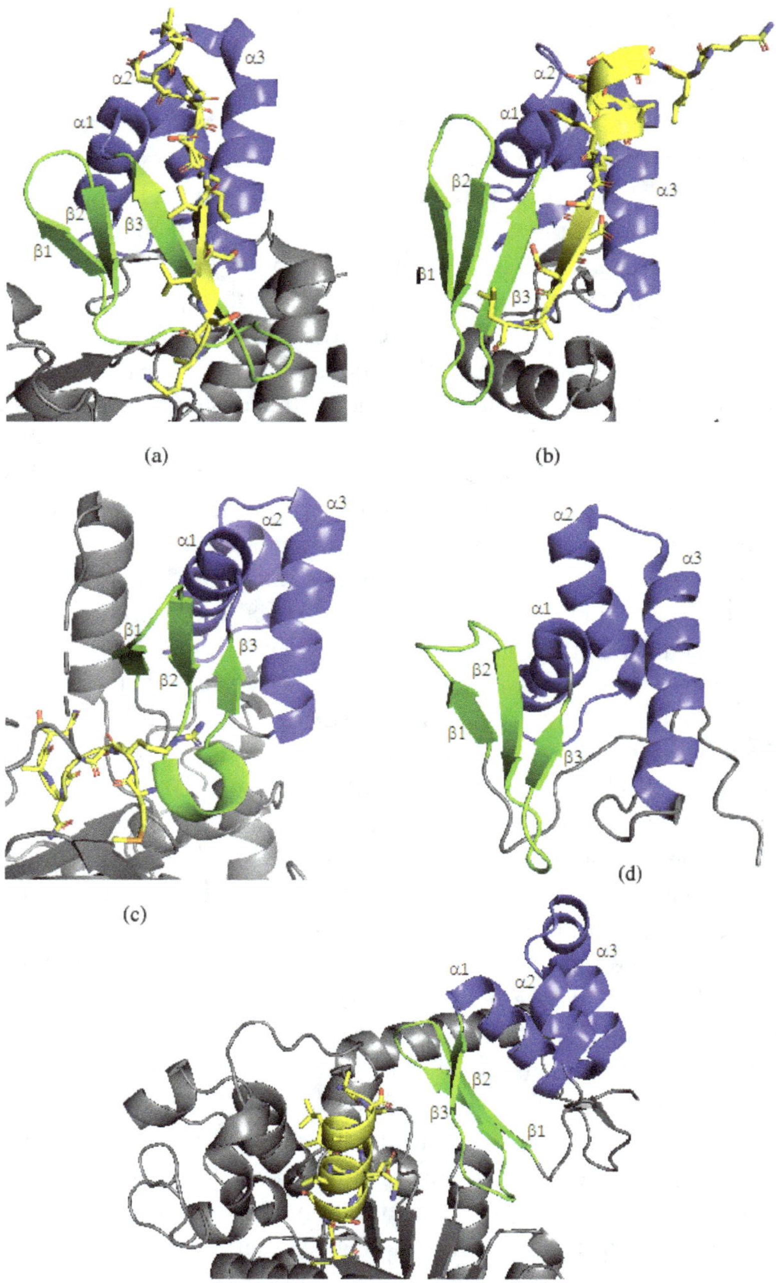
α3
α2
α1
β2
β3
β1
(a)
α2
α1
β2
α3
β1
β3
(b)
α3
α1
α2
β1
β3
β2
(c)
α2
α3
α1
β2
β1
β3
(d)
α3
α1
α2
β2
β3
β1
(e)

ranthipeptide [22–26]. Intriguingly, the elucidation of both structures of the streptide SuiA and its maturation enzyme belonging to the radical-SAM family SuiB revealed a binding of the leader peptide in a location that is distinct from the archetypal PqqD-like RRE domain [28–30] (Figure 2(e)). This unique SuiA-binding mode suggests that the RRE-like domain is involved in an undetected interaction in which it recognizes the peptide and delivers it to the active site but at a certain stage in the catalytic cycle releases the precursor peptide.

It has also been proposed that the leader peptide not only acts as a recognition sequence but might also induce conformational changes on the maturation enzymes, leading to its catalytic activation or increased affinity for the core peptide. This hypothesis is supported by the trans-activity of the leader peptides of some RiPPs. It has been shown that nisin, lacticin, and catenulipeptin, respectively class I, class II and class III lanthipeptides, are modified by their maturation enzymes when the leader sequence is not contained in the precursor peptide but rather expressed or provided by itself. Moreover, studies on nisin and lacticin also revealed low levels of PTMs incorporation even in the absence of the leader sequence. Therefore, a second model was proposed in which the leader peptide would not induce conformational changes but rather trap the enzyme in its active form. In this model, maturation enzymes would exist in multiple evolving conformations, hence the appropriate state for catalytic activity would be in low concentration. Binding of the leader sequence to the enzyme would form a stable complex, and the concentration of active enzyme would then increase as the concentration of leader peptide increases as well. This trans activity of the leader peptide has been proven for other subclasses of RiPPs such as microcin MccJ25 but not for all subclasses. It is possible that this mechanism is specific of a few

←

Fig. 2. Structural comparison of five specific RiPPs precursor peptide Recognition Elements. Structurally equivalent sections of RiPP biosynthetic proteins involved in the biosynthesis of the lantibiotic nisin, NisB dehydratase [4WD9] (a), antitumor cyanobactins, LynD cyclodehydratase [4V1T] (b), the Trojan horse antibiotic microcin C7, MccB adenylating enzyme [3h9J]) (c), bacterial dehydrogenase cofactor PQQ, PqqD rSAM-associated [5SXY] (d), streptide SuiA, SuiB rSAM-enzyme [5V1T] (e). The green β-sheets and marine blue α-helices constitute a conserved RiPP precursor peptide recognition element (RRE). In (a–c, e), the precursor peptide is shown in yellow stick format. Dashed lines indicate missing electron density.

classes of RiPPs or that the region needed for optimal enzyme conformation covers partially the sequences of the leader peptide and of the core peptide. Indeed, in the native biosynthetic pathways of RiPPs the distinction between leader and core peptide only occurs during proteolysis after PTMs incorporation [7,14] (Figure 1). The role of the leader peptide as an anchor, or an activator for maturation enzymes, provides options for the generation of new RiPPs by its fusion to non-natural core peptides or even by designing hybrid RiPP biosynthetic pathways. In that sense, Burkhart and co-workers built a chimeric leader peptide with recognition elements for maturation enzymes from different RiPP biosynthetic pathways, such as thiazoline associated with either lanthipeptide or sactipeptide. After optimization of a non-natural peptide sequence and in the presence of two distinct enzymes, both types of PTMs were successfully introduced on the chimeric precursor [31].

3.2. *Involvement in the producer protection and in secretion*

The second role proposed for the leader peptide is a protective role for the producer. In fact, most RiPPs are inactive when attached to their leader peptide and its removal occurs during or after secretion, thus ensuring that the RiPP is not toxic for the producer strain. From that role, a third one comes up: the function as a secretion signal [14,32]. In the case of nisin, an extracellular protease and an ABC transporter are encoded in the BGC. Diverse modified and unmodified peptides fused to the leader peptide of nisin were successfully exported in the extracellular compartment when co-expressed with the nisin transporter in a heterologous system. Therefore, the leader peptide of the nisin precursor indeed harbors a secretion signal [33]. In the nisin biosynthetic pathway, the protease NisP is exported and bound to the cell-wall of the producing bacterial cells. Other class I lanthipeptides can be cleaved through cytoplasmic proteases or proteases secreted in the extracellular compartment [34]. Whereas for lanthipeptides from class I like nisin a protease is encoded in the genetic cluster, no such protease-encoding sequence is found for class II. However, the transporters encoded in the cluster harbor an N-terminal peptidase domain. *In vitro* incubation of the purified lacticin precursor with the *N*-terminal domain of its ABC transporter (150 out of 691 total amino acid residues) was sufficient to achieve leader peptide removal. Thus, the export and proteolysis of lacticin are coupled and both performed by a bi-functional enzyme. The transmembrane domain of the transporter is not required for leader peptide recognition and cleavage. Proteolysis of the leader peptide of the lacticin precursor occurs after two Gly residues. Mutations of these residues prevent the excision of the leader peptide [35]. Similar Gly-Gly cleavage sites or sometimes a Gly-Ala motif have been identified in other lanthipeptides or RiPPs as well as in class IIb bacteriocins. Class IIb bacteriocins are linear antibacterial peptides produced by Gram-positive bacteria. Likely to the RiPPs, they are ribosomally synthesized as precursors, but unlike RiPPs the core peptide is not subjected to PTMs [36]. Therefore, this conserved motif seems to play an important role in proteolytic processing of the precursor. The ABC transporters processing this Gly-Gly motif were found in multiple classes of RiPPs biosynthetic pathways and renamed Peptidase-Containing ATP-binding Cassette (PCAT). Common features of PCAT include three distinct domains: a transmembrane domain, a *C*-terminal nucleotide-binding domain achieving ATP hydrolysis, and an *N*-terminal cysteine protease domain cleaving the leader peptide after a Gly-Gly motif. The PCAT transporters form dimers and their overall structure resembles ABC transporters lacking the peptidase domain [14]. Although mutation of the Gly-Gly motif prevents cleavage in many RiPPs, it doesn't affect the incorporation of PTMs on the core peptide by maturation enzymes, suggesting that distinct sequences of the leader peptides are involved in different roles [32]. Other motifs necessary for the removal of the peptide leader have been identified. For example, in the class I lanthipeptide epilancin 15X precursor, the excision of the leader peptide is mediated through an Asp-Leu-Asn-Pro-Gln-Ser sequence recognized by the peptidase ElxP. The introduction of this sequence in the NisA precursor allowed the cleavage of NisA by ElxP, whereas the wild-type NisA was not processed by ElxP [37].

The excision of the leader peptide by proteolysis can be a one-step or a multi-step process. For example, the precursor of lichenicidin, a class II lanthipeptide, is partially cleaved after a Gly-Gly motif by the peptidase domain of a transporter, and then the last six amino acid residues of the leader peptide are removed after secretion by an extracellular protease [38]. A similar two-step processing of the leader peptide was also identified for the sactipeptide ruminococcin C. Whereas for lichenicidin, the peptidase transporter and the protease are encoded in the genome of the *Bacillus licheniformis,* in ruminococcin C, the removal of the leader peptide involves a bacterial peptidase form *Ruminococcus gnavus* E1 and the mammalian pancreatic trypsin. *R. gnavus* is a commensal of the gut microbiota of animals and in particular humans. Thus, the latter symbiont and its host have developed a mutualistic relationship to process ruminococcin C into an active antibacterial form [39]

4. Classification

RiPPs are classified according to their PTMs and their related biosynthetic machineries [5]. A brief description of each class of RiPPs is given here and a summary table is included at the end of this subsection. As sactipeptides and ranthipeptides will be further discussed (see Sections 1.5 and 1.6), they are not included in this section.

4.1. *Lanthipeptides*

Lanthipeptide, one of the most studied classes of RiPPS, stands for lanthionine-containing peptide as these RiPPs carry lanthionine (Lan) and/or 3-methylanthionine (MeLan) residues (Figure 3(a)). Lan corresponds to two alanine residues bound by a thioether bridge between their β-carbons and MeLan to a Lan carrying an additional methyl group. In lanthipeptides, the thioether crosslinks of Lan and MeLan are formed by the addition of a Cys onto previously dehydrated amino acids, respectively a Ser in 2,3-dideshydroalanine (Dha) and a threonine (Thr) in 2,3-dideshydrobutyrine (Dhb). In class I lanthipeptides, the formation of Lan and MeLan residues is catalyzed by two enzymes: a dehydratase and a cyclase. For classes II to IV, a single bi-functional enzyme, named lanthionine synthetase, carries out the formation of Lan and MeLan. Class II lanthionine synthetases harbor an N-terminal dehydration domain with no homology among the synthetases from the other classes and a *C*-terminal domain similar to the class I cyclases. Classes III and IV are distinctive in their *C*-terminal cyclase domains but harbor similar phospholyase and kinase domains in the N-terminus both responsible for dehydration. Lanthipeptides can carry dehydrated residues (Dha or Dhb) that are not involved in thioether bridges if the number of Ser and Thr exceeds the number of Cys (Figure 3(a)). Although the identified lanthipeptides are produced by bacteria, putative homologues of lanthipeptide synthetases have been found in the genomes of archaea and eukaryotes including mammals. Lanthipeptide BGCs are found in both Gram-positive and -negative bacteria [5,40].

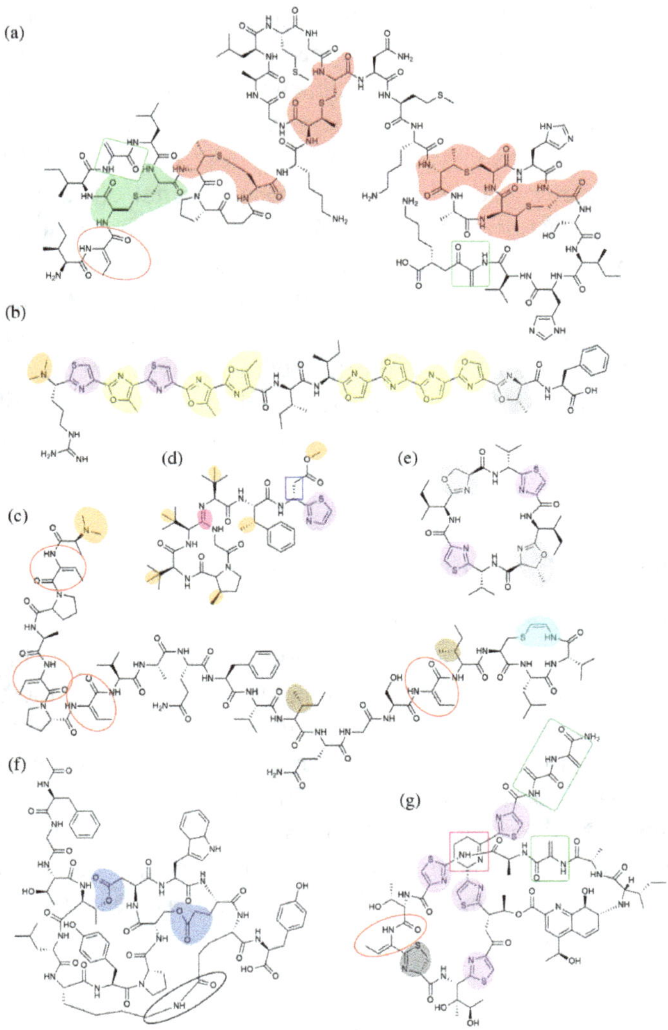

Fig. 3. Structure of prokaryotic RiPPs : Lanthipeptide nisin A (a), LAP plantazolicin (b), linaridin cypemycin (c), bottromycin A2 (d), cyanobactin patellamide A (e), microvirdin B (f) and thiopeptide thiostrepton A (g). Lan and MeLan residues are, respectively, highlighted in green and red while unreactive Dha and Dhb are circled in green and red. Thiazoles; thiazolines; oxazoles and methyloxazoles; oxazolines and methyloxazolines; AviCys are highlighted in lilac, dark grey, light yellow, light grey and light blue, respectively. Methylation, macrocylisation, ester bonds and allo-residues are highlighted in orange, pink, dark blue and brown, respectively. Dark blue, black and pink outlines indicate epimerization, amide bond between side chains and dehydropiperidine residues, respectively.

Lanthipeptides exhibit antibacterial activity but also antifungal and antiviral activities as well as other types of functions than antimicrobial such as pain relief. The identified antibacterial modes of action of lanthipeptides involve binding to the cell membrane resulting in pore formation and inhibition of cell wall synthesis [5,41]. Currently, Re-Tain™, a nisin pre-filled syringe developed by the company ImmuCell, is under FDA approval for the treatment of mastitis [42]. Mastitis is one of the most common afflictions in cows and is linked to bacterial infections caused by a wide range of pathogens, the most frequent being S*treptococcus* spp., *Staphylococcus aureus, Corynebacterium bovis* and *E. coli* [43]. Other lanthipeptides are under pre-clinical or clinical investigations for infectious diseases but also for other medical applications. For example, duramycin entered Phase II trial for the treatment of cystic fibrosis, a genetic disease [44].

4.2. *Linear azol(in)e-containing peptides (LAPs)*

LAPs harbor thiazol(in)e and (methyl)-oxazol(in)e heterocycles resulting from the cyclization of Cys with the side chains of Ser or Thr (Figure 3(b)). LAPs can undergo other PTMs including acetylation, methylation, and dehydration [5]. This subclass of RiPPs is produced by both Gram-negative and positive bacteria. The identified spectra and the modes of action of LAPs differ among them. For example, the LAP microcin B17 inhibits DNA synthesis and especially DNA gyrase with a mechanism similar to the quinolone antibiotic ciprofloxacin, whereas plantazolicin acts by depolarization and phazolicin as well as klebsazolicin inhibit protein synthesis [45–47].

4.3. *Linaridins*

Linear dehydrated peptides (or linaridins) are a small subclass of RiPPs with only three members isolated produced by *Streptomyces* spp., although dozens of putative linaridin BGCs have been identified in both Gram-positive and negative bacteria as well as archaea with genomic tools. The common features of linaridins are the presence of *allo*-isoleucine and Dhb residues (Figure 3(c)). Additional nonproteinogenic residues such as *N,N*-dimethylalanine, *N,N*-dimethylisoleucine and S-[(Z)-2-aminovinyl]-*D*-cysteine (AviCys) can be found in linaridins. The PTMs formation involves an enzyme composed of an *N*-terminal horizontally transferred transmembrane helix (HTTH) domain and a *C*-terminal α/β hydrolase fold or two enzymes carrying each of these domains. So far, the described biological activity of these RiPPs includes anticancer and narrow spectrum antibacterial effects but little is known about their mode of action [48–50].

4.4. *Bottromycins*

This subclass is original in the RiPP classification as the precursors harbor a C-terminal follower peptide instead of an *N*-terminal leader peptide but with similar functions. The core peptide is only composed of 8 residues whereas the follower is large with 35–37 amino acid residues. Additionally, a Met is found at the *N*-terminus of the precursor upstream of the core peptide. PTMs of bottromycins consist of multiple methylations through radical-SAM enzymes in pathways similar to proteusins, amidine macrocycle and thiazole heterocycle formations and finally *C*-terminal decarboxylation (Figure 3(d)). Both the follower peptide and the *N*-terminal Met are removed by proteolysis [5,51,52]. Bottromycins are produced by *Streptomyces* spp. and active against Gram-positive bacteria. They inhibit protein synthesis with a mechanism similar to the antibiotic chloramphenicol, i.e. they block the binding of aminoacyl-tRNA to the site A of the 50S ribosome subunit leading to premature termination of the nascent polypeptide chain [5,53].

4.5. *Cyanobactins*

This subclass of RiPPs is one of the largest, with around 200 members identified, all from cyanobacteria. These RiPPs have a length of 6–20 residues. Most of them form an *N*- to *C*-terminal macrocyclic ring but some are linear. They all contain a heterocycle at their *C*-terminus, either a proline or an azol(in)e (thiazole or oxazole) derived from Cys, Ser or Thr (Figure 3(e)). However, this is the only common chemical feature of cyanobactins, therefore they are defined by their BGCs rather than their structures. Cyanobactins BGCs all harbor a gene encoding a precursor similar to PatE, the precursor of patellamide, and at least one subtilisin-like protease from the PatG family. In addition to the leader peptide, the precursors of cyanobactins carry *N*- and *C*-terminal conserved recognition sequences of 4–5 amino acid residues essential for maturation and in particular cyclization by *N*- to *C*-termini peptidic linkage. The precursors can be composed of multiple core sequences separated by *N*- and *C*-terminal recognition sequences. In these cases, multiple mature cyanobactins are produced from one precursor. Most cyanobactins display an anticancer activity but some of them also have an antimicrobial activity, mainly towards parasite or virus but also in some cases against selective bacteria [5,8].

4.6. *Microviridins*

Identified microviridins are produced mainly by Cyanobacteria although they might be produced by other families. A phylogenetic analysis spotted more than 170 BGCs in Cyanobacteria but also in Bacteroidetes and Proteobacteria. Microviridins are tricyclic *N*-acetylated peptides that harbor an original cage-like structure arising from intramolecular ω-amide and/or ω-ester bonds (Figure 3(f)). Most microviridins contain lactam or lactone rings. The precursor of microvidins comprises a Pro-Phe-Phe-Ala-Arg-Phe-Leu motif involved in a α-helix structure and in interaction with the maturation enzymes. Additionally, many microviridin precursors harbor a Gly-Gly cleavage motif. Another conserved motif is found in the core sequences: Thr-X-Lys-X-Pro-Ser-Asp that is implicated in cyclization. Based on their precursor sequence, microviridins can be divided into three classes. Class I regroups precursor consisting in one leader sequence fused to one core sequence. Class II precursors are composed of one leader sequence fused to up to five core sequences separated by Gly-Gly motifs or Gly-rich domains or lacking spacers. It is unclear to date if multiple mature RiPPs or one RiPP with repeated cage-like structure are produced from these specific precursors. Multiple RiPPs production from one precursor has been identified in other subclasses such as cyanobactins, orbitides and cyclotides. Class III corresponds to precursors with a length similar to class II, however, only one sequence in the *C*-terminus is found to resemble a core sequence. Rather than acting as antimicrobials, microviridins seem to have a selective activity as serine protease inhibitors, in particular their potent activity was demonstrated against trypsin, chymotrypsin and elastase [54].

4.7. *Thiopeptides*

Thiopeptides or “Thiazolyl peptides” also form a large subclass of RiPPs with more than a hundred members, identified from Gram-positive soil and marine bacteria. The common chemical feature of thiopeptides is the presence of a central 6-membered ring containing nitrogen and carrying at least one macrocycle and one tail. The macrocycle and the tail can harbor dehydroamino acids and thiazoles, oxazoles or thiazolines derived from Cys, Ser or Thr. The central 6-membered ring is found in different oxidation states, establishing families of thiopeptides. Group **a** corresponds to a totally reduced piperidine, group **b** to α1,2-dehydropiperidine (Figure 3(g)), group **c** to a piperidine fused with imidazoline, group **d** to a trisubstituted pyridine and finally group **e** to a tetrasubstituted pyridine. Group **d** is the only family with only one macrocycle, whereas other families harbor two macrocycles. Thiopeptides have a wide range of biological activities such as anticancer, antifungal, antiplasmodial, antibacterial and immunosuppressive activities. They show potent activity toward Gram-positive bacteria but not against Gram-negative strains, resulting from the inhibition of protein synthesis with specific mechanisms varying according to the size of the macrocycles [55].

Currently, several semi-synthetic analogs of the thiopeptide GE2270A isolated from *Planobispora rosea* are under clinical trials. GE2270A has a broad spectrum of activity against Gram-positive bacteria including species of *Staphylococcus, Enterococcus, Streptococcus*, *Clostridium* and inhibits protein synthesis by interacting with the Elongation Factor Tu [56,57]. The analog LFF571 is considered as a therapeutic agent for the treatment of *Clostridium difficile* infections (CDIs) which are the most frequent nosocomial infections in the US [58]. A phase I clinical trial showed no adverse effects in subjects treated with LFF571 [59]. Then in a phase II clinical trials, treatment with LFF571 was as effective to cure patients from CDIs than the antibiotic vancomycin commonly used for the treatment of CDIs [60]. Another analog of GE2270A, NAI003, shows a reduce spectrum of action but a potent activity against *Propionibacterium acnes*, which is believed to provoke acne [61]. NAI003 was the subject of a phase II clinical trial in 2019 for the treatment of acne in adult men and a phase III is planned for 2021–2022 (*Source*: AdisInsightTrials).

4.8. *Proteusins*

Currently, only one family of proteusins, the polytheonamides, has been identified and produced by the uncultured sponge symbiont *Candidatus* Entotheonella factor. The polytheonamides are the most extensively modified RiPPs exhibiting nearly 50 PTMs. Their precursor is composed of a large leader sequence and the core peptide of 48 residues is modified by multiple types of enzymes, including radical-SAM enzymes, also involved in the maturation of other RiPPs such as bottromycins and sactipeptides. Among their many PTMs, polytheonamides [62] contain methylations of carbon and nitrogen atoms and in particular epimerization of 18 amino acid residues as shown in Figure 4(a). The structure of polytheonamide B was solved by Nuclear Magnetic Resonance (NMR) and consists in a β-helix stabilized by hydrogen bonds between the alternating *L*- and *D*-amino acids [63] similar to the structure of the antibiotic and non-ribosomal peptide (NRP) gramicidin D [5]. Similar to gramicidin D, polytheonamide B has a cytotoxic activity toward mammalian cells. Polytheonamide B inserts in the cell membrane, mimicking transmembrane ion channel proteins, leading to cell depolarization and affects the lysosomal pH gradient after energy-dependent internalization. Treatment of mammalian cells with this RiPP eventually leads to apoptosis. Hence, it could be developed as a drug for cancer treatment [64].

4.9. *Microcins*

The term microcins regroup unmodified peptides and RiPPs produced by Gram-negative bacteria. RiPPs belonging to microcins are active against Gram-negative bacteria and in most cases specifically against Enterobacteria. They cross the outer membrane of Gram-negative bacteria through specific receptors, and then the inner membrane through ABC transporter or binding to membrane proteins. Class I encompasses RiPPs with a molecular weight lower than 5 kDa and so far regroups three members: MccB17, MccJ25 and MccC. MccB17 and MccJ25 also belong to other RiPP subclasses as their PTMs classify them, respectively, as LAP and lasso peptides. MccC is the only microcin that is not produced as a precursor with a leader peptide. MccC is a heptapeptide with PTMs consisting in formylation of the *N*-terminal Met and covalent *C*-terminal binding to an adenosine monophosphate with a propylamine group on the phosphate. Because of their different chemical compositions and structures, these RiPPs have different mechanisms of action. For example, MccB17 targets DNA gyrase whereas MccJ25 targets RNA polymerase. Class II regroups microcins with a size between 5 and 10 kDa. Microcins from class IIa don't undergo PTMs and are therefore not classified as RiPPs. On the contrary, Class IIb microcins are linear peptides carrying siderophore-type PTMs.

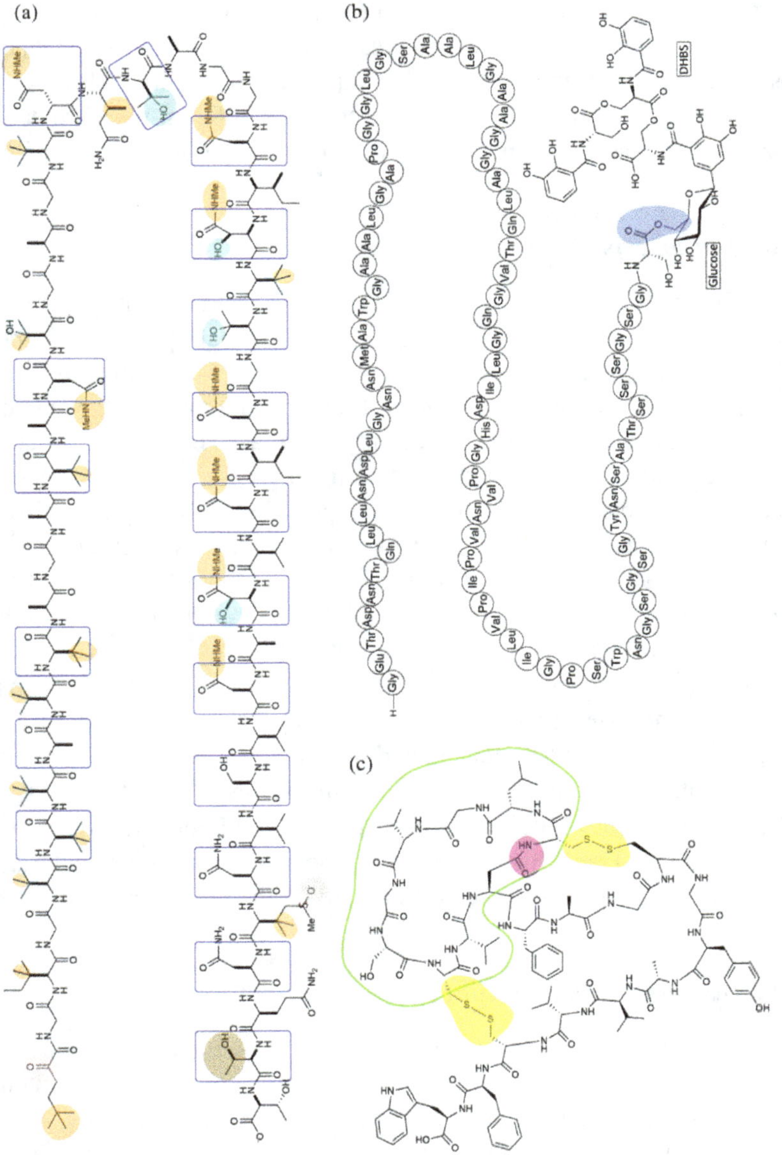

Fig. 4. Structure of prokaryotic RiPPs: Proteusin polytheonamide B (a), microcin E492 (b), and lasso peptide specialicin (c). Methylation, dehydration, hydroxylation, oxidation, allo-residues are highlighted in orange, light pink, teal, beige and brown, respectively. Ester, isopeptide and disulfide bonds are highlighted in dark blue, purple, and yellow, respectively. Dark blue and bright green outlines indicate epimerization and macrolactam ring. Additional PTMs are indicated directly in the figure.

The siderophore is linked to a Ser-rich *C*-terminal domain through a glycosylic bond (Figure 4(b)). These peptides are chromosome-encoded whereas most microcins are encoded on plasmids. Microcins from class IIb can form ion channel or pores in the inner membrane of Gram-negative bacteria or target some bacterial ion channels and impair their activities [5,65,66].

4.10. *Lasso peptides*

These RiPPs are produced by both Gram-positive and negative bacteria. So far, around 50 members have been identified. They are peptides composed of 15–26 amino acid residues harboring 7–9 residues *N*-terminal macrolactam ring with a *C*-terminal tail passing through and trapped in the macrolactam ring. This particular structure resembling a lasso confers great stability to chemical, thermal or proteolytic treatments. Lasso peptides are subdivided into four classes. Class I regroups peptides harboring two disulfide bonds, one linking the *N*-terminal Cys to the ring and one linking the ring to the *C*-terminal tail (Figure 4(c)). Class II corresponds to peptides with no disulfide bonds and a lasso structure stabilized through steric interactions. Classes III and IV both refer to peptide with one disulfide bond, in class III it is located between the macrolactam ring and the tail, whereas it is linking two parts of the *C*-terminal tail in class IV [67]. Lasso peptides have different types of biological activities including anticancer, antiviral and antibacterial activities associated with different mechanisms of actions. As cited earlier, for example, MccJ25 inhibits the RNA polymerase. Antibacterial lasso peptides can be active against Gram-positive or negative bacteria, but they usually have a narrow spectrum regarding the producer strain [5,68].

4.11. *Bacterial head-to-tail cyclized peptides*

Bacterial head-to-tail cyclized peptides are also nominated circular bacteriocins. These peptides produced by Gram-positive bacteria undergo circularization by the formation of a peptide bond between the *N*- and *C*-termini after removal of the leader peptide (Figure 5(a)). They are differentiated from other circular RiPPs like cyanobactins or cyclotides by their large size (between 35 and 70 amino acid residues) and as their lacking a recognition sequence at the *C*-terminus of the precursor. The mechanisms behind circularization remain elusive, although it has been hypothesized that a conserved aromatic residue at the *C*-terminus could play an important role.

Their BGCs, which can be carried on plasmids or chromosomes, encode a heavy biosynthetic machinery with up to 10 genes. So far, a dozen of circular bacteriocins have been purified and they were thought to be produced only by Gram-positive bacteria. No conserved motif or high sequence homology has been identified from these circular bacteriocins. A phylogenetic analysis identified almost 400 BGCs that could be responsible for the production of 59 unique circular bacteriocins. Though most clusters were indeed found in the genome of Gram-positive bacteria and in particular Firmicutes, one of these clusters was found in the genome of the Gram-negative bacteria *Novosphingobium* sp.B-7. Bacterial head-to-tail cyclized peptides can be subclassified: class I corresponds to strongly cationic peptides with 4–5 helices whereas class II regroups acidic peptides. The circular structure provides to these RiPPs increased resistance to thermal, chemical and proteolytic treatments. They show broad spectrum activity mainly against Gram-positive strains but also against Gram-negative bacteria. Identified mechanisms of action of circular bacteriocins consist in cell membrane interaction and pore formation [5,69].

4.12. *Glycocins*

So far, less than 10 glycocins have been purified from Gram-positive bacteria or identified in their genome. These peptides are composed of 37–48 amino acids and they all carry one or two monosaccharides linked to the side chain of a Cys, or a Ser or a Thr. Additionally, glycocins harbor two disulfide bridges (Figure (5b)). Rather than homology in core sequences, glycocins exhibit structural similarity consisting of two helices connected by a loop. These RiPPs have an antibacterial activity and while some have a very narrow spectrum, others can be active against both Gram-positive and negative bacteria. Glycocins can have a bacteriostatic or bactericidal effect and little is known on their mode of action so far except that it doesn't seem to affect membrane integrity. The monosaccharides are not always essential for antibacterial activity, when they are, the glycocins are designated as "glycoactive" [70,71].

4.13. *Methanobactins*

Methanobactins were first identified from methanotroph Gram-negative bacteria. These 11 amino acid residues peptides chelate copper through

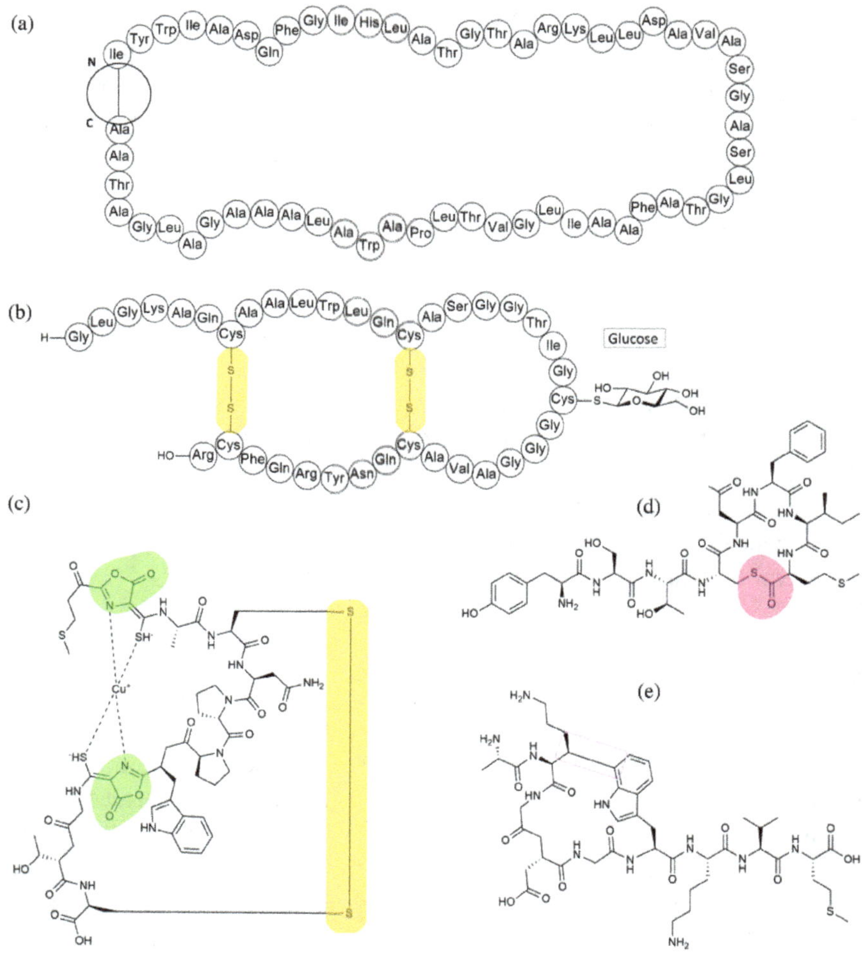

Fig. 5. Structure of prokaryotic RiPPs: Head-to-tail cyclized peptide acidocin B (a), glycocin sublancin 168 (b), methanobactin produced by Methylocystis sp. LW4 (c), autoinducing peptide AIP-1 (d), and streptide StrA (e). Head-to-tail cyclization by amide bond is indicated by a black circle while N and C are each designated as termini. Disulfide bonds and oxazolones are indicated in yellow and bright green, respectively. Pink highlight indicates macrocyclization of cysteine and methionine to thiolactone while lilac outline shows macrocyclization by carbon-carbon linkage.

interactions with two nitrogen heterocycles and adjacent thioamide or enethiol moieties, all derived from modified and conserved Cys (Figure (5c)). Most nitrogen heterocycles found in methanobactins correspond to oxazolone rings. These peptides can chelate copper(I) directly or copper(II) after a reduction process with unknown mechanisms. BGCs were identified in other Gram-negative bacteria like Proteobacteria but also in Gram-positive bacteria like Actinobacteria [72].

4.14. *Autoinducing peptides*

Bacteria live in communities and adapt their gene expression depending on the cell concentration. This process is called Quorum Sensing (QS) and employs different types of molecules for bacteria to communicate and detect the surrounding population level. Autoinducing peptides are part of the QS molecules secreted by at least 48 different species of Gram-positive bacteria. Their common features comprise a lactone or thiolactone macrocycle ring composed of five amino acids and linked to a tail of 2–5 amino acids (Figure (5d)). The only exception so far has been found in *Enterococcus faecalis* with a nine residues lactone macrocycle. The amino acid composition of the core sequences is variable. These autoinducing peptides can be involved in intra- or inter-species communications and have been shown to regulate virulence, therefore they could be exploited in bacterial infection treatment [73]. Another type of autoinducing peptides, ComX, is found in various species of *Bacillus* and corresponds to an isoprenylated and cyclic peptide with 6–10 amino acids and a conserved Trp [5].

4.15. *Streptides*

Streptides have been recently discovered in Streptococcal bacteria, including pathogenic species such as *Streptococcus suis* or *Streptococcus agalactiae*. Only three members have been identified so far: StrA, AgaA and SuiA. The PTM of streptides consists of a cyclization by a carbon-carbon (C-C) linkage between Lys and Trp residues from a Lys-Gly-Asp-Gly-Trp-conserved motif (Figure (5e)). Such as other subclasses of RiPPs like bottromycins or proteusins, the PTM formation is performed by a radical-SAM maturase enzyme. NMR investigations clearly established that the Lys-Trp crosslinks in StrA, SuiA and AgaA connect the β-carbon (Cβ) of Lys and the C-7 of Trp in the core peptides. So far, the biological roles of streptides remain to be characterized but they might be involved in intra-species communication. The regulation of their BGCs is under the control of a QS system and they are likely produced at high cell densities by pathogenic Streptococci; a state associated with virulence [28–30,74,75].

4.16. *Amatoxins and phallotoxins*

These fungal RiPPs are produced by several genera of Basidiomycetes, in particular *Amanita* but also *Galerina*, *Lepiota* and *Conocybe*. They are bicyclic peptides harboring a head-to-tail circularization as well as a tryptathionine resulting from the crosslinking of a Cys and a Trp. Amatoxins are octapeptides (Figure 6(a)) whereas phallotoxins are heptapeptides (Figure 6(b)). Both their precursors comprise a 10 amino acids leader peptide and a *C*-terminal recognition sequence. While the core sequences are diverse the leader and recognition sequences are highly conserved. The core sequences are surrounded by Pro residues targeted by a prolyl protease belonging to the serine protease family for removal of the leader and recognition sequences. The prolyl protease performs both proteolytic cleavage and head-to-tail cyclization by transpeptidation. Amatoxins are actually the agents responsible for the most fatal mushroom poisonings. They act by inhibiting the RNA polymerase II in liver cells, resulting in liver failure and eventually death. Phallotoxins are not as dangerous as they are not active when delivered orally but show toxicity when injected. They have been developed as cytoskeleton dyes as they bind actin [6,76].

4.17. *Borosins*

Borosin is one of the most recently discovered subclasses of RiPPs. So far, only omphalotin A and its derivatives belong to this family. Although omphatolins have been isolated from the Basidiomycetes *Omphatolius oleariusin* 1997, until the identification of their BGCs in 2017, they were thought to be NRPs. These peptides composed of 12 amino acids are head-to-tail circularized and harbor 9–12 *N*-methylation (Figure 6(c)). This recent subclass is rather original from other RiPPs as their precursor is actually fused to the *C*-terminus of their maturation enzyme which displays homology with SAM-methyltransferase. Like amatoxins, cleavage and cyclization of the precursor involve a prolyl oligopeptidase. In addition to the leader peptide, the precursor harbors a *C*-terminal recognition sequence. Omphalotins seem to have a selective nematoxic activity [6,77–79].

4.18. *Dikaritins*

Dikaritins are also fungal RiPPs, however, unlike amatoxins, phallotoxins and borosins, they are produced by Ascomycetes rather than

Basidiomycetes. They are characterized by cyclic structures involving a Tyr residue. Phomopsins have seven amino acid residues and a 13-membered macrocyclic ring resulting from the ether linkage of the phenyl ring of a Tyr to Ile (Figure 6(d)). Ustiloxins have a similar ring but are composed of four amino acids (Figure 6(e)). However, the main difference is that ustiloxins only harbor proteinogenic amino acids whereas phomopsins are composed of dehydroamino acids. Finally, asperipins are composed of six residues and exhibit a bicyclic structure arising from ether linkages of Tyr side chains and β-carbons (Figure 6(f)). The precursors of dikaritins are composed of repeated core sequences surrounded by cleavage recognition motif such as Lys-Arg. Dikaritins have an antimitotic activity and could be used as anticancer drugs [6,80,81].

4.19. *Epichloëcyclins*

Like dikaritins, epichloëcyclins are produced by Ascomycetes. They were first identified in *Epichloë*, a genus of fungi that can be both symbiont or pathogens of temperate grasses. Phylogenetic analyses revealed that they might be produced by other fungi but restricted to the Clavicipitaceae and Ophiocordycipitaceae families. These peptides of a length up to 12 amino acid residues harbor an oxidative cyclization on a conserved Tyr and a methylation on a Lys (Figure 6(g)). Their precursor is composed of multiple repeats of core sequences with some amino acid substitutions and conserved motifs, including Lys-Arg cleavage sites. Therefore, a single precursor is processed in multiple RiPPs. Epichloëcyclins biological activities remain to be characterized. It should be noted that the production of epichloëcyclins has been identified in symbiotic conditions but not in fungal culture and therefore might be involved in mutualistic effects [6,82].

4.20. *Cyclotides*

This subclass is produced by a wide range of plant families such as Rubiaceae, Violaceae, Cucurbitaceae or Fabaceae and hundreds of members have been identified. Cyclotides are composed of around 30 amino acid residues and are characterized by a cyclic cystine knot (CCK) motif and a head-to-tail cyclic backbone (Figure 6(h)). The CCK motif consists of six conserved Cys forming three disulfide bonds. This particular structure provides resistance to thermal, chemical and proteolytic treatments. Cyclotides can be subdivided into three categories: Möbius, bracelets and linear. Möbius and bracelets differ by a 180° twist in the cyclic backbone due to the presence of a conserved Pro residue. Few linear cyclotides with no head-to-tail cyclic backbone but conserved cyclotide sequence have been identified. The precursor of cyclotides harbors an N-terminal signal sequence that addresses the precursor to the endoplasmic reticulum before maturation, then the leader peptide is composed of two domains: an *N*-terminal pro-peptide domain (NTPP) and an *N*-terminal repeat domain (NTR). A small C-terminal sequence (CTR) can be found in the precursors of some cyclotides. NTR, CTR and the core sequence can be repeated in the precursor. Cyclotides can exert many biological activities including but not only insecticidal, antiviral, anticancer, anthelmintic, immunosuppressive and antibacterial activity. Their main mode of action is the interaction with lipids resulting in membrane disruption [83].

4.21. *Orbitides*

Similar to cyclotides, these RiPPs are produced by plants and nine families have been identified yet as cyclotide producers such as Caryophyllaceae, Euphorbiaceae, Lamiaceae, Linaceae, and Rutaceae. These RiPPs are composed of 5–12 amino acid residues and harbor a head-to-tail cyclization (Figure 6(i)). The amino acid composition in this subclass is original as Cys is the least abundant amino acid, whereas it is often conserved and involved in PTMs in lots of other RiPP subclasses. Orbitides display high contents of hydrophobic amino acids. The precursor might carry a recognition sequence depending on the producer family and such as cyclotides might contain multiple sequences of the core peptide. Hence, one single precursor can be processed in multiple cyclic precursors. Orbitides exert many different activities including anticancer, antimalarial, immunosuppressive and antibacterial effects. Regarding the antibacterial activity some orbitides have been identified as active against exclusively Gram-positive or Gram-negative bacteria whereas others can target both. Similarly, some orbitides display a very narrow spectrum of action and seem specific to one specie while others are broad spectrum antimicrobial. Little is known about

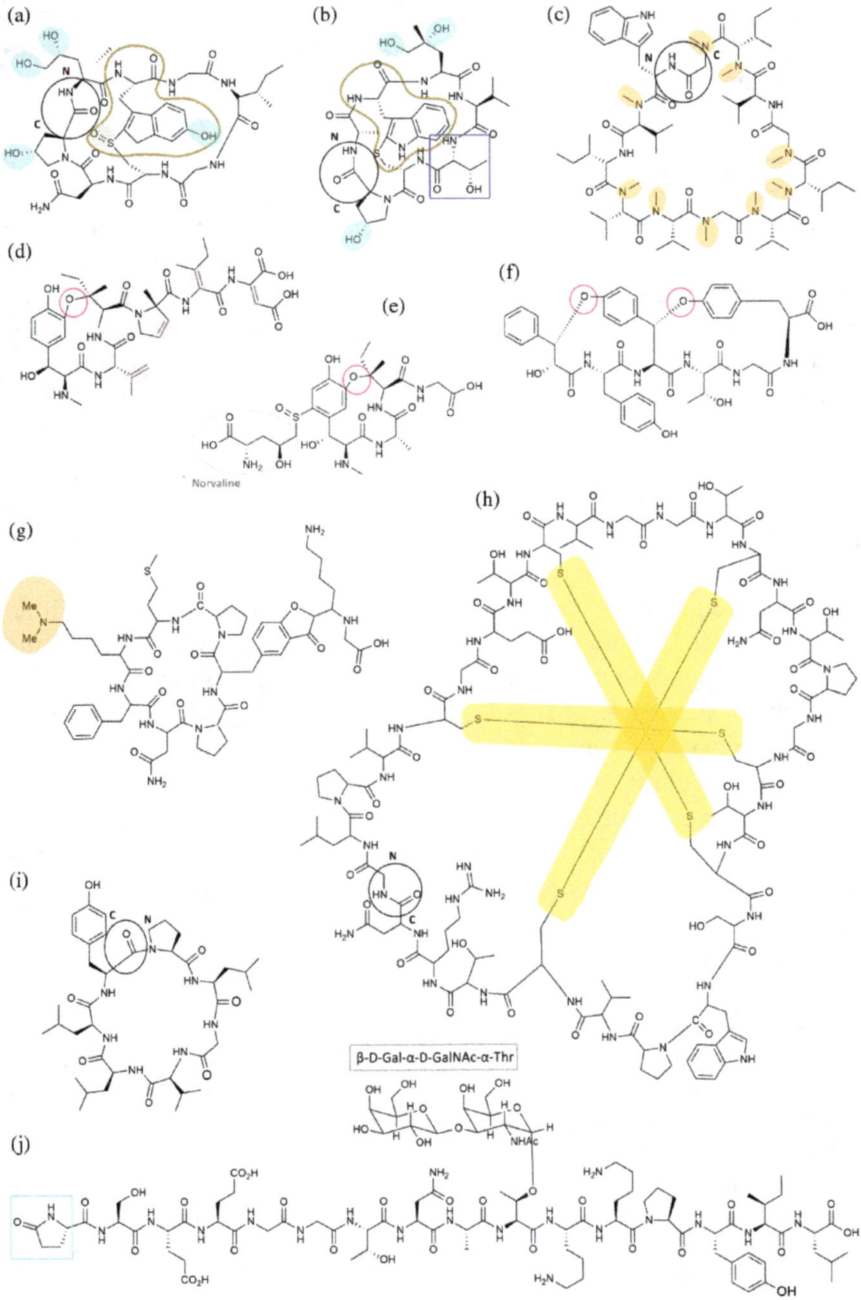
(a)
(b)
(c)
(d)
(e)
(f)
Norvaline
(g)
(h)
(i)
(j)
β-D-Gal-α-D-GalNAc-α-Thr

their mechanisms of action, although some orbitides active against Gram-positive bacteria exclusively are known to form pores in the bacterial membrane [5,6,84].

4.22. *Conopeptides*

These RiPPs are toxins produced in the venom of marine snails. It is estimated that around 500 species of *Conos* are potential producers of conopeptides and hundreds of conopeptides have been identified. These *Conos* toxins differ from venom toxin from other animals as they are smaller, from 10–30 residues compared to 30–90, and harbor many and diverse PTMs. Identified PTMs that might be incorporated on conopeptide precursors so far include the following: C-terminal amidation on Gly; *N*-terminal cyclization on Gln; hydroxylation on Pro, Val, Lys; carboxylation on Glu; sulfation on Tyr; bromination on Trp; oxidation on Cys; glycosylation on Thr; epimerization of Val, Leu, Phe, Trp (Figure 6(j)). Conopeptides usually describe disulfide-poor peptides (none to one disulfide bridge) and conotoxins disulfide-rich peptides (two or more disulfide bridges). Their precursors harbor an extremely conserved endoplasmic reticulum recognition sequence while the core sequences are diverse. The biosynthetic pathways of most conopeptides remain unclear especially since the biosynthetic genes are not clustered and the peptides can be produced concomitantly in their mature form with PTMs or without. While many conopeptides still have unknown functions, others have been identified as interacting with cell membrane or ion channels and have been developed as neurological drugs [5,6,85]. As examples, the conopeptides CGX-1160, ACV1 and ziconitide are, respectively, in Phase I, Phase II or already approved by the FDA for pain management [86].

Fig. 6. Structure of eukaryotic RiPPs: Amatoxin α-amanitin (a), phallotoxin phalloidin (b), borosin omphalotin A (c), dikaritins phomopsin B (d), ustiloxin B (e) and asperipin-2a (f), epichoëcylcin A (g), cyclotide kalata B1 (h), orbitide pohlianin A (i) and conopeptide contulakin-G (J). Methylation, hydroxylation, oxidation, dehydro-residues are highlighted in orange, teal, beige and light pink, respectively. Disulfide bonds are highlighted in yellow. Head-to-tail cyclization by amide bond is indicated by a black circle while N and C are each designated as termini. Brown, dark blue and light blue outlines represent, respectively, trypthationine residues, epimerization and cyclization of glutamine to pyroglutamate. Pink and light pink outlines depict ether linkage or oxidative cyclization both involving tyrosine residues. Additional PTMs are indicated directly on the figure.

Families	Main PTMs	Producers	Identified Activities	Example
Lanthipeptide	Lan, MeLan residues	Gram + Gram -, eukaryotes?	Antibacterial, antifungal, antiviral, pain relief	Fig. X.3.A
LAP	Thiazol(in)e and (methyl)-oxazol(in)e heterocycles	Gram + / -	Antibacterial	Fig. X.3.B
Linaridin	*Allo*-isoleucine, Dhb residues	*Streptomyces* Other Gram +, Gram -?	Antibacterial Anticancer	Fig. X.3.C
Bottromycin	Methylation, amidine macrocyle, thiazole heterocycle	*Streptomyces*	Antibacterial	Fig. X.3.D
Cyanobactin	Heterocycle at C-terminus	Cyanobacteria	Anticancer, antiviral, anti-parasite, antibacterial	Fig. X.3.E
Microviridin	Intramolecular ω-amide and/or ω-ester bonds	Cyanobacteria Other Gram -?	Protease inhibitors	Fig. X.3.F
Thiopeptide	Central 6-membered ring containing nitrogen, at least one macrocycle and one tail	Gram +	Anticancer, antibacterial, antiplasmodial, antifungal, immunosuppressive	Fig. X.3.G
Proteusin	Various (including epimerization)	*Candidatus* Entotheonella factor	Anticancer	Fig. X.4.A

Families	Main PTMs	Producers	Identified Activities	Example
Microcin	Various	Gram -	Antibacterial	Fig. X.4.B
Lasso peptide	N-terminal macrolactam ring with a C-terminal tail passing through	Gram + / -	Anticancer, antiviral, antibacterial	Fig. X.4.C
Head-to-tail cyclized peptide	Circularization by an amide bond between N- and C-termini	Gram + Gram -?	Antibacterial	Fig. X.5.A
Glycocin	Bound to 1 or 2 monosaccharides	Gram +	Antibacterial	Fig. X.5.B
Methanobactin	Nitrogen containing heterocycle, thioamide or enethiol moieties	Methanotroph Gram – bacteria Other Gram -, Gram +?	Chelate copper	Fig. X.5.C
Autoinducing peptide	Lactone or thiolactone macrocycle ring Isoprenylated and cyclic peptide	Gram + *Bacillus spp.*	Bacterial communication	Fig. X.5.D
Streptide	Carbon-carbon linkage	*Streptococcus spp.*	Bacterial communication?	Fig. X.5.E
Sactipeptide	Sulfur-to-α carbon thiother linkage	*Bacillus spp.* Other Gram +, Gram -?	Antibacterial	Fig. X.7-8
Ranthipeptide	Sulfur-to-β or -γ carbon thiother linkage	Gram +	?	Fig. X.12-13

Families	Main PTMs	Producers	Identified Activities	Examples
Amatoxin and Phallotoxin	Circularization by an amide bond between N- and C-termini, tryptathionine	Basidiomycetes	Cytoskeleton dye	Fig. X.6.A-B
Borosin	Circularization by an amide bond between N- and C-termini, N-methylation	*Omphatolius olearius*	Nematoxic	Fig. X.6.C
Dikaritin	Cyclic structure involving a Tyr residue	Ascomycetes	Anticancer	Fig. X.6.D-F
Epichloëcyclin	Oxidative cyclization on Tyr, methylation on Lys	*Epichloë* Other Ascomycetes?	?	Fig. X.6.G
Cyclotide	Cystine Cystic Knot	Various Plants	Insecticidal, antiviral, anticancer, anthelmintic, immunosuppressive, antibacterial	Fig. X.6.H
Orbitide	Circularization by an amide bond between N- and C-termini	Various plants	Anticancer, antimalarial, immunosuppressive, antibacterial	Fig. X.6.I
Conopeptide	Various	*Conos*	Neurological	Fig. X.6.J

5. Sactipeptides

5.1. *Definition and members*

Sactipeptides are RiPPs containing one or multiple sactionine linkages or **s**ulfur-to-***α*** **c**arbon **t**hioether (sacti) linkages, i.e. crosslinks between the sulfur (S) atom of a Cys and the α-carbon (Cα) of an acceptor amino acid residue [5]. In addition to sacti-bridges, sactipeptides can harbor other modifications like head-to-tail linkage by amide bonds or disulfide bridges. So far, six sactipeptides have been identified: subtilosin A [87,88], the sporulation killing factor SKF [89], thurincin H [90], thuricin CD [91], the latter being composed of the two distinct sactipeptides Trn-α and Trn-β, huazacin which is also named thuricin Z [92,93] and finally ruminococcin C which is declined in five isoforms (RumC1–5) [39,94,95]. Subtilosin A has been isolated from different species of *Bacillus* [96]. Thuricins and thurincin H are produced by *Bacillus thurengiensis*, a soil microorganism, whereas SKF is produced by *Bacillus subtilis* which can be found in both soil and human or animal gastrointestinal tracts. Ruminococcin C remains the only sactipeptide identified from a different genus than *Bacillus* so far, indeed it was isolated from the human fecal strain E1 of *Ruminococcus gnavus.* Originally, thermocellin (CteA) and Tte1186a were identified as sactipeptides but were very recently reclassified as ranthipeptides which will be discussed in the following section [93,97].

5.2. *Common chemical features and structures*

The length of the amino acid core sequence of the known sactipeptides varies as well as the number of sactionine linkages and the presence of other modifications (Figure 7).

SKF is the smallest sactipeptide with 26 amino acids and harbors one sactionine linkage, one disulfide bond and a head-to-tail cyclization. The two peptides of Thuricin CD, Trn-α and Trn-β, are both composed of 30 amino acids with a sequence identity of 40% and display three conserved Cys involved in sacti-bridges. The amino acid acceptors of these bridges differ in their nature in Trn-α and Trn-β but are located at the same positions. Thurincin H is composed of 33 amino acid residues and carries four sacti-bridges. Subtilosin A is slightly bigger with 35 amino acids and harbors three sactionine linkages as well as head-to-tail cyclization. Thuricin Z or huazacin is characterized by 39 amino acids and four sacti-bridges. Finally, RumC1–5 are the largest sactipeptides with each isoform being composed of 44 residues and harboring four sacti-bridges as well. RumC1–5 have sequences identity between them ranging from 80–86%. While the sequences in amino acids are slightly different in each isoform, the acceptor residues of the thioether bonds are all located at the same positions, which are depictures for RumC1 in Figure 7.

Based on the known sactipeptides, a wide range of amino acid residues can act as acceptors of the thioether bridges. Indeed, Phe, Met, Asn, Ala, Tyr, Ser, Asp, His, Lys, Arg, Glu have been identified hitherto as partners of Cys in sactionine linkages in one or two sactipeptides. Subtilosin A, thuricins and thurincin H, all harbor at least one sactionine linkage involving a Thr. It is worth noting that at the exception of ruminococcin C in all these sactipeptides, the Cys residues are situated in the *N*-terminal half of the core peptide whereas the acceptor residues are in the *C*-terminal part. This specific distribution of Cys donors and

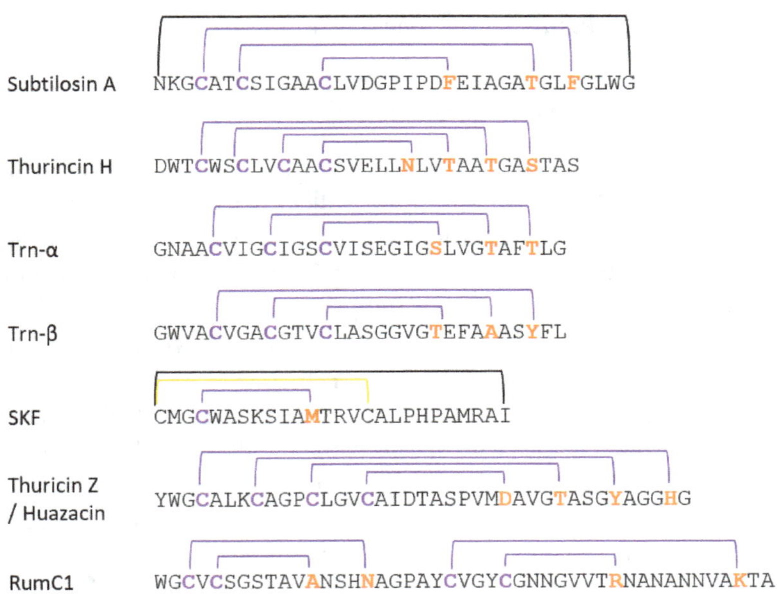

Fig. 7. Sequences and thioether networks of sactipeptides. Thioether, disulfide bonds and head-to-tail cyclization are indicated, respectively, in purple, yellow and black lines. Cys are highlighted in purples and amino acid acceptors of the sacti-bonds in orange.

acceptors folds the sactipeptide backbone in a peculiar hairpin structure maintained by the thioether bridges. Regarding ruminococcin *C*, the Cys display a wider distribution and are present in both *N*- and *C*-terminal half of the core peptide. However, the Cys are still located upstream of their acceptors, thus this hairpin shape is still found in ruminococcin C but in two distinct domains, creating a double-hairpin structure.

The structures of subtilosin A, thurincin H, RumC1, Trn-α and Trn-β were determined by NMR using ^{13}c-and ^{15}N-labeled peptides (Figure 8). Except for RumC1, all these sactipeptides present a net anionic charge at physiological pH with a mostly hydrophobic surface. On the contrary, RumC1 has a net cationic charge and a surface presenting mostly hydrophilic surface. The amino acid acceptors involved in the thioether bonds holding the helical backbone can adopt *L*- or *D*-stereochemistry. The three bridges of Trn-α and Trn-β have a LLD stereochemistry while the three bridges of subtilosin A have an LDD stereochemistry [87,90]. In thurincin H and RumC1, the four sacti-bridges have a *D*-stereochemistry [90,98].

Based on the different distribution of Cys leading to a double-hairpin structure rather than a single hairpin shape and the opposed overall surface structure, it was proposed that ruminococcin *C* and its five isoforms compose a new subfamily of sactipeptides [39,98].

5.3. *Biosynthesis genetic clusters* (*BGCs*)

The BGCs of sactipeptides comprise at least genes encoding: a precursor peptide, a maturation enzyme from the radical-SAM family and an ABC transporter (Figure 9). Except for huazacin, a sequence encoding a signal peptidase has also been found in the BGCs of known sactipeptides. Additionally, genes involved in self-immunity and response regulation are present in some of the clusters. The BGC of SKF also contains a putative thioredoxin. In the BGC of subtilosin A and SKF, only one sequence encodes a precursor, whereas two and three sequences encoding identical precursors are found in the BGC of thuricin Z and thurincin H, respectively. For thuricin CD, two different sequences corresponding to Trn-α and Trn-β are found. Finally, as mentioned previously in the case of ruminococcin C, five distinct sequences encode the precursors of the five isoforms.

Sactipeptides' BGCs can contain more than one gene encoding maturation enzymes but in that case, it is unclear if one or several enzymes perform the PTMs. In vitro incubation of the precursors of thuricin Z with either ThzC and ThzD, two highly divergent putative maturation enzymes encoded

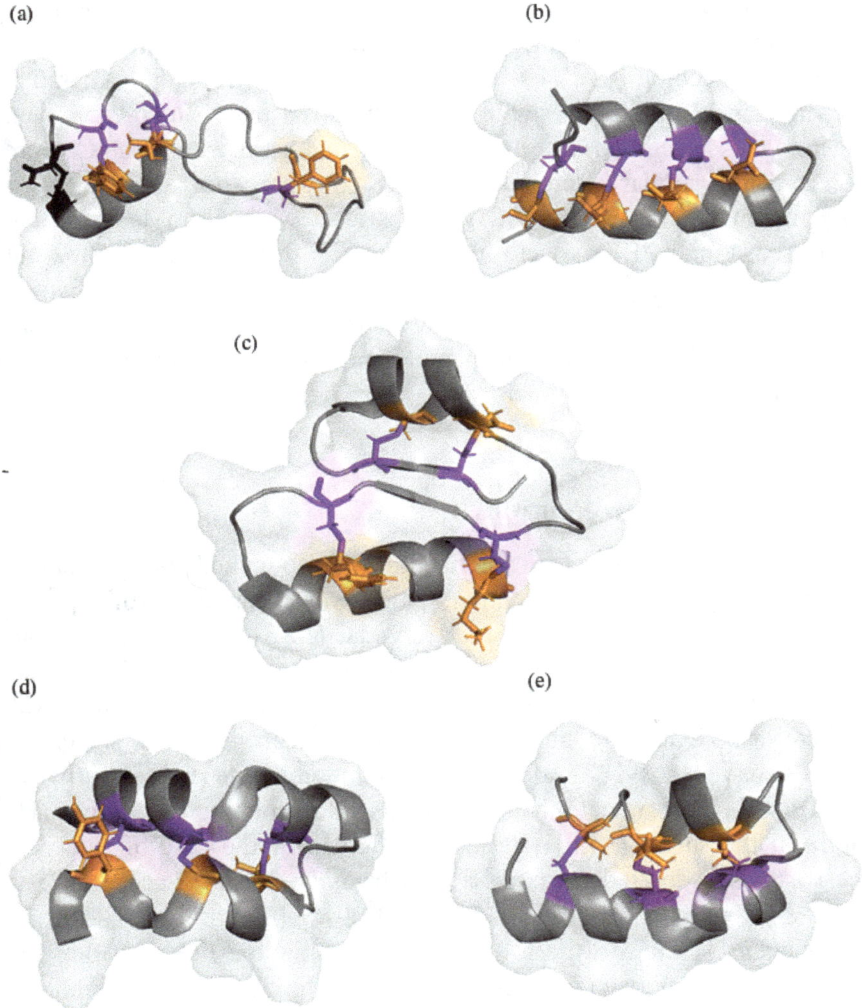

Fig. 8. Three-dimensional structure of sactipeptides. Representation of NMR structures of subtilosin A (a), thurincin H (b), RumC1 (c) and thuricin CD composed of Trn-α (d) and Trn-β (e). Cysteines involved in the sacti-bridges are indicated in purple while the acceptor residues are in orange.

in the BGC of thuricin Z, yielded a precursor with sactionine linkages [92]. Although both of the enzymes were able to incorporate PTMs *in vitro*, it is unknown if this is also true *in vivo*. In the case of ruminococcin C, the genetic sequence corresponding to RumC1 precursor is adjacent to the maturation enzyme RumMc1 gene, the sequences of RumC2-3 are clustered with another gene encoding the maturation enzyme RumMc2 and the sequences encoding RumC4-5 are also clustered but without a maturation enzyme gene. RumMc1 was able to fully modify RumC1 in co-expression heterologous system and *in vitro* [39,98]. Low amounts of mature RumC2 were obtained in a similar heterologous system co-expressing RumMc2, however, no maturation of RumC2 was observed when RumMc1 was co-expressed. Finally, PTMs were incorporated on RumC1 by RumMc2 but with lower efficiency than with RumMc1 [99]. These results are intriguing as the precursors of RumC1 and RumC2 share the exact same leader peptide, conserved Cys in the core peptide and conserved acceptors in two sactionines.

5.4. *Maturation mechanisms*

The maturation enzymes of sactipeptides, also called sactisynthases, belong to the radical S-adenosylmethionine (SAM) enzymes family [100]. Radical-SAM enzymes contain a conserved Cys-X3-Cys-X2-Cys motif in which Cys act as ligands for three iron (Fe) atoms of a [4Fe-4S] cluster (Figure 10(a)). The free fourth Fe of the cluster coordinates the SAM cofactor, which under reductive conditions and electron transfer is cleaved into 5-deoxyadenosyl (5′-Ado•) radical and methionine (Figure 10(b)).

This 5′-Ado• radical initiates catalysis by abstracting a hydrogen (H) atom on the substrate [101,102]. In particular, in the case of sactisynthases, the 5′-Ado• radical extracts an H from the Cα of the acceptor residue, resulting in a substrate radical [103,104] (Figure 11). The exact mechanisms leading to the formation of a sactionine linkage from this substrate radical with a Cys remain to be characterized to date. In addition to the canonical Cys-X3-Cys-X2-Cys motif, sactisynthases are characterized by a Cys-rich C-terminal domain bound to one or two additional [4Fe-4S] clusters, respectively, named Twitch or SPASM (**S**ubtilosin A/ **P**yrroloquinoline quinone/**A**naerobic **S**ulfatase/**M**ycofactocin maturation enzymes) domains. SPASM domains are constituted by a conserved 7 Cys motif and Twitch domains can be found in different truncated versions of SPASM [105]. Surprisingly, in SkfB, the sactisynthase involved in the biosynthesis of SKF, the Twitch domain, is found to coordinate a [2Fe-2S] cluster rather than a [4Fe-4S] [25]. Although the precise role of these domains remains unclear in sactipeptides so far, they are essential for

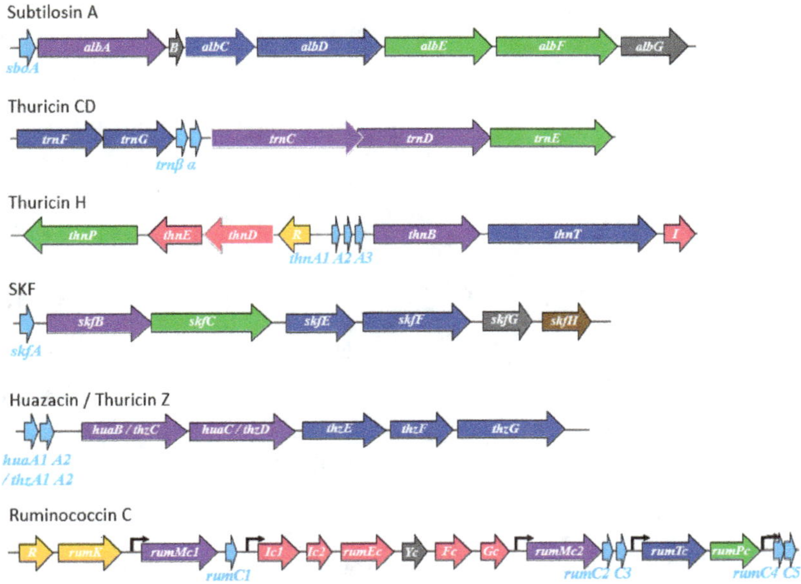

Fig. 9. Biosynthetic genetic clusters of sactipeptides. Representation of the genes involved in the production of subtilosin A, thuricin CD, thurincin H, SKF and huazacin / thuricin Z and ruminococcin C. The colors indicate the identified or putative functions of each gene: light blue corresponds to precursor peptides; purple to radical-SAM enzymes; dark blue to export systems; green to peptidases; yellow to regulators; pink to immunity systems; brown to thioredoxin; grey indicates unknown function.

thioether bond formation. Mutations of the Cys from the SPASM domain involved in the binding of the auxiliary [4Fe-4S] clusters of AlbA, as well as from the SPASM domain of ThnB and from the Twitch domain of SkfB, prevented the formation of sactionine linkages on the precursor of subtilosin A, thurincin H and SKF, respectively. Despite these mutations, SAM was still cleaved in 5′-Ado•. Hence the first [4Fe-4S] cluster performs the reductive cleavage of SAM while the auxiliary clusters are involved in thioether linkage formation [24,106,107]. The proposed roles for the SPASM or Twitch domain involve electron acceptance by the [4Fe-4S] auxiliary cluster during thioether bond formation of the radical substrate with the S of a Cys that might be coordinated by the auxiliary cluster [103,108] (Figure 11).

The core fold of radical-SAM enzymes includes a partial TIM barrel $(\beta/\alpha)_6$ with six α-helices on the outer surface and six parallel β-sheets in

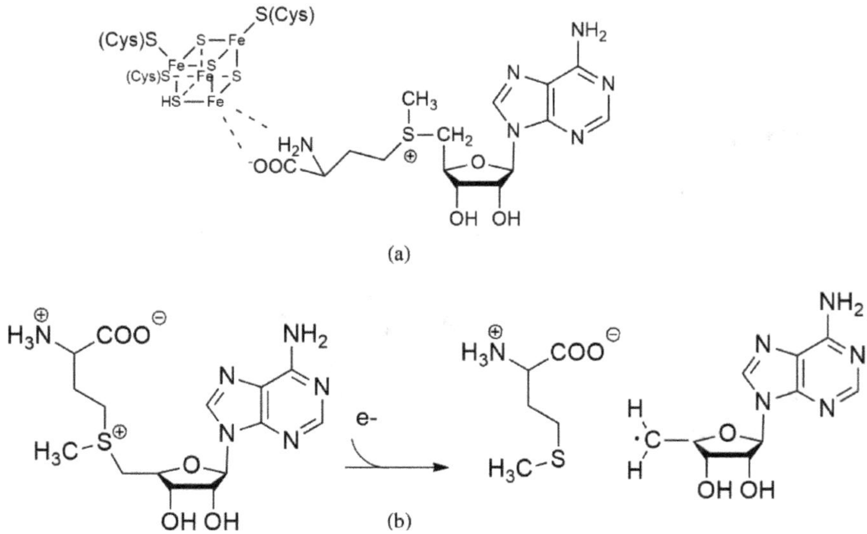

Fig. 10. Radical-SAM-based chemistry. Coordination of a [4Fe-4S] cluster by three Cys and of a SAM molecule by the fourth Fe of the [4Fe-4S] cluster (A). Reduction cleavage upon electron transfer of SAM in 5′-Ado• (B).

the inner face. The canonical Cys-X_3-Cys-X_2-Cys motif is located in the "cluster-binding loop" located after $\alpha 1$ and before $\beta 1$ [105]. The structure of SkfB was resolved by X-ray crystallography and highlighted that SkfB is a modular enzyme composed of N-terminal peptide-binding domain, a core with the TIM barrel structure described above and a C-terminal domain including the Twitch domain [25].

The role of the leader peptide in sactipeptide maturation has been explored on subtilosin A, SKF and RumC1. The formation of sactionine linkages on the precursors of these RiPPs by their respective sactisynthases was shown to be prevented in precursors lacking the leader sequence [98,106,107]. Therefore, the maturation of sactipeptides seems to be leader-dependent. When the leader peptide of the precursor of RumC1 was provided in trans *in vitro*, only 10% of the core peptides were modified with four sacti-bridges whereas full maturation was efficient on 99% of the core peptides attached to their leader peptide in the same conditions. The equivalent maturation rate without the leader attached to the core peptide nor provided in trans was 1% [98]. Therefore, the leader provided in trans helps the maturation process but is not sufficient to obtain full maturation.

A PqqD-like RRE was identified in ThnB and SkfB, as well as HuaB and HuaC, the sactisynthases involved in the maturation of thurincin H, SKF, thuricin Z/huazacin respectively [24,25,93]. Deletion of the RRE of ThnB didn't impair the ability of ThnB to generate 5′-Ado• radical from SAM but prevented the formation of the sacti-bridges on the precursor of thurincin H, proving its essential role for thurincin H maturation [24]. The structure of SkfB shows that the N-terminal peptide-binding domain of the protein sits below the N-terminal region of the radical-SAM domain and the C-terminal Twitch domain [25]. As expected, the RRE motif in SkfB is composed of a three-stranded antiparallel β-sheets and three α-helices (Figure 12(a)). It is predicted that SkfA binds to SkfB using the leader peptide sequence to extend to the antiparallel β-sheet of the RRE. However, the distance between the RRE domain and the active site of about 20 Å is short [25]. To position the 55-mer SkfA precursor peptide in a catalytically competent orientation, it is possible that SkfA adopts an ordered secondary structure and/or the RRE domain of SkfB undergoes a conformational change upon SkfA binding. So far, how the full-length precursor peptides bind to sactisynthases to allow for sactionine linkage

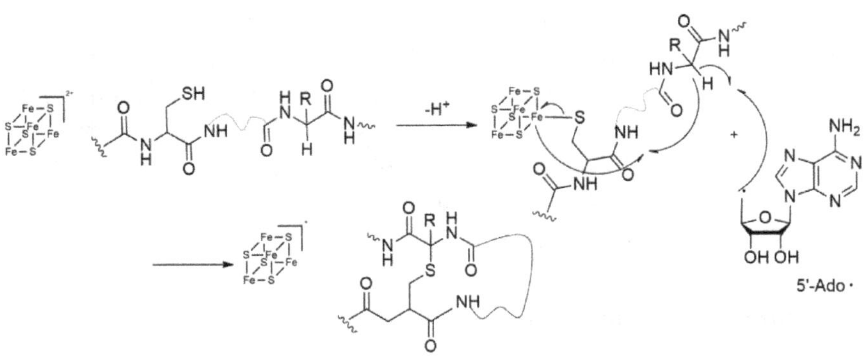

Fig. 11. Radical-based mechanism of thioether formation in sactipeptides. In this proposed mechanism for thioether formation, the precursor peptide is linked by a Cys to an auxiliary [4Fe-4S] cluster found in the SPASM domain of the sactisynthase. The 5′-Ado• radical, generated by cleavage of SAM by the first [4Fe-4S] cluster found at the canonical Cys-X3-Cys-X2-Cys motif of the sactisynthase abstracts an H atom from the acceptor amino acid. An electron from the radical acceptor is transferred to the auxiliary [4Fe-4S] cluster during thioether formation.

formation and possible conformational changes associated with this interaction remain to be determined.

In Trn-α and Trn-β, a Gly-Gly proteolytic motif is found at the C-terminus of the leader peptide like in many RiPPs, although unlike these RiPPs the proteolytic cleavage occurs in between the two Gly residues instead of after them [91]. However, this motif is not found in other sactipeptide precursors in which the cleavage sites involve different amino acid residues. The proteases responsible for leader peptide removal of sactipeptides belong to various families. The BGC of thurincin H encodes a protein with high homology for EpiP, a leader peptide processing serine protease [24], whereas two zinc-dependent proteases are encoded in the subtilosin A BGC and are thought to be responsible for both leader peptide removal and macrocyclization [106]. A putative membrane-bound metalloprotease is also encoded in BGC of SKF, belonging to the Cys-A-A-X (A: an aliphatic amino acid) amino-terminal protease family [109]. The proteolytic cleavage of the precursors of Trn-α and Trn-β might occur in the cytoplasmic compartment as no signal sequence is found in the peptidase TnrE from the S41-type superfamily [91]. As previously mentioned (see Section 1.3.2), the leader peptide removal of RumC1 requires two proteolytic enzymes. First, a zinc-peptidase predicted to be cytoplasmic cleaves partially the leader and then, after export of the rest of the precursor in the extracellular gut compartment of the producer symbiont *R. gnavus* E1, the host trypsin removes the last five residues of the leader [39]. Finally, the removal of the leader peptide of huazacin is unexplained so far, as no peptidase is found in its BGC [92]. In class III lanthipeptides, it has been shown that the processing of the leader peptide involved proteases encoded in the genome of the producer that is located outside of the lanthipeptides BGC [38], a similar processing of huazacin is a possibility.

5.5. *Biological activities*

Regarding the biological roles of sactipeptides, they all exhibit an antibacterial activity. While subtilosin A has a broad spectrum of activity against Gram-positive and negative bacteria, thuricins CD, Z and thurincin H and RumC1 display activity restricted to Gram-positive bacteria. The antibacterial activity of SKF appears to be less potent than other sactipeptides and its use as an alternative to antibiotic unlikely. SKF is produced by *B. subtilis* in a cannibalism process occurring when nutriments are limited. In

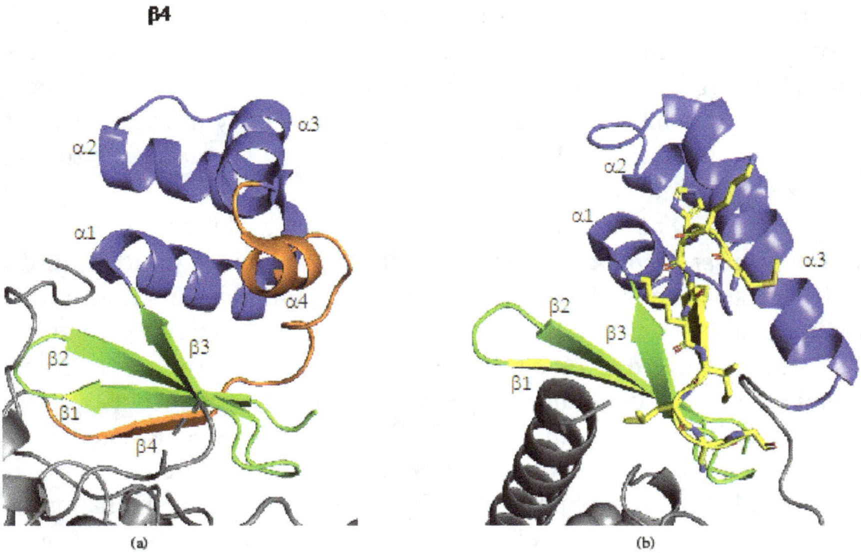

Fig. 12. Structural comparison of specific Sactipeptide and Ranthipeptide RREs. Structurally equivalent sections of RiPP biosynthetic proteins involved in the biosynthesis of the sactipeptide SKF, SkfB rSAM-enzyme [6eFN] (a), and the ranthipeptide CteA, CteB rSAM-enzyme [5WGG] (b). The green β-sheets and marine blue α-helices constitute a conserved RiPP precursor peptide recognition element (RRE), whereas in orange the extra-secondary structures are involved. In (b), the precursor peptide is shown in yellow stick format.

these conditions, to delay the sporulation, *B. subtilis* cells with an active Spo0A protein produce and export SKF while cells with an inactive Spo0A protein are sensitive to SKF and lyse, releasing nutriments [109]. Although the activity of purified SKF against *B. subtilis* was proven on solid media, still, to date, no growth inhibition was observed in liquid culture of any type of bacteria [89].

Subtilosin A is active against Gram-positive bacteria including *Enterococcus faecalis, Listeria monocytogenes, Streptococcus pyogenes* and *Porphyromonas gingivalis* as well as some strains of Gram-negative bacteria among, for example, *Klebsiella pneumoniae* or *Shigella sonnei* [110]. The mode of action of subtilosin A involves bacterial membrane interaction. This sactipeptide partially buries itself in the phospholipid bilayers with the Trp-containing edge situated inside the bilayer while its negative charge groups stay outside, resulting in disturbance of the membrane architecture. At high concentration, subtilosin A forms pores in the membrane resulting in cytoplasm leakages, although it might have a different and unidentified mode of action at lower but effective concentrations [111]. In *Gardnerella vaginalis*, it has been shown that subtilosin A causes efflux of intracellular ATP and ions, most likely through transient pores [112]. In addition to its antibacterial activity, subtilosin A also displays a spermicidal action [113].

Thuricin CD has a narrow spectrum comprising Clostridia and Bacilli as well as *Listeria monocytogenes* with Minimum Inhibitory Concentrations (MIC) under the micromolar range and for lots of strains inferior to conventional antibiotics [91,114,115]. The antibacterial activity of thuricin CD seems restricted to Gram-positive bacteria and inefficient on Gram-negative bacteria. In Gram-positive bacteria, most Lactic Acid Bacteria (LAB) and *Bifidobacterium* spp., which are considered as beneficial for the gut microbiota, are also resistant to thuricin CD. Although Trn-α and Trn-β display antimicrobial activity by themselves, the combination of both results in a synergistic effect with an increase potency by a factor of around 25 [115]. Because of its selectivity and potency against Clostridia, thuricin CD could be used as an alternative to antibiotic for the treatment of *C. difficile* infections (CDIs). Indeed, these infections are associated with dysbiosis, therefore selective antibiotics that wouldn't impair the gut microbiota are actively sought. In an *ex vivo* distal colon model, thuricin CD was shown to be more effective than metronidazole, one of the antibiotics commonly used for the treatment of CDIs, to clear *C. difficile* [91]. No significant alterations of the microbiota from this model was detected with thuricin CD treatment, whereas treatments with metronidazole or vancomycin, another antibiotic used for CDIs, or the lanthipeptide lacticin 3147 led to drastic remodeling of the different microbial communities populating in this *ex vivo* distal colon model [91]. Trn-α and Trn-β used alone or in combination have the same lytic action on bacterial cells which arises from pore formation in the membrane and depolarization of the membrane. Since these sactipeptides have a narrow spectrum, it is very unlikely that the mechanisms leading to pore formation are similar to those of the lanthipeptide nisin targeting lipid II which is present in most Gram-positive bacteria. Thuricin CD most likely targets specific receptors located in the membrane or the cell wall before forming pores [115].

Similar to thuricin CD, thuricin Z has a pore-forming action effective on *Bacillus cereus* and *L. monocytogenes* with respective MIC of 2–8 μM and 4 μM [92,93]. Hardly any information on the biological activity of thurincin H is available but it seems to have a spectrum of activity similar to thuricin Z, that extends to other species of *Listeria* and *B. subtilis*. Gram-negative bacteria as well as some genera of Gram-positive bacteria such as *Lactobacillus* seem resistant to thurincin H. It should be noted that such information on the spectrum of action of thurincin H was collected in assays employing the producer strain and not the purified form of thurincin H [116]. The mode of action of thurincin H remains to be elucidated.

Regarding ruminococcin C, its antibacterial activity was investigated on the isoform RumC1. RumC1 is active against a broad spectrum of Gram-positive bacteria with MIC under the micromolar range for laboratory and clinical strains of *Clostridium perfringens, C. difficile, L. monocytogenes* and *Streptococcus pneumoniae.* Additionally, RumC1 is active against resistant and MDR strains in the micromolar range such as *B. cereus* vancomycin resistant or *Enterococcus faecium* vancomycin and amoxicillin resistant [98]. Finally, RumC1 displays modest activity against other Gram-positive bacteria such as *S. aureus*. RumC1 is not active against Gram-negative bacteria [39]. Unlike most sactipeptides, RumC1 does not have a pore-forming action [39]. The difference of mode of action might arise from the difference of surface hydrophobicity. Indeed, sactipeptides that are pore-forming have mostly hydrophobic surfaces whereas the surface of RumC1 is mostly hydrophilic [98]. Although the precise target of RumC1 is not currently known, it was shown that RumC1 inhibits the synthesis pathways on DNA, RNA, proteins and peptidoglycan as a likely consequence of ATP synthesis inhibition [98].

In order to use sactipeptides as alternatives to antibiotics, supplementary information must be gathered on their antibacterial activity and also on their safety and their stability. Subtilosin A and thuricin Z have been shown to be safe for models of vaginal tissues or some human cell lines, respectively [92,113]. RumC1 has been shown to be safe for intestinal and gastric human cells lines as well as on human ileo-cecal resection at high doses (up to 100–200 μM). Moreover, RumC1 does not induce lysis of human erythrocytes [39,98]. However, the knowledge on sactipeptide cytotoxicity is limited to these experiments.

Similarly, little is known on the sactipeptide stability to chemical, thermal or proteolytic treatments which could restrain their use in the clinic. The supernatant of the producer strain of thuricin CD was shown to keep its antibacterial activity in acidic condition (up to pH2) [91]. However, purified Trn-β is sensitive to the action of trypsin and pepsin. Thus, thuricin CD can't be administrated orally as Trn-β would be degraded. Trn-α is resistant to the action of digestive enzymes, probably because its aromatic residues that could be used as cleavage sites are protected by sacti-bridges whereas they are located outside of the bridges, near the termini, in Trn-β [117]. So far, RumC1 shows the most promising clinical properties among sactipeptides as it is resistant to digestive enzymes and physio-chemical conditions of the gastrointestinal tract, as well as salts at physiological concentrations and human serum. Additionally, the activity of RumC1 wasn't impaired by extreme acidic or basic conditions and RumC1 showed decent resistance to heat with no loss of activity 1 hour at 70°C or 15 minutes at 100°C [98]. Based on these observations, RumC1 could be considered for pharmaceutical development and for both oral and systemic routes administration.

5.6. *Perspectives on sactipeptides discovery*

Currently all known sactipeptides, except ruminococcin C, are produced by *Bacillus* spp. However, putative sactipeptide BGCs have been identified by genome mining in other phyla, thus this subclass of RiPPs could expand rapidly. The vast majority of them were found in Firmicutes but putative sactipeptide BGCs were also found in Actinobacteria or even in Gram-negative Proteobacteria and Bacteroidetes [93]. Another genome mining study found that sactipeptide BGC-like clusters are the second most common RiPP cluster after lanthipeptide in the human gastrointestinal tract [118]. Both thuricin CD and ruminococcin C were isolated from fecal strains, respectively of *B. thurengiensis* and *R. gnavus* [91,119] and the sequence of the precursor of subtilosin A has been identified in metagenomic data from samples collected in the human gut, oral cavity and skin [120]. Therefore, the human microbiota could be a potential source of sactipeptides. Other strategies to expand the class of sactipeptides employ bioengineering of known sactipeptides. As an example, a variant of subtilosin A with Ile instead of Thr at the 6th position was isolated with increased antibacterial potency [96]. Although this variant exhibits hemolytic activity and thus won't be used in a clinical context, point mutation is an interesting lead for variant generation with novel features or increased potency. In that sense, variants of subtilosin A with Cys at different positions or with different amino acid acceptors or even with the introduction of non-proteinogenic amino acids were produced by co-expression of a bio-engineered gene encoding the precursor of subtilosin A and the gene encoding the sactisynthase AlbA in *E. coli* [121].

6. Ranthipeptides

6.1. *Definition and the first identification of ranthipeptides*

The ranthipeptide or **ra**dical **n**on-α **thi**oether (ranthi-) peptide subclass of RiPPs was very recently proposed to classify RiPPs with thioether linkages similar to sactionine but involving the β- or γ-carbon ($C\beta$, $C\gamma$) of the acceptor residue instead of the $C\alpha$ [93,97] (Figure 13). Ranthipeptides were discovered through the study of SCIFFs which stands for precursor peptides with **S**ix **C**ysteines **I**n **F**orty-**F**ive residues. Originally, SCIFFs were identified through genome mining targeting radical-SAM enzyme containing RiPP BGCs. Radical-SAM enzymes next to short sequences encoding putative precursors were classified in five groups, including a group where the precursors corresponded to putative SCIFFs. This group was the most prevalent in Clostridia [122]. Sequence similarities between the precursor and the sactisynthase of subtilosin A with some putative SCIFF precursors and associated radical-SAM enzymes suggested that SCIFFs could harbor PTMs similar to sactipeptides.

One of these SCIFFs, thermocellin CteA encoded in the genome of *Clostridium thermocellum*, was modified *in vitro* after production by heterologous expression in *E. coli* and purification of both the precursor CteA and its associated radical-SAM enzyme CteB. A sactionine linkage was identified on this SCIFF that was classified as a sactipeptide [26]. Another SCIFF, Tte1186a, with a sequence similar to CteA was identified from the genome of *Caldanaerobacter subterraneus* subsp. *tengcongensis* and processed by its corresponding radical-SAM enzyme in a similar way. Analysis of the maturation of Tte1186a revealed the presence of one thioether linkage at the same position of CteA that was assumed to be a sactionine linkage [123]. Tte1186a shows conserved residues with CteA and is therefore part of the thermocellin family. However, no natural SCIFFs were isolated from their producer strains and the studied SCIFFs were reconstituted *in vitro* which can sometimes fail to obtain a full maturation and consequently an active form [93]. Hence, the incorporation of PTMs on SCIFFs and their nature remained speculative.

Later, another genome mining study identified other putative SCIFFs and their associated radical-SAM enzymes. This study revealed that the radical-SAM enzymes found in the BGCs of SCIFFs, including thermocellins, are actually more related to the enzyme QhpD than the known sactisynthases. QhpD performs PTMs formation on quinohemoprotein amine dehydrogenase (QHNDH). The PTMs of QHNDH consist in three thioether linkages essential for QHNDH activity: two between Cys and the Cβ of Asp and one between Cys and the Cγ of Glu. Moreover, it was noted that Asp was a conserved residue in putative SCIFF precursors. Therefore, it was hypothesized that SCIFFs might harbor thioether linkages involving Cβ of Asp in particular and Cγ rather than Cα [93]. Therefore new structural studies were conducted on CteA. A mature and L-[4-^{13}c,2,3-^{2}H2]-Thr labeled CteA was produced by co-expression of the genes encoding the precursor and the radical-SAM maturase CteB in *E. coli*. NMR studies confirmed that CteA harbors a thioether bond between Cys and Thr but also revealed that the linkage involves the Cγ of Thr and not the Cα [93]. Although the precise thioether bond of Tte1186a has not been determined yet, because of the high resemblance of Tte1186a to CteA, it can be expected to involve the Cγ (Figure 14).

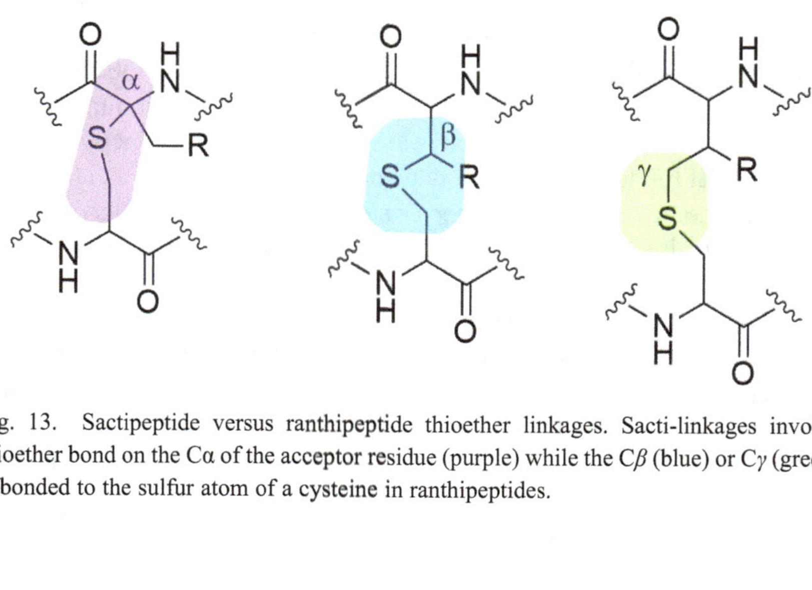

Fig. 13. Sactipeptide versus ranthipeptide thioether linkages. Sacti-linkages involve thioether bond on the Cα of the acceptor residue (purple) while the Cβ (blue) or Cγ (green) is bonded to the sulfur atom of a cysteine in ranthipeptides.

6.2. *Expansion of the ranthipeptides subclass*

Another SCIFF identified in this genome mining study from the genome of *Paenibacillus polymixa* was produced by co-expression of the *papA* and *papB* genes encoding the precursor and the radical-SAM enzyme, respectively, in *E. coli* [93]. PapA has an original sequence as it contains six repeats of Cys-X3-Asp (Figure 14). Mass spectrometry (MS) analyses of PapA revealed a monoisotopic mass 12 Da lighter than the theoretical mass, which is consistent with the formation of six thioether linkages as each thioether bridge results in a loss of two hydrogen atoms and therefore two Da. Tandem Mass spectrometry (MS/MS) analyses of thioether linkages involving Cα or Cβ, respectively, found in sactipeptides and lanthipeptides, reported that collision-induced dissociation causes the thioether bridges involving a Cα to open whereas those involving Cβ stay intact. In the case of PapA, the MS/MS pattern was closer to lanthipeptides than sactipeptides, suggesting that the thioether bonds employ Cβ. NMR studies confirmed that the six Cys of PapA were bound to the six Asp through their Cβ. Other variants of PapA were found with conserved six repeats of Cys-X3-Asp and this subclass of ranthipeptides was named freyrasins [93].

Whereas only one Cys of thermocellin CteA is modified, the six Cys of freyrasin PapA undergo maturation. Therefore, SCIFFs maturation can involve thioether linkages between Cβ and Cγ either on the six Cys or on selective Cys. Because of the distribution of Cys and their amino acid acceptors in freyrasins, they adopt a structure with several loops on the backbone rather than a hairpin structure like sactipeptides (Figure 14). Until now, only one ranthipeptide that doesn't also belong to the SCIFF family has been identified from the genomes of *Streptococcus orisratti* and *Streptococcus porci*, two commensal bacteria of the oral cavity of rats and pigs, respectively. The synthetic precursor NxxcA was processed *in vitro* by the associated radical-SAM enzyme NxxcB after production by heterologous expression in *E. coli*. MS/MS and NMR analyses showed that NxxcA harbors one thioether bond linking a Cys and the Cβ of an Asn. Surprisingly, the thioether bond in this SCIFF involves a Cys situated downstream of acceptor residues whereas in all the other SCIFFs the Cys is always situated closer to C-terminus than the acceptor residues [124] (Figure 14). It should be noted that no natural ranthipeptide has been isolated yet from the producer strain. Although some ranthipeptides

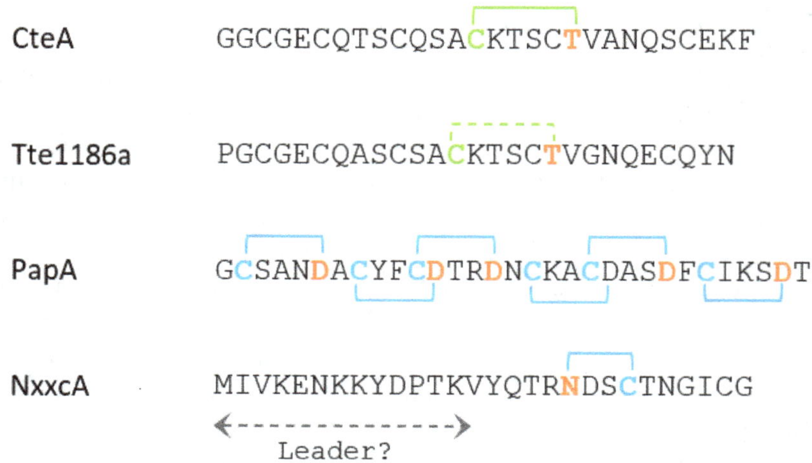

Fig. 14. Sequences and thioether networks of sactipeptides. Thioether linkages involving $C\beta$ and $C\gamma$ are represented in blue and green, respectively. Cys engaged in those bonds are also in blue or green whereas amino acid acceptors are in orange. The green dashed line indicates a thioether bond for which the linkage of S to $C\gamma$ has not been confirmed. For NxxcA, the sequence of the full precursor is provided as the partition between the leader and core sequences has not been identified yet whereas only the core sequences are shown for the other ranthipeptides.

have been produced *in vivo* in *E. coli* rather than reconstituted *in vitro*, there is currently no proof that the mature ranthipeptides observed in the above-mentioned studies fully correspond to natural products.

6.3. *Ranthipeptides' BGC and ranthisynthases*

Regarding the BGC of ranthipeptides, they all contain genes encoding: one precursor, one radical-SAM enzyme also named ranthisynthase and one protein involved in export. Except for freyrasins, a second protein for export and one gene with unknown function are found. In the NxxC cluster, a gene corresponding to a peptidase is found as well as two genes involved in regulation.

Like sactisynthases, ranthisynthases are SAM-dependent. *In vitro* reconstitution of mature PapA with PapB occurred only when SAM was added. In PapB, the mutation of any Cys from the Cys-X3-Cys-X2-Cys motif binding the first [4Fe-4S] cluster prevented the formation of 5′-Ado• [97]. Moreover, all described ranthisynthases harbor a SPASM domain predicted to bind to two auxiliary [4Fe-4S] clusters. Therefore, a mechanism similar to sactisynthase in which the [4Fe-4S] bound by the Cys-X3-Cys-X2-Cys motif activates SAM in 5′-Ado• and the auxiliary clusters are involved in thioether bond formation can be expected. However, it is unclear how the ranthisynthases select Cβ or Cγ rather than Cα for thioether formation. In PapA, the Asp were replaced with Glu. PapB was still able to form thioether bonds on the Cγ instead of the Cβ, meaning that the ranthisynthase can tolerate different substrates and that the carbon of the acceptor involved in the thioether bond depends on the amino acid acceptors as observed for QhpD. However, when Asp were mutated in Ala, no PTMs were incorporated by PapB on PapA, so it seems the ranthisynthase has a substrate specificity. Individual mutation of Cys residues of the precursor PapA revealed that each Cys-X3-Asp repeat is modified independently. In addition, the distance between Cys and the acceptor Asp plays a role in the maturation process as Cys-X4-Asp repeats were not processed by PapB. Finally, the leader peptide rather than the core sequence seems to be essential for the recognition of the precursor by the ranthisynthase. Indeed, a thioether bond was incorporated by PapB on a precursor composed of the leader peptide of PapA fused to a single Cys-X3-Asp motif [97].

Regarding the recognition of the leader peptide by the ranthisynthases, a PqqD-like RRE has been identified in both CteB and PapB. The structure of CteB in the presence of its precursor peptide CteA confirms the presence of an *N*-terminal wHTH RRE motif [26]. Despite sharing only 13% sequence identity to the RRE domains of LynD and NisB, the overall R.M.S.D is strong at 2.16 Å and 3.05 Å, respectively over 71 α-carbons. In CteB, the three stranded β-sheet, or wing, of the RRE hydrogen bonds with the backbone of the *N*-terminus of the CteA fragment in a manner similar to LynD and NisB (Figure 12(b)). A mutant of PapB lacking the RRE was unable of forming PTMs on PapA in the co-expression heterologous system. However, when the RRE was also expressed by itself in trans in this system, PapA was fully modified [26,97]. Thus, recognition of the precursor by an RRE seems to be essential in the maturation of ranthipeptides too.

6.4. *Biological activities*

No biological activity has been linked to ranthipeptides so far, however, they were tested only against few bacteria. They might have a very selective antibacterial activity or a different type of biological activity. Moreover, as no ranthipeptide has been naturally isolated from natural producer, the forms produced in *E. coli* or *in vitro* might lack additional processing essential for biological activity. Therefore, further investigations are needed to determinate the functions of ranthipeptides, including screening for other antimicrobial and biological activities (e.g. anti-inflammatory, and anti-proliferative).

References

1. O'Neill, J. (2016) Tackling Drug-Resistant Infections Globally Final Report and Recommendations. *Publ. Html* The Review on Antimicrobial Resistance.
2. Ventola, C. L. (2015) The Antibiotic Resistance Crisis: Part 1: Causes and Threats. *P T Peer-Rev. J. Formul. Manag.* 40, pp. 277–283.
3. Lewis, K. (2013) Platforms for Antibiotic Discovery. *Nat. Rev. Drug Discov.* 12, pp. 371–387.
4. Ghosh, C., Sarkar, P., Issa, R. and Haldar, J. (2019) Alternatives to Conventional Antibiotics in the Era of Antimicrobial Resistance. *Trends Microbiol.* 27, pp. 323–338.
5. Arnison, P. G., Bibb, M. J., Bierbaum, G., Bowers, A. A., van der Donk, W. A. *et al.* (2013) Ribosomally Synthesized and Post-Translationally Modified Peptide Natural Products: Overview and Recommendations for a Universal Nomenclature. *Nat.Prod. Rep.* 30, pp. 108–160.
6. Luo, S. and Dong, S.-H. (2019) Recent Advances in the Discovery and Biosynthetic Study of Eukaryotic RiPP Natural Products. *Molecules.* 24, pp. 1541.
7. Yang, X. and van der Donk, W. A. (2013) Ribosomally Synthesized and Post-Translationally Modified Peptide Natural Products: New Insights into the Role of Leader and Core Peptides during Biosynthesis. *Chem. Eur. J.* 19, pp. 7662–7677.
8. Gu, W., Sardar, D., Pierce, E. and Schmidt, E. W. (2018) Roads to Rome: Role of Multiple Cassettes in Cyanobactin RiPP Biosynthesis. *J. Am. Chem. Soc.* 140, pp. 16213–16221.
9. Truman, A. W. (2016) Cyclisation Mechanisms in the Biosynthesis of Ribosomally Synthesised and Post-Translationally Modified Peptides. *Beilstein J. Org. Chem.* 12, pp. 1250–1268.
10. Haft, D. H. (2009) A Strain-Variable Bacteriocin in Bacillus Anthracis and Bacillus Cereus with Repeated Cys-Xaa-Xaa motifs. *Biol. Direct.* 4, p. 15.
11. Li, B., Sher, D., Kelly, L., Shi, Y., Huang, K., Knerr, P.J., Joewono, I., Rusch, D., Chisholm, S. W. and van der Donk, W. A. (2010) Catalytic Promiscuity in the Biosynthesis of Cyclic Peptide Secondary Metabolites

in Planktonic Marine Cyanobacteria. *Proc. Natl. Acad. Sci.* 107, pp. 10430–10435.

12. Bartholomae, M., Buivydas, A., Viel, J. H., Montalbán-López, M. and Kuipers, O. P. (2017) Major Gene-Regulatory Mechanisms Operating in Ribosomally Synthesized and Post-Translationally Modified Peptide (RiPP) Biosynthesis: Major Gene-Regulatory Mechanisms. *Mol. Microbiol.* 106, pp. 186–206.
13. Moll, G. N., Kuipers, A. and Rink, R. (2010) Microbial Engineering of Dehydro-Amino Acids and Lanthionines in Non-Lantibiotic Peptides. *Antonie Van Leeuwenhoek.* 97, pp. 319–333.
14. Ortega, M. A. and van der Donk, W. A. (2016) New Insights into the Biosynthetic Logic of Ribosomally Synthesized and Post-translationally Modified Peptide Natural Products. *Cell Chem. Biol.* 23, pp. 31–44.
15. Zhang, Q., Yang, X., Wang, H. and van der Donk, W. A. (2014) High Divergence of the Precursor Peptides in Combinatorial Lanthipeptide Biosynthesis. *ACS Chem. Biol.* 9, pp. 2686–2694.
16. Tang, W. and van der Donk, W. A. (2012) Structural Characterization of Four Prochlorosins: A Novel Class of Lantipeptides Produced by Planktonic Marine Cyanobacteria. *Biochemistry.* 51, pp. 4271–4279.
17. Mavaro, A., Abts, A., Bakkes, P. J., Moll, G. N., Driessen, A. J. M., Smits, S. H. J. and Schmitt, L. (2011) Substrate Recognition and Specificity of the NisB Protein, the Lantibiotic Dehydratase Involved in Nisin Biosynthesis. *J. Biol. Chem.* 286, pp. 30552–30560.
18. Ortega, M. A., Hao, Y., Zhang, Q., Walker, M. C., van der Donk, W. A. and Nair, S. K. (2015) Structure and Mechanism of the tRNA-Dependent Lantibiotic Dehydratase NisB. *Nature.* 517, pp. 509–512.
19. Regni, C. A., Roush, R. F., Miller, D. J., Nourse, A., Walsh, C. T. and Schulman, B. A. (2009) How the MccB Bacterial Ancestor of Ubiquitin E1 Initiates Biosynthesis of the Microcin C7 Antibiotic. *EMBO J.* 28, pp. 1953–1964.
20. Koehnke, J., Mann, G., Bent, A. F., Ludewig, H., Shirran, S., Botting, C., Lebl, T., Houssen, W. E., Jaspars, M. and Naismith, J. H. (2015) Structural Analysis of Leader Peptide Binding Enables Leader-Free Cyanobactin Processing. *Nat. Chem. Biol.* 11, pp. 558–563.
21. Evans, R. L., Latham, J. A., Xia, Y., Klinman, J. P. and Wilmot, C. M. (2017) Nuclear Magnetic Resonance Structure and Binding Studies of PqqD, a Chaperone Required in the Biosynthesis of the Bacterial Dehydrogenase Cofactor Pyrroloquinoline Quinone. *Biochemistry.* 56, pp. 2735–2746.
22. Burkhart, B. J., Hudson, G. A., Dunbar, K. L. and Mitchell, D. A. (2015) A Prevalent Peptide-Binding Domain Guides Ribosomal Natural Product Biosynthesis. *Nat. Chem. Biol.* 11, pp. 564–570.

23. Link, A. J. (2015) Leading the Way to RiPPs. *Nat. Chem. Biol.* 11, pp. 551–552.
24. Wieckowski, B. M., Hegemann, J. D., Mielcarek, A., Boss, L., Burghaus, O. and Marahiel, M. A. (2015) The PqqD Homologous Domain of the Radical SAM Enzyme ThnB is Required for Thioether Bond Formation During Thurincin H Maturation. *FEBS Lett.* 589, pp. 1802–1806.
25. Grell, T. A. J., Kincannon, W. M., Bruender, N. A., Blaesi, E. J., Krebs, C., Bandarian, V. and Drennan, C. L. (2018) Structural and Spectroscopic Analyses of the Sporulation Killing Factor Biosynthetic Enzyme SkfB, a Bacterial AdoMet Radical Sactisynthase. *J. Biol. Chem.* 293, pp. 17349–17361.
26. Grove, T. L., Himes, P. M., Hwang, S., Yumerefendi, H., Bonanno, J.B., Kuhlman, B., Almo, S. C. and Bowers, A. A. (2017) Structural Insights into Thioether Bond Formation in the Biosynthesis of Sactipeptides. *J. Am. Chem. Soc.* 139, pp. 11734–11744.
27. Chekan, J. R., Ongpipattanakul, C. and Nair, S. K. (2019) Steric Complementarity Directs Sequence Promiscuous Leader Binding in RiPP Biosynthesis. *Proc. Natl. Acad. Sci.* 116, pp. 24049–24055.
28. Schramma, K. R., Bushin, L. B. and Seyedsayamdost, M. R. (2015) Structure and Biosynthesis of a Macrocyclic Peptide Containing an Unprecedented Lysine-to-Tryptophan Crosslink. *Nat. Chem.* 7, pp. 431–437.
29. Davis, K. M., Schramma, K. R., Hansen, W. A., Bacik, J. P., Khare, S. D., Seyedsayamdost, M. R. and Ando, N. (2017) Structures of the Peptide-Modifying Radical SAM Enzyme SuiB Elucidate the Basis of Substrate Recognition. *Proc. Natl. Acad. Sci.* 114, pp. 10420–10425.
30. Schramma, K. R. and Seyedsayamdost, M. R. (2017) Lysine-Tryptophan-Crosslinked Peptides Produced by Radical SAM Enzymes in Pathogenic Streptococci. *ACS Chem. Biol.* 12, pp. 922–927.
31. Burkhart, B. J., Kakkar, N., Hudson, G. A., van der Donk, W. A. and Mitchell, D. A. (2017) Chimeric Leader Peptides for the Generation of Non-Natural Hybrid RiPP Products. *ACS Cent. Sci.* 3, pp. 629–638.
32. Oman, T. J. and van der Donk, W. A. (2010) Follow the Leader: The Use of Leader Peptides to Guide Natural Product Biosynthesis. *Nat. Chem. Biol.* 6, pp. 9–18.
33. Kuipers, A., de Boef, E., Rink, R., Fekken, S., Kluskens, L. D., Driessen, A. J. M., Leenhouts, K., Kuipers, O. P. and Moll, G. N. (2004) NisT, the Transporter of the Lantibiotic Nisin, Can Transport Fully Modified, Dehydrated, and Unmodified Prenisin and Fusions of the Leader Peptide with Non-lantibiotic Peptides. *J. Biol. Chem.* 279, pp. 22176–22182.
34. Montalbán-López, M., Deng, J., van Heel, A. J. and Kuipers, O. P. (2018) Specificity and Application of the Lantibiotic Protease NisP. *Front. Microbiol.* 9, pp. 160.

35. Furgerson Ihnken, L. A., Chatterjee, C. and van der Donk, W. A. (2008) *In Vitro* Reconstitution and Substrate Specificity of a Lantibiotic Protease †. *Biochemistry.* 47, pp. 7352–7363.
36. Nissen-Meyer, J., Oppegård, C., Rogne, P., Haugen, H. S. and Kristiansen, P. E. (2010) Structure and Mode-of-Action of the Two-Peptide (Class-IIb) Bacteriocins. *Probiotics Antimicrob. Proteins.* 2, pp. 52–60.
37. Ortega, M. A., Velásquez, J. E., Garg, N., Zhang, Q., Joyce, R. E., Nair, S. K. and van der Donk, W. A. (2014) Substrate Specificity of the Lanthipeptide Peptidase ElxP and the Oxidoreductase ElxO. *ACS Chem. Biol.* 9, pp. 1718–1725.
38. Chen, S., Xu, B., Chen, E., Wang, J., Lu, J., Donadio, S., Ge, H. and Wang, H. (2019) Zn-Dependent Bifunctional Proteases are Responsible for Leader Peptide Processing of Class III Lanthipeptides. *Proc. Natl. Acad. Sci.* 116, pp. 2533–2538.
39. Chiumento, S., Roblin, C., Kieffer-Jaquinod, S., Tachon, S., Leprètre, C., Basset, C., Aditiyarini, D., Olleik, H., Nicoletti, C., Bornet, O., Iranzo, O., Maresca, M., Hardré, R., Fons, M., Giardina, T., Devillard, E., Guerlesquin, F., Couté, Y., Atta, M., Perrier, J., Lafond, M. and Duarte, V. (2019) Ruminococcin C, A Promising Antibiotic Produced by a Human Gut Symbiont. *Sci. Adv.* 5, pp. eaaw9969.
40. Repka, L. M., Chekan, J. R., Nair, S. K. and van der Donk, W. A. (2017) Mechanistic Understanding of Lanthipeptide Biosynthetic Enzymes. *Chem. Rev.* 117, pp. 5457–5520.
41. Bierbaum, G. and Sahl, H.-G. (2009) Lantibiotics: Mode of Action, Biosynthesis and Bioengineering. *Curr. Pharm. Biotechnol.* 10, pp. 2–18.
42. ImmuCell UNITED STATES SECURITIES AND EXCHANGE COMMISSION Washington. DC. (2016).
43. Dufour, S., Labrie, J. and Jacques, M. (2019) The Mastitis Pathogens Culture Collection. *Microbiol. Resour. Announc.* 8, pp. MRA.00133-19, e00133-19.
44. Huo, L., Ökesli, A., Zhao, M. and van der Donk, W. A. (2017) Insights into the Biosynthesis of Duramycin. *Appl. Environ. Microbiol.* 83, pp. e02698-16, e02698-16.
45. Pierrat, O. A. and Maxwell, A. (2003) The Action of the Bacterial Toxin Microcin B17: Insight into the Cleavage-Religation Reaction of DNA Gyrase. *J. Biol. Chem.* 278, pp. 35016–35023.
46. Molohon, K. J., Blair, P. M., Park, S., Doroghazi, J. R., Maxson, T., Hershfield, J. R., Flatt, K. M., Schroeder, N. E., Ha, T. and Mitchell, D. A. (2016) Plantazolicin Is an Ultranarrow-Spectrum Antibiotic That Targets the *Bacillus anthracis* Membrane. *ACS Infect. Dis.* 2, pp. 207–220.
47. Travin, D. Y., Watson, Z. L., Metelev, M., Ward, F. R., Osterman, I. A., Khven, I. M., Khabibullina, N. F., Serebryakova, M., Mergaert, P., Polikanov,

Y. S., Cate, J. H. D. and Severinov, K. (2019) Structure of Ribosome-Bound Azole-Modified Peptide Phazolicin Rationalizes its Species-Specific Mode of Bacterial Translation Inhibition. *Nat. Commun.* 10, pp. 4563.

48. Tietz, J. I. and Mitchell, D. A. (2016) Using Genomics for Natural Product Structure Elucidation. *Curr. Top. Med. Chem.* 16, pp. 1645–1694.
49. Claesen, J. and Bibb, M. (2010) Genome Mining and Genetic Analysis of Cypemycin Biosynthesis Reveal an Unusual Class of Posttranslationally Modified Peptides. *Proc. Natl. Acad. Sci.* 107, pp. 16297–16302.
50. Mo, T., Liu, W.-Q., Ji, W., Zhao, J., Chen, T., Ding, W., Yu, S. and Zhang, Q. (2017) Biosynthetic Insights into Linaridin Natural Products from Genome Mining and Precursor Peptide Mutagenesis. *ACS Chem. Biol.* 12, pp. 1484–1488.
51. Mann, G., Huo, L., Adam, S., Nardone, B., Vendome, J., Westwood, N. J., Müller, R. and Koehnke, J. (2016) Structure and Substrate Recognition of the Bottromycin Maturation Enzyme BotP. *ChemBioChem* 17, pp. 2286–2292.
52. Schwalen, C. J., Hudson, G. A., Kosol, S., Mahanta, N., Challis, G. L. and Mitchell, D. A. (2017) In Vitro Biosynthetic Studies of Bottromycin Expand the Enzymatic Capabilities of the YcaO Superfamily. *J. Am. Chem. Soc.* 139, pp. 18154–18157.
53. Otaka, T. and Kaji, A. (1976) Mode of Action of Bottromycin A2. Release of Aminoacyl- or Peptidyl-tRNA from Ribosomes. *J. Biol. Chem.* 251, pp. 2299–2306.
54. Ahmed, M. N., Reyna-González, E., Schmid, B., Wiebach, V., Süssmuth, R. D., Dittmann, E. and Fewer, D. P. (2017) Phylogenomic Analysis of the Microviridin Biosynthetic Pathway Coupled with Targeted Chemo-Enzymatic Synthesis Yields Potent Protease Inhibitors. *ACS Chem. Biol.* 12, pp. 1538–1546.
55. Just-Baringo, X., Albericio, F. and Álvarez, M. (2014) Thiopeptide Antibiotics: Retrospective and Recent Advances. *Mar. Drugs* 12, pp. 317–351.
56. Goldstein, B. P., Berti, M., Ripamonti, F., Resconi, A., Scotti, R. and Denaro, M. (1993) *In Vitro* Antimicrobial Activity of a New Antibiotic, MDL 62,879 (GE2270 A). *Antimicrob. Agents Chemother.* 37, pp. 741–745.
57. LaMarche, M. J., Leeds, J. A., Amaral, A., Brewer, J. T., Bushell, S. M., Deng, G., Dewhurst, J. M., Ding, J., Dzink-Fox, J., Gamber, G., Jain, A., Lee, K., Lee, L., Lister, T., McKenney, D., Mullin, S., Osborne, C., Palestrant, D., Patane, M. A., Rann, E. M., Sachdeva, M., Shao, J., Tiamfook, S., Trzasko, A., Whitehead, L., Yifru, A., Yu, D., Yan, W. and Zhu, Q. (2012) Discovery of LFF571: An Investigational Agent for *Clostridium difficile* Infection. *J. Med. Chem.* 55, pp. 2376–2387.

58. Nowak, A., Hedenstierna, M., Ursing, J., Lidman, C. and Nowak, P. (2019) Efficacy of Routine Fecal Microbiota Transplantation for Treatment of Recurrent *Clostridium difficile* Infection: A Retrospective Cohort Study. *Int. J. Microbiol.* 2019, pp. 1–7.
59. Ting, L. S. L., Praestgaard, J., Grunenberg, N., Yang, J. C., Leeds, J. A. and Pertel, P. (2012) A First-in-Human, Randomized, Double-Blind, Placebo-Controlled, Single- and Multiple-Ascending Oral Dose Study To Assess the Safety and Tolerability of LFF571 in Healthy Volunteers. *Antimicrob. Agents Chemother.* 56, pp. 5946–5951.
60. Mullane, K., Lee, C., Bressler, A., Buitrago, M., Weiss, K., Dabovic, K., Praestgaard, J., Leeds, J. A., Blais, J. and Pertel, P. (2015) Multicenter, Randomized Clinical Trial To Compare the Safety and Efficacy of LFF571 and Vancomycin for Clostridium difficile Infections. *Antimicrob. Agents Chemother.* 59, pp. 1435–1440.
61. Fabbretti, A., He, C.-G., Gaspari, E., Maffioli, S., Brandi, L., Spurio, R., Sosio, M., Jabes, D. and Donadio, S. (2015) A Derivative of the Thiopeptide GE2270A Highly Selective against Propionibacterium Acnes. *Antimicrob. Agents Chemother.* 59, pp. 4560–4568.
62. Helf, M. J., Jud, A. and Piel, J. (2017) Enzyme from an Uncultivated Sponge Bacterium Catalyzes *S*-Methylation in a Ribosomal Peptide. *ChemBioChem.* 18, pp. 444–450.
63. Hamada, T., Matsunaga, S., Fujiwara, M., Fujita, K., Hirota, H., Schmucki, R., Güntert, P. and Fusetani, N. (2010) Solution Structure of Polytheonamide B, a Highly Cytotoxic Nonribosomal Polypeptide from Marine Sponge. *J. Am. Chem. Soc.* 132, pp. 12941–12945.
64. Hayata, A., Itoh, H. and Inoue, M. (2018) Solid-Phase Total Synthesis and Dual Mechanism of Action of the Channel-Forming 48-mer Peptide Polytheonamide B. *J. Am. Chem. Soc.* 140, pp. 10602–10611.
65. Baquero, F., Lanza, V.F., Baquero, M.-R., del Campo, R. and Bravo-Vázquez, D. A. (2019) Microcins in Enterobacteriaceae: Peptide Antimicrobials in the Eco-Active Intestinal Chemosphere. *Front. Microbiol.* 10, pp. 2261.
66. Duquesne, S., Destoumieux-Garzón, D., Peduzzi, J. and Rebuffat, S. (2007) Microcins, Gene-Encoded Antibacterial Peptides from Enterobacteria. *Nat. Prod. Rep.* 24, pp. 708.
67. Martin-Gómez, H. and Tulla-Puche, J. (2018) Lasso Peptides: Chemical Approaches and Structural Elucidation. *Org. Biomol. Chem.* 16, pp. 5065–5080.
68. Kaweewan, I., Hemmi, H., Komaki, H., Harada, S. and Kodani, S. (2018) Isolation and Structure Determination of a New Lasso Peptide Specialicin Based on Genome Mining. *Bioorg. Med. Chem.* 26, pp. 6050–6055.

69. van Heel, A. J., Montalban-Lopez, M., Oliveau, Q. and Kuipers, O. P. (2017) Genome-Guided Identification of Novel Head-to-Tail Cyclized Antimicrobial Peptides, Exemplified by the Discovery of Pumilarin. *Microb. Genomics.* 3.
70. Norris, G. E. and Patchett, M. L. (2016) The Glycocins: In a Class of Their Own. *Curr. Opin. Struct. Biol.* 40, pp. 112–119.
71. Kaunietis, A., Buivydas, A., Čitavičius, D. J. and Kuipers, O. P. (2019) Heterologous Biosynthesis and Characterization of a Glycocin from a Thermophilic Bacterium. *Nat. Commun.* 10, p. 1115.
72. Kenney, G. E., Dassama, L. M. K., Pandelia, M.-E., Gizzi, A. S., Martinie, R. J., Gao, P., DeHart, C. J., Schachner, L. F., Skinner, O. S., Ro, S. Y., Zhu, X., Sadek, M., Thomas, P. M., Almo, S. C., Bollinger, J. M., Krebs, C., Kelleher, N. L. and Rosenzweig, A. C. (2018) The Biosynthesis of Methanobactin. *Science.* 359, pp. 1411–1416.
73. Gordon, C. P. (2020) Synthetic Strategies to Access Staphylococcus Auto-Inducing Peptides as Quorum Sensing Modulators. *Org. Biomol. Chem.* 18, pp. 379–390.
74. Ibrahim, M., Guillot, A., Wessner, F., Algaron, F., Besset, C., Courtin, P., Gardan, R. and Monnet, V. (2007) Control of the Transcription of a Short Gene Encoding a Cyclic Peptide in *Streptococcus thermophilus*: A New Quorum-Sensing System? *J. Bacteriol.* 189, pp. 8844–8854.
75. Bushin, L. B., Clark, K. A., Pelczer, I. and Seyedsayamdost, M. R. (2018) Charting an Unexplored Streptococcal Biosynthetic Landscape Reveals a Unique Peptide Cyclization Motif. *J. Am. Chem. Soc.* 140, pp. 17674–17684.
76. Walton, J. D., Hallen-Adams, H. E. and Luo, H. (2010) Ribosomal Biosynthesis of the Cyclic Peptide Toxins of Amanita Mushrooms. *Biopolymers.* 94, pp. 659–664.
77. Sterner, O., Etzel, W., Mayer, A. and Anke, H. (1997) Omphalotin, A New Cyclic Peptide with Potent Nematicidal Activity from *Omphalotus Olearius* II. Isolation and Structure Determination. *Nat. Prod. Lett.* 10, pp. 33–38.
78. Ramm, S., Krawczyk, B., Mühlenweg, A., Poch, A., Mösker, E. and Süssmuth, R. D. (2017) A Self-Sacrificing *N*-Methyltransferase Is the Precursor of the Fungal Natural Product Omphalotin. *Angew. Chem. Int. Ed.* 56, pp. 9994–9997.
79. van der Velden, N. S., Kälin, N., Helf, M. J., Piel, J., Freeman, M. F. and Künzler, M. (2017) Autocatalytic Backbone *N*-Methylation in a Family of Ribosomal Peptide Natural Products. *Nat. Chem. Biol.* 13, pp. 833–835.
80. Ding, W., Liu, W.-Q., Jia, Y., Li, Y., van der Donk, W. A. and Zhang, Q. (2016) Biosynthetic Investigation of Phomopsins Reveals a Widespread Pathway for Ribosomal Natural Products in Ascomycetes. *Proc. Natl. Acad. Sci.* 113, pp. 3521–3526.

81. Nagano, N., Umemura, M., Izumikawa, M., Kawano, J., Ishii, T., Kikuchi, M., Tomii, K., Kumagai, T., Yoshimi, A., Machida, M., Abe, K., Shin-ya, K. and Asai, K. (2016) Class of Cyclic Ribosomal Peptide Synthetic Genes in Filamentous Fungi. *Fungal Genet. Biol.* 86, pp. 58–70.
82. Johnson, R. D., Lane, G. A., Koulman, A., Cao, M., Fraser, K., Fleetwood, D. J., Voisey, C. R., Dyer, J. M., Pratt, J., Christensen, M., Simpson, W. R., Bryan, G. T. and Johnson, L. J. (2015) A Novel Family of Cyclic Oligopeptides Derived from Ribosomal Peptide Synthesis of an in Planta-Induced Gene, gigA, in Epichloë Endophytes of Grasses. *Fungal Genet. Biol.* 85, pp. 14–24.
83. Park, S., Yoo, K.-O., Marcussen, T., Backlund, A., Jacobsson, E., Rosengren, K. J., Doo, I. and Göransson, U. (2017) Cyclotide Evolution: Insights from the Analyses of Their Precursor Sequences, Structures and Distribution in Violets (Viola). *Front. Plant Sci.* 8, p. 2058.
84. Ramalho, S., Pinto, M., Ferreira, D. and Bolzani, V. (2018) Biologically Active Orbitides from the Euphorbiaceae Family. *Planta Med.* 84, pp. 558–567.
85. Lebbe, E. K. M. and Tytgat, J. (2016) In the Picture: Disulfide-Poor Conopeptides, A Class of Pharmacologically Interesting Compounds. *J. Venom. Anim. Toxins Trop. Dis.* 22, p. 30.
86. Gao, B., Peng, C., Yang, J., Yi, Y., Zhang, J. and Shi, Q. (2017) Cone Snails: A Big Store of Conotoxins for Novel Drug Discovery. *Toxins.* 9, p. 397.
87. Kawulka, K. E., Sprules, T., Diaper, C. M., Whittal, R. M., McKay, R. T., Mercier, P., Zuber, P. and Vederas, J. C. (2004) Structure of Subtilosin A, A Cyclic Antimicrobial Peptide from *Bacillus subtilis* with Unusual Sulfur to α-Carbon Cross-Links: Formation and Reduction of α-Thio-α-Amino Acid Derivatives † , ‡. *Biochemistry* 43, pp. 3385–3395.
88. Kawulka, K., Sprules, T., McKay, R. T., Mercier, P., Diaper, C. M., Zuber, P. and Vederas, J. C. (2003) Structure of Subtilosin A, An Antimicrobial Peptide from *Bacillus subtilis* with Unusual Posttranslational Modifications Linking Cysteine Sulfurs to *α*-Carbons of Phenylalanine and Threonine. *J. Am. Chem. Soc.* 125, pp. 4726–4727.
89. Liu, W.-T., Yang, Y.-L., Xu, Y., Lamsa, A., Haste, N. M., Yang, J. Y., Ng, J., Gonzalez, D., Ellermeier, C. D., Straight, P. D., Pevzner, P. A., Pogliano, J., Nizet, V., Pogliano, K. and Dorrestein, P. C. (2010) Imaging Mass Spectrometry of Intraspecies Metabolic Exchange Revealed the Cannibalistic Factors of *Bacillus subtilis*. *Proc. Natl. Acad. Sci.* 107, pp. 16286–16290.
90. Sit, C. S., van Belkum, M. J., McKay, R. T., Worobo, R. W. and Vederas, J. C. (2011) The 3d Solution Structure of Thurincin H, *a* Bacteriocin with Four Sulfur to *α*-Carbon Crosslinks. *Angew. Chem. Int. Ed.* 50, pp. 8718–8721.

91. Rea, M. C., Sit, C. S., Clayton, E., O'Connor, P. M., Whittal, R. M., Zheng, J., Vederas, J. C., Ross, R. P. and Hill, C. (2010) Thuricin CD, A Posttranslationally Modified Bacteriocin with a Narrow Spectrum of Activity Against *Clostridium difficile*. *Proc. Natl. Acad. Sci.* 107, pp. 9352–9357.
92. Mo, T., Ji, X., Yuan, W., Mandalapu, D., Wang, F., Zhong, Y., Li, F., Chen, Q., Ding, W., Deng, Z., Yu, S. and Zhang, Q. (2019) Thuricin Z: A Narrow-Spectrum Sactibiotic that Targets the Cell Membrane. *Angew. Chem. Int. Ed.* 58, pp. 18793–18797.
93. Hudson, G. A., Burkhart, B. J., DiCaprio, A. J., Schwalen, C. J., Kille, B., Pogorelov, T. V. and Mitchell, D. A. (2019) Bioinformatic Mapping of Radical *S*-Adenosylmethionine-Dependent Ribosomally Synthesized and Post-Translationally Modified Peptides Identifies New Cα, Cβ, and Cγ-Linked Thioether-Containing Peptides. *J. Am. Chem. Soc.* DOI: 10.1021/jacs.9b01519
94. Crost, E. H., Pujol, A., Ladiré, M., Dabard, J., Raibaud, P., Carlier, J. P. and Fons, M. (2010) Production of An Antibacterial Substance in the Digestive Tract Involved in Colonization-Resistance Against *Clostridium perfringens*. *Anaerobe* 16, pp. 597–603.
95. Pujol, A., Crost, E. H., Simon, G., Barbe, V., Vallenet, D., Gomez, A. and Fons, M. (2011) Characterization and Distribution of the Gene Cluster Encoding RumC, An Anti-*Clostridium perfringens* Bacteriocin Produced in the Gut. *FEMS Microbiol. Ecol.* 78, pp. 405–415.
96. Huang, T., Geng, H., Miyyapuram, V.R., Sit, C. S., Vederas, J. C. and Nakano, M. M. (2009) Isolation of a Variant of Subtilosin A with Hemolytic Activity. *J. Bacteriol.* 191, pp. 5690–5696.
97. Precord, T. W., Mahanta, N. and Mitchell, D. A. (2019) Reconstitution and Substrate Specificity of the Thioether-Forming Radical-Adenosylmethionine Enzyme in Freyrasin Biosynthesis. *ACS Chem. Biol.* 14, pp. 1981–1989.
98. Roblin, C., Chiumento, S., Bornet, O., Nouailler, M., Müller, C., Jeannot, K., Basset, C., Kieffer-Jaquinod, S., Couté, Y., Torelli, S., Le Pape, L., Schüneman, V., Olleik, H., De La Villeon, B., Sockeel, P., Di Pasquale, E., Nicoletti, C., Vidal, N., Poljak, L., Iranzo, O., Giardina, T., Fons, M., Devillard, E., Polard, P., Maresca, M., Perrier, J., Atta, M., Guerlesquin, F., Lafond, M. and Duarte, V. (2020) The Unusual Structure of Ruminococcin C1 Antimicrobial Peptide Confers Clinical Properties. *Proc. Natl. Acad. Sci. USA*. 117, pp. 19168–19177.
99. Balty, C., Guillot, A., Fradale, L., Brewee, C., Boulay, M., Kubiak, X., Benjdia, A. and Berteau, O. (2019) Ruminococcin C, An Anti-Clostridial Sactipeptide Produced by a Prominent Member of the Human Microbiota Ruminococcus Gnavus. *J. Biol. Chem.* 294, pp. 14512–14525.
100. Mahanta, N., Hudson, G. A. and Mitchell, D. A. (2017) Radical *S* - Adenosylmethionine Enzymes Involved in RiPP Biosynthesis. *Biochemistry.* 56, pp. 5229–5244.

101. Broderick, J. B., Duffus, B. R., Duschene, K. S. and Shepard, E. M. (2014) Radical *S*-Adenosylmethionine Enzymes. *Chem. Rev.* 114, pp. 4229–4317.
102. Fontecave, M., Atta, M. and Mulliez, E. (2004) *S*-Adenosylmethionine: Nothing Goes to Waste. *Trends Biochem. Sci.* 29, pp. 243–249.
103. Flühe, L. and Marahiel, M. A. (2013) Radical *S*-Adenosylmethionine Enzyme Catalyzed Thioether Bond Formation in Sactipeptide Biosynthesis. *Curr. Opin. Chem. Biol.* 17, pp. 605–612.
104. Bruender, N. A. and Bandarian, V. (2016) SkfB Abstracts a Hydrogen Atom from Cα on SkfA To Initiate Thioether Cross-Link Formation. *Biochemistry.* 55, pp. 4131–4134.
105. Grell, T. A. J., Goldman, P. J. and Drennan, C. L. (2015) SPASM and Twitch Domains in *S*-Adenosylmethionine (SAM) Radical Enzymes. *J. Biol. Chem.* 290, pp. 3964–3971.
106. Flühe, L., Knappe, T. A., Gattner, M. J., Schäfer, A., Burghaus, O., Linne, U. and Marahiel, M. A. (2012) The Radical SAM Enzyme AlbA Catalyzes Thioether Bond Formation in Subtilosin A. *Nat. Chem. Biol.* 8, pp. 350–357.
107. Flühe, L., Burghaus, O., Wieckowski, B. M., Giessen, T. W., Linne, U. and Marahiel, M. A. (2013) Two [4Fe-4S] Clusters Containing Radical SAM Enzyme SkfB Catalyze Thioether Bond Formation during the Maturation of the Sporulation Killing Factor. *J. Am. Chem. Soc.* 135, pp. 959–962.
108. Benjdia, A., Guillot, A., Lefranc, B., Vaudry, H., Leprince, J. and Berteau, O. (2016) Thioether Bond Formation by SPASM Domain Radical SAM Enzymes: Cα H-Atom Abstraction in Subtilosin A Biosynthesis. *Chem. Commun.* 52, pp. 6249–6252.
109. Gonzalez-Pastor, J. E. (2003) Cannibalism by Sporulating Bacteria. *Science.* 301, pp. 510–513.
110. Shelburne, C. E., An, F. Y., Dholpe, V., Ramamoorthy, A., Lopatin, D. E. and Lantz, M. S. (2006) The Spectrum of Antimicrobial Activity of the Bacteriocin Subtilosin A. *J. Antimicrob. Chemother.* 59, pp. 297–300.
111. Thennarasu, S., Lee, D.-K., Poon, A., Kawulka, K. E., Vederas, J. C. and Ramamoorthy, A. (2005) Membrane Permeabilization, Orientation, and Antimicrobial Mechanism of Subtilosin A. *Chem. Phys. Lipids* 137, pp. 38–51.
112. Sutyak Noll, K., Sinko, P. J. and Chikindas, M. L. (2011) Elucidation of the Molecular Mechanisms of Action of the Natural Antimicrobial Peptide Subtilosin Against the Bacterial Vaginosis-Associated Pathogen *Gardnerella vaginalis*. *Probiotics Antimicrob. Proteins.* 3, pp. 41–47.
113. Sutyak, K. E., Anderson, R. A., Dover, S. E., Feathergill, K. A., Aroutcheva, A. A., Faro, S. and Chikindas, M. L. (2008) Spermicidal Activity of the Safe Natural Antimicrobial Peptide Subtilosin. *Infect. Dis. Obstet. Gynecol.* 2008, pp. 1–6.

114. Mathur, H., O'Connor, P. M., Hill, C., Cotter, P. D. and Ross, R. P. (2013) Analysis of Anti-*Clostridium difficile* Activity of Thuricin CD, Vancomycin, Metronidazole, Ramoplanin, and Actagardine, both Singly and in Paired Combinations. *Antimicrob. Agents Chemother.* 57, pp. 2882–2886.
115. Mathur, H., Fallico, V., O'Connor, P. M., Rea, M. C., Cotter, P. D., Hill, C. and Ross, R. P. (2017) Insights into the Mode of Action of the Sactibiotic Thuricin CD. *Front. Microbiol.* 8, pp. 696.
116. Lee, H., Churey, J. J. and Worobo, R. W. (2009) Biosynthesis and Transcriptional Analysis of Thurincin H, A Tandem Repeated Bacteriocin Genetic Locus, Produced by *Bacillus thuringiensis* SF361. *FEMS Microbiol. Lett.* 299, pp. 205–213.
117. Rea, M. C., Alemayehu, D., Casey, P. G., O'Connor, P. M., Lawlor, P. G., Walsh, M., Shanahan, F., Kiely, B., Ross, R. P. and Hill, C. (2014) Bioavailability of the Anti-Clostridial Bacteriocin Thuricin CD in Gastrointestinal Tract. *Microbiology* 160, pp. 439–445.
118. Walsh, C. J., Guinane, C. M., Hill, C., Ross, R. P., O'Toole, P. W. and Cotter, P. D. (2015) In Silico Identification of Bacteriocin Gene Clusters in the Gastrointestinal Tract, Based on the Human Microbiome Project's reference Genome Database. *BMC Microbiol.* 15, pp. 183.
119. Crost, E. H., Ajandouz, E. H., Villard, C., Geraert, P. A., Puigserver, A. and Fons, M. (2011) Ruminococcin C, A New Anti-*Clostridium perfringens* Bacteriocin Produced in the Gut by the Commensal Bacterium *Ruminococcus gnavus* E1. *Biochimie.* 93, pp. 1487–1494.
120. Zheng, J., Gänzle, M. G., Lin, X. B., Ruan, L. and Sun, M. (2015) Diversity and Dynamics of Bacteriocins from Human Microbiome: Bacteriocins of Human Microbiome. *Environ. Microbiol.* 17, pp. 2133–2143.
121. Himes, P. M., Allen, S. E., Hwang, S. and Bowers, A. A. (2016) Production of Sactipeptides in *Escherichia coli:* Probing the Substrate Promiscuity of Subtilosin A Biosynthesis. *ACS Chem. Biol.* 11, pp. 1737–1744.
122. Haft, D.H. and Basu, M.K. (2011) Biological Systems Discovery In Silico: Radical *S*-Adenosylmethionine Protein Families and Their Target Peptides for Posttranslational Modification. *J. Bacteriol.* 193, pp. 2745–2755.
123. Bruender, N. A., Wilcoxen, J., Britt, R. D. and Bandarian, V. (2016) Biochemical and Spectroscopic Characterization of a Radical *S*-Adenosyl-l-Methionine Enzyme Involved in the Formation of a Peptide Thioether Cross-Link. *Biochemistry.* 55, pp. 2122–2134.
124. Caruso, A., Bushin, L. B., Clark, K. A., Martinie, R. J. and Seyedsayamdost, M. R. (2019) Radical Approach to Enzymatic β-Thioether Bond Formation. *J. Am. Chem. Soc.* 141, pp. 990–997.

https://doi.org/10.1142/9789811261664_0004

Chapter 4

Peptide Nanotubes as Dynamic Materials

Federica Novelli and Juan R. Granja*

Centro Singular de Investigación en Química Biolóxica e Materiais Moleculares (CIQUS) and Departamento de Química Orgánica, Universidade de Santiago de Compostela, Compostela, Spain

**juanr.granja@usc.es*

1. Introduction

In nature, self-assembly and self-organization of monomeric units into a hollow tubular structure is a process that often occurs to perform different biological functions [1]. The formation of transmembrane ion channels, cytoskeleton proteins, oligomeric enzyme, and viral capsids represent some examples of cellular components made by this strategy. In all these systems, self-assembled arrangements and functionalities are strongly related and involve multiple intermolecular interactions such as hydrophobic effects, hydrogen bonds, or electrostatic forces. Rational control over these weak non-covalent interactions is essential to achieve precise structural and functional optimization. Nature uses the supramolecular processes not only to form large aggregates built-up by thermodynamically driven self-assembling processes but also to construct the structural components of living organisms. Consequently, the dynamic behavior of these structures is the most important property by which external factors or media conditions can control their formation or dissociation. Such dynamic behavior is what makes the function of, for example, DNA so important. Although DNA structure is able to store the genetic information essential for cell functions, its dynamic character that allows self-replication, i.e., make copies of itself, or transferring the stored information to functional proteins, is the really amazing feature of nucleic acids. All these functions are regulated by proteins capable of recognizing specific sections of DNA to trigger some of the properties mentioned above. Therefore, the very essence of life is the dynamism that enables controlling the key processes and their regulation but is also the masterpiece of survival and evolution. These dynamic concepts have also evolved supramolecular chemistry, from molecular recognition and self-assembling process to more sophisticated processes based on reversibility, adaptability, and kinetic-driven methods.

Inspired by the role of tubular structures in nature, the preparation of synthetic organic nanotubes has significantly gained attention due not only to their potential applications in biological systems but also in materials science and nanotechnology [2]. Although several advances have been made in the area of covalently assembled nanotubes [3–7], supramolecular chemistry provides a powerful method, by a bottom-up approach, for the development of nanoscale tubular structures in which small building blocks are combined in an encoded way through non-covalent interactions [1,8,9]. Key advantages of this approach are high synthetic convergence, built-in error correction, and easy control of self-assembly through sub-assembly design.

In pursuing this strategy, a variety of biomolecules (e.g., peptides, proteins, lipids, oligonucleotides, or carbohydrates, among others) have been devoted to the production of synthetic nanotubular structures [10,11]. Among these, self-assembling cyclic peptide nanotubes (SCPNs) are notable building blocks for the preparation of such materials due to the ease with which they may be endowed with structural and functional properties in the supramolecular assemblies, the biocompatibility, and their dynamic behavior [2,12–14]. Nanotube formation is driven by stacking on top of each other of cyclic peptide (CP) units via β-sheet-type hydrogen-bonding interactions (Figure 1) [2,13,14]. Appropriate CPs containing an even number of amino acids (AA) with alternating chirality can adopt a flat, ring-shaped conformation in which the amide C=O and NH groups are oriented perpendicular to the ring plane, while the amino acid side chains point outwards in a pseudo-equatorial orientation. These structural features enable the formation of extensive hydrogen-bond networks among CPs due to the complementarity between the donors (NH) and the acceptors (C=O) on both sides of the pleated structure, thus driving the assembly in a hollow

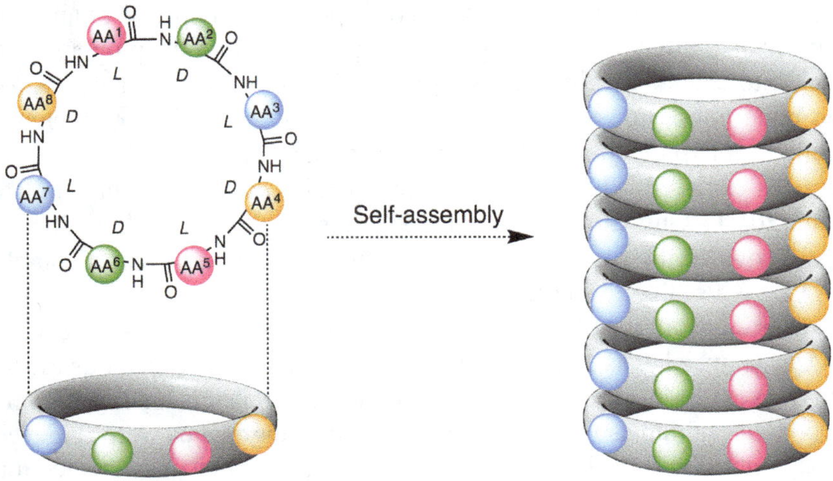

Fig. 1. Schematic representation of nanotube formation by stacking of CPs driven by the formation of hydrogen bonds.

tubular architecture. According to this approach, the number and type of amino acids can be used to define and control the internal diameter and properties of the nanotubes, while the amino acid side chains determine the outer surface characteristics [13]. It is important to note that their self-assembly processes are highly reversible, allowing the exchange of CP units among nanotubes or rapid adaptation to environmental conditions.

Hence, careful design of the CP unit, together with the straightforward synthesis, can provide complete control over the self-assembly, diameter, and functionality of the side chain to tailor their properties for specific applications ranging from electronics to nanomedicine [15–18].

This chapter will describe the theoretical and experimental efforts made for the design and synthesis of self-assembling cyclic peptide nanotubes (SCPNs) with special attention on their dynamic behavior. In particular, we will focus on the bio- and nanotechnology applications developed by exploiting the self-assembly properties of peptide nanotube supramolecular hybrids.

2. Self-Assembling Nanotubes from *D,L*-α-CPs

In the context of a theoretical analysis of cylindrical α-helical conformations accessible to linear poly-*D,L*-α-peptides, such as gramicidin, in 1974

De Santis and co-workers stated that cyclic peptides comprised of an even number of alternating *D*- and *L*-amino acids would have the propensity to stack into extended cylindrical structures via backbone-backbone hydrogen bond interactions [19]. However, the first attempts to verify experimentally this prediction were inconclusive due to the insolubility of the peptides explored, which required strong acidic conditions to manipulate them [20,21]. Only 20 years later, in 1993, the pioneering work of Ghadiri *et al.* provided the first evidence of nanotube formation by self-assembly of *D,L*-*α*-CPs (Figure 2) [22].

Starting from the pH-responsive octapeptide *c*-[(*L*-Gln-*D*-Ala-*L*-Glu-*D*-Ala-)$_2$], which was selected to confer solubility in basic aqueous media and prevent association through electrostatic repulsion among anionic carboxylates, high aspect ratio microcrystalline aggregates were achieved upon controlled acidification of the basic solution. Transmission electron microscopy, electron diffraction, FT-IR spectroscopy, and molecular

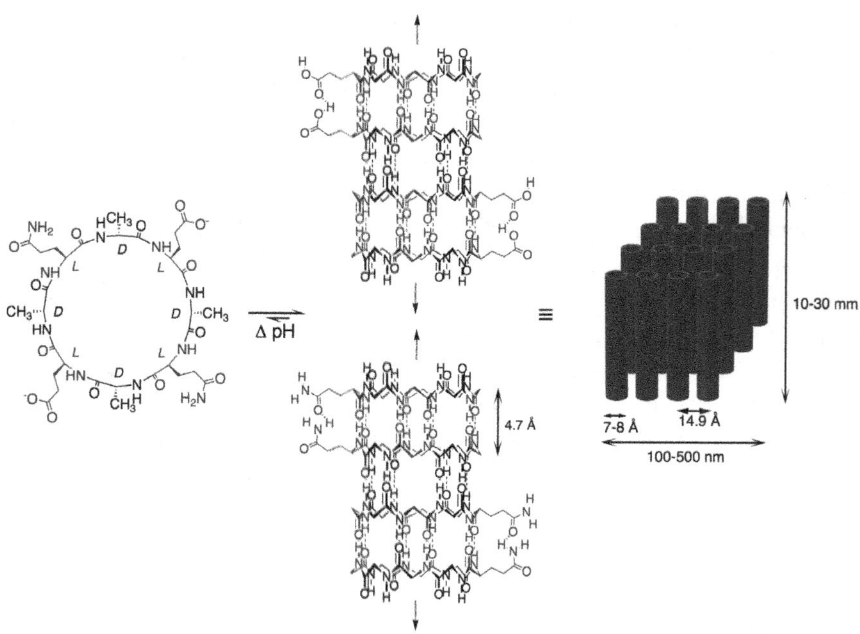

Fig. 2. pH-trigger self-assembly process of *D,L*-*α*-CPs, highlighting the antiparallel stacking and the widespread network of intermolecular hydrogen bonds (only the backbone structure is shown for clarity).

modeling studies of the resulting microcrystals unequivocally confirmed the formation of hollow tubes with an internal diameter of 7.5 Å and distance of 4.73 Å among CP units staked in an antiparallel hydrogen-bonded β-sheet-like structure.

Subsequent work demonstrated the design flexibility by the preparation of *c*-[(*D*-Ala-*L*-Glu-*D*-Ala-*L*-Gln-)$_3$] that undergoes similar proton-triggered assembly into nanotubes with an expanded inner diameter of 13 Å [23]. This finding validated the ability to control the internal diameter of the tube by altering the number of residues in the cyclic subunits (from 2 Å for a tetramer to 13 Å for a dodecamer). Therefore, the possibility of modulating the chemical profile of the outer surface and inner diameter can be fine-tuned by merely adjusting the type and number of amino acids employed in the CP. It is worth noting that the dynamic response to external stimuli of these systems, such as pH variation, is an attractive feature that can be exploited to build smart materials able to undergo proper changes in structure or size depending on the specific applications [24,25].

Taking advantage of these principles, several types of nanotubular assemblies have been prepared using neutral amino acids [26–28], combining basic/cationic and hydrophobic residues [29–31], or even amphiphilic or hydrophobic peptides [12,32]. Depending on the above-mentioned orientation of the side chains towards the outer surface, the resulting nanotubes exhibit different properties and characteristics.

The self-assembly of CP units by antiparallel β-sheet-hydrogen bonding in water was firstly investigated by Karlström *et al.* by fluorescence quenching assay [33]. Their results demonstrated that this type of association occurs not only as a result of the crystallization process but also in the strongly competing aqueous medium. In principle, the build-in of the nanotubes can be determined by either antiparallel or parallel β-sheet-like arrangements. However, preliminary computational and experimental findings suggested the thermodynamic bias for the antiparallel pattern [34,35]. The rationale for this preference is not completely clear. Employing different computational methods with the CP *c*-[(*L*-Phe-*D*-Ala-)$_4$], Liu *et al.* proposed that the difference in energetics among parallel and antiparallel arrangements is mainly ascribed to the steric interactions between cross-strand lateral chains, promoting the antiparallel stacking mode [34]. The authors suggested a new self-assembling mechanism in which the antiparallel dimer, the one formed by the interactions among *L*-*L*-faces, instead of the usually alleged monomer, acts as an essential building block in the self-assembly process. As stated above, the differences between *L-L-* and *D-D-*faces can be explained by the cross-strand steric interactions, which also would be the key factor for the preference for antiparallel stacking patterns over the parallel one (Figure 3(a)).

Recently, Silk and co-workers reported the first crystal structures made by either parallel or antiparallel SCPNs [35]. They suggest that both intra- and inter-nanotubular interactions can dictate the peptide stacking in the solid-state formation of nanotubes. However, the X-ray crystal structure showed a less preferred parallel stacking of one of the CPs, presumably because of lateral chain interactions and distortions of the peptide backbone to an ovular pore shape, which may offset the lower stability of this configuration.

To better understand the thermodynamic basis for the CP self-assembly, the simplest nanotubes, i.e., toroidal dimers, have been prepared [36,37]. In these systems, selective alkylation of the amino groups of the amino acids with the same chirality was performed. As a result, the alkyl groups point to the same face of the peptide ring, thus hindering the

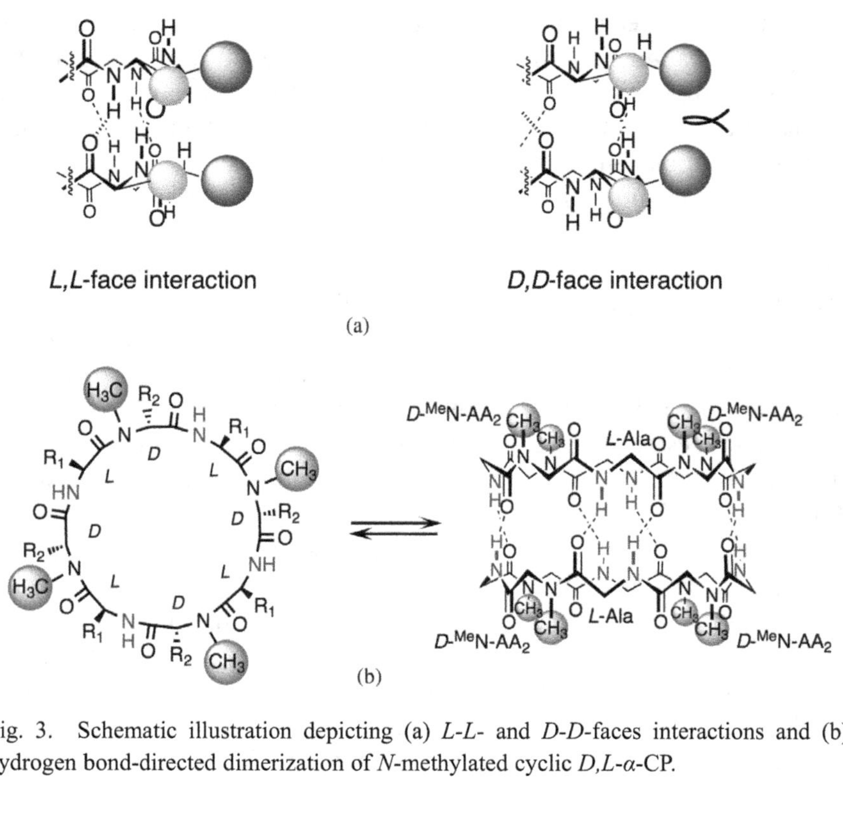

Fig. 3. Schematic illustration depicting (a) *L-L-* and *D-D-*faces interactions and (b) hydrogen bond-directed dimerization of *N*-methylated cyclic *D,L-α*-CP.

assembly properties through this face and restricting the equilibrium to the formation of dimeric nanocylinders (Figure 3(b)).

In 1995, Ghadiri *et al.* reported X-ray crystallography and NMR analysis of the *N*-methylated octapeptide *c*-[(*L*-Phe-*D*-^{Me}*N*-Ala-)$_4$], demonstrating its ability to self-assemble into the cylindrical dimeric antiparallel β-sheet structure previously proposed, with an association constant of Ka = 2540 M^{-1} in nonpolar organic solvents. Dimerization studies of several *D,L*-α-CPs (changing AA composition, location of backbone alkyl substituents, and ring size) established that cyclic octapeptides show the optimal rigidity and predisposition to stack into nanotubular assemblies [37]. In contrast, deca- and dodeca-peptides fail to dimerize due to the difficulty of adopting the required flat conformation, partly as a consequence of the steric interactions caused by the methyl group. In fact, the reported differences in association constants observed for the stacking of N-methylated and non-methylated CPs have been justified by these steric interactions that make it difficult for the peptide to adopt the required flat conformation [38,39]. CPs with less than six residues did not lead to the respective dimer because of conformational restrictions that do not allow the nanotube formations. Moreover, these extensive investigations assessed that the choice of alkyl chains was not trivial since unfavorable steric interactions with the carbonyl group occur due to the incorporation of long chains on the peptide skeleton [37].

The self-assembly of toroidal dimers also led to the first experimental model for the evaluation of the relative stability of parallel and antiparallel β-sheet structures (Figure 4) [40]. ^{1}H-NMR studies, combining *c*-[(*L*-Phe-*D*-^{Me}*N*-Ala-)$_4$] and its enantiomeric peptide, *c*-[(*D*-Phe-*L*-^{Me}*N*-Ala-)$_4$], allowed to estimate that the antiparallel β-sheet structure was 0.8 kcal·mol^{-1} more stable than the parallel one.

Further corroboration of the β-sheet-type hydrogen-bonding interactions was achieved by covalent capture of non-covalent cyclic peptide dimers [41,42]. For instance, Clark and collaborators have shown that specific orientations among *N*-methylated cyclic peptide dimers can be captured by olefinic metathesis of CPs composed by two homoallylglycines (Hag) [41]. In this process, the covalent capture not only stabilizes the dimeric form but also restricts the dynamic process to the dimer in which both Hag are hydrogen-bonded while the dimer in which the Hag is hydrogen-bonded to the Phe has to equilibrate towards the reactive form for the metathesis reaction to take place (Figure 5).

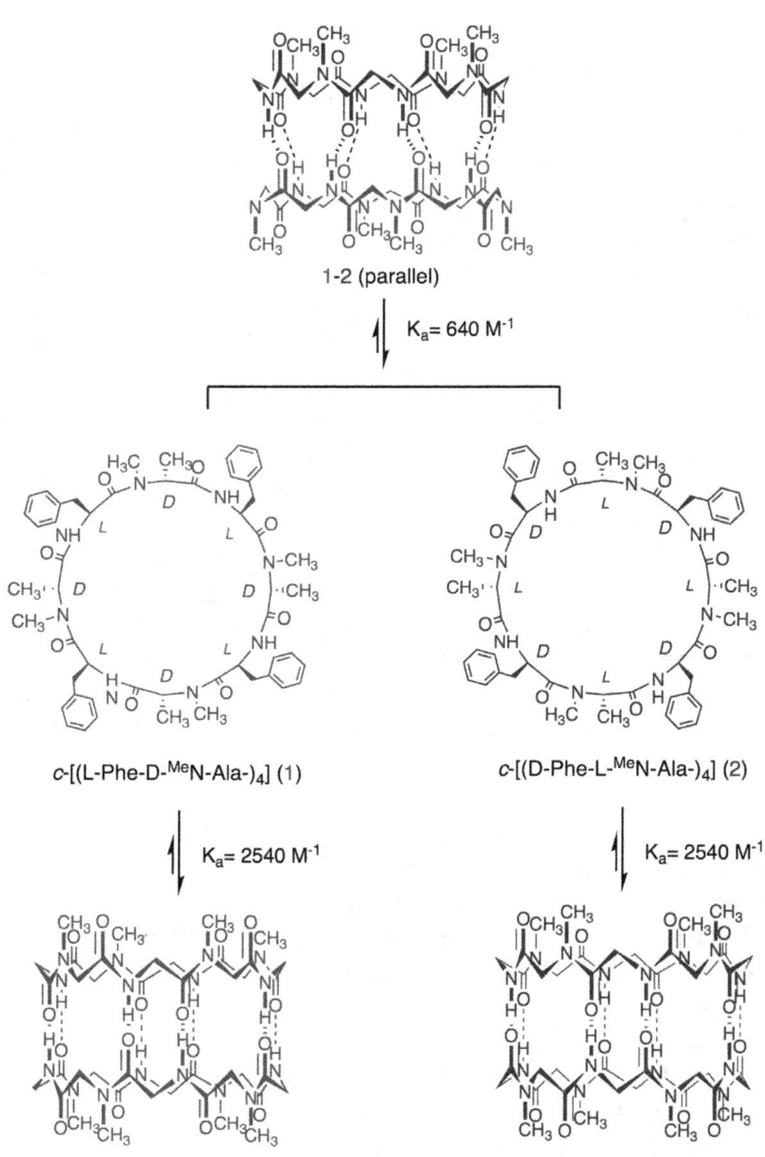

Fig. 4. Schematic representation of the formation of homodimers and heterodimers used for assessing the relative stability of parallel (heterodimer) and antiparallel (homodimers) β-sheet structures.

In later studies, the same authors extended the investigations to CP containing two Cys residues for reversible disulfide isomerization (Figure 5) [42]. The oxidation of acetamidomethyl protected cysteine [Cys(Acm)] provided a mixture of folded and polymeric aggregates that can be equilibrated under reduced conditions to form the corresponding covalently linked dimer.

A covalently linked dimer was also used as a photoswitchable responsive material (Figure 6) [43]. In this case, both peptides are linked through an azobenzene moiety. While the *cis*-isomer stabilized the discrete dimeric form, the *trans*-form induced the formation of a supramolecular polymer. The isomerization by ultraviolet or visible light, or heating, between both forms resulted in photoswitchable hydrogen bonding, which allows the controlled conversion between inter- and intramolecularly assembled structures. This process can not only be carried out in solution but also in films at the air–water interface.

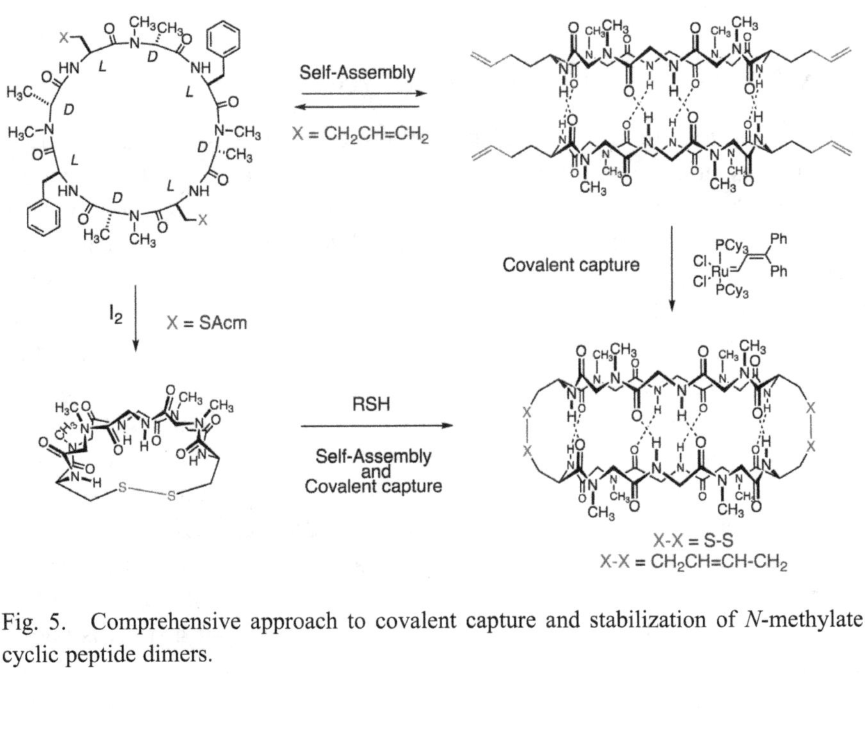

Fig. 5. Comprehensive approach to covalent capture and stabilization of *N*-methylate cyclic peptide dimers.

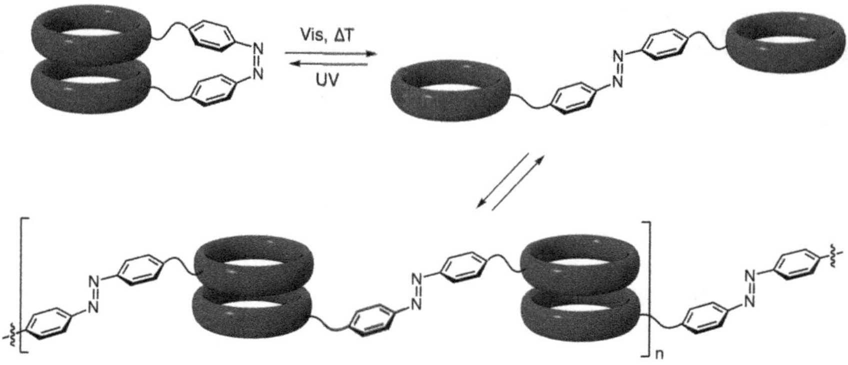

Fig. 6. Photoswitchable system based on cyclic peptide dimers that are linked through an azobenzene moiety. The visible light isomerization of the azobenzene induced the disassembling of the intramolecular dimer that subsequently assembles into intermolecular aggregates resulting in the formation of supramolecular polymers. Alternatively, the UV irradiation of this polymer induced the formation of the *Z*-isomer that results in the formation of discrete dimers with 100% efficiency. The process is fully reversible.

3. Self-Assembling Nanotubes from *β*-CPs

Cyclic peptide nanotubes can also be obtained using chiral β^3-amino acid residues, as first demonstrated by Seebach *et al.* in 1997 [44]. Molecular modeling based on X-ray powder diffraction analysis has shown that cyclic tetrapeptides comprising only chiral β^3-residues can adopt a flat disk-like conformation and stack through backbone-backbone hydrogen bonds in the solid state to form hollow tubular assemblies, as described above for *D,L-α*-CPs. Nevertheless, as a result of the extra carbon atom in the backbone of these amino acids, multiple CP conformations allow to achieve hydrogen-bonded tubular nanostructures from CP units composed of homochiral *β*-AA residues aside from CPs of alternating chirality [44].

Like the *D,L-α*-CPs, the amino acid side chains radiate equatorially from the peptide ring. However, due to the additional CH_2 units in the *β*-AA residues, the C=O and N–H groups adopt an opposite unidirectional orientation along the tubular structure. As a result, only parallel *β*-sheet stacking of the *β*-CPs can form the nanotube [44,45]. This packing implies that the formed nanotube exhibits a net macrodipole moment, which has been shown to be beneficial in gating, current rectification, and ion transport applications [45]. Indeed, Ghadiri and co-workers examined the self-assembly process of some β^3-CPs equipped with hydrophobic residues (tryptophan and leucine) to screen their application as ion channels in planar lipid bilayers (**CP1-3**, Figure 7). Conductance measurements and fluorescence couple proton transport assays reveal an ion channel activity similar to the *D,L*-α-CPs counterparts, with a K^+ transport rate of $1.9 \cdot 10^7$ ion$\cdot s^{-1}$. There were multiple conductance levels and channel gating, which were assigned to changes in the number of CP units, assembly/disassembly processes, and ring flexibility, thus supporting the model of dynamic transporting nanotubes [45]. Regrettably, the current rectification behavior of such ion channels has not been established so far due to the difficulty in inducing a specific nanotube orientation in the lipid bilayer.

Kimura *et al.* synthesized and studied a new class of sugar-containing β-CPs capable to self-assemble into bundles of nanotubes with higher rigidity and hydrophilicity [46,47]. The resulting columnar assembly was able to interact with lectin, leading to the formation of a protein nanotube after lectin cross-linking [47]. More recently, the same group also investigated the self-assembly properties of a novel pseudo-β-CP composed of

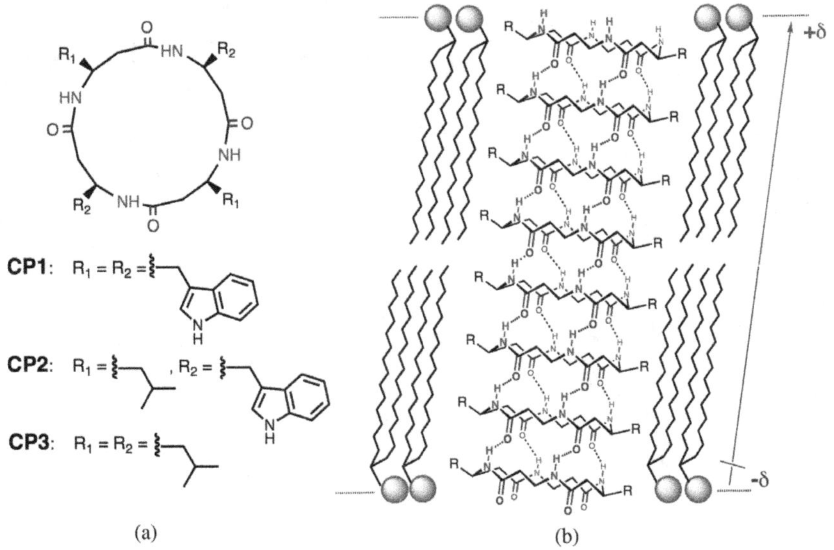

(a) (b)

Fig.7. (a) β^3-CP structures and (b) the resultant membrane β^3-SCPN. The alignment of carbonyl and amide groups creates a net dipole moment.

an ethylenediamine-succinic acid sequence (ED-SA) able to form peptide nanotubes [48]. The authors suggested that the insertion of this succinic acid derivative into the β-amino acid skeleton provides a way to align the side chains on one side of the SCPN, due to the maximization of the number of hydrogen bonds formed between the CP subunits.

To prepare two one-dimensional-(1D) arrays of aromatic groups along the SCPNs, Kimura and co-workers designed a hexa-β-CP composed of α-AAs of opposite chirality (i.e., *L*-α-naphthlalanine and *D*-α-anthrylalanine) and four β-alanines (Figure 8) [49]. Upon SCPN formation, the occurrence of higher photo-excited energy transfer, induced Cotton effects, and a higher rate of photo-dimerization reaction supported the 1D topological assembly of the anthryl groups. Besides, AFM and piezo-force microscopy (PFM) analysis revealed that nanotube bundles with diameters between 5 and 15 nm are dielectric microcrystals with a piezoelectric coefficient of 2–6 pC/N. Hence, the strategy of combining α- and β-AAs in the peptide backbone offers a promising approach in obtaining functional arrays with specific electronic properties.

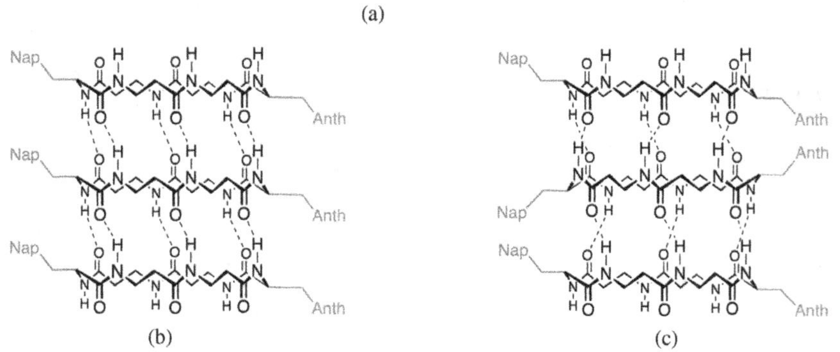

Fig. 8. (a) Chemical structure of the hexa-β-CP composed of α-AAs of opposite chirality, i.e., *L*-α-naphthlalanine (orange) and *D*-α-anthrylalanine (green). SCPN formation upon molecular stacking in either (b) parallel or (c) antiparallel orientation.

4. Self-Assembling Nanotubes from α,γ-CPs

The self-assembling *D,L*-α-CP and β-CP nanotubes described above show structural and functional features suitable for their application in various fields ranging from materials science to nanomedicine [2,13–17]. Most of their characteristics rely on the hydrophilic character of the internal cavity, which cannot be modified or improved by introducing functional groups on the inner face since any further modification in Cα or Cβ would inhibit the nanotube formation. To overcome this drawback, Granja's group has developed a new family of hybrid cyclic peptides, called α,γ-CPs, combining an equal number of natural α-AAs with artificial γ-AAs residues, more specifically *cis*-3-aminocycloalkanecarboxylic acids (γ-Aca, $n = 1$ in Figure 9(a)) [50–54]. The cycloalkane ring of the γ-amino acids preserves the rigidity and flat conformation of α,γ-CPs, thus ensuring the ideal conditions for the stacking of the peptide rings (Figure 9(a)). Besides, in these structures, the methylene group (β-C) of the γ-Acas is projected towards the lumen of the assembly, creating a hydrophobic region that can be functionalized to alter the behavior of the inner cavity of the ensemble. The hydrophobic character of the lumen was confirmed by the ability to encapsulate chloroform molecules in the cavity of cyclic hexapeptides [50,58]. Computational studies have also shown that such encapsulation provides additional stability to the nanotube [55]. In fact, MD simulations envisaged a possible control of the nanotube length through the encapsulation of oligomers of 1,2-bis[2-(2,2,2-trichloroethoxy)ethoxy]ethane, in which the number of ethylene glycol units of the oligomer could control the number of stacked CP units. Recently, our group, in collaboration with Pierangelo Metrongolo's team, demonstrated the ability to encapsulate Xenon (Xe) atom in the dimer cavity of cyclic α,γ-hexapeptides by displacing the previously captured chloroform molecules [56]. The dimer imprints its shape and symmetry to the trapped Xe atom, providing a new tool to build supramolecular nanostructures that take advantage of the properties of cyclic rings and their directional interactions to construct tailored porous crystals. However, further work revealed disorderly water molecules in the inner core of the dimer, revealing a certain amphiphilic behavior of the cavity [53].

The most straightforward way to design self-assembling α,γ-CPs is to replace any α-AA residue of a *D,L*-α-CPs with a γ-Aca of equivalent chirality. In this regard, (*1R,3S*)- and (*1S,3R*)-γ-Aca residues can be considered as structural equivalents of the *L*- and *D*-α-amino acids, respectively, when adopting the conformation required for nanotube formation (Figure 9(b)) [38].

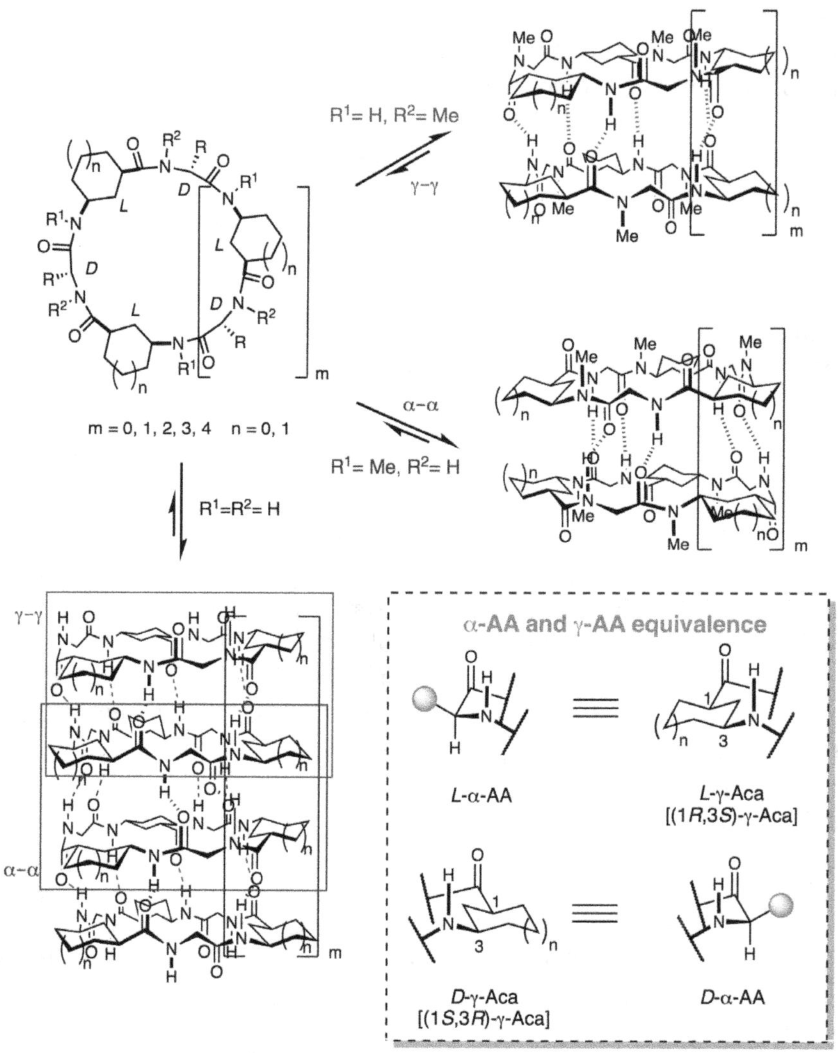

Fig. 9. Design for self-assembling nanotubes from α,γ-CP. Representation of the two different sets of hydrogen-bonding networks along the SCPN structure (γ–γ in red and α–α in blue, bottom left) and the respective N-methylated dimers are also shown (top right). Equivalence between *D*-α-AAs and (*1S,3R*)-γ-Acas or *L*-α-AAs with (*1R,3S*)-γ-Acas (insert).

Due to the odd number of carbon atoms between the C = O and NH groups of both types of residues, the combination of *α*- and *γ*-AAs of alternating chirality gives rise to a flat-disc conformation with non-equivalent faces, i.e., the *α*- and *γ*-faces, according to which amide group is projected on each side. Thus, the construction of self-assembling nanotubes from *α*,*γ*-CPs involves two different sets of antiparallel *β*-sheet-like hydrogen bonds along the SCPN structure (Figure 9(a)): one comprises only the NH and C = O groups of the *γ*-amino acid (*γ*–*γ* interactions) and the other, those of the *α*-amino acid (*α*–*α* interactions) [50]. More recently, our group discovered that this type of CPs could also form parallel *β*-sheets in which the *γ*-faces are hydrogen-bonded to the α-faces [57]. Surprisingly, in some cases, this interaction is even stronger than the antiparallel arrangement.

To evaluate the thermodynamic properties and the feasibility of these types of interactions, *N*-methylated CPs composed of alternating *α*-AAs and *cis*-3-aminocyclohexanecarboxylic acid (*γ*-Ach, $n=1$ in Figure 9(a)), and featuring only the two hydrogen-bonding patterns already described, were investigated [50]. In all cases, the *γ*–*γ* interactions were not as strong as the *α*–*α*. As mentioned above, this can be ascribed to the steric interactions among the carbonyl and methyl groups in the *N*-methylated *α*-amino acids [51–53]. Furthermore, the cyclic *γ*-residue significantly rigidifies the peptide backbone compared to the more flexible *α*-CPs, giving rise to larger association constants. The ability to control the nanotube inner diameter by this approach was confirmed by the synthesis and study of tetra- [52,54], hexa- [50,53], and octa-peptides [51]. All of them can form the corresponding dimers in non-polar solvents, except for the tetrapeptides that are not able to self-assemble through their *γ*-face and showed a small K_a (15 M^{-1}) for the *α*–*α* interactions [52,54].

By expanding this methodology, Granja and collaborators also synthesized and studied *α*,*γ*-CPs in which the *γ*-Ach is replaced by the five-member ring residue (*1R*,*3S*)-3-aminocyclopentanecarboxylic acid (*γ*-Acp, $n=0$ in Figure 9(a)). In this amino acid, the angle defined in the plane of the CP ring by the O=C–C and C–N bonds radiating from the cycloalkane ring is wider than that of *γ*-Ach (140° versus 120°), which favors the construction of CPs with large internal diameter. It also has a smaller hydrophobic outer surface (two methylene for *γ*-Acp versus three for *γ*-Ach), which influences the properties of the structure.

In an attempt to control the inner diameter of the resultant nanotubes, tetra- [52,54], hexa- [58], octa- [59] deca-, [59] and dodecapeptides [59] were prepared made up of alternating α-AAs and *N*-methyl γ-Acp residues. The inner diameter of these CPs ranged from 4 to 17 Å and all form the expected dimers through their α-face with a high association constant ($K_a > 10^5\ M^{-1}$) in non-polar solvents, except for the 4-residue γ-Acp-based CP, whose constants are smaller than 100 M^{-1}. [52,54] However, unlike the γ-Ach derivatives, the CPs formed by γ-Acp and *N*-methyl-α-AAs did not form the corresponding dimers, adopting folded conformations likely due to the greater flexibility of the 5-member ring and the formation of intramolecular hydrogen bonds among the carbonyl group and amide proton of the γ-residues [60].

Lately, Granja *et al.* reported a novel approach for the design and production of highly stable heterodimeric assemblies based on the combination of cyclic α,γ-(Acp)-based and cyclic α,γ-(Ach)-based peptides (Figure 10) [58]. Interestingly, the heterodimeric assemblies are more stable than the corresponding homodimers (about 30 times) and the selective heterodimerization is mainly driven by backbone-to-backbone dynamic hydrogen-bonded interactions, rather than the van der Walls interactions between the lateral chains employed. This high propensity for the heterodimer formation enables the modification of the side-chains

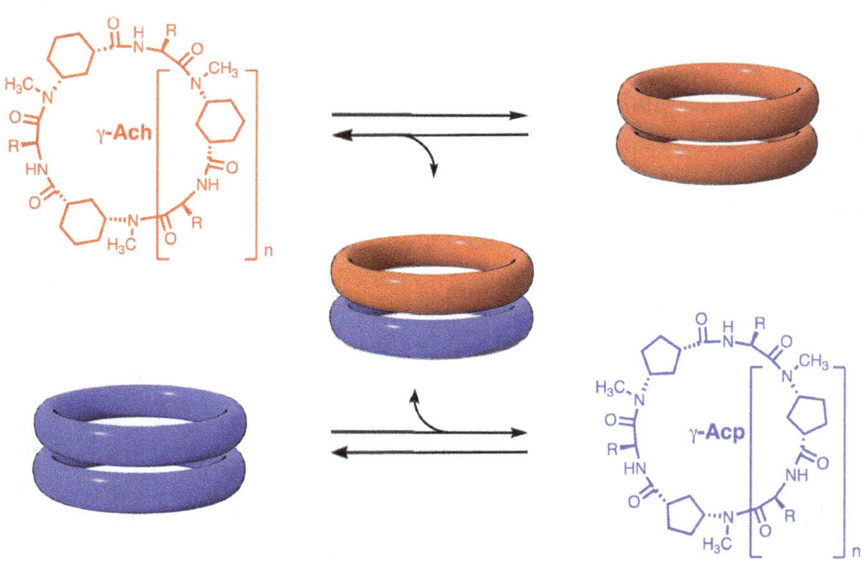

Fig. 10. Schematic depiction of the favored heterodimers formation between γ-Ach and γ-Acp-based CPs over the respective homodimers ($n = 0$ or 1).

properties with different functionalities to generate novel functional systems, such as electron or energy transfer active arrays, without affecting the self-association properties of heterodimer structures [61–63]. Based on the analysis of X-ray data, it was proposed that the heterodimer is more stable due to the better alignment of hydrogen-bond donors and acceptors, as well as the mixing entropy (ΔS_{mix}) [58]. Although an increase in ΔS_{mix} is an expected outcome, the formation of heterodimer would not vary the overall trend in association constants significantly [55].

According to the mentioned correspondence between *α*- and *γ*-amino acids, further classes of SCPN-forming CPs were prepared, such as those in which the two types of residues were arranged in a 3:1 ratio (3*α*,*γ*-CP, Figure 11(a)) [38]. NMR, IR, MS, and X-ray diffraction studies have shown that depending on the backbone *N*-methylation patterns and the medium, monomers of eight-residue 3*α*,*γ*-CPs can adopt a flat ring conformation or fold into double reverse turns. The flat rings can dimerize through antiparallel *β*-sheet-type hydrogen bonding while the monomers forming double turns associate to form helical supramolecular structures.

Finally, CPs comprising only *γ*-amino acids of alternating chirality were synthesized (*γ*-CP, Figure 11(b)). Remarkably, the self-assembly properties of the *γ*-CPs showed a strong correlation with the ring size. While the

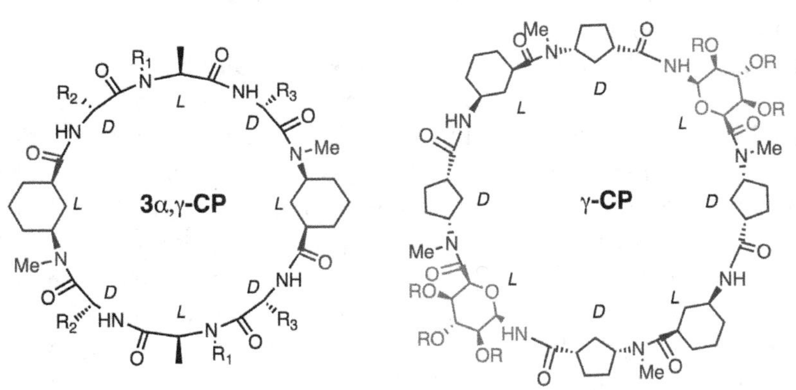

(a) (b)

Fig. 11. CPs formed alternating *α*- and *γ*-amino acids in (a) a 3:1 ratio (3*α*,*γ*-**CP**) and (b) comprising only *γ*-residues (*γ*-**CP**, 1-aminoglucuronic acid residues (*γ*-Aga) are highlight in green).

γ-octapeptides dimerize through hydrogen-bonded antiparallel interactions [64], the tetrapeptides associate through parallel β-sheet-like stacking [65].

Not surprisingly, the α,γ-SCPNs were able to insert into a lipid bilayer and efficiently transport ions [66]. Transport studies (H^+ migration) on dye-entrapped liposomes (LUVs) showed activity of both tryptophan-rich hexa- and octameric α,γ-CP {*c*-[*L*-Gln-*D*-γ-Ach-(*L*-Trp-*D*-γ-Ach-)$_2$] and *c*-[*L*-Gln-*D*-γ-Ach-(*L*-Trp-*D*-γ-Ach-)$_3$] (**CP4**, Figure 12)}. However, ion conductance experiments using patch-clamp techniques confirmed that only the octamer has a pore diameter large enough to allow the transport of metal ions with rates in the order of 10^7 ions·s^{-1}. The average open time was slightly shorter than that of *D,L*-α-SCPNs, and the overall ion transport efficiency was five times lower. The selectivity among alkali metal ions was minimal and followed the order $Cs^+ > K^+ > Na^+$ [66]. In any case, no transport of divalent cations (Ca^{2+}) or chloride (Cl^-) was observed. The transport rates of the alkali metal ions display the same order as their mobility in solution, although Na^+ flux was 30–40% greater than expected based on their relative bulk diffusion coefficients. These differences might account for the influence of ion dehydration on the transport rate. Once again, the dynamic behavior of the nanotubes can be visualized in the planar lipid bilayer experiments. Most of the recording showed, in addition to the open and closed events characteristic of ion channels, events with different conductivity. These quantified events were assigned to nanotubes with different lengths. The most predominant events are those ascribed to nanotubes made of 5–6 CPs. The changes in length can derive from the incorporation or disassembly of one of the CP units at the edge of the nanotube. Alternatively, these changes may also be due to exchange between shorter nanotube subunits that are not able to expand the membrane bilayer, as illustrated in Figure 12. The nanotube breaking/forming at their central part might also explain the gaiting mechanism. This process must be accelerated by the membrane pressure in which each of the membrane layers can move independently of each other [66].

The influence of the nanotube on the dynamic behavior of the membrane was investigated using molecular dynamics calculations [67]. These studies revealed periodic spatial distributions of different lipid properties as a function of the distance from the nanopore. This was mainly observed for carbon nanotubes and to a lesser extent for SCPNs. Such findings suggested that nanotubes with rougher surfaces would insert into a membrane without perturbing the structure and dynamics of a membrane, something that should be considered in the design of membrane-active components.

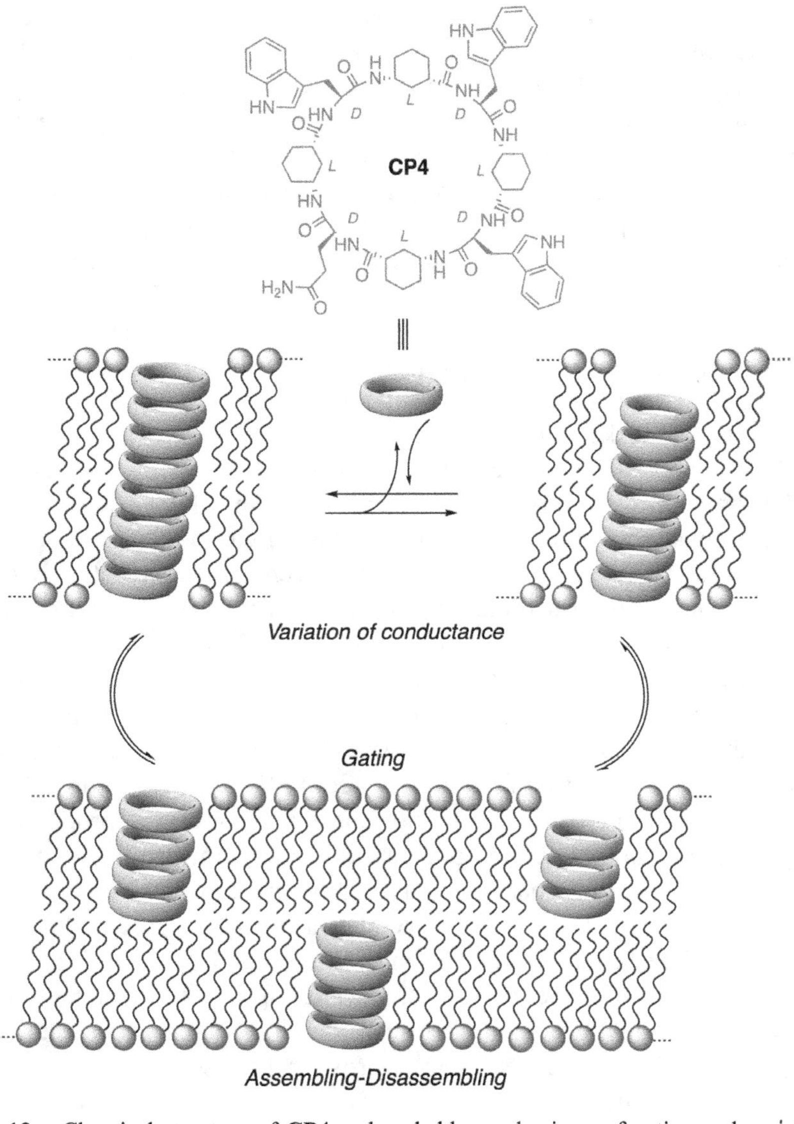

Fig. 12. Chemical structure of **CP4** and probable mechanisms of gating and variable conductance resulting from variations in the number of CP units or assembly/disassembly processes of one single CP at the edge of the nanotube.

As stated above, the main advantage of using γ-AAs in CP sequences is the projection of the C2 methylene of each cycloalkane moiety towards the lumen of the cylindrical structure, generating a partially hydrophobic internal cavity. X-ray data proved that the resulting dimeric structures possess cavities with amphipathic properties, as non-polar ($CHCl_3$) or polar (H_2O) molecules have been identified within the dimers [50,53]. State-of-art theoretical calculations revealed that partially ordered water molecules were present along the axial axis of the SCPN cavity [68]. Likewise, density functional theory (DFT) calculations showed that in the presence of non-polar molecules (i.e., $CHCl_3$), the interior remains fully hydrophobic and the dimer assembly is stabilized through van der Waals interactions with the methylene group of the γ-AA [65]. On the other hand, *D,L*-α-SCPNs have a hydrophilic inner surface, and any change of the non-cyclic AAs would significantly affect the nanotube formation, thus limiting their applications in different fields.

In 2000, Roeske *et al.* presented an alternative strategy to obtain functionalized cavities by synthesizing a CP with an $(LLLD)_3$ pattern capable of self-assembling into artificial transmembrane ion channels with hydrophilic groups arrayed in the inner channel and hydrophobic residues projected outwards (Figure 13(a)) [69]. The proven pH-dependent activity of the ion channel confirmed that the side chain of the central amino acid of the three homochiral residue motif is projected into the pore.

More recently, Helms and co-workers reported the design and synthesis of a self-assembling eight-residue α-CP containing a benzimidazole group in the skeleton (**Bzim-CP**, Figure 13(b)), in which one nitrogen group is projected towards the inner cavity [70]. The resemblance to the imidazole group of the histidine introduces pH-responsive properties to the resulting nanotube lumen, opening a new path toward functionalized sub-nanometer porous channels with biomimetic transport properties.

In the case of the α,γ-CPs, several strategies have been adopted to modify the inner cavity of the CP rings. The suitable functionalization of the C2-methylene of the γ-residues, substituting it with a heteroatom or different functional groups in this position, allows tailoring of the inner properties of the nanotube without destroying the assembly.

The first example of this kind of modification was described in 2009, when the 4-amino-3-hydroxytetrahydrofuran-2-carboxylic acid (γ-Ahf) residue, prepared from D-xylose, was included in the sequence of an α, γ-cyclic tetrapeptide (Figure 14) [71]. In the γ-Ahf derivatives, which can be considered an equivalent of the *L*-residues, the hydroxyl group is *trans*-oriented relative to the α-carboxylic and γ-amino groups. As a result of the flat conformation of the CP, the hydroxylic group would be projected into the cavity in a pseudo-equatorial orientation modifying the internal

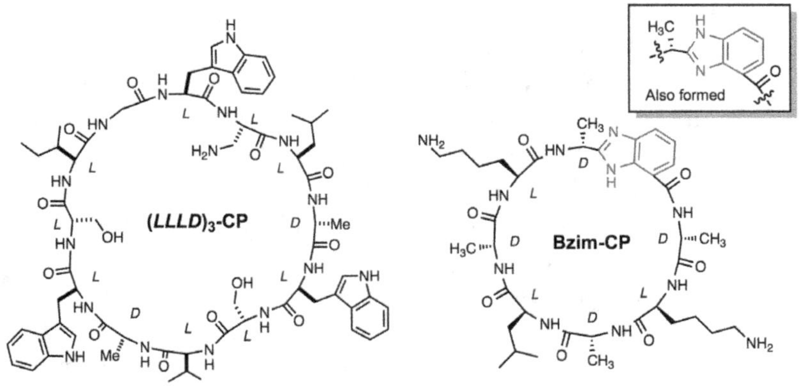

(a) (b)

Fig. 13. Representation of CP with a $(LLLD)_3$ pattern capable of self-assembling into artificial transmembrane ion channel (a) and self-assembling α-cyclic octapeptide containing a benzimidazole group in the skeleton (b).

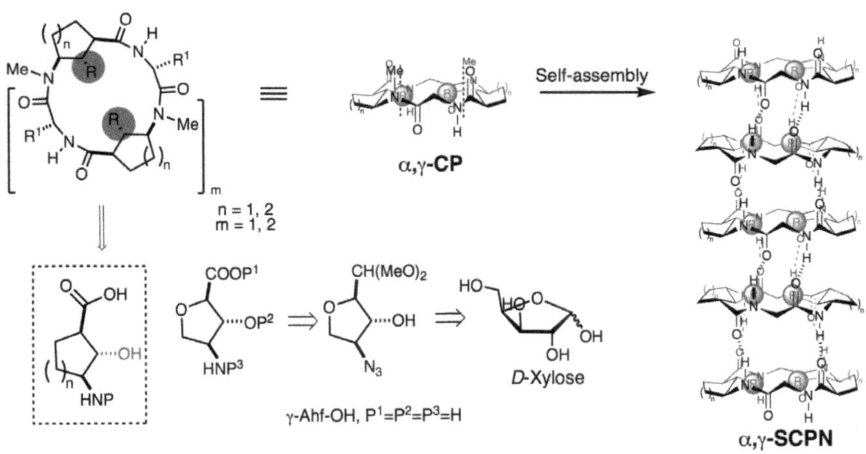

Fig. 14. Schematic illustration of SCPNs formation and synthetic strategy for the functionalization of the C2-methylene of the γ-residues (γ-Ahf-OH).

properties of the nanotube when combined with other residues of appropriate configuration, i.e., *D*-α-residues.

Dimerization studies on *c*-[*D*-Leu-γ-Ahf-*D*-Tyr(Me)-γ-^{Me}N-Acp-] showed the crucial role of the hydroxy groups in directing the self-assembly process, not only stabilizing the ensemble but also shifting the equilibrium towards the formation of the dimer in which the two hydroxyl groups are hydrogen-bonded [71].

Following the same strategies, the hydroxy-functionalized γ-amino acids were incorporated in larger CPs (Figure 15), such as the octapeptides *c*-[(*D*-Leu-γ-Ahf-*D*-Tyr(Me)-*L*-^{Me}N-Acp-)$_2$] (**CP5**) and *c*-[(*D*-Leu-^{Me}N-γ-Ahf(X)-*D*-Leu-*L*-^{Me}N-Acp-)$_2$] (**CP6**) [72,73]. In the former case, the CP folds into a 'V-shaped' conformation in which the carbonyl group and amide proton of the Ahf residue are hydrogen-bonded rather than adopting the flat conformation needed for the dimer formations [72]. However, this conformation was able to dynamically self-assemble in pseudo-spherical aggregates upon recognition of biologically relevant anions (i.e., chloride, nitrate, and carbonate), in which six CPs and four anions are arranged in a tetrahedral geometry. Interestingly, the resulting clusters were capable of selectively transporting anions through lipid membranes in an antiporter fashion [72]. In the second case, ^{Me}N-Ahf residues were employed to prevent the formation of the folded shape [73]. The resulting protected CP (**CP6a**, X=Bn) is able to self-assemble into the respective dimers, whereas the hydroxyl-free CP (**CP6b**, X=H) can only dimerize in chloroform by addition of a small amount of polar and protic solvents as methanol or water molecules (5%). This result suggests that

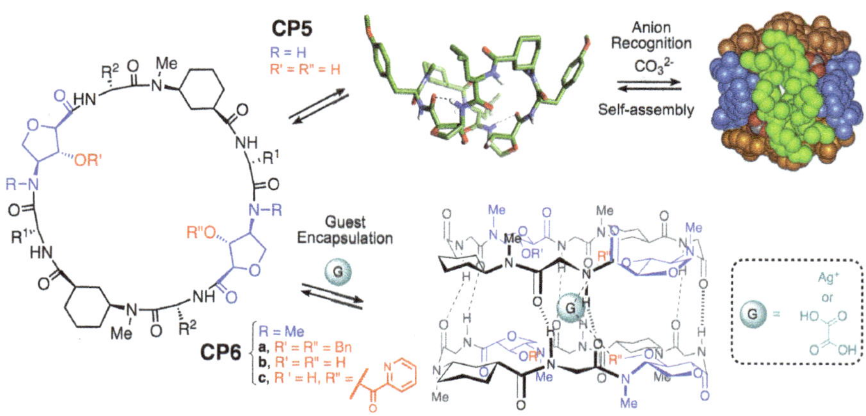

Fig. 15. Structures of CPs incorporating the γ-Ahf residues. According to the N-methylation of this amino acid, the CP (CP5) can adopt a "V" conformation that self-assembles into pseudo-spherical aggregates upon recognition of biologically relevant anions, or self-assembles to form dimers that can encapsulate different guests (CP6a-c).

the hydrophilic cavity must encapsulate protic molecules to induce and stabilize the dimer formation. Another interesting characteristic of these ensembles is their simple chemical modification, which can further be used to tune the cavity properties. For this purpose, the incorporation of a picolinic acid unit through a simple ester linkage allows entrapping silver ions (Ag^+) or dicarboxylic acids (e.g., oxalic acid) within the dimeric structure (Figure 15) [73].

Under the same strategy, Granja's group also reported the development of cytotoxic agents based on the cyclodecapeptide *c*-[^{Me}N-Ahf(CH2COOH)-*D*-Ala-*L*-^{Me}N-Acp-*D*-Ala-*L*-^{Me}N-Acp-*D*-Ach-*L*-^{Me}N-Acp-*D*-Prg-*L*-^{Me}N-Acp-*D*-Ala-] (**CP7**) [74]. The presence of the carboxylate group pointing towards the lumen allowed the efficient encapsulation of analogs of *cis*-platinum complexes in its inner cavity (Figure 16). The **CP7⊃Pt** complex showed cytotoxicity activity against A2780 ovarian cancer cell lines independent of acquired platinum resistance.

Recently, Granja's group reported a molecular dynamics investigation on the effect of the presence of different numbers of hydroxyl groups in various positions of the pore of the SCPNs when they are placed into a lipid bilayer to assess how they can influence their dynamical behavior as well as the transmembrane transport of different ions [75]. The findings provided atomic insights into the impact of polar groups on the dynamical, structural, and transport properties of this type of peptide channel when embedded in lipid bilayers, suggesting a promising future for their use as biomimetic channels.

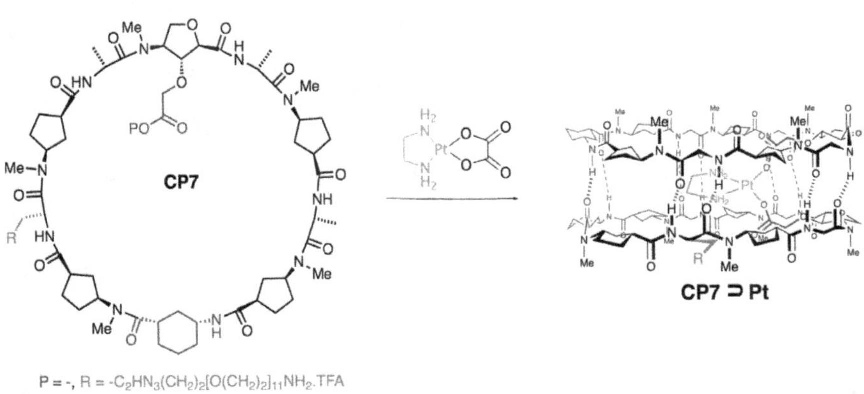

Fig. 16. Chemical structure of CP7 and the resultant dimeric complex (**CP7⊃Pt**).

With a slightly different approach, our group also prepared a sugar derived of 1-aminoglucuronic acid (γ-Aga), which was incorporated into the sequence of a CP composed exclusively by cyclic γ-AAs (γ-CP in Figure 11(b)) [64]. In this AA, the hemiaminal oxygen would be projected into the assembly, thus modifying the cavity properties, while the remaining hydroxyl groups are outwardly projected, providing a saccharide-like outer surface to the nanotube. NMR, FT-IR, and X-ray structural analyses revealed that the dimeric structure, which formed preferentially, was the one in which the γ-Aga residues were not staked on top of each other. This was related to a possible repulsive interaction among oxygen lone pairs present in the other dimer.

Recently, Dhavale *et al.* reported the syntheses of a novel class of fluorinated sugar amino acid-derived α,γ-cyclic tetra- and hexapeptides capable of self-assembling into β-sheet-like hydrogen-bonded nanotubes with a fluorinated interior (Figure 17) [76]. In this case, the fluorine atom is projected into the cavity as a consequence of adopting a distorted partially flat oval- or triangular-ring-shaped conformation based on the PM6 modeling studies. Apparently, nanotube formation takes place by a parallel-like stacking of CPs. The fluorinated hexapeptide acts as an

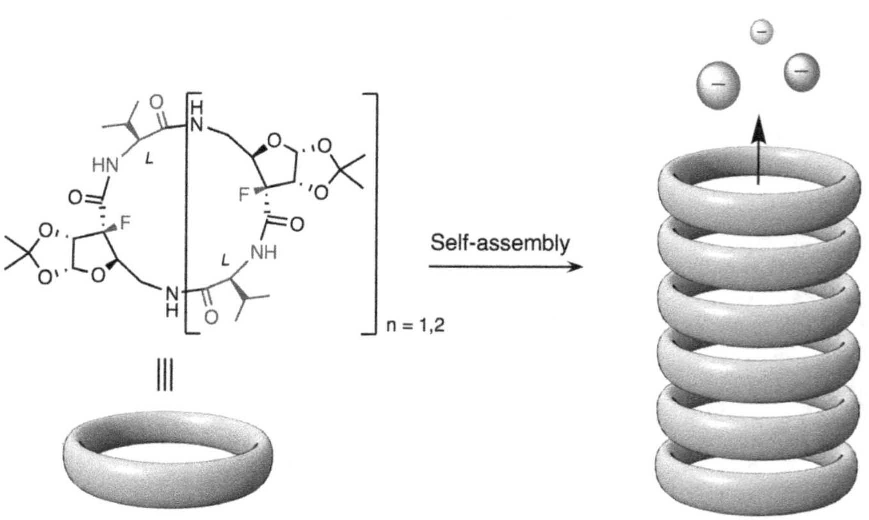

Fig. 17. Chemical structures of α,γ-cyclic tetra- (n = 1) and hexapeptides (n = 2) comprising fluorinated sugar amino acid-derived and the corresponding SCPN model as transporting agent for anions.

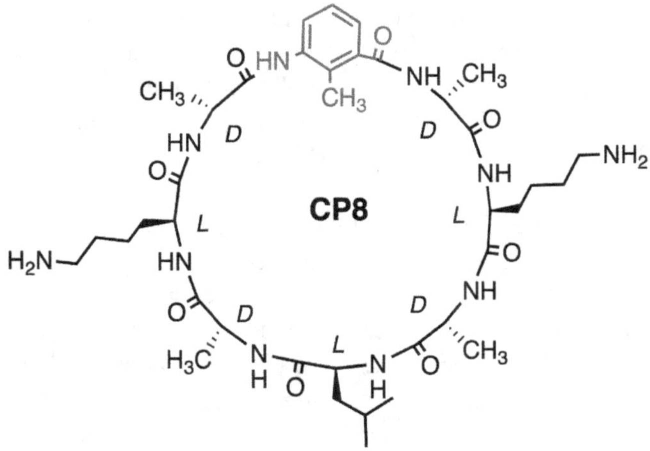

Fig. 18. Chemical structure of **CP8** that integrates an aromatic γ-Mba-OH residue (green).

artificial transporting agent for anions and might find various biomedical applications as a possible therapeutic tool.

Xu and collaborators also prepared nanotubes with tunable lumen properties integrating an aromatic γ-AA (3-amino-2-methylbenzoic acid, γ-Mba-OH) in a *D,L*-CP skeleton (**CP8**, Figure 18) [31,77]. With this approach, the methyl substituent in the aromatic ring (C2) points towards the interior of the cavity, giving it a partial hydrophobic character despite the drastic reduction of the inner diameter (from 7.6 to 4.7 Å). The incorporation of Mba residue reduced the stability of the nanotube since some of the amide protons cannot participate in the formation of hydrogen bonds with the neighboring CPs. The functionalization of the CP with PEG polymer enables to modulate the nanotube formation to be compatible with the processing window of polymeric membranes, without affecting the growth of high-aspect-ratio nanotubes. This allows for the embedding of short nanotubes into a polymer matrix to fabricate functional membranes *in situ*.

5. Self-assembling Nanotubes from Other CPs

Peptide tubular assemblies constitute a novel class of supramolecular structures with promising biotechnological applications. However, the CPs based on α-, β- and γ-amino acids already described do not cover all the various types of CPs that have been developed as basic units for nanotube preparation. Some examples of other cyclic platforms designed to spontaneously self-assemble into nanotubes are given in what follows.

Dory *et al.* developed new CPs formed by α,β-unsaturated δ-AA that crystallized as bundles of nanotubes (δ-CP (**CP9**), Figure 19(a)) [78]. Because of the *trans* geometry of the vinyl groups, the CPs adopt a flat conformation necessary for the molecular self-assembly. As in the case of β-amino acids, all carbonyl groups are oriented in the same direction leading to parallel β-sheet stacking of the CP units. These structural features give rise to a significant dipole moment along the nanotubes of around 9 D, according to the authors' DFT calculations [79]. Surprisingly, the resulting nanotubes pack parallel into the crystals, with all the dipoles pointing toward the same direction. As a result, the crystals are anisotropic forming highly polar crystals. Besides, the δ-CP nanotubes self-organize to form liquid crystals, in which each ensemble acts as a fundamental component in the more complex supramolecular structures [80]. Recently, to increase the cavity size, the same authors have added an extra double bond in the structure, using the (E,E)-6-aminohex-2,4-dienoic acid as a

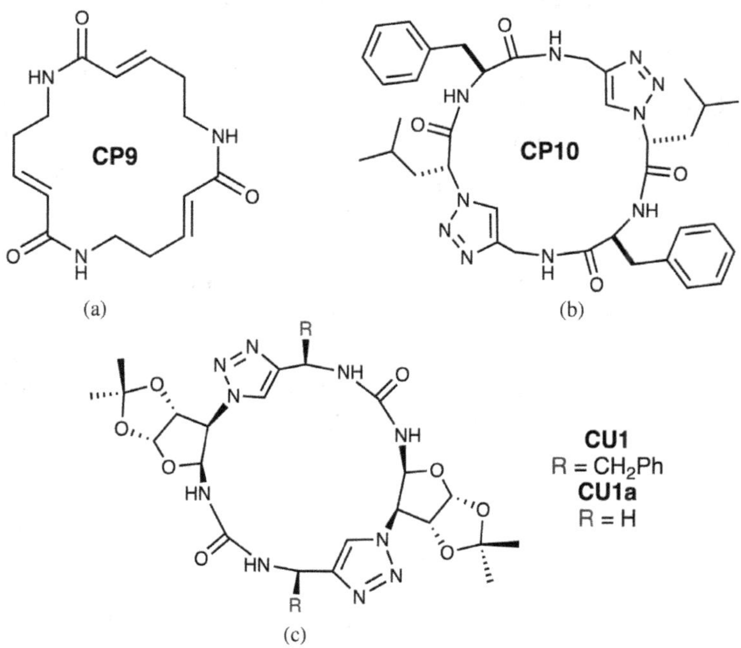

Fig. 19. Chemical structure of (a) **CP9**, (b) **CP10**, (c) **CU1** and **CU1a**.

basic component [79]. The tubes formed with this derivative, although providing the dipoles aligned, do not form an infinite triangular prism. Instead, they form, seen along the nanotube axis, a kind of a star of David. The inner channel occupies almost 15% of the total volume and is filled with water molecules. Interestingly, all the nanotubes pack in a similar manner, which might explain the macrodipole formation. Each nanotube is surrounded by six tubular structures that are shifted with respect to each other. Those places at 0, 120, and 240° stabilize the lattice by favorable electrostatic interactions, while the remaining tubes, positioned at 60, 180, and 300°, do not have any effect.

Ghadiri and co-workers reported a peptide-based macrocycle that incorporates 1,2,3-triazole ε-amino acids in the skeleton via a Cu(I) catalyzed azide/alkyne cycloaddition reaction (α,ε-CP **(CP10)**, Figure 19(b)) [81]. The presence of the triazole ring modified the properties of the internal cavity of the tubular structure resulting in a 5.2 Å elliptical pore between the triazole ring and 6.8 Å across the perpendicular axis. More recently, Granja's group proposed rigid 4-aminocyclohexanecarboxylic acid (δ-Ach) as a promising building block for the preparation of nanotubes with large diameter and hydrophobic properties of the internal cavity (Figure 20) [82]. For this purpose, α,δ-hybrids were prepared by combining α-AA and δ-Ach residues of alternating chirality in octa-, dodeca- (**CP11**) and

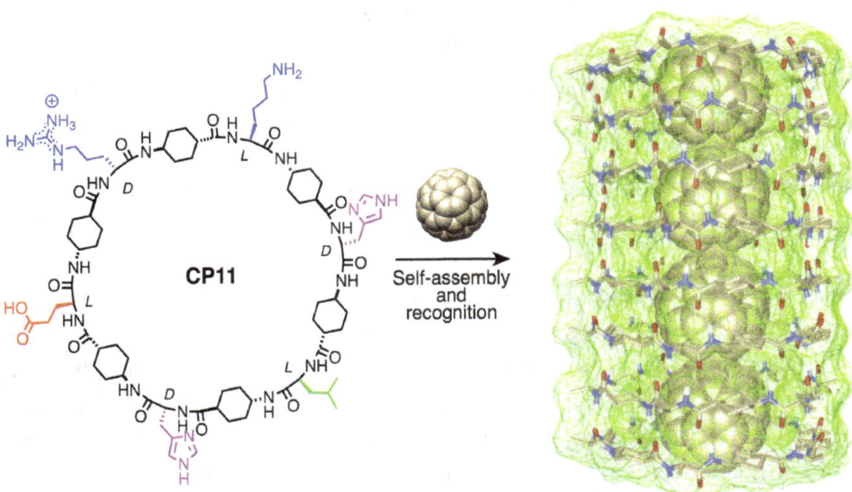

Fig. 20. Chemical structures of dodeca- α,δ-CP (**CP11**) and a computer-assisted model of C_{60} encapsulated in the inner cavity of the corresponding SCPN.

hexadeca-peptides. The resultant CPs can stack through antiparallel-like interactions. Further, due to hydrophobic properties and the appropriate size of the lumen, the encapsulation of C_{60} moieties has been successfully achieved to form a new type of bionanopeapod structure.

Based on the peptide nanotube formation model, cyclic ureas and urea/amide hybrids (**CU**) have also been used as precursors to obtain tubular structures [83–85]. Guichard *et al.* have reported the use of cyclic oligoureas, consisting of homochiral residues bearing proteinogenic side chains, capable of crystallizing as hydrogen-bonded polar nanotubes with electron density inside the tubular cavity [83]. Hydrophobic oligourea/amide macrocycles were also studied as ion carriers. The resulting tubular transporter systems were anion-selective as a result of the anion — macrodipole interactions observed in these assemblies. However, the transport cannot be correlated with the migration through the nanotube pore, as the anion diameter was too large compared to the size of the nanotube lumen [84]. In 2009, López *et al.* employed a combination of π–π stacking interactions and urea–urea hydrogen bonds to prepare electroactive self-assembling nanotubes decorated with the electron-donor di(methylthio)tetrathiafulvalene groups on the periphery [85].

More recently, ureas have also been used to prepare triazole/urea-based peptidomimetic macrocycles using carbohydrate precursors [86]. According to the chirality introduced in the peptide skeleton, the macrocycle **CU1** self-assembles into antiparallel dimers while **CU1a** stacks in a parallel-like β-sheet structure that provides a large dipole moment (Figure 19(c)). Similarly, C2-symmetric pseudo-peptides, containing bis furanoid triazole moieties as di-β-peptides surrogates linked to a *D*-α-AA or a β-AA in each half, have been studied. The *D*-α-AA-derived macrocycle showed the ability to assemble into parallel tubular stacks with high dipole moments, while β-AA-derived products did not undergo self-assembly [87].

Ranganathan and colleagues explored the self-assembly properties of a new class of cystine-based nanotubes composed of n-alkanes that connect a cysteine moiety as bisureas [88] or bisamides. [89] Although these macrocycles showed great flexibility, they were able to crystallize in nanotubes of uniform shape and internal diameter by means of hydrogen bond interactions between adjacent rings (two hydrogen bonds in the bisamides and four in the bisurea). Further stabilization of the ensembles may be due to the hydrophobic collapse of the alkyl chains. Ranganathan *et al.* also investigated the nanotube-forming possibilities of aromatic cyclodepsipeptides [90] in which the amide hydrogen-bonding groups lie in the plane of the ring. In this case, the main organizing forces for ring-ring stacking are aromatic π–π interactions between phenyl and pyridyl rings. Recently, bisurea macrocycles, composed of *C*-shaped phenylethynylene spacers connecting two urea motifs, have also shown the ability to self-assemble into fiber-like single crystals with 1D microchannels of around 9 Å in diameter [91]. Greytak *et al.* investigated the capability of such channels to encapsulate and orient the fluorescent push-pull dye 5-(dimethylamino)-5′-nitro-2,2′-bithiophene [92]. Polarized fluorescence microscopy experiments revealed that the guest fluorescence is polarized along the fiber axis, suggesting a high degree of orientational order inside the 1D channels. These findings may help to optimize reactions, energy transfer, and electron transfer between guest molecules within confined nanospaces.

6. Peptide Nanotubes Hybrids

6.1. *Primary sequence dictates function and properties*

The unique features of the CPs, along with their simple synthesis, biocompatibility, and the precise control over the internal pore size and external properties, make them particularly well suited to the development of new biomaterials. Additionally, the right choice of primary amino acid sequence can be critical in determining the final function and properties of the resulting nanotubes. For instance, the use of hydrophobic residues such as tryptophan and leucine can result in SCPNs capable of interacting with the phospholipid bilayer to form active ion channels. In 1994, Ghadiri *et al.* reported the first octapeptide *c*-[*L*-Gln-*D*-Leu-(*L*-Trp-*D*-Leu-)$_3$] (**CP12**, Figure 21(a)) able to spontaneously self-assemble in an artificial ion channel in lipid bilayers [16,22]. The tubular ensemble was long enough to span across the thickness of the membrane and exhibited good transport activities for K^+ and Na^+ ions (transport rate > 10^7 ions·s^{-1}). Typically, all records displayed different conductance levels and open and closed events, suggesting the presence of dynamic transporting nanotubes formed by a distinct number of CP subunits [16].

Later work showed that the selective transport of polar molecules across the channel strongly depends on the size of the peptide ring. Therefore, a slight elongation of the peptide mentioned above resulted in the achievement of the decapeptide *c*-[*L*-Gln-*D*-Leu-(*L*-Trp-*D*-Leu-)$_4$]

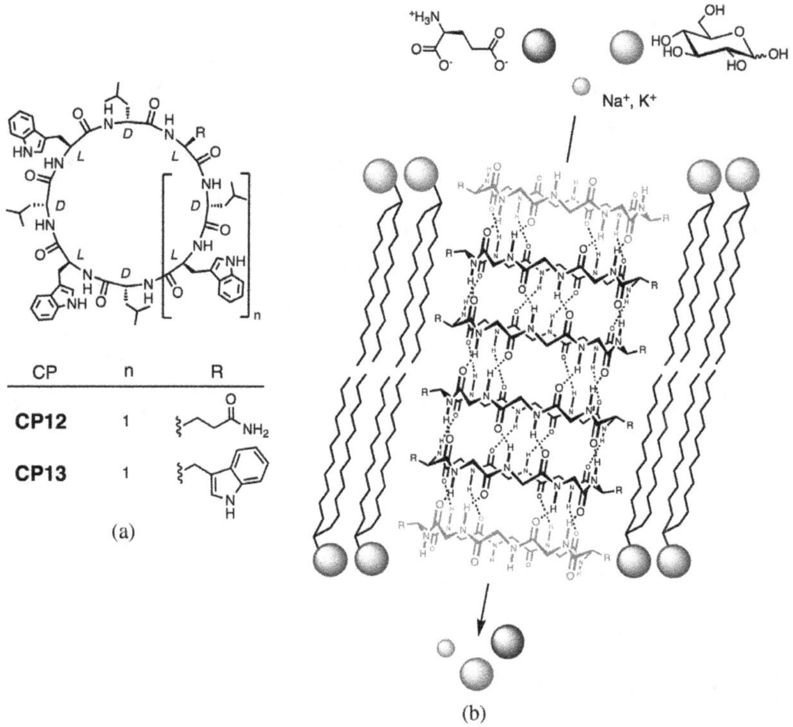

Fig. 21. (a) Structures of **CP12** and **CP13**; (b) model of the transmembrane channels in the lipid bilayer (the lateral chains are omitted for clarity), which were able to transport ions (orange), glucose (green), or glutamic acid (violet).

(**CP13**, Figure 21(a)) with an inner diameter of 10 Å, capable of effectively transporting hydrophilic molecules (i.e., glucose or glutamic acid) through the lipid bilayers (Figure 21(b)) [28,93].

The same CP was also explored for the delivery of small hydrophilic anticancer drugs across the membrane [94,95]. *In vitro* studies on unilamellar liposomes revealed that hydrophilic molecules smaller than 1 nm could be efficiently transported upon the addition of the SCPNs in a size-selective and dose-dependent manner. The smallest 5-FU molecule showed the fastest rate of diffusion. A synergistic antitumor effect was achieved by the combinatory use of CP and 5-FU *in vitro* and *in vivo.* On the basis of computational studies, the authors suggested that 5-FU is transported through the hollow nanotube cavities via a hopping mechanism.

Validation of transport activities through SCPNs fostered the development of heteromeric nanotubes with altered transport capacities [96]. For this purpose, ionic amphiphilic CPs containing ammonium (**CP14**), guanindinium (**CP16**) and carboxylate (**CP15**, **CP17**) moieties were designed for assembling as molecular caps at the end of the ion channel-forming peptide **CP13**, regulating the access of ions in the nanotube lumen (Figure 22).

Non-ohmic current rectification was observed upon the addition of the charged peptides on one side of the membrane, thus demonstrating the dynamic binding of the peptide caps to the channel edge.

More recently, Perrier and co-workers investigated the effect of the amino acid sequence of CPs on the formation of transmembrane channels in lipid bilayers [97]. The six self-assembling octapeptides examined consisted of a constant number of *D*-leucine residues alternated with different combinations of *L*-residues. Employing fluorescence LUV assays and DLS analysis, they established that charged CPs tended to form large pore (barrel stave) while non-charged CPs form single tubes. They also found that the amphiphilicity of the peptide plays a crucial role in the selective partitioning between zwitterionic and anionic bilayers.

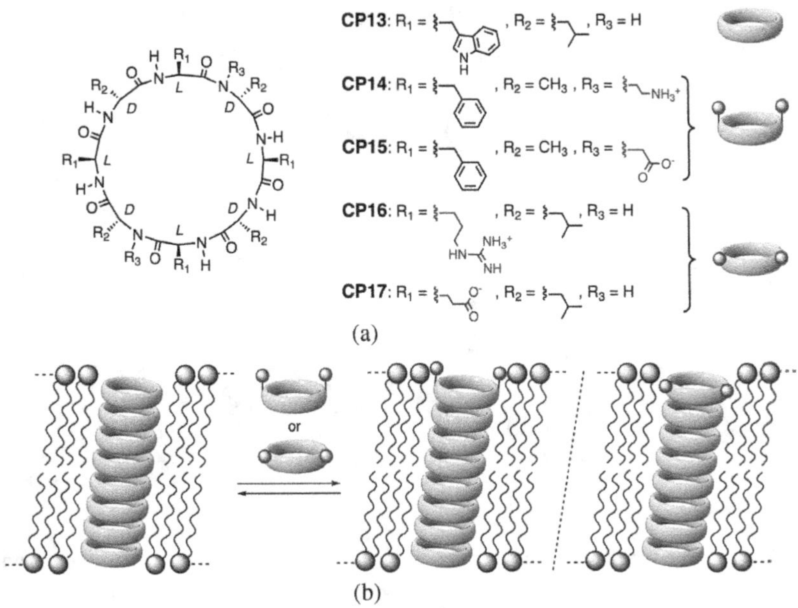

Fig. 22. (a) Chemical structures of **CP13-17**. (b) Schematic mode of interaction of the molecular caps with **CP12** to afford heteromeric transmembrane channels.

These findings highlighted that depending on the peptide structure the resulting nanotubes are oriented differently (Figure 23). CPs consisting mainly of hydrophobic residues could form ion channel embedded approximately perpendicular to the lipid bilayer. On the other hand, peptide nanotubes made up of amphiphilic CPs can form barrel-stave pores or lay parallel to the membrane surface [17,32].

This latter orientation provides the possibility of disrupting the membrane via a carpet-like mechanism, thus leading to their application as antibacterial therapeutic agents [17,32]. In this regard, Fernández-López *et al.* reported the preparation of a series of amphiphilic CPs that presented a significant *in vitro* activity against gram-negative (*E. Coli*) and gram-positive bacteria (methicillin-resistant *S. aureus*, MRSA) [32]. ATR-FTIR studies in synthetic lipids were consistent with a carpet-like mode of action for these antibacterial peptides with a tilt angle of 70° ± 5 in oriented DMPC bilayer. Interestingly, the antibacterial activity was strongly related with the ring sizes and AA compositions. Eight-residues CPs displayed a preference for gram-positive bacteria, whereas hexamers are also effective against gram-negative bacteria. Enhancement of the antibacterial activity was observed by increasing the number of basic residues (such as lysine) in the CPs, although the replacement of lysine with

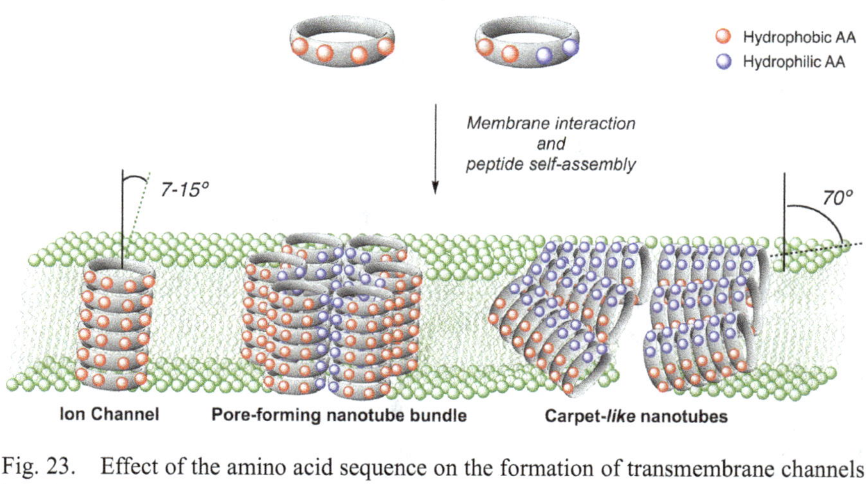

Fig. 23. Effect of the amino acid sequence on the formation of transmembrane channels in lipid bilayers. Hydrophilic regions are shown in blue and hydrophobic regions in red. The hydrophobic CPs form single transmembrane channels, while amphipathic CPs can form nanotube barrel-stave pores or lie parallel to the membrane surface in a carpet-like structure.

histidine resulted in a drastic loss of the activity. Adopting a similar strategy, Fletcher and collaborators developed a combinatorial library of six-residues CPs with different activity towards prokaryotic bacteria (MRSA and *E. coli*) and eukaryotic marine algae, *Ulva linza* and *Navicula perminuta* [98]. Sequence optimization studies resulted in the discovery of a phenylalanine-rich peptide (*c*-[*L*-Lys-*D*-Trp-*L*-Phe-*D*-Phe-*L*-Phe-*D*-His-]) with a 100-fold selectivity towards *U. linza.* Likewise, Ghadiri *et al.* demonstrated that membrane-selective amphiphilic *D,L*-α-CPs with similar structure and properties have great potential as novel supramolecular assemblies for the development of broad-spectrum antiviral agents [99,100].

These amphiphilic peptide architectures also found application for the treatment of neurodegenerative diseases such as Alzheimer and Parkinson [101,102]. Due to their strong structural and functional resemblances with amyloid fibrillar aggregates, self-assembling CPs can modulate aggregation and toxicity of Aβ and α-Synuclein proteins *in vitro* by interacting with appropriate sequences of hydrogen-bond donors and acceptors. More recently, dynamic supramolecular *D,L*-α-CP nanotubes were exploited to alter and remodel the morphologies and functions of high-density lipoprotein complexes (HDLs) of human and mouse plasma for treating atherosclerosis [103]. Through a series of functional assays with different control peptides, including peptide sequences that cannot self-assemble into nanotubular structures, these studies proved that only the dynamic supramolecular assemblies could be effective therapeutic supramolecular agents [104].

All these outcomes outlined above establish the role of the interaction of the peptides and their subsequent supramolecular nanotubes with the membrane interface or protein compartments. While hydrophobic side chains allow the insertion of the peptide in lipophilic regions (i.e., the phospholipid membrane or the hydrophobic protein pockets), hydrophilic residues might guide the surface recognition by electrostatic interactions. It is worth noting that due to the dynamic character of hydrogen-bonding networks between CP units, the rotation of a single CP unit in the nanotubes can result in different SCPN assemblies with distinct surface properties, thus enhancing their structural diversity and therapeutic activity (Figure 24).

The recently reported small differences between parallel and antiparallel stacking bring even further diversity by forming stacks of parallel oriented CPs. In any case, it should be pointed out that the structural

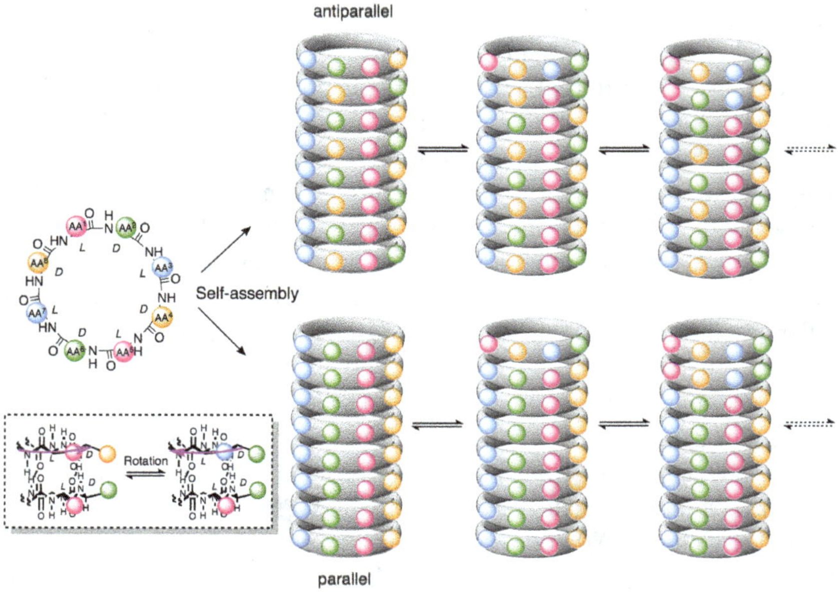

Fig. 24. Nanotube diversity generated by a single CP of symmetry C2 from the relative rotation of each CP in the nanotube.

diversity is limited by the own characteristic of these assemblies, since *L*-AAs can only stack on top of *L*-residues and *D*- with *D*-AAs.

6.2. *SCPN-small molecule supramolecular hybrids*

In addition to the ability to modulate the properties of the SCPNs outer surface through appropriate peptide sequence selection, the covalent functionalization of reactive groups placed at the side chain of any residue of the CP with different functionalities or nanostructures provides an alternative strategy for obtaining new building blocks with function-based properties. In fact, without affecting the self-assembly process, this approach allows the modification of the chemical profile of the nanotube outward, paving the way toward new possible applications.

For instance, the specific functionalization of amphiphilic antimicrobial CPs with sugar moieties on the lateral chains significantly reduces toxicity in mammalian cells while preserving strong bactericidal activities against multidrug-resistant gram-positive bacteria [105].

Similarly, the incorporation of 1,4,5,8-naphthalenetetracarboxylic diimide (NDI) units on the lysine side chains of an eight-residues *N*-methylated CP results in an electronically active dimeric assembly [106]. Structural and fluorescence studies revealed that hydrogen-bonded intermolecular interactions between CPs are an effective method for templating productive aromatic interactions and efficient charge transfer between NDI units. Expanding this methodology, the same group also prepared a nanotube-forming cyclic octapeptide bearing four NDI moieties that undergoes redox-triggered self-assembly in the first electronic delocalized nanotubes hundreds of nanometers in length [107].

For the formulation of nanosize 1D wires with possible applications in molecular electronic components, Granja and co-workers reported the synthesis and characterization of α,γ-SCPN bearing fullerene side chains (C_{60}) [108]. AFM, STM, and TEM studies showed that antiparallel-like peptide–peptide interactions could promote and template the arrangements of C_{60} units on both sides of the SCPNs on solid supports, resulting in 1D supramolecular wires (Figure 25). Such disposition is possible thanks to the alignment of the positively charged Arg residues on the same side of the tube, establishing favorable interactions with the anionic surface of the mica.

Later work based on the dynamic self-sorting of *N*-methylated CP homodimers into heterodimeric ensembles enables the development of

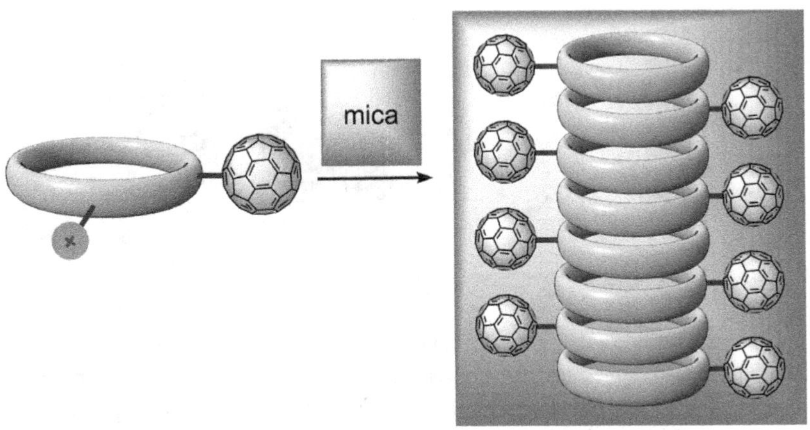

Fig. 25. Model for SCPN formation from α,γ-CPs bearing fullerene side chains in which the dynamic self-assembly process is induced by the surface properties.

artificial photosystem-like arrangements. To this end, β-sheet-like hydrogen-bonded CP heterodimers incorporating electron acceptor (C_{60}) and electron donor (tetrathiafulvalene derivative, TTF) chromophores on the outer surface have been prepared (Figure 26(a)) [63]. The dynamic control of inter-conversion between the electro-active heterodimers and the inactive homodimers was used to build light-harvesting/light-converting

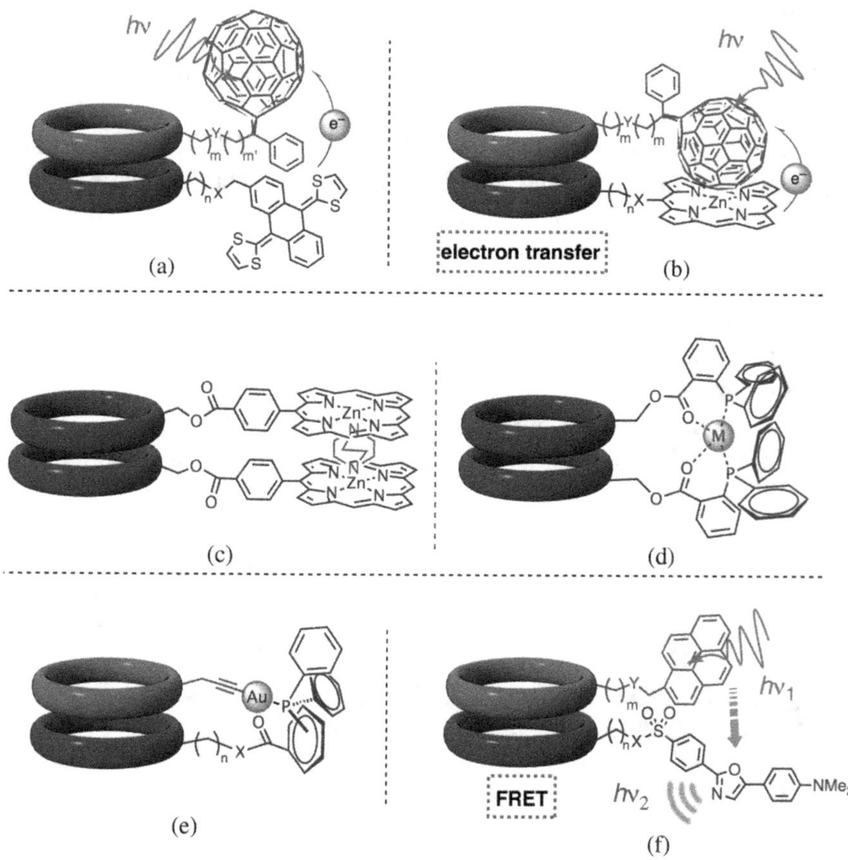

Fig. 26. Structural model of the supramolecular donor–acceptor systems (a) tetrathiafulvalene-fullerene and (b) Zn-porphyrin-fullerene based on heterodimeric self-assemblies in electron transfer processes. (c) Model of the selective recognition of diamines (i.e., DABCO) with homodimer molecular tweezers. Models of the homo- (d) and heterodimer (e) formation stabilized by coordination with metals (Pd, Au). (f) Model of CP heterodimers bearing pyrene and dapoxyl moieties for efficient FRET process.

hybrid nanostructures with great potential as efficient artificial photosystems. In an analogous system, the combination of C60 unit with a Zn–porphyrin as electron-donor residue resulted in thermodynamically stable heterodimeric assemblies in which both groups are nearby and exhibit an efficient intramolecular photoinduced electron-transfer (PET) process (Figure 26(b)) [109].

Cyclic peptides decorated with Zn–porphyrin groups on the periphery were also described to obtain molecular tweezers capable of controlling the formation of only one dimeric structure via an external molecular trigger (Figure 26(c)) [110]. Through the coordination of diamine molecules, such as DABCO, Granja *et al.* successfully achieved the exclusive formation of dimeric species where the porphyrin units are overlaid, forming a sandwich complex with potential applications as light-induced energy and electron-transfer switches. All these systems are very dynamic and the equilibria between homo- and heterodimers can be shifted between them according to the type of CPs (Ach-based versus Acp-based derivatives) or the small substituent attached to them. Alternatively, metal coordination (Pd or Au) to ligands, such as phosphines or alkynes covalently linked to a CP, allowed precise control over the interaction and switching among homo- or heterodimer species (Figures 26(d)–(e)) [111]. For instance, a mixture of CPs bearing acetylene or phosphine moieties can be switched from a statistic mixture of homo- and heterodimers to the heterodimer by Au addition or to the homodimers by Pd addition.

The dynamic self-sorting over the homo-/heterodimer equilibria has also been used to design a multi-signal system whose light emission depends on the type of aggregate formed in solution, such as those formed by pyrene-based and dapoxyl-based *N*-methylated α,γ-CP dimers (Figure 26(f)) [62]. By exploiting the homo- and heterodimers formation and excimer/fluorescence resonance energy transfer (FRET) effects, extensive fluorescence studies provided a detailed characterization of the dynamic self-assembling process of different supramolecular combinations. In particular, the intermolecular FRET process between pyrene and dapoxyl pairs enabled to evaluate the different equilibria involved in the formation of the heterodimeric ensembles. Similarly, the selective heterodimer formation from α,γ-cyclic octapeptides bearing pyrene/perylene pair was also explored. However, in both cases, dynamic backbone-to-backbone hydrogen-bonding interactions determine the selective formation of the heterodimeric species rather than lateral chain interactions. This controlled homo/hetero equilibrium allows the preparation of a broad range of supramolecular assemblies with potential applications such as biosensors or electronic/optical devices.

With a slightly different approach and in an attempt to obtain supramolecular cages [112], a Zn-porphyrin cap was linked via dynamic covalent bonds to the substituents attached to the nitrogen of the γ-AA of an eight-residue CP [113]. The resulting self-assembled dimer forms a molecular capsule with a large empty cavity capable of recognizing and encapsulating bipyridine-based ligands with possible applications as drug delivery systems or light-induced energy- and electron-transfer switches (Figure 27).

More recently, to investigate the dynamic self-assembling process in confined space, Mendez-Ardoy *et al.* reported on pH-controlled nanotube formation and fibrillation from *D,L*-CPs within water micro-droplet containers [114]. The CPs used incorporate histidine residues to confer pH-responsive dynamic self-assembling properties to the system and were decorated with a pyrene fluorescence probe to follow the fibrillation process (**CP18**, Figure 28(a)). Upon increasing the solution pH, fluorescence, FT-IR, and CD experiments revealed that the peptides cooperatively self-assembled in nanotubes with an antiparallel β-sheet arrangement in a reversible manner. Moreover, increasing the peptide concentration, viscoelastic hydrogels were obtained whereby the one-dimensional molecular array was fully retained from nanoscale to microscale. The pH-triggered self-assembly strategy could also be performed in the confined space of water in oil drops, resulting in 1D fibril-like structures whose

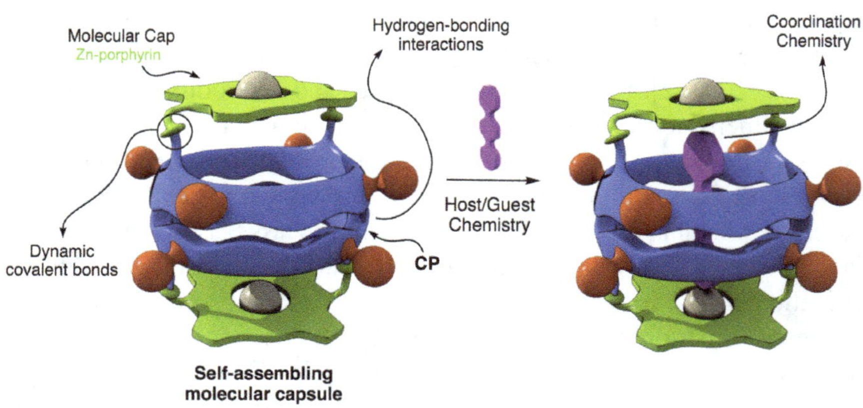

Fig. 27. Schematic representation of the dynamic covalent bonds involved in capsule formation.

self-assembly process could be tracked by fluorescence spectroscopy (Figure 28(b)). The confined fibrillation spanned and impacted the shape of the droplets confirming the strong directionality of the 1D supramolecular polymerization. Such a breakthrough can enable a better insight into the mechanisms involved in the self-assembly of tubular networks in confined environments or biological systems and lead to pH-responsive materials for several biomedical applications (i.e., drug delivery or tissue engineering).

In an effort to precisely direct and control nanotube assembly, Silk and co-workers described the construction of heterogeneous, covalently linked CP tetramers that provide improved control over nanotube composition and length. For this purpose, two cyclic peptides were coupled through their side chains employing copper-activated azide-alkyne cycloaddition followed by a self-dimerization through disulfide bond formation

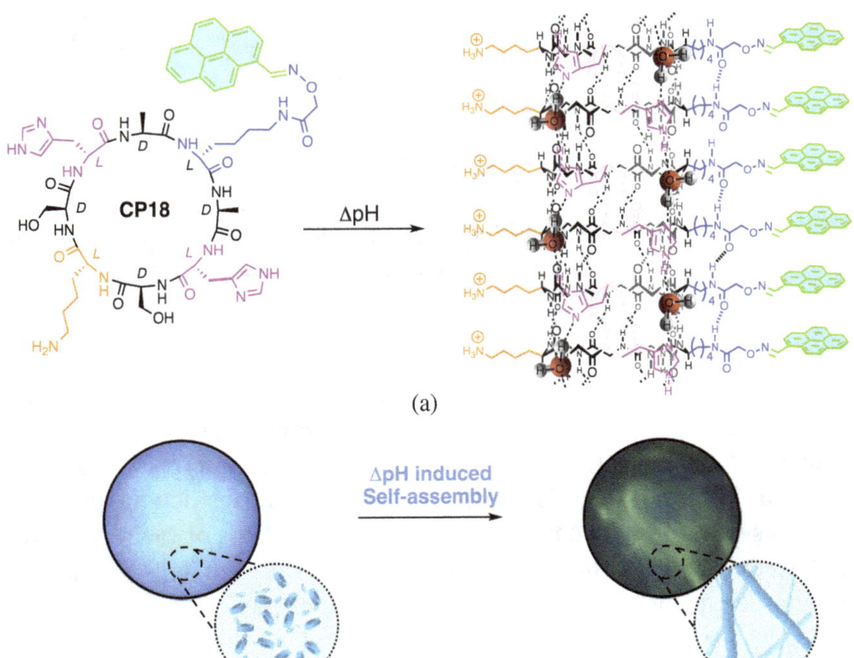

Fig. 28. (a) Chemical structure and pH-dependent self-assembly of **CP18**; (b) Supramolecular polymerization of **CP18** within the confined space of water in oil microdroplet containers.

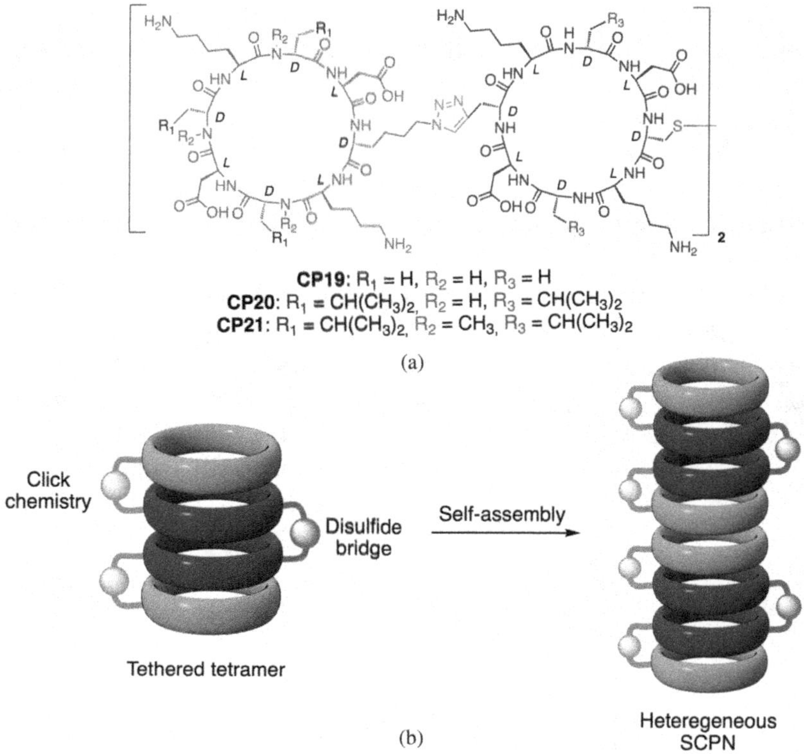

Fig. 29. Schematic representation of (a) covalently tethered CP tetramers **CP19**, **CP20**, and **CP21** and (b) formation of heterogeneous SCPNs with controlled CP order resulting from self-assembly of tetramers.

(Figure 29(a)) [115]. The covalent chemistry described generates heteromeric nanotubes in which two subunits of each CP are alternated along the nanotube (Figure 29(b)). The lack of such covalent restrictions provides nanotubes with different combinations and organizations of each CP. Cryo-TEM studies revealed the capability of these systems to self-assemble in highly ordered fibrous structures. The dynamic character of the tetrameric species was studied by NMR experiments, showing that the backbone of **CP19** is more solvent-accessible than **CP20** or **CP21**, as these peptides contain bulkiest side chains that shield them from the solvent. The N-methylated derivative (**CP21**) did not provide any evidence of extended nanostructures, confirming the preference of forming discrete tetramers instead of large nanotube bundles in which the non-N-alkylated peptides are participating in different nanotubes. Overall these studies support the CP tethering as a versatile method to build precisely functionalized dynamic nanomaterials with controllable chemical properties.

Aiming to prepare bundles of nanotubes with a defined diameter in an aqueous environment, Kimura and colleagues reported on β-CPs composed of β-glucosamino acids and a β-glutamic acid decorated with guanine moiety on the side chain (**CP22**, Figure 30) [116]. CD and TEM analyses revealed that in the presence of potassium ions, the CPs self-assembled into nanofibers with a uniform diameter of 7–8 nm that corresponds to a four-peptide-nanotube bundle construct by the formation of guanine quadruplex (G-quartet, Figure 30). Therefore, the introduction of natural motifs in CP self-assembling systems allowed to control in water media the dynamic processes of nanotube formation and their subsequent association in well-defined bundles through the G-quartet patterns. Previous studies with other

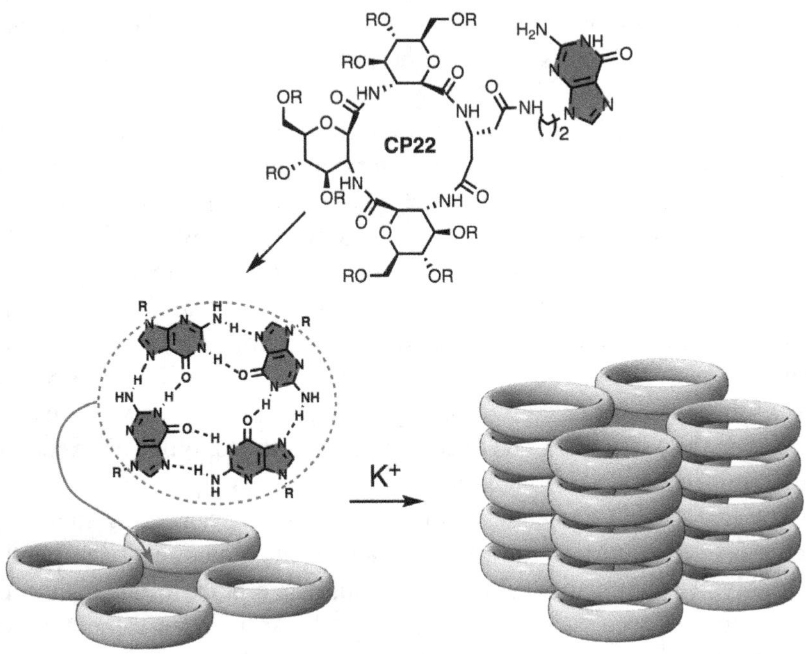

Fig. 30. Model for the self-assembly of β-CPs (**CP22**) decorated with a guanine moiety on the lateral chain. Four-peptide-nanotube bundle construct by the formation of guanine quadruplex.

G-quartet derivatives suggested that these dynamic tetrameric bundles could be used in the design of new metal ion transporters [117,118].

DNA bases pairing was also used in the recognition of different types of dimers and aggregates [119]. In this study, CPs bearing a thymine base covalently attached to a serine side chain formed β-sheet-based dimers that further self-assembled into tetrameric aggregates. The tetrameric entities can be recognized by a PNA-based diguanine dinucleotide through the nucleobase pairing forming supramolecular ternary species in which the cross-strand interactions are controlled by the selective base recognition process.

6.3. *SCPN-polymer supramolecular hybrids*

Although the outer surface of SCPN can be altered by conjugation with small functional molecules, one alternative way to fine-tune the outward chemistry is through the attachment of synthetic macromolecules to their surface, thus embedding the SCPN in a polymer shell. This strategy offers the possibility to generate bio-inspired nanomaterials with the potential to synergistically combine the advantages of their constituents and avoid their respective liabilities. The CPs provide the precise structural, chemical, and functional specificity that synthetic polymers lack. However, due to the peptide sensitivity to external stimuli (i.e., temperature, pH, ionic strength, etc.) and the occurrence of lateral aggregation among nanotubes that reduce their solubility, the attachment of appropriate synthetic polymers could provide biomolecular mimics with improved processability and stability. Hence, the conjugation of synthetic polymers to the CPs could be used to prevent nanotube aggregation, control the nanotube length at the nanometer scale, expand their functionality, as well as allow a comprehensive study of the dynamic mechanism of self-assembly.

On the other hand, the cyclic peptides, due to the structural features encoded in their sequence, can exert control over the topological orientation of the built-in polymeric functionalities, thus templating the self-assembly of these larger macromolecules. However, the key to achieving successful assemblies relies on preserving the structure and function of the peptide upon polymer conjugation. For this reason, it is crucial to understand the interactions between each building block to balance and manipulate them without interfering with the designed structures and functionalities.

Typically, cyclic peptide–polymer conjugate nanotubes can be synthesized following two different synthetic routes, the so-called *grafting from* (divergent growth, Figure 31(a)) and *grafting to* (convergent growth,

Figure 31(b)) approaches [120–123]. In the *grafting from* approach, the peptide surface can act as a macroinitiator from which the polymer chains grow via a variety of polymerization methods (ATRP, RAFT, ROP, NMP, etc.). On the contrary, in the *grafting to* approach, end-functionalized polymers are synthesized and then coupled to the peptide. Both strategies can be performed either before or after the formation of SCPNs.

In 2005, Couet *et al.* reported on the first examples of divergent growth of *D*,*L*-CP-polymer conjugate (Figure 31(a)) [124]. Taking advantage of the ability of the CPs to dynamically self-organize into tubular structures, nanotubes obtained from self-assembled cyclic octapeptides bearing ATRP initiators at specific side-chain positions were used as a template to polymerize *N*-isopropylacrylamide (NIPAAM) monomers in aqueous dispersion. The resulting CP-polymer hybrid nanotubes presented a single rod-like peptide core wrapped in a covalently attached soft polymeric shell, as evidenced by AFM analysis. Later studies from the same group revealed that as the molecular weight of the grafted chains growths, the outer diameter of the CP-polymer hybrids increase while the length decreases. This reduction in nanotube length is independent of the chemical characteristics of the attached polymer (i.e., styrene (S), *n*-butyl acrylate (nBA), or *N*-isopropylacrylamide (NIPAAM)) and can be ascribed to the increased bulkiness of the end-grafted chains [125]. However, the strategy of using SCPNs as a template for *in-situ* ATRP polymerization of monomers could not ensure a high graft density of the polymer chains due to the constrained nature of the grafting sites on the surface of the peptide nanotube [126].

Following another synthetic strategy, the same octapeptide *c*-[*L*-Asp-*D*-Ala-(*L*-Lys-*D*-Ala-)$_3$] was used as initiator for divergent growth of poly(butylacrylate) (pBA) in DMSO, which was shown to disaggregate the CPs completely [127]. Similar structures were obtained from the two synthetic approaches. The new hybrid macromolecule showed solvent-induced self-assembly in *core-shell* type nanorods similar to those obtained from CP grafting after nanotube formation.

For the preparation of other peptide-polymer conjugates, Borner and collaborators were the first to employ the *grafting to* approach for the preparation of novel SCPN/polymer structures (Figure 31(b)) [128]. To this end, the octapeptide *c*-[(*L*-Gln-*D*-Ala-*L*-Lys-*D*-Ala-)$_2$] was selected as aggregator domain and functionalized on opposite sides with two poly(butylacrylate) chains via an amide linkage. The resulting peptide-polymer conjugates exhibited a strong tendency to form uniform tubular

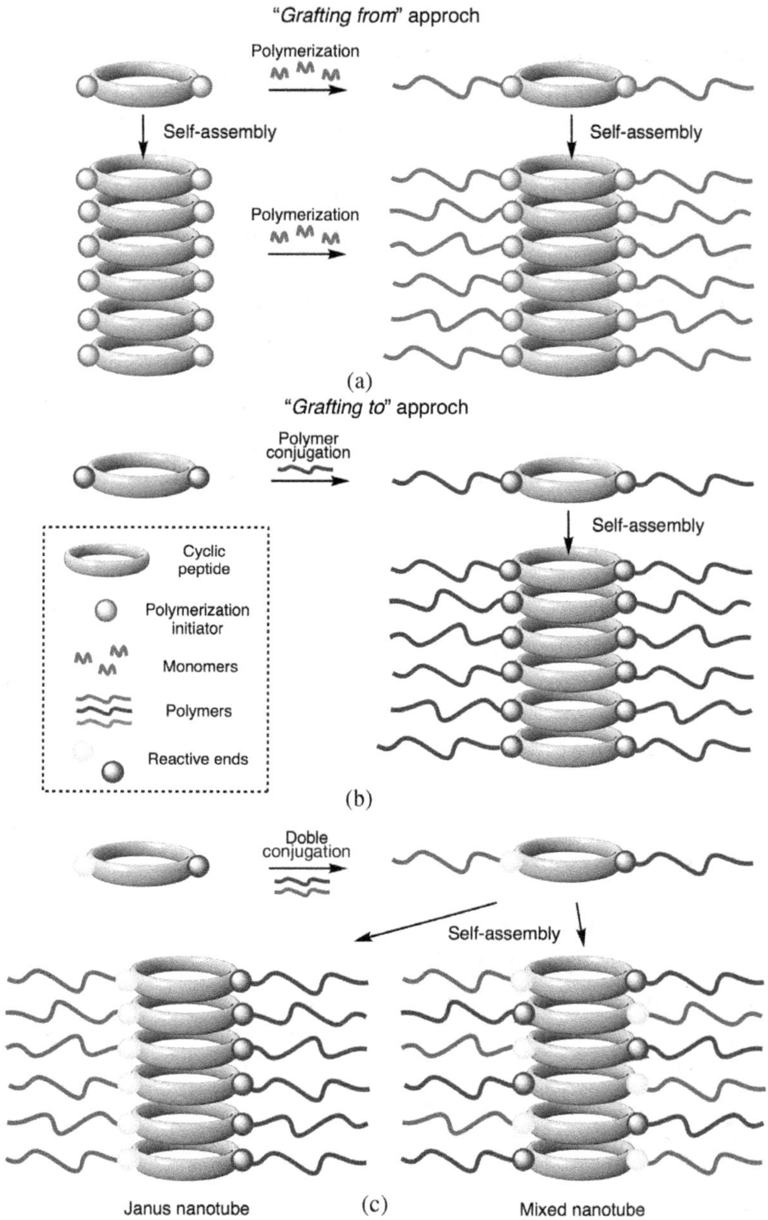

Fig. 31. Strategies for the synthesis of CP–polymer hybrid conjugates following (a) *grafting from* or (b) *grafting to* approaches; (c) model for the formation of self-assembling CP–polymer nanotubes with dual functionality in the form of Janus or mixed polymeric corona.

structures with a *core-shell* morphology. In general, the hybrid conjugates achieved by the *grafting to* technique are analogous to those obtained by the *grafting from* method [123]. However, the *grafting to* approach provides access to well-defined conjugates with higher efficiency, which suggests greater flexibility of this strategy as regards bulky monomers.

More recently, Perrier's group reported the use of copper-catalyzed azide-alkyne click reaction to couple a guiding *D,L-α*-CP motif to polymers, resulting in well-defined conjugates with various degrees of functionalization and sensitivity to the external stimuli [129–139]. Starting from the CP *c*-[(*L*-Trp-*D*-Leu-*L*-Lys(N_3)-*D*-Leu-)$_2$] (**CP23**), functional SCPN hybrids have been developed from a range of polymers comprising pBA, poly(dimethylamino ethyl acrylate) (pDMAEA), poly(acrylic acid) (pAA), poly(styrene) (pS), and poly(hydroxyl ethyl acrylate) (pHEA), as well as tubular architectures with mixed chemical properties by self-assembly of conjugates bearing different polymeric components [122]. The straightforward characterization by DLS and SANS measurements *in situ* allowed studying the resulting nanotube structures and the dynamic mechanism of self-assembly in solution [130]. By controlling the solvent mixture and the polymer length, direct observation of the nanotube formation and fine control over the SCPN length were obtained. Moreover, the examination of the self-assembly process with temperature enabled to probe the strength of the assembly, supporting the idea that these systems associate via a cooperative self-assembly process [130]. In this context, the dynamic self-assembly process in water was also assessed, and further control over the aggregation of such supramolecular assemblies was achieved through the introduction of pH- and thermo-responsive polymeric units [132–134]. The achievement of water-soluble CP-polymer nanotubes responsive to their environment provides a significant advance towards their use in biological applications, such as gene or drug delivery carriers and antimicrobials agents.

Another feature of the CP-polymer conjugates is the possibility of the subsequent modification of the conjugated polymers leading to the achievement of functional drug delivery systems. Attempting to transport therapeutic ruthenium anticancer drugs (RAPTA-C), p(HEA_{58}-co-$CEMA_{10}$) copolymer was coupled to the octapeptide **CP23** and functionalized with RAPTA-C [135]. Self-assembly into nanotubes of the resulting structures led to efficient carriers with high activity against cisplatin-resistant ovarian cancer cell lines. Recently, the same octapeptide was conjugated to biocompatible polymer poly(2-hydroxypropyl methacrylamide) (pHPMA), and the resulting hybrids were loaded with organoiridium anticancer complexes in the polymer shell [136]. Scattering analysis confirmed their ability to self-assemble into nanotubes in solution. The drug-loaded conjugates showed a more potent antiproliferative activity against human cancer cell lines than the drug-bearing polymers or free-drug used as control. The enhanced potency of the drug-bearing conjugate could be related, through studies of iridium-cellular accumulation, to a more effective mode of action rather than an increase in cellular accumulation.

To prepare self-assembling CP–polymer nanotubes with dual functionality in the form of either a Janus or mixed polymeric corona (Figure 31(c)), Perrier's group developed a two-step convergent synthetic strategy to link two different immiscible and phase-separating polymers, such as pS and pBA, to the **CP23** [137]. The novel conjugates are able to self-assemble in tubular architectures with well-defined sub-nanometer pore and hybrid polymer corona. LUV fluorescence assays enabled the evaluation of the capability of the Janus CP–polymer SCPNs to form artificial macropores in model phospholipid bilayers *via* phase segregation. The unique feature of such supramolecular ensembles may pave the way for the design of *trans*-bilayer protein channel mimics through a bottom-up approach.

Phospholipid bilayer partitioning and self-assembly in transmembrane channels could be improved and modulated by combining the CP with a series of hydrophilic and hydrophobic polymers [138]. Fluorescence experiments on dye-entrapped liposomes (LUVs) allowed for an extensive elucidation of structure-channel formation relationships. Hydrophobic conjugates form well-defined single channels, while hydrophilic conjugates form monomeric channels to a much lesser extent. Moreover, the conjugation of a thermo-responsive polymer such as pNIPAAM enabled on-demand control over the formation and transport of the resulting transmembrane channels by tuning of the temperature.

To further develop this strategy and avoid unspecific interactions between SCPNs, the same group envisioned a stimuli-responsive activation mechanism to induce membrane activity of SCPN-polymer hybrids [140]. For this purpose, poly(2-ethyl-2-oxazoline) (PEtOx) chains of different lengths and bearing cleavable disulfide connectors were attached to the CP through an amide linkage. Upon cleavage of the disulfide linker between polymer and peptide by the addition of chemical stimulus (i.e., 1,4-dithiothreitol (DTT) as reducing agent), an on-demand membrane activity was generated, while initial conjugates remain inactive, shielded by the polymer shell (Figure 32). Also, control over the dynamic stacking of the CPs in longer nanotubes was obtained by the cleavage of a predefined share of the polymer shell, as proven by DLS experiments. The ability of the CP–polymer conjugates to permeabilize synthetic liposomes as well as mammalian cell membranes when triggered has also been evaluated. This feature, combined with biocompatibility, makes these systems very attractive for biomedical applications.

More recently, the same group developed a supramolecular strategy for switching the dynamic self-assembly of CP–polymer conjugates using cucurbit[n]urils (CB[n]s) host–guest chemistry (Figure 33) [139]. For this purpose, a CP-poly(ethylene glycol) (PEG) conjugate capable of self-assembling into a tubular supramolecular polymer and bearing two phenylalanine residues as binding sites of CB[7] was synthesized.

By exploiting host–guest interactions, the introduction of bulky CB[7] hosts onto the conjugate led to the disassembly of the tubular structure due to the steric hindrance of CB[7] among the CPs, as evidenced by

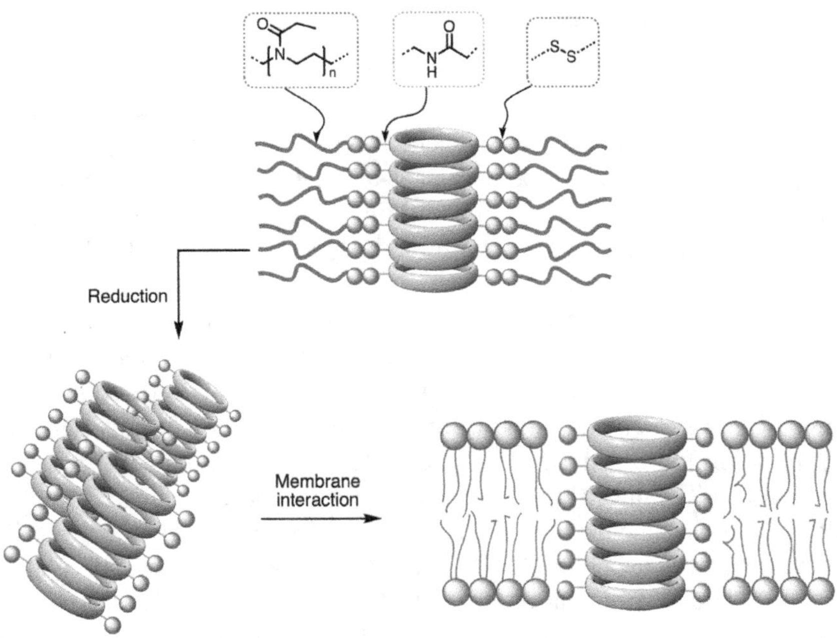

Fig. 32. Schematic illustration of CP–polymer conjugates linked by reversible covalent connectors and reduction produced membrane interaction.

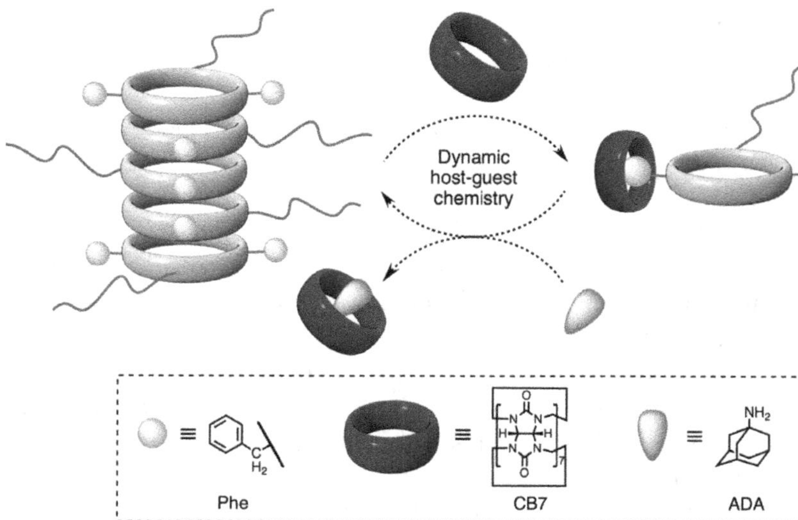

Fig. 33. Schematic illustration of the dynamic self-assembly of CP-polymer conjugates through host–guest chemistry.

NMR, SANS and isothermal titration calorimetry (ITC) analysis. Interestingly, because of the dynamic nature of the host–guest strategy, the tubular supramolecular polymers can be reversibly refolded by adding a competitive guest molecule, such as 1-adamantanamine (ADA). In this way, the possibility of controlling and fine-tuning the structure and function of these tubular ensembles through dynamic host–guest chemistry was successfully demonstrated.

It is well known that the supramolecular nature of SCPNs allows them to exchange subunits and adapt to environmental conditions quickly. Therefore, to probe the dynamic character of such supramolecular systems, Perrier and collaborators have designed modified CP-polymer conjugates with fluorescent dyes to investigate *in-situ* their dynamic behavior through FRET studies (Figure 34) [141]. For this purpose, an asymmetric CP bearing two anchor points on opposite sides was functionalized with the donor Cy3 or acceptor Cy5 dyes as a FRET pair and with a PEG chain to avoid lateral aggregation (i.e., PEG–CP–Cy3 and PEG–CP–Cy5). SANS, SLS, and TEM analysis confirmed the formation of a 1D structure with a *core-shell* morphology. FRET studies carried out on a mixture of readily assembled nanotubes in various solvents of different polarities

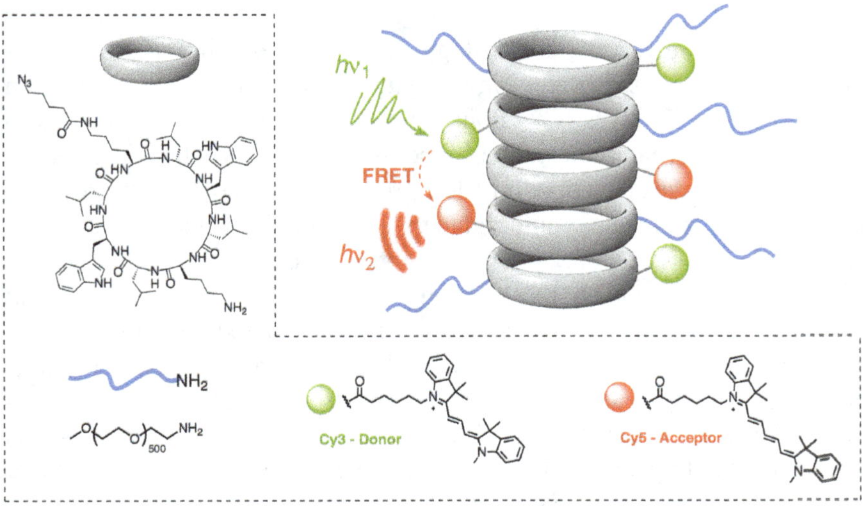

Fig. 34. Schematic depiction of the CP–dye–polymer conjugates (insert) and the FRET effect occurring in SCPNs containing donor (Cy3) and acceptor (Cy5) dyes.

revealed a time-dependent increase in energy transfer associated with FRET, which proved the exchange of monomer units or peptide segments among the formed nanotubes. The obtained results demonstrated for the first time that the self-assembly of these systems is extremely dynamic, not kinetically trapped, and highly solvent-dependent. The use of FRET enabled the examination of the dynamic exchange of these supramolecular ensembles in mammalian cells *in vitro* by fluorescence confocal microscopy, proving their integrity and dynamic character even in a highly complex environment such as living cells.

These findings provide the basis for further investigation on the manipulation of the dynamic nature of these supramolecular systems for their possible use as biological sensors or trackers.

Recently, Perrier's group reported on the introduction of secondary hydrophobic interactions close to the CP core to induce control and stabilization over the highly dynamic behavior of the CPs in water [142]. For this purpose, an amphiphilic diblock copolymer poly(*n*-butyl acrylate)-*b*-poly(N,N-dimethylacrylamide) (pBA-*b*-pDMA) was coupled to the CP *c*-[(*L*-Trp-*D*-Leu-*L*-Lys-*D*-Leu-)$_2$] in order to form a hydrophobic core around the peptide and a hydrophilic shell that stabilizes the nanostructure in an aqueous environment. TEM, SANS, and SLS measurements assessed the tubular morphology of the resulting CP-(pBA-*b*-pDMA)$_2$ aggregates. Then, to investigate the dynamic behavior of such hybrids, the FRET dyes (Cy3 donor and Cy5 acceptor) were attached to the CP-polymer nanotubes. The outcomes revealed a small increase in energy transfer associated with FRET, providing proof of a slow exchange among CP units in the nanotubes due to the stabilizing effect of the hydrophobic pBA core-region. Stochastic optical reconstruction microscopy (STORM) studies corroborate the achievement of a less dynamic system since the FRET dyes Cy3 and Cy5 cannot be visualized randomly distributed within the supramolecular assemblies. Therefore, these findings demonstrate that an additional hydrophobic driving force next to the peptide core can contribute to controlling the dynamic nature of such systems in water, resulting in functional supramolecular polymers with defined nanostructures useful for biomedical applications.

6.4. *SCPN supramolecular hybrids through non-covalent interactions*

Another approach for altering the inward and outward properties of SCPNs is the non-covalent attachment of functional molecules to provide nanotubular functional supramolecular hybrids for various types of biomedical and technological applications. Interesting features of the non-covalent conjugation are the straightforward synthesis, its reversible nature, and the ability to maintain the tubular structure integrity during the conjugation process.

Recently, our group reported on the preparation of hybrid nanotubular architectures derived from the coupling of SCPNs and single-walled carbon nanotubes (SWCNTs) [143]. To engage the SWCNTs via water-enhanced π–π interactions, an eighth-residue α,γ-CP was functionalized with a pyrene moiety on a lysine side chain (Figure 35(a)). The resulting pyrene "paddle" was employed to engage the SWCNTs and assist their dispersion in water media. The SWCNTs/SCPNs hybrids obtained formed highly ordered oriented arrays (as revealed by TEM and AFM analysis) and combined the properties of both components, such as the electrical conductivity and robustness of the SWCNTs and the solubility and biocompatibility of the SCPNs counterpart. The supramolecular nature of this methodology allows SWCNT properties to be preserved and provided

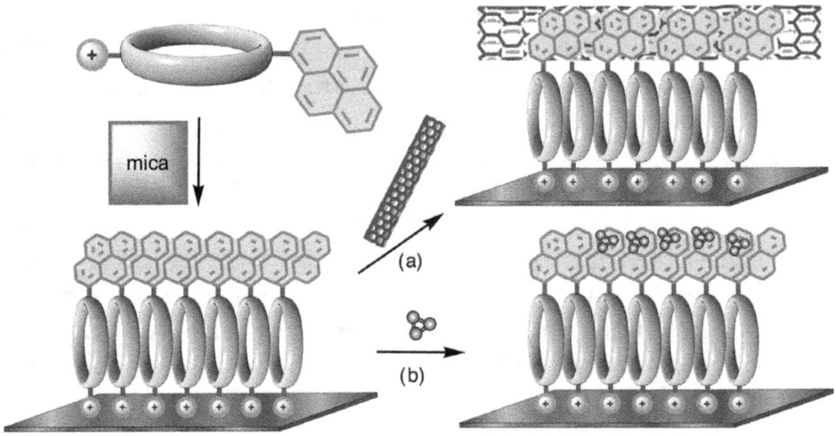

Fig. 35. Schematic representation of the hierarchical surface deposition of (a) CP/SWCNT and (b) CP/subnanometric Ag_3 metal clusters.

knowledge on novel methods for their controlled deposition and manipulation.

Subsequently, the same α,γ-CP equipped with the pyrene "paddle", was also used for the alignment of subnanometric silver clusters (Ag_3) through non-covalent interactions at the metal/organic interfaces (Figure 35(b)) [144]. The resulting self-assembled hybrid architectures displayed a 1D array of Ag_3 clusters aligned on top of SCPNs over long distances (μm), as demonstrated by AFM analysis. Fluorescence experiments of SCPN solutions titrated with Ag_3 corroborated the occurrence of non-covalent interactions and the synergistic stabilization of the peptide/Ag_3 supramolecular hybrids by cluster intercalation among pyrene excimers. These outcomes delineate the potential of this approach to exploit the excellent properties of the metal clusters in combination with supramolecular hosts.

The possibility of non-covalently functionalizing SCPNs with multiple components opens up the opportunity to exploit them for the intracellular delivery of bio-functional compounds. In this regard, Wang and co-workers designed and prepared SCPN bundles loaded with doxorubicin (DOX) and modified with polyethylene glycol (PEG) chains as drug carriers for cancer therapy [145]. The resulting nanotubular supramolecular aggregates exhibited increased cytotoxicity, enhanced DOX uptake, and altered the intracellular DOX distribution in human breast cancer

MCF-7/ADR cells. Alternatively, a positively charged CP *c*-[(*L*-Lys-*D*-Ala-)$_4$] modified with a guanidiniocarbonyl pyrrole moiety (GPC), a weakly basic but efficient Arg analog, has resulted in cationic nanorods capable of interacting and delivering DNA under physiological condition (Figure 36) [146]. A detailed study of the transfection mechanism revealed that DNA molecules could enter the cells via an uptake mediated by the tubular assemblies rather than an endocytotic pathway. Similarly, Hsieh *et al.* utilized a neutral CP of alternating chirality *c*-(*D*-Trp-*L*-Tyr-)$_2$ as an oral gene delivery carrier [147]. The resulting nanotubes were able to complex plasmid DNA, improved its duodenal permeability *in vitro*, and successfully deliver it by oral administration *in vivo* through an energy-dependent process.

Aiming to obtain artificial ionophores able of translocating anions and cations (symport transport) across lipid bilayers, Fuertes *et al.* developed

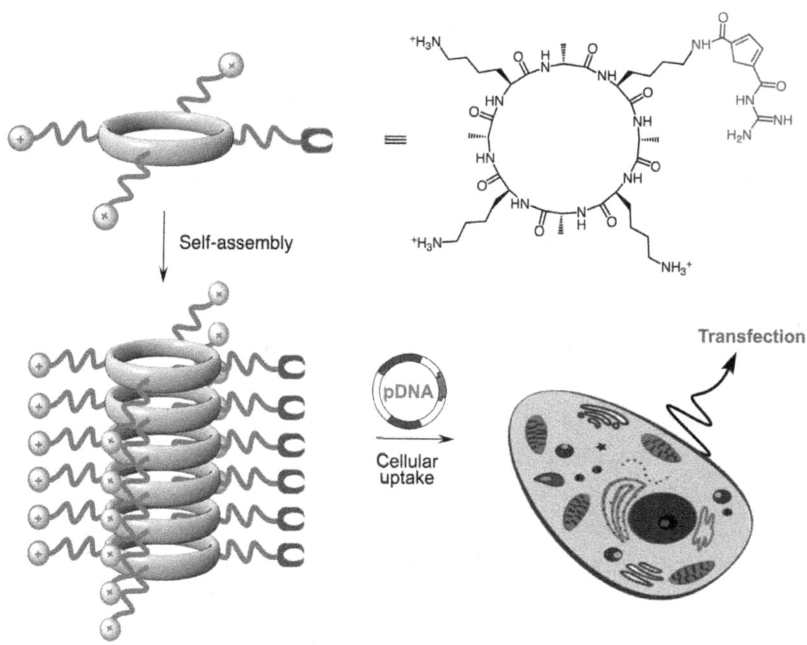

Fig. 36. Positively charged CP *c*-[(*L*-Lys-*D*-Ala-)$_4$] modified with a guanidiniocarbonyl pyrrole moiety (GPC, red) able to self-assemble in cationic nanorods capable of delivering DNA into cells.

a novel family of transmembrane carriers based on tris-pyridine-decorated α,γ-CPs (Figure 37) [148]. ^{1}H-NMR and FT-IR experiments confirmed the ability of the CPs to self-assemble into dimeric structures in non-polar solvents through antiparallel β-sheet-type interactions. Thanks to the coordination capabilities of the pyridine rings and their topological arrangement at the entrance of the dimer cavity, LUVs fluorescence assays revealed that these molecules effectively act as ion shuttles for both cations and anions across model lipid bilayers. *Ortho*-pyridine-substituted transporter outperformed the *meta*-substituted isomer, particularly for Cl^- transport, proving that the position of the nitrogen atom at the entrance or pointing towards the inner cavity plays a pivotal role in the binding mode of the different ionic species. Each carrier showed a reversed anion selectivity trend in the HPTS rectification assay, in which ionic radius and hydration energy were crucial parameters that determine the transport efficiencies. Control experiments with CP scaffolds lacking pyridine moieties or bearing only one tris-pyridine cap indicated the significant role of

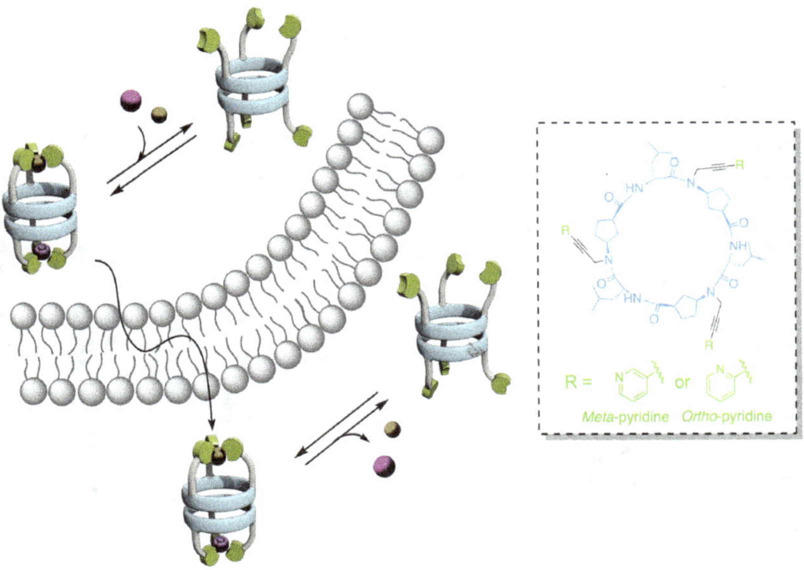

Fig. 37. Schematic illustration of the proposed ion complexation model and transport across lipid bilayers by the tris-pyridine-substituted α,γ-CPs. Chemical structures of tris-pyridine-decorated α,γ-CPs (insert).

the CP skeleton in the transport, displaying a cooperative behavior, and that both pyridine caps are needed for the transmembrane activity. Hence, such supramolecular assemblies represent new appealing systems for design artificial transmembrane carriers as new biomedical therapeutics.

Recently, our group reported on Venturi-*like* peptide nanotubes with an internal constricted area based on a covalently linked CP dimer functionalized with a complementary CP [149]. In this system, the dimeric peptide was constructed by click conjugation of two CPs of different diameters and supramolecular properties. By controlling the dynamic homo- and heterodimer equilibria and media conditions (i.e., concentration and solvent properties), the combination of the covalent dimer with a second CP with complementary assembly characteristics lead to different nanostructures with excellent control over nanotube length (Figure 38). In this way, SCPNs consisting of three, four, or six subunits and controlled internal diameter were precisely prepared. The shape of the resulting nanotubes mimics the structure of natural ion channels. Therefore, such a strategy can be applied for engineering novel transmembrane channels or porous membranes with enhanced transport properties.

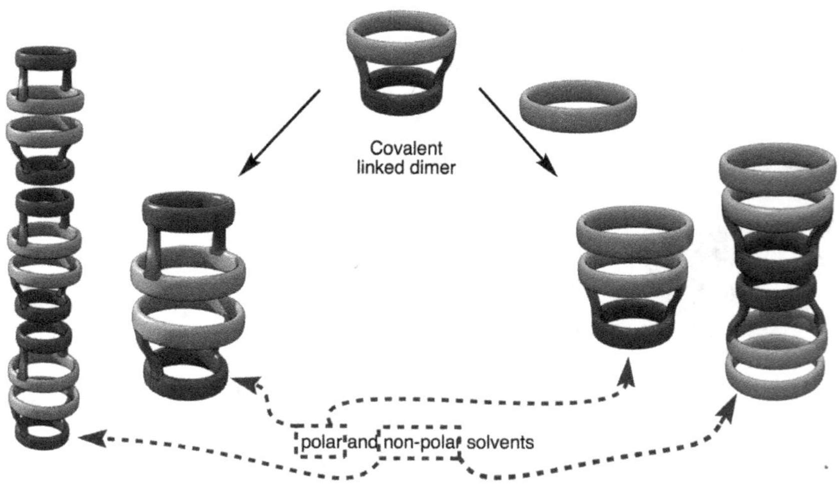

Fig. 38. Venturi-*like* peptide nanotubes with an internal constricted area based on a covalently linked CP dimer functionalized with a complementary CP.

To achieve hierarchically organized two-dimensional (2D) peptide-based materials, Montenegro *et al.* reported on the design of the first CP that can undergo sequential 1D-to-2D self-assembly in water to yield dynamic and giant 2D supramolecular nanosheets in the mesoscale (Figure 39) [150]. The authors demonstrate the specificity of this particular CP sequence for the initial adoption of its nanotubular (1D) structure and successive self-organization into 2D nanosheets comprised of nanotubular bilayers. These micrometric 2D nanosheets are established by a key interplay of attractive H-bonded β-sheets, hydrophobic effects (i.e., Leu zippers and Trp stacks), and repulsive anionic interactions. Due to the presence of pH-sensitive residues in the CP, the 2D supramolecular nanosheets exhibited dynamic behavior in response to external stimuli (i.e., pH and temperature) by reversibly switching their structure between 1D and 2D arrangement. Overall, this pioneering work provides a novel strategy for obtaining giant 2D materials with hierarchical organization and controlled self-assembly with possible applications as responsive surfaces, molecular transporters, and biocompatible sensors, among others.

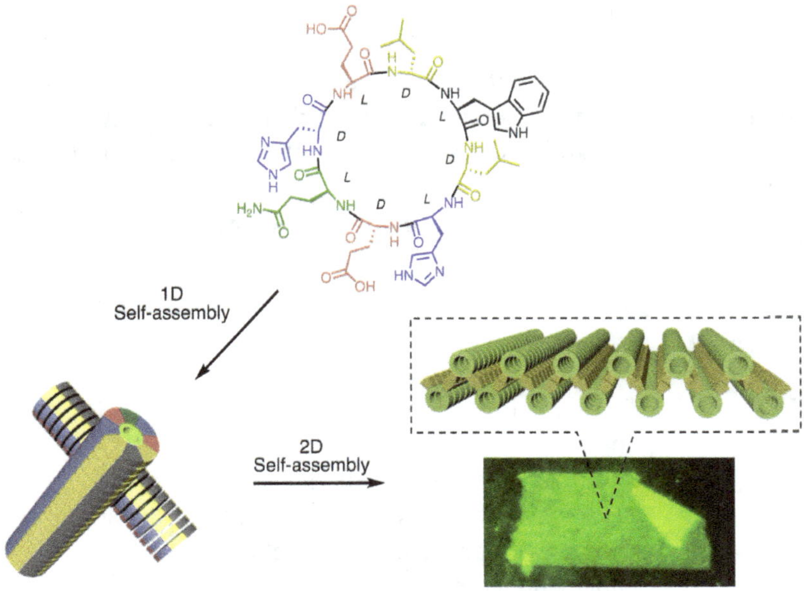

Fig. 39. Schematic illustration of CP sequential 1D-to-2D self-assembly to yield giant 2D supramolecular nanosheets.

7. Conclusion

Inspired by the approaches that nature explores in constructing complex supramolecular tubular assemblies, mainly relying on bottom-up and self-assembly paths, SCPNs act as excellent and powerful building blocks to create novel nanostructures with existing applications or for future developments. For this reason, in recent years, research efforts have focused on implementing efficient synthetic strategies to gain precise control over their properties, such as nanotubes length, inner diameter, internal pore chemistry, and external functionalities. Some exhaustive examples outlined in this chapter provide a unique insight into the corresponding molecular packaging, intermolecular interactions, self-assembly process, as well as their dynamic behavior. Such knowledge enables us to understand the basic principles for engineering smart self-assembled supramolecular tubular architectures with advanced applications in biology, chemistry, and materials science. Besides, the possibility of functionalizing the nanotube periphery with functional molecules (i.e., small molecules, polymers, drugs, and dyes) provides a unique way to develop multi-responsive hybrid self-assemblies otherwise challenging to achieve. Importantly, due to the highly dynamic nature of hydrogen-bonding networks among CP units, the hierarchical self-assembly process can result in a strong structural diversity that makes them the ideal candidates for obtaining new bioactive materials. However, there are still many fascinating challenges to be addressed in exploiting the dynamic nature of such supramolecular systems to build cutting-edge nanotechnologies that will facilitate human progress. We are eagerly awaiting new discoveries as this field progresses.

List of abbreviations

5-FU	Fluorouracil
AA	Amino acid
Aca	3-aminocycloalcanecarboxylic acid
Ach	3-aminocyclohexanecarboxylic acid
Acp	3-aminocyclopentanecarboxylic acid
ADA	1-adamantanamine
AFM	Atomic force microscopy
Ahf	4-amino-3-hydroxytetrahydrofuran-2-carboxylic acid
Ala	Alanine

Arg	Arginine
ATR-IR	Attenuated total reflection infrared
ATRP	Atom transfer radical polymerization
Bn	Benzyl
CB[7]	Cucurbit[7]urils
Cys	Cysteine
Cy	Cyanine
co	Copolymer
CP	Cyclic peptide
CU	Cyclic ureas
DABCO	1,4-diazabicyclo[2.2.2]octane
DLS	Dynamic light scattering
DNA	Deoxyribonucleic acid
DTT	1,4-dithiothreitol
ED-SA	Ethylenediamine-succinic acid sequence
FRET	Fluorescence resonance energy transfer
Gln	Glutamine
Glu	Glutamic acid
GPC	Guanidiniocarbonyl pyrrole moiety
G-quartet	Guanine quadruplex
Hag	Homoallylglycine
HPTS	8-hydroxypyrene-1,3,6-trisulfonic acid trisodium salt
IR	Infrared
ITC	Isothermal titration calorimetry
Leu	Leucine
LUVs	Large unilamellar vesicles
Mba	3-amino-2-methylbenzoic acid
NDI	1,4,5,8-naphthalenetetracarboxylic diimide
NIPAAM	N-isopropylacrylamide
NMP	Nitroxide-mediated radical polymerization
NMR	Nuclear magnetic resonance
pAA	Poly(acrylic acid)
pBA	Poly(butylacrylate)
pDMAEA	Poly(dimethylamino ethyl acrylate)
pHEA	Poly(hydroxyl ethyl acrylate)
pHPMA	Poly(2-hydroxypropyl methacrylamide)
pS	Poly(styrene)
PEtOx	Poly(2-ethyl-2-oxazoline)
PEG	Polyethylene glycol

PFM	Piezo-force microscopy
Phe	Phenylalanine
PNA	Peptide nucleic acid
RAFT	Reversible addition-fragmentation chain transfer polymerization
ROP	Ring-opening polymerization
SANS	Small-angle neutron scattering
SCPN	Self-assembling cyclic peptide nanotube
SLS	Static light scattering
STM	Scanning tunneling microscope
STORM	Stochastic optical reconstruction microscopy
SWCNT	Single-walled carbon nanotubes
TEM	Transmission electron microscopy
Trp	Tryptophan
Tyr	Tyrosine
Val	Valine

References

1. Whitesides, G. M., Mathias, J. P., and Seto, C. T. (1991) Articles Molecular and A Chemical Strategy for the Synthesis of Nanostructures. *Science* 254, pp. 1312–1319.
2. Bong, D. T., Clark, T. D., Granja, J. R. and Ghadiri, M. R. (2001) Self-Assembly Organic Nanotubes. *Angew. Chem. Int. Ed.* 40, pp 988–1011.
3. Eder, D. (2010) Carbon Nanotube-Inorganic Hybrids. *Chem. Rev.* 110, pp. 1348–1385.
4. Baughman, R. H. (2007) Carbon Nanotubes — The Route Toward. *Science* 297, pp. 787–793.
5. Tenne, R. and Redlich, M. (2010) Recent Progress in the Research of Inorganic Fullerene-like Nanoparticles and Inorganic Nanotubes. *Chem. Soc. Rev.* 39, pp. 1423–1434.
6. Huo, Q., Margolese, D. I., Ciesla, U., Feng, P., Gier, T. E., Sieger, P., Leon, R., Petroff, P. M., Schüth, F. and Stucky, G. D. (1994) Generalized Synthesis of Periodic Surfactant/Inorganic Composite Materials. *Nature* 368, pp. 317–321.
7. Patzke, G. R., Krumeich, F. and Nesper, R. (2002) Oxidic Nanotubes and Nanorods - Anisotropic Modules for a Future Nanotechnology. *Angew. Chem. Int. Ed.* 41, pp. 2446–2461.
8. Steed, J. W. and Atwood, J. A. (2009) *Supramolecular Chemistry*, 2nd edn. Chichester: John Wiley & Sons Ltd.
9. Varshey, D. B., Sander, J. R. G., Friščić, T. and MacGillivray, L. R. (2012) Supramolecular interactions. In *Supramolecular Chemistry: From*

Molecules to Nanomaterials, Gale, P. A. and Steed, J. W., eds., vol. 1, p. 9. New York, NY: John Wiley & Sons Ltd.

10. García-Fandiño, R., Amorín, M. and Granja, J. R. (2012) Synthesis of supramolecular nanotubes. In *Supramolecular Chemistry: From Molecules to Nanomaterials*, Gale, P. A. and Steed, J. W., eds., vol. 5, p. 2149. New York, NY: John Wiley & Sons Ltd.
11. Hamley, I. W. (2014) Peptide Nanotubes. *Angew. Chem. Int. Ed.* 53, pp. 6866–6881.
12. Brea, R. J., Reiriz, C. and Granja, J. R. (2010) Towards Functional Bionanomaterials Based on Self-Assembling Cyclic Peptide Nanotubes. *Chem. Soc. Rev.* 39, pp. 1448–1456.
13. Rodríguez-Vázquez, N., Amorín, M. and Granja, J. R. (2017) Recent Advances in Controlling the Internal and External Properties of Self-Assembling Cyclic Peptide Nanotubes and Dimers. *Org. Biomol. Chem.* 15, pp. 4490–4505.
14. Chapman, R., Danial, M., Koh, L. M., Jolliffe, K. A. and Perrier, S. (2012) Design and Properties of Functional Nanotubes from the Self-Assembly of Cyclic Peptide Templates. *Chem. Soc. Rev.* 41, pp. 6023–6041.
15. Novelli, F., De Santis, S., Morosetti, S., Titubante, M., Masci, G. and Scipioni, A. (2018) Peptides with Regularly Alternating Enantiomeric Sequence: From Ion Channel Models to Bioinspired Nanotechnological Applications. *Pept. Sci.* 110, p.e24043. doi: 10.1002/pep2.24043.
16. Montenegro, J., Ghadiri, M. R. and Granja, J. R. (2013) Ion Channel Models Based on Self-Assembling Cyclic Peptide Nanotubes. *Acc. Chem. Res.* 46, pp. 2955–2965.
17. Rodríguez-Vázquez, N., Ozores, H., Guerra, A., Gonzalez-Freire, E., Fuertes, A., Panciera, M., Priegue, J., Outeiral, J., Montenegro, J., García-Fandiño, R., Amorín, M. and Granja, J. R. (2014) Membrane-Targeted Self-Assembling Cyclic Peptide Nanotubes. *Curr. Top. Med. Chem.* 14, pp. 2647–2661.
18. Hsieh, W. H. and Liaw, J. (2018) Applications of Cyclic Peptide Nanotubes (CPNTs). *J. Food Drug Anal.* 27, pp. 32–47.
19. De Santis, P., Morosetti, S. and Rizzo, R. (1974) Conformational Analysis of Regular Enantiomeric Sequences. *Macromolecules*. 7, pp. 52–58.
20. Tomasic, L. and Lorenzi, G. P. (1987) Some Cyclic Oligopeptides with S2n Symmetry. *Helv. Chim. Acta*. 70, pp. 1012–1016.
21. Pavone, V., Benedetti, E., Di Blasio, B., Lombardi, A., Pedone, C., Tomasich, L. and Lorenzi, G. P. (1989) Regularly Alternating *L,D*-Peptides. III. Hexacyclic Peptides from Valine or Phenylalanine. *Biopolymers*. 28, pp. 215–223.
22. Ghadiri, M. R., Granja, J. R., Milligan, R. A. and McRee, D. E. (1993) Self-Assembling Organic Nanotubes Based on a Cyclic Peptide Architecture. *Nature*. 366, pp. 324–327.
23. Khazanovich, N., Granja, J. R., McRee, D. E., Milligan, R. A. and Ghadiri, M. R. (1994) Nanoscale Tubular Ensembles with Specified Internal

Diameters. Design of a Self-Assembled Nanotube with a 13-Å Pore. *J. Am. Chem. Soc.* 116, pp. 6011–6012.

24. Adler-Abramovich, L. and Gazit, E. (2014) The Physical Properties of Supramolecular Peptide Assemblies: From Building Block Association to Technological Applications. *Chem. Soc. Rev.* 43, pp. 7236–7236.
25. Polaskova, M. E., Ede, N. J. and Lambert, J. N. (1998) Synthesis of Nanotubule-Forming Cyclic Octapeptides via an Fmoc Strategy. *Aust. J. Chem.* 51, pp. 535–540.
26. Hartgerink, J. D., Granja, J. R., Milligan, R. A., Ghadiri, M. R. (1996) Self-Asembling Peptide Nanotubes. *J. Am. Chem. Soc.* 118, pp. 43–50.
27. Ghadiri, M. R., Granja, J. and Buehler, L. K. (1994) Artificial Transmembrane Ion Channels from Self-Assembling Peptide Nanotubes. *Nature* 369, pp. 301–304.
28. Granja, J. R. and Ghadiri, M. R. (1994) Channel-Mediated Transport of Glucose across Lipid Bilayers. *J. Am. Chem. Soc.* 116, pp. 10785–10786.
29. Sanchez-Quesada, J., Ghadir, M. R., Bayley, H. and Braha, O. (2000) Cyclic Peptides as Molecular Adapters for a Pore-Forming Protein. *J. Am. Chem. Soc.* 122, pp. 11757–11766.
30. Rosenthal-Aizman, K., Svensson, G. and Unden, A. (2004) Self-Assembling Peptide Nanotubes from Enantiomeric Pairs of Cyclic Peptides with Alternating *D* and *L* Amino Acid Residues. *J. Am. Chem. Soc.* 126, pp. 3372–3373.
31. Hourani, R., Zhang, C., Van Der Weegen, R., Ruiz, L., Li, C., Keten, S., Helms, B. A. and Xu, T. (2011) Processable Cyclic Peptide Nanotubes with Tunable Interiors. *J. Am. Chem. Soc.* 133, pp. 15296–15299.
32. Fernández-López, S., Kim, H.-S., Choi, E. C., Delgado, M., Granja, J. R., Khasanov, A., Kraehenbuehl, K., Long, G., Weinberger, D. A., Wilcoxen, K. M. and Ghadiri, M. R. (2001) Antibacterial Agents Based on the Cyclic *D,L-α*-Peptide Architecture. *Nature* 412, pp. 452–455.
33. Karlström, A. and Undén, A. (1997) Association of Cyclic Peptides in Aqueous Solution Measured by Fluorescence Quenching. *Biopolymers* 41, pp. 1–4.
34. Qu, W., Tan, H., Chen, G. and Liu, R. (2010) The Self-Assembled of Cyclic *D,L-α*-Peptide Systems: Insights Into the Structure and Energetics. *Int. J. Quant. Chem.* 110, pp. 1648–1659.
35. Silk, M. R., Newman, J., Ratcliffe, J. C., White, J. F., Caradoc-Davies, T., Price, J. R., Perrier, S., Thompson, P. E. and Chalmers, D. K. (2017) Parallel and Antiparallel Cyclic *D/L* Peptide Nanotubes. *Chem. Commun.* 53, pp. 6613–6616.
36. Ghadiri, M. R., Kobayashi, K., Granja, J. R., Chadha, R. K. and McRee, D. E. (1995) The Structural and Thermodynamic Basis for the Formation of Self-Assembled Peptide Nanotubes. *Angew. Chemie Int. Ed.* 34, pp. 93–95.

37. Clark, T. D., Buriak, J. M., Kobayashi, K., Ister, M. P., McRee, D. E. and Ghadiri, R. M. (1998) Cylindrical β-Sheet Peptide Assemblies. *J. Am. Chem. Soc.* 120, pp. 8949–8962.
38. Amorín, M., Castedo, L. and Granja, J. R. (2008) Folding Control in Cyclic Peptides through N-Methylation Pattern Selection: Formation of Antiparallel β-Sheet Dimers, Double Reverse Turns and Supramolecular Helices by $3\alpha,\gamma$ Cyclic Peptides. *Chem. Eur. J.* 14, pp. 2100–2111.
39. Chou, K.-C., Pottle, M., Némethy, G., Ueda, Y. and Scheraga, H. A. (1982) Structure of β-Sheets: Origin of the Right-Handed Twist and of the Increased Stability of Antiparallel over Parallel Sheets. *J. Mol. Biol.* 162, pp. 89–112.
40. Kobayashi, K., Granja, J. R. and Ghadiri, M. R. (1995) β-Sheet Peptide Architecture: Measuring the Relative Stability of Parallel vs. Antiparallel *B*-Sheets. *Angew. Chemie Int. Ed. Engl.* 34, pp. 95–98.
41. Clark, T. D. and Ghadiri, M. R. (1995) Supramolecular Design by Covalent Capture. Design of a Peptide Cylinder via Hydrogen-Bond-Promoted Intermolecular Olefin Metathesis. *J. Am. Chem. Soc.* 117, pp. 12364–12365.
42. Clark, T. D., Kobayashi, K. and Ghadiri, M. R. (1999) Covalent Capture and Stabilization of Cylindrical β-Sheet Peptide Assemblies. *Chem. Eur. J.* 5, pp. 782–792.
43. Vollmer, M. S., Clark, T. D., Steinem, C. and Ghadiri, M. R. (1999) Photoswitchable Hydrogen-Bonding in Self-Organized Cylindrical Peptide Systems. *Angew. Chemie - Int. Ed.* 38, pp. 1598–1601.
44. Seebach, D., Matthews, J. L., Meden, A., Wessels, T., Baerlocher, C. and McCusker, L. B. (1997) Cyclo-β-Peptides: Structure and Tubular Stacking of Cyclic Tetramers of 3-Aminobutanoic Acid as Determined from Powder Diffraction Data. *Helv. Chim. Acta* 80, pp. 173–182.
45. Clark, T. D., Buehler, L. K. and Ghadiri, M. R. (1998) Self-Assembling Cyclic β^3-Peptide Nanotubes as Artificial Transmembrane Ion Channels. *J. Am. Chem. Soc.* 120, pp. 651–656.
46. Fujimura, F., Hirata, T., Morita, T., Kimura, S., Horikawa, Y. and Sugiyama, J. (2006) Columnar Assembly of Cyclic β-Amino Acid Functionalized with Pyranose Rings. *Biomacromolecules*. 7, pp. 2394–2400.
47. Fujimura, F., Horikawa, Y., Morita, T., Sugiyama, J. and Kimura, S. (2007) Double Assembly Composed of Lectin Association with Columnar Molecular Assembly of Cyclic Tri-β-Peptide Having Sugar Units. *Biomacromolecules*. 8, pp. 611–616.
48. Tabata, Y., Mitani, S. and Kimura, S. (2016) Peptide Nanotube Aligning Side Chains onto One Side. *J. Pept. Sci.* 22, pp. 391–396.
49. Tabata, Y., Uji, H., Imai, T. and Kimura, S. (2018) Two One-Dimensional Arrays of Naphthyl and Anthryl Groups along Peptide Nanotubes Prepared

from Cyclic Peptides Comprising α- And β-Amino Acids. *Soft Matter* 14, pp. 7597–7604.

50. Amorín, M., Castedo, L. and Granja, J. R. (2003) New Cyclic Peptide Assemblies with Hydrophobic Cavities: The Structural and Thermodynamic Basis of a New Class of Peptide Nanotubes. *J. Am. Chem. Soc.* 125, pp. 2844–2845.
51. Amorín, M., Castedo, L. and Granja, J. R. (2005) Self-Assembled Peptide Tubelets with 7 Å Pores. *Chem. Eur. J.* 11, pp. 6543–6551.
52. Amorín, M., Brea, R. J., Castedo, L. and Granja, J. R. (2005) The Smallest α,γ-Peptide Nanotubulet Segments: Cyclic α,γ-Tetrapeptide Dimers. *Org. Lett.* 7, pp. 4681–4684.
53. Amorín, M., Villaverde, V., Castedo, L. and Granja, J. R. (2005) New α,γ-Peptide Tubulets. *J. Drug Deliv. Sci. Technol.* 15, pp. 87–92.
54. Amorín, M., Brea, R. J., Castedo, L. and Granja, J. R. (2006) Self-assembling cyclic α,γ-tetrapeptides. *Heterocycles.* 67, pp. 575–583.
55. García-Fandiño, R. and Granja, J. R. (2013) Effect of Organochloride Guest Molecules on the Stability of Homo/Hetero Self-Assembled α,γ-Cyclic Peptide Structures: A Computational Study toward the Control of Nanotube Length. *J. Phys. Chem. C.* 117, pp. 10143–10162.
56. Pizzi, A., Ozores, H. L., Calvelo, M., García-Fandiño, R., Amorín, M., Demitri, N., Terraneo, G., Bracco, S., Comotti, A., Sozzani, P., Bezuidenhout, C. X., Metrangolo, P. and Granja, J. R. (2019) Tight Xenon Confinement in a Crystalline Sandwich-like Hydrogen-Bonded Dimeric Capsule of a Cyclic Peptide. *Angew. Chemie Int. Ed.* 58, pp. 14472–14476.
57. Calvelo, M., Lamas, A., Guerra, A., Amorín M., Garcia-F andino, R., and Granja J. R. (2020) Parallel Versus Antiparallel β-Sheet Structure in Cyclic Peptide Hybrids Containing γ- or δ-Cyclic Amino Acids. *Chem. Eur. J.* 26, pp. 5846–5858.
58. Brea, R. J., Amorín, M., Castedo, L. and Granja, J. R. (2005) Methyl-Blocked Dimeric α,γ-Peptide Nanotube Segments: Formation of a Peptide Heterodimer through Backbone-Backbone Interactions. *Angew. Chemie Int. Ed.* 44 (35), pp. 5710–5713.
59. Brea, R. J., Castedo, L. and Granja, J. R. (2007) Large-Diameter Self-Assembled Dimers of α,γ-Cyclic Peptides, with the Nanotubular Solid-State Structure of Cyclo-[(*L*-Leu-*D*-^{Me}N-γ-Acp)4]·4CHCl2COOH. *Chem. Commun.* pp. 3267–3269.
60. Reiriz, C., Castedo, L. and Granja, J. R. (2008) New α,γ-Cyclic Peptides-Nanotube Molecular Caps Using α,α-Dialkylated α-Amino Acids. *J. Pept. Sci.* 14, pp. 241–249.
61. Brea, R. J., Pérez-Alvite, M. J., Panciera, M., Mosquera, M., Castedo, L. and Granja, J. R. (2011) Highly Efficient and Directional Homo And

Heterodimeric Energy Transfer Materials Based on Fluorescently Derivatized α,γ-Cyclic Octapeptides. *Chem. Asian J.* 6, pp. 110–121.

62. Brea, R. J., Eugenio Vázquez, M., Mosquera, M., Castedo, L. and Granja, J. R. (2007) Controlling Multiple Fluorescent Signal Output in Cyclic Peptide-Based Supramolecular Systems. *J. Am. Chem. Soc.* 129, pp. 1653–1657.
63. Brea, R. J., Castedo, L., Granja, J. R., Herranz, A. M., Sanchez, L., Martin, N., Seitz, W. and Guldi, D. M. (2007) Electron Transfer in Me-Blocked Heterodimeric α,γ-Peptide Nanotubular Donor–Acceptor Hybrids. *Proc. Natl. Acad. Sci.* 104, pp. 5291–5294.
64. Guerra, A., Brea, R. J., Amorín, M., Castedo, L. and Granja, J. R. (2012) Self-Assembling Properties of All γ-Cyclic Peptides Containing Sugar Amino Acid Residues. *Org. Biomol. Chem.* 10, pp. 8762–8766.
65. Li, L., Zhan, H., Duan, P., Liao, J., Quan, J., Hu, Y., Chen, Z., Zhu, J., Liu, M., Wu, Y. D. and Deng, J. (2012) Self-Assembling Nanotubes Consisting of Rigid Cyclic γ-Peptides. *Adv. Funct. Mater.* 22, pp. 3051–3056.
66. García-Fandiño, R., Amorín, M., Castedo, L. and Granja, J. R. (2012) Transmembrane Ion Transport by Self-Assembling α,γ-Peptide Nanotubes. *Chem. Sci.* 3, pp. 3280–3285.
67. García-Fandiño, R., Piñeiro, Á., Trick, J. L. and Sansom, M. S. P. (2016) Lipid Bilayer Membrane Perturbation by Embedded Nanopores: A Simulation Study. *ACS Nano* 10, pp. 3693–3701.
68. García-Fandiño, R., Granja, J. R., D'Abramo, M. and Orozco, M. (2009) Theoretical Characterization of the Dynamical Behavior and Transport Properties of α,γ-Peptide Nanotubes in Solution. *J. Am. Chem. Soc.* 131, pp. 15678–15686.
69. Wang, D., Guo, L., Zhang, J., Jones, L. R., Chen, Z., Pritchard, C. and Roeske, R.W. (2001) Artificial Ion Channels Formed by a Synthetic Cyclic Peptide. *J. Pept. Res.* 57, pp. 301–306.
70. Darnall, S. M., Li, C., Dunbar, M., Alsina, M. A., Keten, S., Helms, B. A. and Xu, T. (2019) Organic Nanotube with Subnanometer, PH-Responsive Lumen. *J. Am. Chem. Soc.* 141, pp. 10953–10957.
71. Reiriz, C., Amorín, M., García-Fandiño, R., Castedo, L. and Granja, J. R. (2009) α,γ-Cyclic Peptide Ensembles with a Hydroxylated Cavity. *Org. Biomol. Chem.* 7, pp. 4358–4361.
72. Rodríguez-Vázquez, N., Amorín, M., Alfonso, I. and Granja, J. R. (2016) Anion Recognition and Induced Self-Assembly of an α,γ-Cyclic Peptide to Form Spherical Clusters. *Angew. Chem. Int. Ed.* 55, pp. 4504–4508.
73. Rodríguez-Vázquez, N., García-Fandiño, R., Amorín, M. and Granja, J. R. (2016) Self-Assembling α,γ-Cyclic Peptides That Generate Cavities with Tunable Properties. *Chem. Sci.* 7, pp. 183–187.
74. Rodríguez-Vázquez, N., García-Fandiño, R., Aldegunde, M. J., Brea, J., Loza, M. I., Amorín, M. and Granja, J. R. (2017) Cis-Platinum Complex

Encapsulated in Self-Assembling Cyclic Peptide Dimers. *Org. Lett.* 19, pp. 2560–2563.

75. Calvelo, M., Vázquez, S. and García-Fandiño, R. (2015) Molecular Dynamics Simulations for Designing Biomimetic Pores Based on Internally Functionalized Self-Assembling α,γ-Peptide Nanotubes. *Phys. Chem. Chem. Phys.* 17, pp. 28586–28601.
76. Burade, S. S., Saha, T., Bhuma, N., Kumbhar, N., Kotmale, A., Rajamohanan, P. R., Gonnade, R. G., Talukdar, P. and Dhavale, D. D. (2017) Self-Assembly of Fluorinated Sugar Amino Acid Derived α,γ-Cyclic Peptides into Transmembrane Anion Transport. *Org. Lett.* 19, pp. 5948–5951.
77. Ruiz, L., Benjamin, A., Sullivan, M. and Keten, S. (2015) Regulating Ion Transport in Peptide Nanotubes by Tailoring the Nanotube Lumen Chemistry. *J. Phys. Chem. Lett.* 6, 15141520.
78. Gauthier, D., Baillargeon, P., Drouin, M. and Dory, Y. L. (2001) Self-Assembly of Cyclic Peptides into Nanotubes and Then into Highly Anisotropic Crystalline Material. *Angew. Chem. Int. Ed.* 40, pp. 4635–4638.
79. Marmin, T. and Dory, Y. L. (2019) Self-Assembly of C3 Symmetric Rigid Macrolactams into Very Polar and Porous Trigonal Crystals. *Chem. A Eur. J.* 25, pp. 6707–6711.
80. Leclair, S., Baillargeon, P., Skouta, R., Gauthier, D., Zhao, Y. and Dory, Y. L. (2004) Micrometer-Sized Hexagonal Tubes Self-Assembled by a Cyclic Peptide in a Liquid Crystal. *Angew. Chem. Int. Ed.* 43, pp. 349–353.
81. Horne, W. S., Stout, C. D. and Ghadiri, M. R. (2003) A Heterocyclic Peptide Nanotube. *J. Am. Chem. Soc.* 125, pp. 9372–9376.
82. Lamas, A., Guerra, A., Amorín, M. and Granja, J. R. (2018) New Self-Assembling Peptide Nanotubes of Large Diameter Using δ-Amino Acids. *Chem. Sci.* 9, pp. 8228–8233.
83. Semetey, V., Didierjean, C., Briand, J., Aubry, A. and Guichard, G. (2002) Self-Assembling Organic Nanotubes from Enantiopure Cyclo-N,N'-Linked Oligoureas: Design, Synthesis, and Crystal Structure. *Angew. Chem. Int. Ed.* 41, pp. 1895–1898.
84. Hennig, A., Fischer, L., Guichard, G. and Matile, S. (2009) Anion-Macrodipole Interactions: Self-Assembling Oligourea/Amide Macrocycles as Anion Transporters That Respond to Membrane Polarization. *J. Am. Chem. Soc.* 131, pp. 16889–16895.
85. López, J. L., Pérez, E. M., Viruela, P. M., Viruela, R., Ortí, E. and Martín, N. (2009) Controlled Self-Assembly of Electron Donor Nanotubes. *Org. Lett.* 11, pp. 4524–4527.
86. Ghorai, A., Reddy K, S., Achari, B. and Chattopadhyay, P. (2014) Rational Construction of Triazole/Urea Based Peptidomimetic Macrocycles as

Pseudocyclo-β-Peptides and Studies on Their Chirality Controlled Self-Assembly. *Org. Lett.* 16, pp. 3196–3199.

87. Kulsi, G., Ghorai, A., Achari, B. and Chattopadhyay, P. (2015) Design and Synthesis of Conformationally Homogeneous Pseudo Cyclic Peptides through Amino Acid Insertion: Investigations on Their Self Assembly. *RSC Adv.* 5, pp. 64675–64681.
88. Ranganathan, D., Lakshmi, C. and Karle, I. L. (1999) Hydrogen-Bonded Self-Assembled Peptide Nanotubes from Cystine-Based Macrocyclic Bisureas. *J. Am. Chem. Soc.* 121, pp. 6103–6107.
89. Ranganathan, D., Haridas, V., Sundari, C. S., Balasubramanian, D., Madhusudanan, K. P., Roy, R. and Karle, I. L. (1999) Design, Synthesis, Crystal Structure, and Host-Guest Properties of Polymethylene-Bridged Cystine-Based Cyclobisamides: A Facile Entry into Hydrogen-Bonded Peptide Nanotubes. *J. Org. Chem.* 64, pp. 9230–9240.
90. Ranganathan, D., Haridas, V., Gilardi, R. and Karle, I. L. (1998) Self-Assembling Aromatic-Bridged Serine-Based Cyclodepsipeptides (Serinophanes): A Demonstration of Tubular Structures Formed through Aromatic π-π Interactions. *J. Am. Chem. Soc.* 120, pp. 10793–10800.
91. Dawn, S., Dewal, M. B., Sobransingh, D., Paderes, M. C., Wibowo, A. C., Smith, M. D., Krause, J. A., Pellechia, P. J. and Shimizu, L. S. (2011) Self-Assembled Phenylethynylene Bis-Urea Macrocycles Facilitate the Selective Photodimerization of Coumarin. *J. Am. Chem. Soc.* 133, pp. 7025–7032.
92. Kittikhunnatham, P., Som, B., Rassolov, V., Stolte, M., Würthner, F., Shimizu, L. S. and Greytak, A. B. (2017) Fluorescence Polarization Measurements to Probe Alignment of a Bithiophene Dye in One-Dimensional Channels of Self-Assembled Phenylethynylene Bis-Urea Macrocycle Crystals. *J. Phys. Chem. C* 121, pp. 18102–18109.
93. Sánchez-Quesada, J., Kim, H. S. and Ghadiri, M. R. (2001) A Synthetic Pore-Mediated Transmembrane Transport of Glutamic Acid. *Angew. Chem. Int. Ed.* 40, pp. 2503–2506.
94. Liu, H., Chen, J., Shen, Q., Fu, W. and Wu, W. (2010) Molecular Insights on the Cyclic Peptide Nanotube-Mediated Transportation of Antitumor Drug 5-Fluorouracil. *Mol. Pharm.* 7, pp. 1985–1994.
95. Chen, J., Zhang, B., Xia, F., Xie, Y., Jiang, S., Su, R., Lu, Y. and Wu, W. (2016) Transmembrane Delivery of Anticancer Drugs through Self-Assembly of Cyclic Peptide Nanotubes. *Nanoscale* 8, pp. 7127–7136.
96. Sánchez-Quesada, J., Isler, M. P. and Ghadiri, M. R. (2002) Modulating Ion Channel Properties of Transmembrane Peptide Nanotubes through Heteromeric Supramolecular Assemblies. *J. Am. Chem. Soc.* 124, pp. 10004–10005.
97. Danial, M., Perrier, S. and Jolliffe, K. A. (2015) Effect of the Amino Acid Composition of Cyclic Peptides on Their Self-Assembly in Lipid Bilayers. *Org. Biomol. Chem.* 13, pp. 2464–2473.

98. Fletcher, J. T., Finlayc, J. A., Callow, E. M., Callowc, J. A. and Ghadiri, M. R. (2007) A Combinatorial Approach to the Discovery of Biocidal Six-Residue Cyclic *D,L-α*-Peptides Against Bacteria MRSA and *E. Coli.* and the Biofouling Algae Ulva Linza and Navicula Perminuta James. *Chem. Eur. J.* 13, pp. 4008–4013.
99. Horne, W. S., Wiethoff, C. M., Cui, C., Wilcoxen, K. M., Amorín, M., Ghadiri, M. R. and Nemerow, G. R. (2005) Antiviral Cyclic *D,L-α*-Peptides: Targeting a General Biochemical Pathway in Virus Infections. *Bioorg. Med. Chem.* 13, pp. 5145–5153.
100. Montero, A., Gastaminza, P., Law, M., Cheng, G., Chisari, F. V. and Ghadiri, M. R. (20111) Self-Assembling Peptide Nanotubes with Antiviral Activity against Hepatitis C Virus. *Chem. Biol.* 18, pp. 1453–1462.
101. Richman, M., Wilk, S., Chemerovski, M., Wärmländer, S. K. T. S., Wahlström, A., Gräslund, A. and Rahimipour, S. (2013) *In Vitro* and Mechanistic Studies of an Antiamyloidogenic Self-Assembled Cyclic *D,L-α*-Peptide Architecture. *J. Am. Chem. Soc.* 135, pp. 3474–3484.
102. Chemerovski-Glikman, M., Rozentur-Shkop, E., Richman, M., Grupi, A., Getler, A., Cohen, H. Y., Shaked, H., Wallin, C., Wärmländer, S. K. T. S., Haas, E., Gräslund, A., Chill, J. H. and Rahimipour, S. (2016) Self-Assembled Cyclic *D,L-α*-Peptides as Generic Conformational Inhibitors of the *α*-Synuclein Aggregation and Toxicity: *In vitro* and Mechanistic Studies. *Chem. Eur. J.* 22, pp. 14236–14246.
103. Zhao, Y., Leman, L. J., Search, D. J., Garcia, R. A., Gordon, D. A., Maryanoff, B. E. and Ghadiri, M. R. (2017) Self-Assembling Cyclic *D,L-α*-Peptides as Modulators of Plasma HDL Function. A Supramolecular Approach toward Antiatherosclerotic Agents. *ACS Cent. Sci.* 3, pp. 639–646.
104. Cui, H. and Xu, B. (2017) Supramolecular Medicine. *Chem. Soc. Rev.* 46, pp. 6430–6432.
105. Motiei, L., Rahimipour, S., Thayer, D. A., Wong, C. H. and Ghadiri, M. R. (2009) Antibacterial Cyclic *D,L-α*-Glycopeptides. *Chem. Commun.* pp. 3693–3695.
106. Horne, W. S., Ashkenasy, N. and Ghadiri, M. R. (2005) Modulating Charge Transfer through Cyclic *D,L-α*-Peptide Self-Assembly. *Chem. A Eur. J.* 11, pp. 1137–1144.
107. Ashkenasy, N., Horne, W. S. and Ghadiri, M. R. (2006) Design of Self-Assembling Peptide Nanotubes with Delocalized Electronic States. *Small*2, pp. 99–102.
108. Reiriz, C., Brea, R. J., Arranz, R., Carroscosa, J. L., Garibotti, A., Manning, B., Valpuesta, J. M., Eritija, R., Castedo, L. and Granja, J. R. (2009) *α,γ*-Peptide Nanotube Templating of One-Dimensional Parallel Fullerene. *J. Am. Chem. Soc.* 131, pp. 11335–11337.

109. Aragay, G., Ventura, B., Guerra, A., Pintre, I., Chiorboli, C., García-Fandiño, R., Flamigni, L., Granja, J. R. and Ballester, P. (2014) Self-Sorting of Cyclic Peptide Homodimers into a Heterodimeric Assembly Featuring an Efficient Photoinduced Intramolecular Electron-Transfer Process. *Chem. Eur. J.* **2014**, 20, pp. 3427–3438.
110. Hernández-Eguía, L. P., Brea, R. J., Castedo, L., Ballester, P. and Granja, J. R. (2011) Regioisomeric Control Induced by DABCO Coordination to Rotatable Self-Assembled Bis-and Tetraporphyrin α,γ-Cyclic Octapeptide Dimers. *Chem. Eur. J.* **2011**, 17, pp. 1220–1229.
111. Panciera, M., Amorín, M., Castedo, L. and Granja, J. R. (2013) Design of Stable β-Sheet-Based Cyclic Peptide Assemblies Assisted by Metal Coordination: Selective Homo- and Heterodimer Formation. *Chem. Eur. J.* 19, pp. 4826–4834.
112. Rizzuto, F. J., von Krbek, L. K. S. and Nitschke, J. R. (2019) Strategies for Binding Multiple Guests in Metal–Organic Cages. *Nat. Rev. Chem.* 3, pp. 204–222.
113. Ozores, H. L., Amorín, M. and Granja, J. R. (2017) Self-Assembling Molecular Capsules Based on α,γ-Cyclic Peptides. *J. Am. Chem. Soc.* 139, pp. 776–784.
114. Méndez-Ardoy, A., Granja, J. R. and Montenegro, J. (2018) pH-Triggered Self-Assembly and Hydrogelation of Cyclic Peptide Nanotubes Confined in Water Micro-Droplets. *Nanoscale Horizons* 3, pp. 391–396.
115. Silk, M. R., Mohanty, B., Sampson, J. B., Scanlon, M. J., Thompson, P. E. and Chalmers, D. K. (2019) Controlled Construction of Cyclic *D/L* Peptide Nanorods. *Angew. Chem. Int. Ed.* 58, pp. 596–601.
116. Ishihara, Y. and Kimura, S. (2013) Four-Peptide-Nanotube Bundle Formation by Self-Assembling of Cyclic Tetra-β-Peptide Using G-Quartet Motif. *Biopolymers* 100, pp. 141–147.
117. Matile, S., Vargas Jentzsch, A., Montenegro, J. and Fin, A. (2011) Recent Synthetic Transport Systems. *Chem. Soc. Rev.* 40, pp. 2453–2474.
118. Rodríguez-Vázquez, N., Fuertes, A., Amorín, M. and Granja, J. R. (2016) Bioinspired artificial sodium and potassium Ion channels. In: *The Alkali Metal Ions: Their Role for Life. Metal Ions in Life Sciences*, Sigel, A., Sigel, H. and Sigel, R., eds., vol. 16, pp. 485–556. Springer International, Cham, Switzerland.
119. Panciera, M., González-Freire, E., Calvelo, M., Amorín, M. and Granja, J. R. (2019) Induced α,γ-Cyclic Peptide Rotodimer Recognition by Nucleobase Scaffolds. *Pept. Sci.* 108. doi: 10.1002/pep2.24132.
120. Gauthier, M. A. and Klok, H. A. (2008) Peptide/Protein-Polymer Conjugates: Synthetic Strategies and Design Concepts. *Chem. Commun.* pp. 2591–2611.

121. Dehn, S., Chapman, R., Jolliffe, K. A. and Perrier, S. (2011) Synthetic Strategies for the Design of Peptide/Polymer Conjugates. *Polym. Rev.* 51, pp. 214–234.
122. Chapman, R., Jolliffe, K. A. and Perrier, S. (2011) Modular Design for the Controlled Production of Polymeric Nanotubes from Polymer/Peptide Conjugates. *Polym. Chem.* 2, pp. 1956–1963.
123. Larnaudie, S. C., Brendel, J. C., Jolliffe, K. A. and Perrier, S. (2016) Cyclic Peptide-Polymer Conjugates: Grafting-to vs Grafting-From. *J. Polym. Sci. Part A Polym. Chem.* 54, pp. 1003–1011.
124. Couet, J., Samuel, J. D. J. S., Kopyshev, A., Santer, S. and Biesalski, M. (2005) Peptide-Polymer Hybrid Nanotubes. *Angew. Chem. Int. Ed.* 44, pp. 3297–3301.
125. Couet, J. and Biesalski, M. (2008) Polymer-Wrapped Peptide Nanotubes: Peptide-Grafted Polymer Mass Impacts Length and Diameter. *Small* 4, pp. 1008–1016.
126. Couet, J. and Biesalski, M. (2006) Surface-Initiated ATRP of N-Isopropylacrylamide from Initiator-Modified Self-Assembled Peptide Nanotubes. *Macromolecules* 39, pp. 7258–7268.
127. Loschonsky, S., Couet, J. and Biesalski, M. (2008) Synthesis of Peptide/Polymer Conjugates by Solution ATRP of Butylacrylate Using an Initiator-Modified Cyclic *D-Alt-L*-Peptide. *Macromol. Rapid Commun.* 29, pp. 309–315.
128. Ten Cate, M. G. J., Severin, N. and Börner, H. G. (2006) Self-Assembling Peptide-Polymer Conjugates Comprising (*D-Alt-L*)- Cyclopeptides as Aggregator Domains. *Macromolecules* 39, pp. 7831–7838.
129. Chapman, R., Jolliffe, K. A. and Perrier, S. (2010) Synthesis of Self-Assembling Cyclic Peptide-Polymer Conjugates Using Click Chemistry. *Aust. J. Chem.* 63, pp. 1169–1172.
130. Chapman, R., Koh, M. L., Warr, G. G., Jolliffe, K. A. and Perrier, S. (2013) Structure Elucidation and Control of Cyclic Peptide-Derived Nanotube Assemblies in Solution. *Chem. Sci.* 4, pp. 2581–2589.
131. Chapman, R., Jolliffe, K. A. and Perrier, S. (2013) Multi-Shell Soft Nanotubes from Cyclic Peptide Templates. *Adv. Mater.* 25, pp. 1170–1172.
132. Catrouillet, S., Brendel, J. C., Larnaudie, S., Barlow, T., Jolliffe, K. A. and Perrier, S. (2016) Tunable Length of Cyclic Peptide-Polymer Conjugate Self-Assemblies in Water. *ACS Macro Lett.* 5, pp. 1119–1123.
133. Chapman, R., Warr, G. G., Perrier, S. and Jolliffe, K. A. (2013) Water-Soluble and pH-Responsive Polymeric Nanotubes from Cyclic Peptide Templates. *Chem. Eur. J.* 19, pp. 1955–1961.
134. Chapman, R., Bouten, P. J. M., Hoogenboom, R., Jolliffe, K. A. and Perrier, S. (2013) Thermoresponsive Cyclic Peptide-Poly(2-Ethyl-2-Oxazoline) Conjugate Nanotubes. *Chem. Commun.* 49, pp. 6522–6524.

135. Blunden, B. M., Chapman, R., Danial, M., Lu, H., Jolliffe, K. A., Perrier, S. and Stenzel, M. H. (2014) Drug Conjugation to Cyclic Peptide-Polymer Self-Assembling Nanotubes. *Chem. Eur. J.* 20, pp. 12745–12749.
136. Larnaudie, S. C., Brendel, J. C., Romero-Canelón, I., Sanchez-Cano, C., Catrouillet, S., Sanchis, J., Coverdale, J. P. C., Song, J. I., Habtemariam, A., Sadler, P. J., Jolliffe, K. A. and Perrier, S. (2018) Cyclic Peptide-Polymer Nanotubes as Efficient and Highly Potent Drug Delivery Systems for Organometallic Anticancer Complexes. *Biomacromolecules* 19, pp. 239–247.
137. Danial, M., Tran, C. M., Young, P. G., Perrier, S. and Jolliffe, K. A. (2013) Janus Cyclic Peptide-Polymer Nanotubes. *Nat. Commun.* 4, 2780. doi: 10.1038/ncomms3780.
138. Danial, M., Tran, C. M. N., Jolliffe, K. A. and Perrier, S. (2014) Thermal Gating in Lipid Membranes Using Thermoresponsive Cyclic Peptide-Polymer Conjugates. *J. Am. Chem. Soc.* 136, pp. 8018–8026.
139. Song, Q., Yang, J., Rho, J. Y. and Perrier, S. (2019) Supramolecular Switching of the Self-Assembly of Cyclic Peptide-Polymer Conjugates: Via Host-Guest Chemistry. *Chem. Commun.* 55, pp. 5291–5294.
140. Hartlieb, M., Catrouillet, S., Kuroki, A., Sanchez-Cano, C., Peltier, R. and Perrier, S. (2019) Stimuli-Responsive Membrane Activity of Cyclic-Peptide-Polymer Conjugates. *Chem. Sci.* 10, pp. 5476–5483.
141. Rho, J. Y., Brendel, J. C., MacFarlane, L. R., Mansfield, E. D. H., Peltier, R., Rogers, S., Hartlieb, M. and Perrier, S. (2018) Probing the Dynamic Nature of Self-Assembling Cyclic Peptide–Polymer Nanotubes in Solution and in Mammalian Cells. *Adv. Funct. Mater.* 28, 1704569.
142. Rho, J. Y., Cox, H., Mansfield, E. D. H., Ellacott, S. H., Peltier, R., Brendel, J. C., Hartlieb, M., Waigh, T. A. and Perrier, S. (2019) Dual Self-Assembly of Supramolecular Peptide Nanotubes to Provide Stabilisation in Water. *Nat. Commun.* 10, 4708. doi:10.1038/s41467-019-12586-8.
143. Montenegro, J., Vázquez-Vázquez, C., Kalinin, A., Geckeler, K. E. and Granja, J. R. (2014) Coupling of Carbon and Peptide Nanotubes. *J. Am. Chem. Soc.* 136, pp. 2484–2491.
144. Cuerva, M., García-Fandiño, R., Vázquez-Vázquez, C., López-Quintela, M. A., Montenegro, J. and Granja, J. R. (2015) Self-Assembly of Silver Metal Clusters of Small Atomicity on Cyclic Peptide Nanotubes. *ACS Nano* 9, pp. 10834–10843.
145. Wang, Y., Yi, S., Sun, L., Huang, Y., Lenaghan, S. C. and Zhang, M. (2014) Doxorubicin-Loaded Cyclic Peptide Nanotube Bundles Overcome Chemoresistance in Breast Cancer Cells. *J. Biomed. Nanotechnol.* 10, pp. 445–454.
146. Li, M., Ehlers, M., Schlesiger, S., Zellermann, E., Knauer, S. K. and Schmuck, C. (2016) Incorporation of a Non-Natural Arginine Analogue

into a Cyclic Peptide Leads to Formation of Positively Charged Nanofibers Capable of Gene Transfection. *Angew. Chem. Int. Ed.* 55, pp. 598–601.

147. Hsieh, W., Chang, S., Chen, H., Chen, J. and Liaw, J. (2012) Oral Gene Delivery with Cyclo-(*D*-Trp-*L*-Tyr-) Peptide Nanotubes. *Mol. Pharm.* 9, pp. 1231–1249.
148. Fuertes, A., Amorin, M. and Granja, J. R. (2019) Versatile Symport Transporters Based on Cyclic Peptide Dimers. *Chem. Commun.* 56, pp. 46–49.
149. Fuertes, A., Ozores, H. L., Amorín, M. and Granja, J. R. (2017) Self-Assembling Venturi-like Peptide Nanotubes. *Nanoscale* 9, pp. 748–753.
150. Insua, I. and Montenegro, J. (2019) 1D to 2D Self Assembly of Cyclic Peptides. *J. Am. Chem. Soc.* 142, pp. 300–307.

https://doi.org/10.1142/9789811261664_0005

Chapter 5

Peptide- and Protein-based Nanomaterials for Theranostics

Pascal Tomasella, Lorena Maria Cucci, Vanessa Sanfilippo, and Cristina Satriano*

Laboratory of Nano Hybrid BioInterfaces (NHBIL), Department of Chemical Sciences, University of Catania, Catania, Italy

**cristina.satriano@unict.it*

1. Introduction: Nanotechnology for Biomedical Engineering

Nanotechnology is a multidisciplinary field that combines various disciplines including chemistry, bioengineering, biology and medicine, and is defined as the understanding and application of knowledge tools from nanosciences to manipulate the matter on a molecular and atomic scale [1,2].

At the nanoscale level, the material's properties are different than at the 'bulk' scale, resulting in new and interesting applications. For instance, the application of nanotechnology to medicine, commonly namely 'nanomedicine', has the potential to improve therapy and medical treatments [2]. The continued development of nanomedicines has the potential to provide numerous benefits, including improved efficacy, bioavailability, dose response, targeting ability, personalization, and safety compared to conventional medicines as well as the ability to facilitate controlled drug release [2].

Rapid advances and emerging technologies in nanoscale systems, particularly nanoparticles (NPs), are having a profound impact on cancer diagnosis, treatment and monitoring, because of their ability to detect cancer cells, provide chemotherapeutic agents and monitor treatment response [3]. In recent years, hybrid nano-biomaterials have received significant attention in the biomedical field for various approaches such as delivery of active molecules and imaging agents for diagnosis, monitoring, control, prevention, and treatment of diseases [4,5].

Nanomaterials (NMs) fall into a size range similar to proteins and other macromolecular structures found inside living cells. As such, NMs easily pass through physiological barriers increasing specificity to desired cell types, tissue or other compartments and gaining access to intracellular structures thereby mediating molecular interactions [6].

Proteins and peptides are essential molecules for life and play a pivotal role in regulating and integrating vital processes, by acting with high specificity and potency. Due to their biocompatibility and biodegradability as well as their involvement in physio-pathological processes, proteins and peptides can be attractive therapeutic agents for development of delivery systems [7,8]. In addition, proteins such as fibrin, collagen, silk fibroin, keratin, casein and albumin are also the main candidates for tissue engineering materials, owing to their features, including the high biodegradation and bioresorbability as well as their intrinsic physicochemical and biological properties, such as (visco)elasticity adhesiveness, flexibility, and mechanical strength [9]. Peptides and proteins have been used as biorecognition elements in biological analysis and fabrication of efficient biosensors due to their different structures which allow to selectively bind to analytes including proteins, nucleic acid, bacteria, metal ions, enzymes and antibodies [10].

Hence, manifold opportunities emerge by the use of protein and peptide-based materials in nanomedicine for the development of unusually versatile composites. Also, their assembly in hybrid peptide/protein-nanomaterials (P-NM) composites allows the engineering, in a medically-oriented exploitable way, of the interplay between the protein biological activity and the nanomaterial features, including optical, electric, magnetic properties mechanic properties.

We revise here the fundamental classification and properties of protein and peptide-based NMs as well as the diverse applications of nanomedicine where they are used on the basis of their advanced and versatile ability to interact with or modify substrates or biological targets.

2. Nanomaterials and Nanomedicine

In consideration of what has been said about the exact definition of NMs and their importance in biotechnology, there is a need to classify nano-sized materials for a better understanding of their properties. Two possible ways to do this are to differentiate them according to their dimensionality and their chemical structure.

2.1. *NMs classification: Dimensionality*

The first categorization of NMs can be made on the basis of their dimensionality [11] (Figure 1).

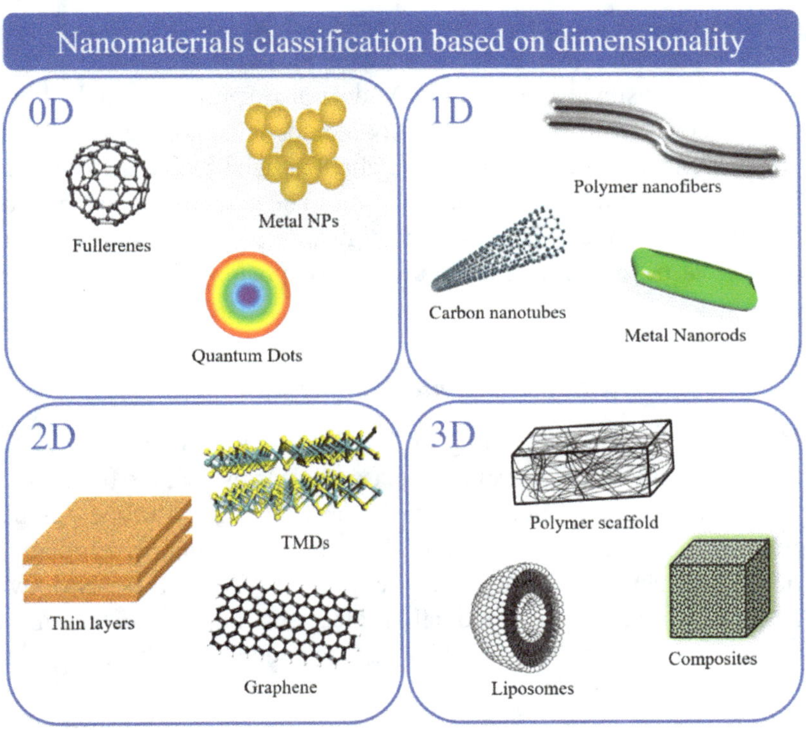

Fig. 1. Dimensionality-based classification of NMs (0D, 1D, 2D and 3D).

Materials that have all three dimensions in the nanoscale range, that is generally from 1 to 100 nm, are classified as zero-dimensional (0D). Here, we can include small organic molecules, fullerenes [12], semi-conductor quantum-dots [13] and various shaped NPs such as nano-spheres, nanocubes, nanotriangles and nanostars [14].

One-dimensional (1D) nanostructures are characterized by exhibiting the size-effects only in two of the three dimensions, while the third is generally of few micrometers. This includes nanoribbons [15], fibers, single wall or multi-wall carbon nanotubes (SWCNT or MWCNT) and metal nanorods.

Systems where the quantum size-related effects are confined only in one dimension are classified as two-dimensional (2D) NMs. They may comprise polymeric, ceramic or composites thin films and nanocoatings. Another class of 2D materials is nanoplates that have seen growing interest in biotechnological applications, especially for graphene and graphene-like materials such as graphene oxide (GO) [16,17], boron nitride nanosheets (BN) and transition metal dichalcogenides (TMDs) like MoS_2 [18] or WS_2 [19]. TMDs are made of a single layer crystal that is described by the formula MX_2, where M is a transition metal (Mo, W, Zr and so on) and X is a chalcogen (S, Se and Te).

Three-dimensional materials (3D) do not display 'external' dimensions at the nanoscale but may certainly include nanostructured and composites materials. Nanocomposites are characterized by having one phase with at least one dimension at the nanoscale. The main difference between composites and nanocomposites is the high surface-to-volume ratio of the nanofillers dispersed in the matrix of nanocomposites [20].

2.2. *NMs classification: Chemical structure*

NMs can be classified according to their chemical structure. Metal NPs represent probably the most relevant class of NMs used at the biointerface and they have received great attention due to the novel properties they show at the nanoscale. In particular, they are extraordinarily efficient ad absorbing and scattering light. The strong interaction of these NMs with light occurs because the conduction electrons on the metal surface undergo a collective oscillation when excited by light at specific wavelengths.

Such phenomenon is known as surface plasmon resonance (SPR) [21], and it is the most investigated property for biotechnological applications because of its easy tunability according to shape, size and surface modification of metal NPs [22].

Gold nanoparticles (AuNPs) are used in nanoelectronics, biosensing, imaging, heat generation (photothermal effect), drug delivery and cancer therapy [14,23,24]. To note, nanogold is intrinsically anti-angiogenic, and the surface tailoring of the metal nanoparticle by proteins and/or peptides has been demonstrated to be a promising strategy to enhance selective cytotoxicity against cancer cells [25–27]. Nanosilver is utilized in antibacterial, medical diagnostic, electrochemical biosensor, catalysis, and optical application [28]. Peptide-tailored silver nanoparticles (AgNP) have been demonstrated to be very promising as a multifaceted platform in applications with cells and bacteria [29]. Copper is applied as antimicrobial and antifungal agent [30] and as bioinorganic catalyst [31];

The second class of NMs is constituted of metal oxides which includes zinc oxide, copper oxide, titanium oxide, cerium oxide and aluminium oxide, which have been largely exploited in conjugation with proteins and peptide for biological applications.

Iron and its oxides (FeO, Fe_2O_3) have been witnessing great interest due to the unique property that they have at the nanosize, known as supermagnetism. For instance, peptide-based functionalization of Fe_3O_4 magnetic NPs can be used for enhanced cell internalization [32]. The biotechnological and biomedical applications that exploit iron, as well as platinum and cobalt magnetic nanosystems, can be counted for magnetic separation of biological materials, drug delivery, for magnetic resonance imaging (MRI) contrast agent and hyperthermia treatment [33,34]. A detailed discussion on peptide- and protein-based metal nanoparticles for drug delivery and biosensing applications is provided in Sections 1.4.1 and 1.4.3, respectively.

Zinc(II) oxide (ZnO) is used as an antibacterial agent [35] and in cosmetic applications, such as UV filter [36], or in biosensing, tissue regeneration, bioimaging and drug delivery. Zou *et al.* for instance, have synthetized silk-fibroin covered Co-doped-ZnO NPs with high magnetization and cellular compatibility for MRI application [37]. Also, ZnO NPs conjugated with hydrophobic peptides have been developed as high efficient anticancer drugs against human colon adenorectal carcinoma cells [38].

Copper(II) oxide (CuO), known for its antifungal and antimicrobial activity, is commonly used in the cosmetic and textile industries as well as in tissue regeneration therapy [39]. For instance, peptide-coated CuO nanoparticles, using a novel cyclic peptide i.e., the CuO-binding peptide 1 (CuBP1), have been synthetized by Ishida *et al.* as potential safe antimicrobial agents with low cytotoxic activity against beneficial microflora (e.g., *E. coli* and *Lactobacillus helveticus*) and human cells [40]. Titanium(IV) dioxide (TiO_2), also known as titania, exhibits bio-related applications such as phototherapy for cancer treatment, drug delivery system, cell imaging and biosensing, genetic engineering as well as biomedical implant for which peptide surface modification has been demonstrated to enhance cell attachment biocompatibility [41,42]. Cerium oxide is used as an antioxidant agent thanks to its enzyme-mimetic activity due to the coexistence of both Ce(III) and Ce(IV) ions on the nanoparticle surface [43]. Cerium oxide NPs were successfully conjugated with antibodies for specific targeting of Aβ aggregates with high capability to modulate neuronal survival pathways [44]. Aluminium oxide or nanoalumina (Al_2O_3) is employed in protein/drug delivery system, cancer therapy as well as in bone tissue engineering [45]. In this regard, α-alumina nanoparticles when functionalized with the vasoactive intestinal peptide (VIP) have been proven effective for the treatment of asthma [46].

Surface functionalized silica nanoparticles were also employed as drug delivery platforms for targeted drug release, biosensor and imaging agent [47–49].

As an example, peptide-decorated doxorubicin (DOX)-loaded mesoporous silica nanoparticles have been proven to be highly efficient as targeted drug delivery system for bladder cancer therapy [50]. For instance, Slowing *et al.* developed cytochrome *c*-encapsulated silica nanoparticles as a transmembrane delivery vehicle for a controlled release of impermeable proteins in living cells for theranostics and metabolic manipulation of cells [51].

Bioceramics are at the center of the research for bones tissues' regenerative therapy and prothesis. They conventionally belong to the class of materials such as alumina, zirconium dioxide (ZrO_2), better known as zirconia, titania, hydroxyapatite (HA) ($Ca_{10}(PO_4)(OH)_2$), calcium silicate ($CaSiO_3$) calcium carbonate ($CaCO_3$) and silica (SiO_2) [52].

Very often, these materials are used in conjugation with proteins and peptides. For instance, it was reported that human bone morphogenetic protein-2 (rhBMP-2) was successfully loaded on calcium/magnesium-doped mesoporous silica scaffolds and preliminarily applied for bone regeneration [53]. Shin-Hee Jun *et al.* developed silica xerogel-chitosan hybrid as a coating material to incorporate bone morphogenic protein-2

(BMP-2) on porous HA scaffold for bone tissue engineering [54]. Porous alumina substrates functionalized with BMP2 protein were also proved beneficial for cell growth and osteogenic differentiation [55]. Self-assembled peptide-HA composites have been extensively used as carriers for protein immobilization in biosensing and as enzyme-stabilizing agents [56]. Besides, typical natural polymers like collagen, gelatine, alginate and chitosan have been incorporated into HA obtaining scaffolds to improve tissue regeneration and repair [57].

Carbon-based nanomaterials (CBNs) represent, probably, one of the most important classes of nanomaterials due to their unique physical and chemical properties (e.g., electric and thermal conductivity, mechanical strength and optical properties). Herein, we can mention graphene, consisting of a single layer of hexagonal arrays of sp^2 carbon atoms and its derivates graphene oxide and reduced graphene oxide (rGO); carbon nanotubes (CNT) and carbon nanofibers made up by cylindrical carbon structure whose properties depend on length, diameter, chirality and single or multi-walled; and fullerenes, characterized by symmetric close-caged of sp^2 carbon structure whose properties depend on the number of carbon atoms. The most common CBNs are spherical C_{60} and elliptical C_{70} fullerenes. Carbon nanodiamonds, unlike other CBNs, are characterized by nanocluster of sp^3 carbon atoms and have similar optical properties than the bulk material. CBNs are gaining importance in biomedical and biotechnological research including drug delivery system, tissue 3D scaffold, biosensing and imaging. Promising applications are expected also in the field of bio-mechatronic [58]. As to GO, it has been largely used as a matrix for protein immobilization in different biotechnological applications such as fluorescence- or electrochemical-based sensors, labeling and imaging, therapy, and targeted delivery [59]. For instance, Guo *et al.* developed a complex of GO and the protein Herceptin, with high stability under ionic conditions as well as near-infrared excitation properties and non-photobleaching features, as excellent bio-probe for live cell imaging [60]. Moreover, it has been demonstrated that GO sheets coated with serum proteins upon their entrance into a biological matrix (corona) delay the Aβ fibrillation in neurodegenerative diseases *via* adsorption of amyloid monomers, thus decreasing the kinetic reaction [61]. A high capability to locally dissociate amyloid peptide aggregates has been found by using thioflavin-modified GO and NIR laser irradiation [62]. Similarly, CNT–protein conjugates have been found very advantageous in biosensor fabrication, drug delivery, and cancer therapy.

For example, streptavidin-coated CNT were successfully used for cancer therapy, with no cytotoxic effects to the nearby normal cells [63]. As to fullerene, its derivatives with amino acids and peptides are of great interest as antiviral, antibacterial, antiapoptotic, neuroprotective, antitumor agents. For instance, Kotelnikova *et al.* have demonstrated *in vitro* that amino acid derivatives of fullerene can penetrate through biological membranes and get inserted into hydrophobic domains of proteins, thus altering the function of membrane-bound enzymes and the rate of redox processes, which determines the pharmacological activities of these compounds. In particular, a study on the anti-HIV effect of sodium C_{60} fullerene-ε-aminocaprote demonstrated its inhibition property on the activity of HIV protease which is crucial for the synthesis and assembly of viral particles [64].

Similar to GO nanosheets, also, TMDs have been shown intriguing properties as 2D NMs, such as the tunability of plasmonic and vibrational properties depending on the number and dimensions of layers, thermal- and thermoelectrical control, exceptional strain limit, high elastic modulus, piezoelectric behavior and, additionally to these, greater biocompatibility than many other nanostructures, making these valuable candidates to future applications in the field of biosensing, imaging, drug delivery system and tissue engineering [65].

The last class includes polymeric NMs whose applications have witnessed a growing development in all areas of nanotechnology. According to their origins, polymers can be divided into natural polymers (e.g., chitosan, alginate, cellulose, starch, lignin, proteins, DNA, RNA) biosynthetic polymers (e.g., polyhydroxyl butyrate, PHB) and chemosynthetic polymers (e.g., poly ε-caprolactone, PCL; poly lactic acid, PLA, poly urethane, PU; polylactic-co-glycolic acid, PLGA, polymethylmethacrylate, PMMA; poly-*N*-isopropylacrylamide, PNIPAM). The increasing interest of polymer-based nanomaterials in biomedicine and biotechnology can be attributed to their easily tailorable properties according to the physical and chemical properties of constituent monomers, size and shape of macromolecules and the possibility to chemically or physically functionalize polymer chain with organic or inorganic bioactive molecules. For example, hybrid molecule-nanoparticle systems based on PEGylate porphyrins suitable for applications in the biomedical field were developed thanks to the solubility of the porphyrinic systems in the biological environment [66]. The main fields of applicability for polymer-based NMs comprise nanoporous membranes for bioanalytic [67], vaccines and drugs delivery systems [68], self-standing scaffold for tissue and bonds engineering (see Section 1.4.2 for a more detailed discussion), and bio-compatible thin films for biomedical implants [69].

3. Nanomedicine: The Application of Nanoscience and Nanotechnology to the Biomedical Field

Nanomedicine involves the development and application of materials and technologies with nanometer length scales for the diagnosis, monitoring, control, prevention, and treatment of disease (Figure 2). In particular, it is especially promising in drug delivery targeted at specific sites in the body, for the delivery of compounds applied in tissue engineering and to

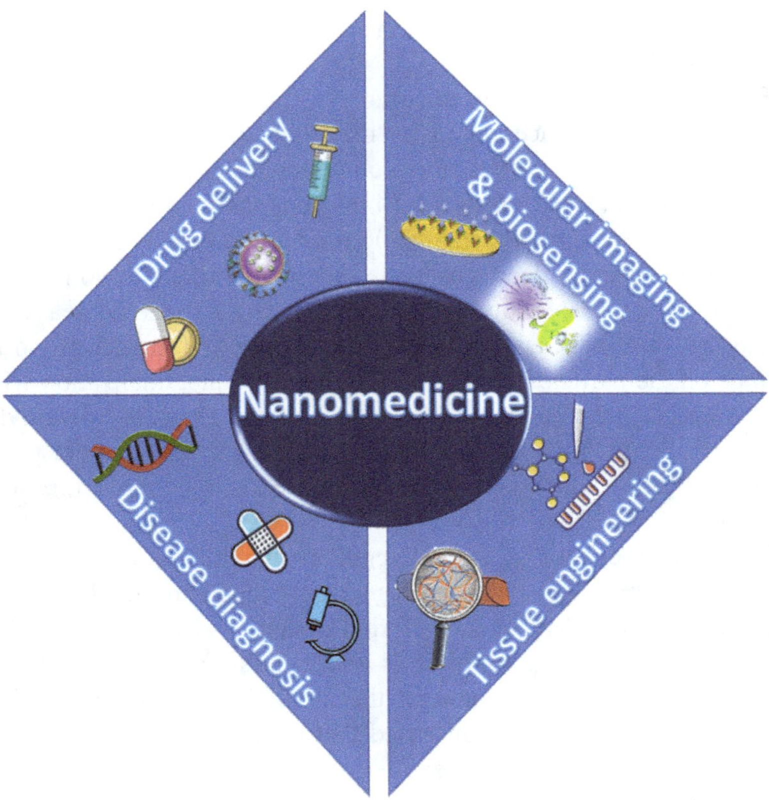

Fig. 2. Schematic illustration of the present applications of nanomedicine.

develop new biosensing and molecular imaging tools [70–72]. Indeed, nanomedicine aims to develop multifaceted systems that are able to load a cargo of hydrophobic and/or hydrophilic drugs and deliver it in a way that improves their biodistribution, pharmacokinetics and side effects.

Specifically for drug delivery, one can use different strategies, including passive targeting, active targeting and triggered drug release, i.e., 'smart' stimuli responsive materials [73]. Such strategies allow for decreasing the accumulation in off-target tissues, hence lead to an improved therapeutic index. On the contrary, conventional anticancer chemotherapeutics may present several issues, including poor specificity, high toxicity and induction of drug resistance.

It is noteworthy that the nanosystems, such as polymeric or metallic NPs, liposomes, quantum dots (QDs), carbon dots (C-dots) and CNTs, can improve the accumulation, internalization and therapeutic efficacy of the drugs allowing for a controlled release of the active compounds, improving their bioavailability, pharmacokinetics and also protecting them from degradation [74–76].

For an efficient targeting, nanocarriers require specific features such as dimension and surface chemistry including surface charge and functionalization, which also affect the blood circulation time.

Indeed, particles with a size $\leq$ 5 nm are quickly eliminated via renal filtration while those with a size $\geq$ 200 nm tend to rapidly accumulate in organs such as liver, spleen and lungs. The high surface-to-volume ratio is an intrinsic characteristic of NMs: as the particle size decreases, the total surface area increases exponentially leading to a greater proportion of atoms on the particle surface. This allows the functionalization with a variety of molecules, polymer-like dextran, starch, citrate or polyethylene glycol (PEG) which also ensure steric stabilization and prevent plasma protein adsorption which can further influence the targeting ability of the nanosystem [2,77,78].

The surface charge of an NM regulates its ability to cross the cell membrane and biological barriers (e.g., brain-blood barrier, BBB) as well as its biodistribution and the adsorption of ions and biomolecules [79]. For instance, surface coating of NMs with neutral hydrophilic polymers, such as PEG, is necessary to increase the circulation half-life times of NPs [78,80]. Soo Choi *et al.* demonstrated that core-shell QDs of CdSe-ZnS coated with anionic, cationic, zwitterionic or neutral small molecules exhibit an increased urinary excretion and prevent the unspecific adsorption of serum proteins [81].

Furthermore, NMs can be functionalized with recognition motifs, like ligands including small molecules, peptides and proteins (e.g., folic acid, RGD and transferrin, respectively), allowing for a specific binding to receptors expressed at the target site, such as the tumor cells [82–84]. For instance, the anti-angiogenic gold nanoparticles functionalized with angiogenin mimicking-peptides are able to modulate the angiogenic processes for brain cancer treatment [27]. Liposomes are a class of NMs that can be used for the targeted release of therapeutic agents. Tan *et al.* used immunosuppressive neuropeptides encapsulated within liposomes as a promising system to treat ocular inflammation [85]. Also, self-assembling peptide nanostructures may offer several potentialities as delivery systems. Alves *et al.* demonstrated that diphenylalanine (FF)-based microtubes perform as good drug delivery vehicles, due to their low *in vitro* toxicity, the very high thermal stability (up to 120°C) and resistance towards protease degradation [86]. Moreover, FF peptide-based nanofibers have also been proposed as vehicles of hydrophobic drugs, like hydroxycamphothecin, for cancer therapy [87]. Similarly, GO nanosheets tailored with the dipeptides of phenylalanine and tyrosine have been recently set up as nanoassemblies for a tunable interaction with (model and true) cell membranes [17,88].

Tissue engineering is the discipline that uses cells, bioengineering, biochemical, physicochemical and materials methods to repair, improve or replace biological tissues (i.e., bone, cartilage, blood vessels, skin, and muscle). Tissue engineering generally requires the application of combinations of biomaterials, cells and biochemically active factors whose purpose is to gain tissue formation both for *in vitro* or *ex vivo* growth in tissue culture or for *in vivo* tissue regeneration [89]. In recent years, NMs have been increasingly studied for tissue engineering and regenerative medicine.

Many NMs can be used as carriers and/or scaffolds for tissue regeneration and fabrication of hybrid biocomposites with multifunctional features depending on the different 'bricks' used to assemble the bioengineered nanoconstruct. Polymeric 3D scaffolds (e.g., proteins) play an essential role in tissue engineering because they provide structure to support cell differentiation and subsequent tissue growth. An ideal scaffold is a transient structure that must have definite properties such as biodegradability, i.e., must be controlled degraded or resorbed within a certain amount of time and replaced by the tissue of interest; must be easily tailored to provide mechanical support and biological signals to promote and increase cells attachment and growth and must seek to mimic ECM (Extra Cellular Matrix) microenvironment to induce or support tissue formation [90]. To this purpose, it is possible to functionalize the material in such a way to incorporate a peptide that displays a specific binding sequence such as arginine-glycine-aspartic acid (RGD) and RGDS motifs, which are prominent in adhesion proteins like fibronectin and fibrinogen, but also structural proteins such as collagen and laminin [91].

Several different methods of synthesis have been described in the literature for preparing porous structures to be employed as scaffolds for tissue engineering including nanofiber self-assembly [92], solvent casting and particulate leaching [93], thermally induced phase separation [94] and electrospinning [95]. Ulijn *et al.* selected FF dipeptides linked to fluorenylmethoxycarbonyl (FF-Fmoc) as scaffold materials in 3D cell culture because is one of the first dipeptides able to form a homogeneous, transparent, self-supporting hydrogel with fibrous nanostructure under physiological conditions for potential use in biological applications, such as tissue engineering and cell culture [96].

Moreover, synthetic polymers such as PLA, PGA, PCL and PHB have also emerged as potential sources for nanocomposite scaffolds due to their good mechanical strength and amiable nature enabling desired shape and degradation rate [97].

Another area of application of NMs is biosensing. Indeed, a new promising trend for the development of biosensing devices is the use of nanoscale materials due to their unique physical and chemical properties.

According to IUPAC, a biosensor is an analytical device characterized by a sensitive biological recognition component and a physicochemical transducer capable of providing specific qualitative, quantitative or semi-quantitative analytical information about target molecules [98,99] (Figure 3). In general, the response arises from the transformation of biological reactions into a detectable and measurable signal that is used for qualitative and quantitative analysis.

A biological element typically includes proteins, nucleic acids, receptors as well as cells, tissue, biomimetic structures or even living microorganisms, such as viruses and bacteria. On the other hand, the transducer depends on the signal that is required to quantify and mainly uses optical and electrochemical systems. It could be electric current, intensity and phase of electromagnetic radiations, electric potential, mass, conductance,

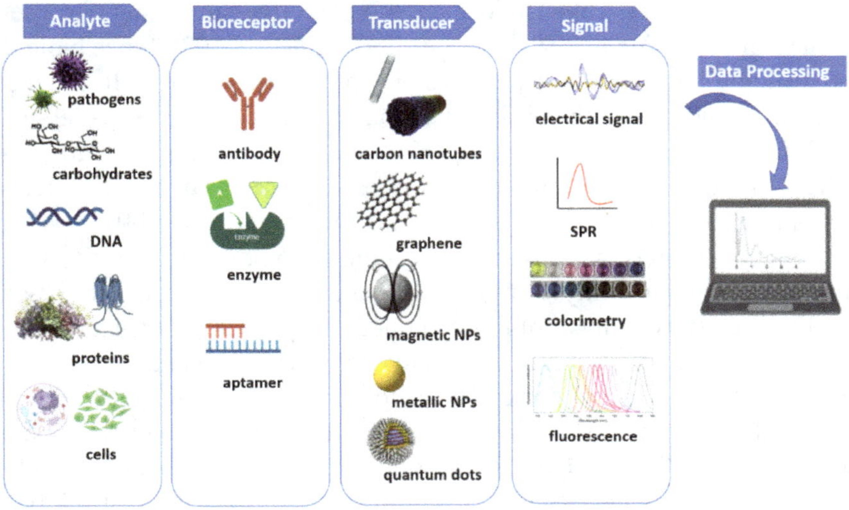

Fig. 3. Schematic diagram of nanomaterial-based biosensors for detection of analytes.

temperature but also viscosity. The produced signal can be directly or inversely proportional to the concentration of the target analyte [98].

Typical characteristics of biosensors include: (i) linearity, which is defined as the maximum output signal that can be detected by the sensor; (ii) sensitivity, which is related to the magnitude of electrode response *per* unit of analyte concentration; (iii) selectivity, which is defined as the ability of the sensor to discriminate the target compound from other interfering molecules, chemicals and materials; (iv) stability, which is related to the response of the sensor over a period of time; and (v) low limit of detection (LOD), which is the smallest amount of molecule that can be detected with respect to the control by the sensor. Moreover, cost-saving, simple operation and real-time analysis are other additional features that should characterize a worthy biosensor.

Wang and co-workers designed a novel electrochemical biosensor, based on zwitterionic peptide anchored to a conducting polymer, for the determination of breast cancer marker BRCA1 [100], while Arya *et al.* proposed the use of a coiled-coil peptide (CCP)-modified microelectrode array to develop an electrochemical biosensor for antibody detection [101]. Moreover, self-assembled hydrogels generated from FF-Fmoc can encapsulate various enzyme bioreceptors like glucose oxidase and fluorescent reporters, like CdTe and CdSe QDs, for biosensing purposes, such as the detection of analytes for example glucose [102]. Since biological building blocks such as peptides or proteins are able to self-organize into nanostructures with particular properties, there are also several possibilities for their use to develop high sensitive biosensing platforms, other than medical applications such as cardiovascular disease, diabetes, wound healing, cancer diagnosis, and prosthesis fabrication [103,104].

The spectrum of biosensors application, owing to their multifunctionality and high versatility, is rather wide and includes agriculture for the quality and safety analysis of food products, but also environmental monitoring of toxic compounds and above all medicine and heath care. Biosensors indeed allow for the detection of specific biological markers that hold promise in earlier diagnosis, indicating the pathological state and providing for a focused treatment. Moreover, biosensors should be useful for drug discovery and straightforward detection of disease-causing bacteria and viruses [105]. In this regard, biosensors have been fabricated for the biological detection of serum antigens and carcinogens [106], for the detection of glucose in diabetic patients [107] or allergic responses [108], as well as to reveal the presence of bacterial infections in the urinary tract [109] and even the HIV virus in the human blood serum [110].

The integration of NMs in a sensing platform can enhance the basic analytical features of biosensors as to the sensitivity, the LOD, the selectivity and reproducibility, thus leading to improved biological signaling and transduction mechanisms [111]. In particular, the high surface-to-volume ratio may offer a significant increase of sensing surface compared to the conventional transducers, which results into a more effective analyte immobilization. Moreover, nanomaterials can enhance the transfer of electrons, which are formed or used in the enzymatic reaction, between the transducer surface and the enzyme as well as enhance the enzyme stability and even allow for the catalysis of additional chemical reactions [112]. Furthermore, their high electrical conductivity, magnetic properties and catalytic activity provide advantageous features for biosensor fabrication and applications [113].

Among the NMs most employed for biosensor fabrication are nanoparticles, nanotubes, nanowires, nanorods and thin films made up of nanocrystallites [114]. NP-based biosensors include all the sensors which use metallic nanoparticles as enhancers of the sensing biochemical signals and are the best studied and employed till date. Nanotube-based sensors mainly involve carbon-based materials as enhancers of the reaction selectivity and efficiency; nanowire biosensors typically use nanowires as charge transport and carriers while QDs-based biosensors employ QDs as contrast agents to enhance the optical responses.

Surface functionalized NMs can provide an alternative way to obtain sensors combining an easy detection method, cost-saving and high effectiveness. It is possible to synthetize nanostructure based-devices, able to form colored complexes with the analytes, which can be detected with the naked eye [115] or by using NMs to achieve the separation of molecules in complex matrixes [116]. It is noteworthy that the nanomaterial surface can be easily functionalized with chemical groups or small molecules that are essential for a selective and highly sensible interaction with biomolecules in several biotechnological assays [117]. In this regard, efficient methods for the functionalization and immobilization of molecules on the nanomaterial surface include non-covalent and covalent approaches. The non-covalent method or physical adsorption is based on non-specific interactions between the materials and the biological entity such as electrostatic and π–π stacking interactions as well as van der Waals forces and has the advantage of maintaining all the specific chemical and physical properties of both the NMs and the biomolecule. On the other hand, the covalent immobilization uses the covalent-binding strategy to link the biomolecule on the material surface showing the advantage of higher stability and reproducibility as well as lower unspecific adsorption with respect to the physisorption. Some of the most employed covalent links are the classic coupling reactions and cross-linking chemistry. Affinity-systems are also used in the field of biosensor engineering to immobilize biomolecules on the surface of nanostructures. The most common method uses the biotin/avidin (or streptavidin) interaction for the detection biotinylated analytes via avidin bridges by binding to biotinylated molecules adsorbed on the material surface [118] (Figure 4).

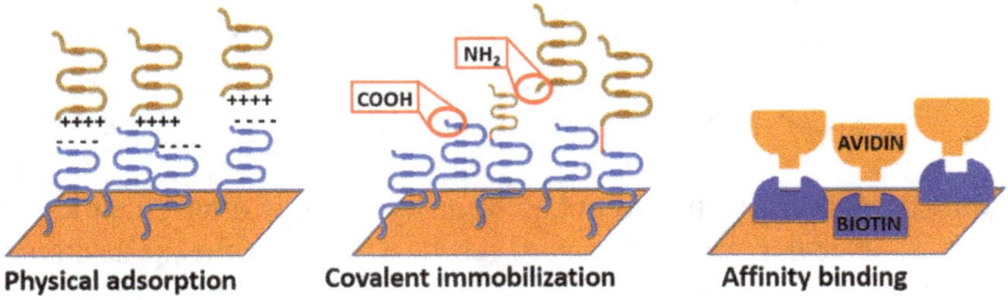

Fig. 4. Non-covalent and covalent interaction of biomolecules on the NM surface.

4. Protein- and Peptide-Based (Nano)Materials (P-NM) for Biotechnology and Therapy Applications

4.1. *P-NM in drug delivery*

Peptides and proteins have great potential as therapeutics and compared with the typical small-molecule drugs that currently make up the majority of the pharmaceutical market, they can be highly selective since they have multiple points of contact with their targets [119]. The advantages of using proteins to prepare NMs for drug delivery applications include their abundance in natural sources, biocompatibility, biodegradability, the easy and cost-effectiveness synthesis. Moreover, protein-based NPs offer the opportunity for surface modification by conjugation of other protein and carbohydrate ligands [120].

Globular proteins were used to associate with anionic polysaccharides to form particulate structures in the nanometer scale as potential delivery devices [121]. Other nanoformulations for drug delivery starting from a material of natural origin include silk protein, used for a sustained release and enhanced insulin stability in a covalently bound silk protein-insulin nanoassembly [122], vascular endothelial growth factor (VEGF) [123] and gelatin, a natural polymer derived from collagen, which is widely used as a biodegradable and biocompatible starting material [124–126].

Recently, peptide self-assembled nanostructures have attracted increasing attention for anticancer drug delivery to develop new paradigms in cancer treatments, because they have the ability to both enhance the therapeutic efficiency and decrease unwanted side reactions [127]. Indeed, small peptides can self-assemble into various morphologies (tubular, fibrillar or vesicular nanostructures) with the advantage of simultaneous enhanced stability and drug delivery capability, both *in vivo* and *in vitro* conditions [102]. In general, self-assembly of peptides can yield an array of well-defined nanostructures that are highly attractive NMs for many biomedical applications such as drug delivery, as they have several advantages including chemical diversity, good biocompatibility, high loading capacity for both hydrophobic and hydrophilic drugs, their ability to target molecular sites and stimuli responsive drug delivery at disease sites [128,129]. For example, Fan *et al.* exploited the amphiphilic properties of peptides that self-assemble into nanovesicles to deliver hydrophobic anticancer agents [127]. In another study, injectable *in situ*-forming hydrogel formulations were developed based on self-assembled KLD peptide motifs to control the delivery of a conventional cytotoxic drug (doxorubicine) for enhanced efficacy and safer tumor therapy compared to the traditional delivery route [130]. Also, Zhang *et al.* developed a series of surfactant peptides composed of a hydrophobic tail attached to a polar head group at the *C*- or *N*-terminus; such peptides self-assembled into nanovesicles and nanotubes act as DNA delivery vehicles to improve the cell growth [102].

Although nanostructures of proteins and peptides may offer significant advantages, they are generally labile for enzymatic degradation and, due to instability in the environment of the gastrointestinal tract, they are not suitable for oral administration. In addition, the dimensions and the hydrophilicity of proteins and peptides often cause poor oral bioavailability and intravenous administration may not be sufficient to obtain optimal therapeutic effects since many proteins and peptides suffer from low circulation half-lives [131].

To this regard, in the past decade, extensive studies have focused on the development of hybrid systems of protein and peptide biomolecules integrated into an NM platform, as novel drug delivery systems that circumvent most of the problems associated with the use of proteins and peptides alone. Various chemical approaches aimed at modifying the original peptide sequences can improve the biomolecule metabolic stability and pharmacokinetic profile [102,131,132] still preserving their pharmacologic properties. For instance, Hamman *et al.* demonstrated that the grafting of polymers can improve the pharmacokinetic properties of the biomolecules. In particular, PEG possesses remarkable properties that make it very suitable in the development of carriers for peptide delivery [133].

In addition to the chemical modification, the integration of a nanostructured carrier has been extensively studied to design protein and peptide-based NMs for drug delivery. Examples of synthetic macromolecules used as nanocarriers for drug delivery include PLA, PLGA and PCL, often featuring a core shell structure, sized in the nanometer range and surface tailored with targeting moieties, such as a cyclic RGD peptide [134]. Polyelectrolytes have been used for pH-triggered drug release, for instance, the chitosan polysaccharide was investigated as a suitable nanoparticle basic material [135] to carry proteins [136]. Also, nanoparticles made of chitosan allow for the penetration of proteins and peptides across the membranes [137,138].

Metal NPs constitute another class of inert but not biodegradable carriers e.g., for anti-cancer drug delivery [139]. For instance, AuNPs were functionalized with peptide sequences mimicking angiogenin (Ang), a protein constituent of the human plasma but also a pathological marker of different cancer types.

Experiments with human neuroblastoma cells demonstrated promising potential in cancer therapy [140]. Also, hybrid nanoassemblies of AuNPs with Ang fragments containing the 60–68 sequence (the putative site of interaction with actin, an essential step in the cellular cytoskeleton reorganization) obtained by different immobilization approaches (i.e., physisorption vs. chemisorption), demonstrated different levels of interaction between the hybrid assemblies and cell membranes of fibroblasts and neuroblastoma [26]. Furthermore, results on cell viability/proliferation, cytoskeleton actin, angiogenin translocation and VEGF release in two brain cell lines, namely tumor glioblastoma (A172 line) and neuron-like differentiated neuroblastoma (d-SH-SY5Y line), pointed to the promising potentialities of Ang protein- and Ang peptide-functionalized AuNPs as anti-angiogenic tunable nanoplatforms in cancer cell treatment [27].

Another class of NPs widely investigated as protein- and peptide-based delivery system is that of inorganic nanoparticles, where the encapsulated therapeutic biomolecules are protected against denaturation of the proteins and possible enzymatic hydrolysis in the gastrointestinal tract [141].

Liposomes and microspheres are another class of carrier system largely used for the delivery of proteins and peptides. Solid lipid nanoparticles (SLNs) have been used to entrap hydrophilic peptide drugs by combining hydrophobic ion-pairing and non-aqueous oil-in-oil emulsion-evaporation methods, which showed improved uptake by the intestinal epithelial cells owing to their high hydrophobic character [142]. Liposomes are mainly used in the oral delivery of the insulin hormone to enhance its absorption in the small intestine [143], whereas microspheres based on pH-sensitive polymers are used for a controlled release of the incorporated therapeutic protein or peptide at specific areas in the gastrointestinal tract [144].

4.2. *P-NM in tissue engineering*

Protein-based biomaterials show promising properties for future application in biomedical devices for tissue regeneration. The long-term biodegradability, mechanical strength, elasticity and biocompatibility designate a perfect biomaterial especially for bone, cartilage and blood vessels tissues reparation.

Peptide-based biopolymers that are well known to be softer and more wet than synthetic polymers, except hydrogels, show several attractive features as bioactive domains that promote cell adhesion [145], spreading [146], biomineralization [147] and proteases control for cell migration [148,149]. In this regard, natural protein and peptide-based polymers, including elastin, collagens, silk and their derivates, have been tested and exploited extensively for tissue engineering applications [150–155].

4.2.1. *Collagen-based NMs*

Collagen is the major protein in the ECM of bone, skin and ligaments. Nowadays, 29 different collagen types are known, and all display a triple-helix structure made up of three α-helix chains. Every α-helix chain is based on the common amino acids sequence $(\text{Gly-X-Y})_n$ where X and Y are generally occupied by Proline (Pro) and 4-Hydroxyproline (Hyp) and 'n' is the degree of polymerization. Different assemblies of three α-helix chains bring several conformations, each produced by its own unique gene [152]. Collagen types I, II, III and V, which are found to be fibril-forming, are the main components of skin, bone, cartilage and muscle [156]. Collagens play an important role in 3D scaffold for tissue engineering due to its high swelling ability, low antigenicity, tissue regeneration potential, biodegradability and cells adhesion enhancement. The latter can be explained by the presence of adhesion domains (Gly-Pro-Hyp) that bind glycoproteins cell receptors and integrin and discoidin domain receptor [157].

Despite its intrinsic attracting properties, natural collagen cannot be used in scaffold preparation because the chemical treatment of the extractive procedures leads to degradation of cross-linkages and subsequently loss of mechanical properties and structural stability.

Physical treatment and chemical cross-linkers can be used to restore and tailor mechanical properties of 3D scaffolds. Chemical cross-linkers such as glutaraldehyde, isocyanate or carbodiimide are the most frequently used agents, they have been demonstrated to be excellent because they increase the tensile strength, avoid the rapid enzymatic degradation and promote linkages with some marginal substances as AuNPs or epoxy [158,159]. However, all chemical techniques leave potential toxic residues that increase antigenicity and cytotoxicity [160,161].

Physical techniques have been demonstrated to be a good alternative to chemical cross-linking: UV irradiation or de-hydrothermal treatment promote cross-link formation in collagen 3D scaffold. In comparison, UV irradiation in the presence of glucose is a faster and more suitable technique to promote cross-linking with no toxic by-products [162].

An alternative to chemical and physical techniques is enzymatic crosslinking, with the use of transglutaminase, that enhances mechanical properties and enzymatic resistance [163]. For skin tissue engineering, 3D nanocomposite scaffolds were prepared using a mixture of type I collagen and polyvinylpyrrolidone (PVP)-coated TiO_2 NPs. The ultimate tensile strength of the scaffolds was improved by hydrogen bond formation between collagen, PVP and TiO_2 [164]. In another study, a highly porous collagen-alginate(-GO) aerogel-based scaffold was demonstrated to promote osteoblast cell attachment and proliferation [165].

Electrospun nanofibers of Type I collagen and gelatin exhibited unique biological properties, very promising in a variety of tissue engineering applications, including endothelial cell–scaffold interactions, the onset of bone mineralization, dermal reconstruction, and the fabrication of skeletal muscle prosthetics [166]. The nanostructure–property relationships of natural materials such as bone can guide the design of synthetic composites. In a biomimetic approach, hybrid scaffolds of hydroxyapatite (HA) and collagen can be designed to reproduce the mineral crystals in bone (platelet-shaped HA particles) as well as the soft, hydrated (collagenous) aligned fiber matrix as clustered helical arrays, 20–30 nm wide and a few nanometers in thickness [167]. Hence, biomaterials that are present in native bone (e.g., HA and collagen) are commonly used to fabricate multiple scale architectures in scaffolds to provide a biomimetic niche for stimulating bone repair and regeneration [168].

4.2.2. *Elastin and elastin-like-based NMs*

Elastin is a water insoluble protein made up of 36 domains of alternating hydrophobic and cross-linked features mainly found in large arteries, elastic ligaments and lung parenchyma ECM, where they provide elasticity and resilience [169]. Natural elastin, biosynthesized from a soluble precursor known as tropoelastin, has received less attention than native collagen because of the difficulty in purification and its tendency in calcifying in implantations due to the association with glycoprotein fibrillin [170]. Therefore, soluble recombinant forms of elastin such as tropoelastin, α-elastin and elastin-like proteins (ELPs) are viable alternatives to form fibers and scaffold for tissue engineering. Specifically, there are many reports showing the great potential of ELPs in tissue regeneration scaffold production for both *in vitro* and *in vivo* applications.

Palumbo *et al.* demonstrated the possibility to create 3D scaffold using hyaluronic acid-ethylenediamine grafted with α-elastin hydrogel. The presence of α-elastin improves cell attachment and proliferation on rat dermal fibroblast and human muscle cells [171]. Also, intriguing mechanical and biophysical properties, such as high elastic modulus, antibacterial effect and triggered cell differentiation and growth, were demonstrated for collagen-ELP blends in a nanohydrogel formulation, upon the loading with the antibacterial drug Doxycycline and human bone recombinant morphogenetic proteins-2 rhBMP-2, to promote the human adipose stem cells (hASC) differentiation in osteoblasts [172]. Recombinant ELPs scaffold based on VPGVG sequence and incorporated into a copolymer with GRGDSP fibronectin-targeting sequence promoted cell adhesion and exhibited elastomeric properties [173]. An electrospun 3D scaffold for *in vitro* keratinocytes and fibroblasts growth was produced by Gonzàlez de Torre *et al.* using multicomponent recombinant ELPs [174]. Recently, recombinant ELPs containing IKVAV and VKAIV laminin-motifs for cell attachment and spreading were crosslinked with PEG to obtain hydrogels suitable for the *in vivo* growth of neuronal tissues [175]. Another example of *in vivo* testing was performed by Mahara *et al.* who used polymers with elastin-like VPGIG hydrophobic domain, the RDG motif and a crosslinker to obtain a hydrogel able to promote rapid tissue regeneration and, at the same time, to maintain a normal blood flow without inflammatory response or thrombogenesis [176].

4.2.3. *Silk and silk-like-based NMs*

Silks are natural protein polymers produced by some insects and spiders. Several forms of silk are known, whose structures and properties are tailored with the role that protein plays in each animal [177]. Native silk is generally composed of two structures: an inner filament protein called fibroin and a glue-coating of a sericin-family protein. The mainly used silk proteins come from the cocoon of silkworm *Bombyx mori* and from spider *Nephila clavipes* [178]. Despite that, several origins of silks correspond in a wide variety of amino acids sequence, all silk fibroins show a common well-defined organization: the largest part of the primary sequence is composed by hydrophobic amino acids domains of GAGAGX (where X=A, S, V or T) that gives tensile strength to the fibers while the rest is composed of more complex hydrophilic blocks that confer elasticity and stiffness [179]. Naturally occurring silk is insoluble in almost all common solvents such as water, ethanol or dilute acids and bases, and only a good solubility is gained in a concentrated solution of sulfuric acid, formic acid, HFIP, LiBr or ionic liquids [180].

Biotechnological applications of silk and silk-like materials for tissue engineering were widely studied and tested both *in vivo* and *in vitro* showing great biocompatibility, low cytotoxicity and low inflammatory response [88,181]. Several strategies and methods were developed for silk biomedical applications, for instance, Ni *et al.* evaluated the cytocompatibility of regenerated fibroin film on chondrocytes for cartilage tissue repairing. The results show an excellent biocompatibility, characterized by the maintenance of normal cell morphology and functionalities, good adhesion, differentiation and growth. Moreover, the secretion of extracellular Collagen II was found on or within the regenerated silk fibroin film, which further confirmed that this biomaterial is feasible and functional for repairing clinical cartilage defects [182]. A different approach was developed by Wang *et al.* in the production of 3D scaffolds for cartilage repairing. The group tested a collagen/silk fibroin scaffold incorporated with PLGA microspheres. The obtained scaffold showed enhanced proliferation, adhesion, great cytocompatibility and histocompatibility in both *in vivo* and *in vitro* experiments [183].

Multicomponent 3D scaffolds of fibroin/hydroxyapatite were developed for bone tissue growth and regeneration. Sofia *et al.* tested osteoblast activity on a decorated silk-based film. Both RGD integrin recognition sequence and a modified parathyroid were used to decorate fibroin regenerated fibers. The *in vitro* biomineralization studies showed a great production of procollagen after four weeks of incubation and calcium deposition only on RGD-decorated fibroin scaffold. The results suggest a promising future use of silk-based biomaterial for cartilage and bone tissue regeneration [184]. Transgenic silkworms were fabricated to functionalize silk proteins with human platelet-derived growth factor and assembled to a bioceramic-modified silk into 3D textile implants by using the 'fiber-assisted molding' technology. The composite biomaterial was shown to be very promising for bone regeneration, since the silk fiber-based 3D textile implant showed good cytocompatibility and stem cells differentiation into bone cells prompted by the bioceramic material functionalized silk implants [185].

4.3. *P-NM in biosensing*

The fabrication of peptide and/or protein-based NMs for biosensing application is a central direction of bioanalytical device research, since the combination of protein and nanomaterial clearly enhances the biosensor performance in terms of sensitivity, selectivity, storage stability and LOD. NMs, indeed, improve the condition of protein immobilization and stability as well as allow to catalyze electrochemical and biochemical reactions.

Moreover, the current progress and exhaustive exploitation of NMs with specific chemical features have made the sensing technology more versatile and robust, offering also novel alternative methods of transduction compared to the conventional mechanisms. Such improvements make protein-NM-based biosensors more efficient and certainly may provide significant advances and a major step forward changes in biological analysis and clinical diagnosis. Various NMs have been exploited for biosensing applications due to their functional electrical and mechanical features. Considering the chemical properties of the NMs employed to improve the sensing mechanism, such devices can be distinguished into plasmonic and magnetic sensors, QD-based, carbon-based (e.g., nanotubes, graphene), and peptide-based sensing devices.

4.3.1. *Plasmonic NMs for protein and peptide detection*

Noble metal NPs are widely used as sensors for biomedical applications due to their unique physicochemical properties which allow us to improve both the sensitivity and the power of these biodetection devices [186]. Among the different metal NPs, the most commonly used for biomedical applications are probably AuNPs, owing to their high biocompatibility, optical and electronic properties as well as their rather simple synthesis and straightforward surface modification [187,188]. The prominent spectroscopic feature of AuNP is the SPR, which gives rise to an intense absorption band in the visible region. This phenomenon was described by the Mie theory [189] and is dependent on the size and shape of the nanoparticle as well as the dielectric constant of the environment surrounding the nanosystems [190]. This environmental dependency represents a great advantage for the biodetection since the recognition event can result in a change of the oscillation frequency of the plasmon and therefore to a color change of

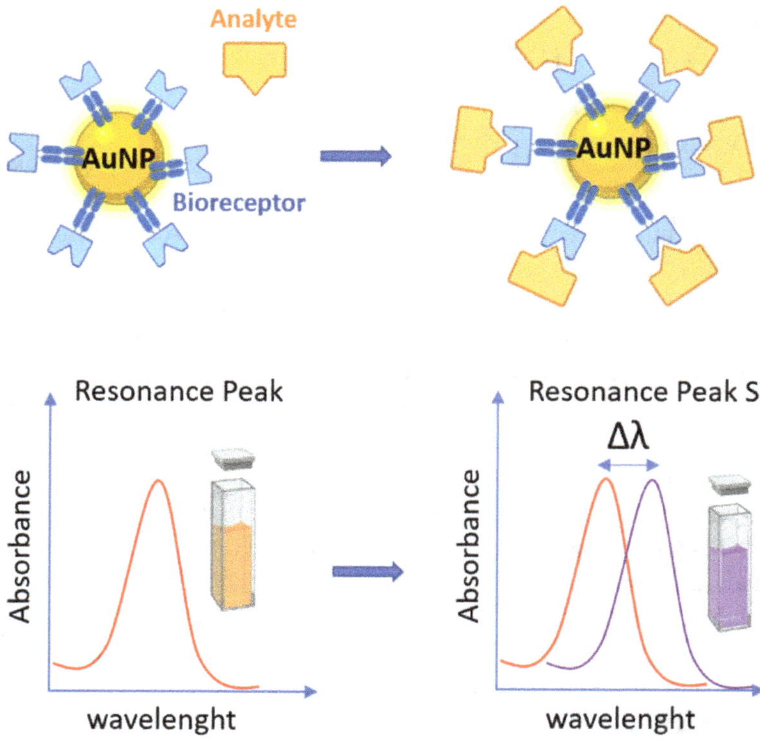

Fig. 5. Surface plasmon resonance-based spectrophotometric determination of analytes using surface-modified gold nanoparticles.

AuNP also observable with the bare eye. In this context, a wide number of colorimetric biosensors have been developed for DNA or oligonucleotide detection or protein detection [191–193] (Figure 5).

SPR has been also used, as transduction element, for the protein/peptide detection. This approach is based on the variation of the dielectric constant of the propagating surface plasmon environment of gold films which causes changes of the angle, intensity, or phase of the reflected light [194,195]. Interestingly, an SPR signal enhancement can be achieved when gold films and AuNPs are used in a sandwich configuration. To this respect, the surface plasmons on AuNPs induce a perturbation of the evanescent field of the gold film in addition to the immobilized bioreceptor unit and the detected analyte (Figure 6). The optimal configuration of this method was fixed by Zeng *et al.* and uses spherical AuNPs with a diameter smaller than 40 nm at a distance to the

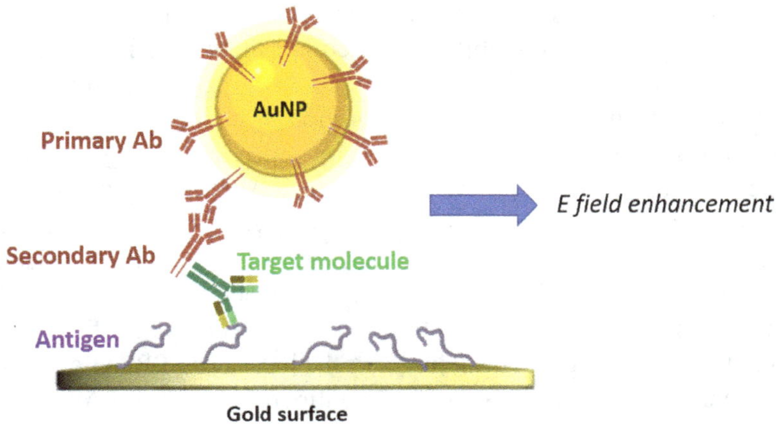

Fig. 6. Schematic illustration of an AuNP-based biosensor.

gold film surface of 5 nm, as labels attached to the secondary antibodies.

AuNPs have been also used in biodetection applications as electron transfer between electroactive biological molecules (enzymes, co-factors) and the electrode. This biosensing approach is based on the catalyzes of the analyte oxidation or reduction by the enzymatic unite and the further oxidation or reduction of the formed species by the electrode, which gives rise to the electrochemical signal. The disadvantage of this method is that the analytes have to diffuse to the electrode where a part of it is unavoidably lost in solution.

AuNPs act as electron shuttles to the catalytic center of the enzyme, regenerating this biocatalyst by transferring the electrons involved in the redox reaction to the electrode and so inducing a strong increase of the electrochemical signal [196]. Based on this method, Xiao *et al*. developed a sensor for the efficient detection of glucose using the glucose oxidase enzyme. As discussed above, glucose oxidase catalyzes the oxidation of glucose to gluconic acid by releasing two electrons which reduce oxygen molecules to hydrogen peroxide. This process involves the natural cofactor flavin adenine dinucleotide (FAD^+), which, after the glucose oxidation, is reduced to $FADH_2$. The goal of this method is the quick regeneration of FAD^+ with favored kinetics by means of FAD^+- modified AuNPs as electron carrier [197].

Although less extensively than AuNPs, AgNPs with a size in the range of 1 to 100 nm have been also exploited for the development of novel and high-tech diagnostic instruments due to their physicochemical properties including the SPR and the large effective scattering cross-section. Interestingly, hydrophobic Ag–Au composite nanoparticles are also widely used for the fabrication of biosensors with high sensitivity and low detection limit due to the strong adsorption associated to the surface-enhanced Raman scattering (SERS) process which produces great electromagnetic fields [198]. Thus, triangular-shaped AgNPs on glass substrate devices were employed for the selective streptavidin-biotin couple detection based on the SPR optical biosensing, with a LOD in the low-picomolar to the high-femtomolar region [199]. Such detection method was then optimized using AuNP-labeled antibodies, which allowed for the amplification of the wavelength shift induced by the localized SPR. After binding the antigen, i.e., the target protein, the antibody-conjugated Ag nanotriangles, in a sandwich configuration, bind to the secondary antibody attached on the gold surface resulting in a plasmonic coupling which leads to a reduction of the LOD by even three orders of magnitude with respect to the classical method [200].

Another recent approach which allowed to enhance the sensitivity of the SPR optical sensor uses AgNPs deposited on optical fibers in order to make the plasmon resonance more sensitive to the variations in the surrounding medium. In this regard, Chen *et al.* developed a localized surface plasmon resonance (LSPR) optical AgNP-fiber sensor using antibody functionalized particles to monitor the antigen-antibody binding process by measuring the plasmon shift in real time, which linearly moves to longer wavelength as the refractive index of the surrounding medium increases [201].

It is noteworthy that AgNP dispersion has also been employed to develop nanoparticle aggregation-based colorimetric assays. Indeed, a decrease in the interparticle distance, triggered by interactions, mainly electrostatic and hydrogen bond as well as donor–acceptor chemical reactions, with the target analytes, leads to an overlap of the plasmon fields of the nearby particle thus inducing a red-shift of the plasmon peak and a further observable variation in the color of the particle dispersion [202]. Colorimetric sensor highly selective for tryptophan and histidine or small peptides tryptophan and histidine-rich were fabricated using organic-coated AgNPs, namely 4.4-bipyridine (4-DPD) and p-sulfonatocalixarene (p-SC4)-modified AgNPs, respectively. As to the tryptophan, it interacts with the pyridine ring of the 4-DPD by π–π stacking interactions and hydrogen bonds resulting in the AgNPs aggregation and a color change from yellow to red, with a LOW of 20 μM [203]. As to the histidine, the interaction involves the electron-rich cyclic cavity of p-SC4 which fit with the imidazole and the side chain of histidine through host–guest electrostatic and cation–π interactions causing a color change from yellow to light red with a LOD of 5 μM [204] (Figure 7).

4.3.2. *Magnetic NMs for protein and peptide detection*

Magnetic NPs are also promising alternatives in biosensor devices due to their superparamagnetic behavior [205]. This means that magnetization can flip the direction randomly within a very short time. Moreover, the magnetization is zero in the absence of an external magnetic field while the magnetic moments align after applying it thus avoiding the attractive or repulsive forces between the magnetic NPs as long as no external magnetic field is applied. Even if this effect seems to be comparable to that of classic paramagnetic materials, the magnetic susceptibility of these superparamagnet NM is quite higher [206]. Magnetic particles are particularly interesting for biosensing applications since biological molecules do not show any magnetic properties or susceptibility, hence no interference or noise is expected during signal capturing [16].

Among the wide range of magnetic materials, iron oxide NPs are mostly employed for biosensing applications [207]. A simple approach uses receptor unit-modified particles that specifically interact with the analyte molecules, i.e., the protein molecule, in solution. An applied external magnetic field leads to the nanoparticle agglomeration that can be then easily separated from the solution. In this way, efficient isolation of DNA strands as well as protein purification was achieved [208,209] (Figure 8).

Moreover, due to the control by an external magnet, these systems are largely used in hybrid catalysts and reusable platforms [210]. For instance, Kamikawa *et al.*, used polyaniline-coated magnetic NPs to detect the

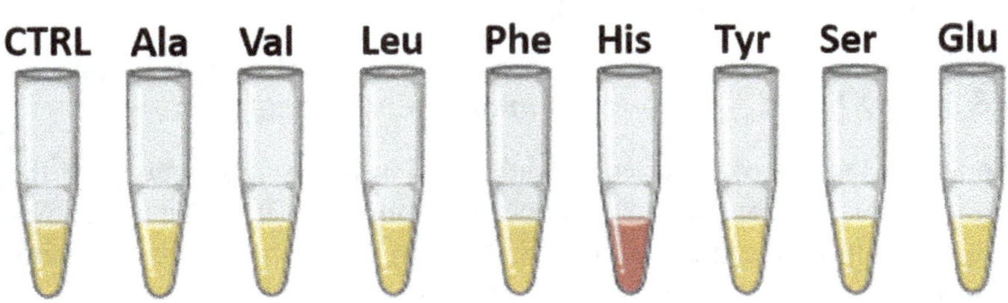

Fig. 7. AgNP aggregation-based colorimetric assays for Histidine detection.

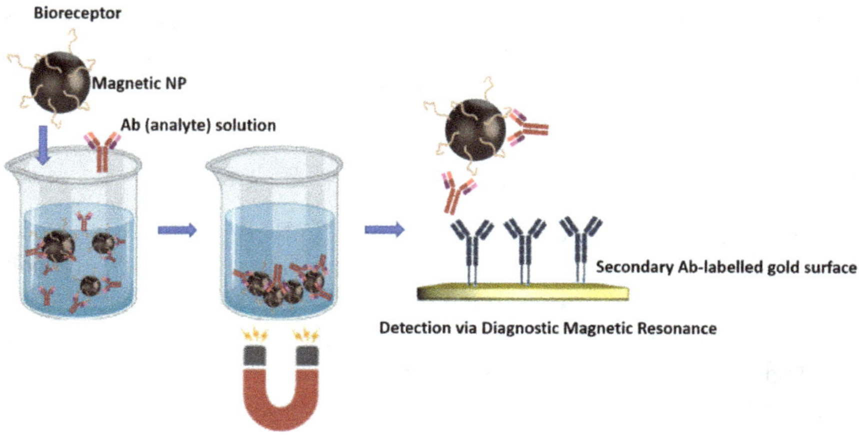

Fig. 8. Schematic illustration of bioreceptor-modified magnetic NPs for the analyte detection.

surface glycoprotein hemagglutinin from the virus H5N1 [211]. The obtained systems provided increased assay kinetics due to the close proximity to the analytes, the magnetic control of the NPs and the high selectivity [212].

Among the NP-based biosensors, acoustic wave biosensors have been also extensively used. These kinds of devices are mainly based on the mass changes of a quartz-based electrode upon the conjugation of antibody-labeled NPs with other antibody molecules immobilized on the electrode surface via the analyte, in a sandwiched assay. This conjugation results in a variation of the vibrational frequency of the sensor that is used for the analyte quantification. These kinds of biosensors typically use gold, platinum, cadmium sulphide and titanium dioxide particles with a diameter in the range of 5 and 100 nm [213].

4.3.3. *QD-based NMs for protein and peptide detection*

Another example of NMs employed for biosensing application are the luminescent semiconducting nanocrystals, known as QDs. The most studied are cadmium chalcogenides (S, Se, Te) QDs which show a large absorption spectrum together with a size-dependent narrow emission spectrum [214,215]. This phenomenon is related to the variation of the band gaps of the semiconductors with the dimension of the particles which further leads to different emission wavelengths (the bigger the particle, the lower the band gap) [216].

This large range of emission wavelengths is exploited for the fabrication of efficient biosensors based on the classic optical transduction [217]. This is noteworthy since structural defects in the crystals can block the exited electrons leading to non-radiative relaxation, core/shell nanocomposites which use another semiconductor material with a larger band gap (e.g., ZnS) have been developed to overcome this issue, thus also enhancing the quantum yields and the photostability [218,219]. Moreover, to provide functional groups for the ease and straightforward interaction with bioreceptors and molecules as well as to minimize possible toxicity and make them suitable in biological environments, QDs can be synthesized with inert or biocompatible coating, which can increase their biocompatibility and hydrophilicity [220].

QDs have been employed for the fabrication of biosensors based on the Fluorescence Resonance Energy Transfer (FRET) process, involving the non-radiative energy transfer between the exited QD (donor) and a quencher (acceptor), for instance, an organic molecule. Thus, when the quenching molecule is in close contact with the QD, its emission is strongly reduced, while reappearing when the quencher is removed (Figure 9).

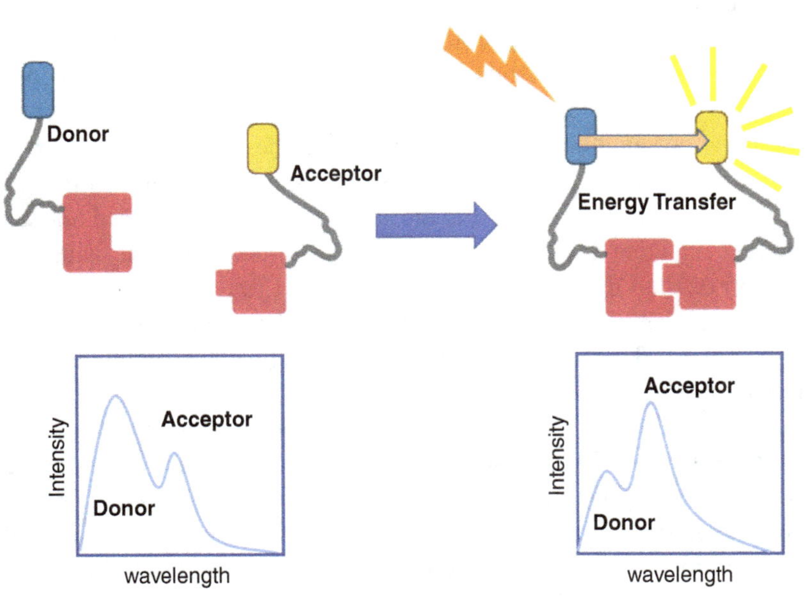

Fig. 9. Schematic illustration of FRET process.

The strategy of donor–acceptor spatial modulation has been widely used for both the optical protein detection and the measurement of the proteolytic enzyme activity. In this latter case, QDs are functionalized with a peptide linker terminating with an energy-accepting fluorescent dye. The ratio of the emission intensities (I_{QD}/I_{dye}) of this hybrid system is altered by the addition of a target analyte, which, cleaving the linker, causes the diffusion of the dye from the QD, resulting in a dominant emission of the nanocrystal.

Boeneman *et al.* synthetized hybrids core/shell semiconductor QDs conjugated to the fluorescent protein mCherry for the *in vitro* biosensing of the caspase-3 enzymatic activity [221]. Similarly, Medintz *et al.* employed this approach for sensing caspase-1, thrombin, chymotrypsin, and collagenase. Specifically, they synthesized QDs functionalized with a peptide containing a polyhistidine unit, a protease-specific cleavage sequence and a terminal cysteine for the dye conjugation. Addition of the dye functionalized peptides to aqueous dots resulted in enhanced dye emission and QD quenching due to energy transfer. Enzyme addition cleaves the peptides, causing QD-dye displacement and a loss of FRET process that causes an increase of the QD emission [222].

Another common non-radiative energy transfer process in biosensing application which uses QD as optical transducer is the Bioluminescence Resonance Energy Transfer (BRET). This phenomenon is based on the presence of a light-emitting protein label that transfers the energy to the QDs crystals, thus avoiding the presence of an external excitation source [223,224]. For instance, Kumar *et al.* fabricated a biosensor based on DNA probe conjugated-QDs and oligonucleotides linked with a protein, the Renilla luciferase (Rluc) that emits blue light at 480 nm. In the presence of the target DNA molecule, the annealing of the two used antisense sequences adjacent to each other in a head-to-head scheme causes the excitation of the QDs and the BRET emission [225]. Similarly, Yu *et al.* developed a BRET immunoassay to detect small molecules i.e., fluoroquinolones (FQs). This detection assay uses norfloxacin conjugated-QDs which in the absence of FQs molecules conjugates with the scFv fragment linked to the Rluc protein, leading to an energy transfer. Whereas, in the presence of the free FQs, these molecules impede the interaction between QDs and Rluc, thus preventing the BRET emission [226]. Another recently developed bio-detection system uses CdSe/ZnS core-shell QDs conjugated to the nanoLuciferase (Nluc) protein that emits blue light at 460 nm and the cyclic RGD (cRGD) for *in vivo* imaging of tumors. Such a peptide sequence is known to exhibit a high affinity for the integrin $\alpha_v\beta_3$ which is mostly expressed on the membrane of various tumor cells. The injection of this construct into mice with integrin expressing glioblastoma tumor demonstrated the high capabilities of this sensor to target the tumor cells after 2 h [227].

4.3.4. *Carbon-based NMs for protein and peptide detection*

The excellent biocompatibility and the electronic properties of carbon-based NMs, such as CNT or graphene sheets, make them suitable as electronic or electrochemical transducer for the fabrication of biosensor devices [228]. CNTs possess mechanical stability and remarkable electrical conductivity related to the sp^2 hybridization of the adjacent carbon atoms [229]. Moreover, CNTs exhibit a high electroactive surface owing to the natural formation of porous three-dimensional networks, which can be used to anchor a high amount of bioreceptors, thus enhancing the biosensor sensitivities [230]. Besides, their nanowire morphology allows the nanostructures to easily approach the active sites of enzymes, leading to a fast and efficient electron transfer and improving the sensitivity of electrochemical enzyme-based biosensors. In this regard, the driving forces are mostly hydrophobic interactions, hence to ensure an efficient electron transfer, the hydrophobic domain of the protein has to be close to the active site. In this respect, CNTs were used to enhance the direct electron transfer and consequently the sensitivity to nitrate of the nitrite reductase, an enzyme presenting a catalytic site nearby the hydrophobic domain and that catalyzes the reduction of nitrite ions to ammonia. After the redox reaction, the oxidized form of the enzyme is regenerated by the CNTs structures [231].

However, this optimal condition cannot be achieved with most of the studied enzymes. To overcome this issue, CNTs are functionalized with carboxylic or amino groups or synthesized in combination with other materials, like polymers, to easily interact with enzymes or redox active species establishing the so-called "mediated electron transfer". For instance, Patolsky *et al.* developed a high performant glucose sensor using AuNPs as electron transfer and FAD co-enzymes anchored to CNTs [232]. Moreover, Kucherenko *et al.* fabricated an enzyme-based biosensor using the horseradish peroxidase and CNTs for the detection of hydrogen peroxide reaching a LOD of 0.22 nM. In this case, the enzyme was modified with a 4-aminothiophenol group and then immobilized into a CNT-polyaniline matrix [233]. Other biosensors used CNTs with urease for the urea determination in the range from 0.1 to 11 μM, which cover the typical urea concentration in blood [234]. Other examples include laccase to reveal phenolic compounds with useful application in the beverage industry, healthcare, and for monitoring environmental pollution [235] and lysine oxidase as l-lysine biosensors [236].

As mentioned in Section 1.2.2, graphene is a 2D NM made of one-atom thick sheets of sp^2 carbon atoms arranged into a hexagonal pattern, which is also used as electrode due to the higher specific surface area compared to the CNTs, fast electron transfer, excellent thermal conductivity and high mechanical stiffness [237]. However, its hydrophobicity limits its application in biosensor devices [238]. The graphene derivatives GO and rGO overcome this problem by increasing the graphene hydrophilicity, maintaining the electrical conductivity of the graphene sheets and improving the surface immobilization capabilities of biomolecules [239]. Graphene and GO electrodes can be fabricated by direct printing of graphene ink or by deposition of the NM after printing a sacrificial polymer pattern [240,241]. On the other hand, graphene-based electrodes can be developed from carbon-based polymers such as polyimide by irradiation with CO_2 laser [242].

The hybridization of graphene and its derivatives with different types of organic polymers, metal NPs and in particular surface functionalities linked to different enzymes and proteins is largely used for the fabrication of efficient biosensors [238]. Biosensors based on GO sheets and proteins include the amperometric devices for the determination of phenolic compounds. They are characterized by GO sheets functionalized with glutaraldehyde moieties also linked through covalent bond to the tyrosinase and are able to detect catechol in the concentration range from 50 nM to 50 μM with a LOD of 30 nM [243]. Chae *et al.* fabricated a successful biosensor based on acetylcholinesterase and rGO to determine the acetylcholinesterase activity and the concentration of the enzyme drug inhibitors i.e., donepezil and rivastigmine for monitoring drug effects in Alzheimer's disease treatment [244]. Moreover, a biosensor based on soybean peroxidase and rGO was proposed to determine hydrogen peroxide with LOD of 50 nM avoiding interference with substances such as ascorbic and uric acids and dopamine which do not affect the results of H_2O_2 quantification [245].

It is noteworthy that it is possible to co-immobilize enzymes on the nanosheet surface. For instance, Bhardwaj *et al.* proposed a bi-enzymes biosensor for the triglyceride and glycerol determination in human blood serum. In this device, lipase and glycerol dehydrogenase proteins were co-immobilized on the surface of rGO sheets modified with a mediator i.e., toluidine blue. Once lipase cleaves triglycerides to glycerol and fatty acids, the glycerol dehydrogenase oxidizes glycerol with the subsequent reduction of the mediator, which is finally oxidized on the electrode surface. Such a system shows high selectivity, fast response (12 s) and long-time stability being able to maintain 90% of the initial sensitivity after 11 weeks [246].

Graphene, due to its excellent optical properties, such as broadband absorption, saturation absorption, and fluorescence can also act as transduction element into an optical or colorimetric biosensor of small molecules, protein and even cells. In this regard, rGO was used to develop a biosensor for the selective binding of proteins in a configuration based on a balanced photodetector able to measure variations in the polarization-dependent absorption related to changes in the refractive index, after the interaction between antigen adsorbed on the sheet surface and antibody. This sensor has the advantages of real-time detection, no covalent labeling, ease of integration and low cost [247].

High efficient FRET biosensors, based on graphene and organic dyes or QDs, were fabricated for proteins detection [248]. For instance, Shi *et al.* developed a rGO-peptide-based FRET biosensor for the selective detection of the botulinum neurotoxins protease activity. This device was fabricated by immobilizing on rGO sheets, a fluorescent protein (SNAP-25-GFP) that includes a specific sequence recognized by the enzyme. In the presence of the neurotoxin, the enzyme specifically cleaves the SNAP-25-GFP substrate leading to its release and diffusion away from the sheets resulting in a fluorescence signal recovery which allows for the quantification of the analyte [249]. Based on the same approach, a GO-peptide conjugate biosensor has been developed for imaging caspase-3 activity in living cells. In this device, a caspase-3-cleavable peptide sequence conjugated with the carboxyfluorescein (FAM) moiety was covalently bound to the GO surface. The cleavage by caspase-3 of the peptide sequence releases the fluorescent peptide restoring its fluorescent emission [250].

4.3.5. *Peptide-based biosensor*

Peptides, such as aromatic diphenylalanine (the core recognition motif of the Alzheimer's β-amyloid peptide) or diphenylglycine dipeptides or more complex linear peptides have the intrinsic ability to self-organize under mild conditions (room temperature, aqueous media) [251] into nanostructures like nanowires, nanotubes, or nanoparticles.

Such self-assembled peptide nanostructures (SAPNs) have shown high chemical and thermal stability as well as high resistance against the attack of proteolytic enzymes [252]. Accordingly, these peptides have been widely used in several applications including drug delivery, tissue engineering as well as in biosensing [253].

Furthermore, SAPNs can be easily assembled, through chemical modifications, with other NMs such as conductive polymer or metallic NPs, organic acids as well as antibody and enzymes, thus providing new possibilities for the fabrication of efficient biosensing devices [254]. The assembling approach depends on the type of peptide used and the functional groups available on its surface. For example, it is possible to employ the amino groups on the surface of diphenylalanine nanotubes to bind to biotin moieties thus allowing the assembly of these SAPNs with gold-labeled streptavidin NPs [255]. In another work, antibodies were linked through hydrogen bonds with the amide groups of self-assembled peptide nanotubes formed by an *L*-glutamic acid-based bolaamphiphile [256]. The same peptide was used to encapsulate *Candida rugose* lipase into the nanotube structure, for the potentiometric measurement of pesticides [257].

Yang *et al.* developed a biosensor for the detection of glucose by using peptide EAK16-II nanofibers covalently functionalized with glucose oxidase via 1-ethyl-3-(3-dimethylaminopropyl) carbodiimide hydrochloride (EDC)/*N*-hydroxysuccinimide (NHS) coupling thus enhancing the activity and the stability of the enzyme. Such modified fibers were then deposited on pyrolytic graphite allowing for the amperometric detection of the monosaccharide [258]. Similarly, EDC was used as a linker to attach folic acid on the surface of diphenylalanine peptide nanotubes. The obtained nanostructures were deposited on graphene electrodes to detect cancer cells which overexpress the folate receptors [259]. Electrochemically active SAPNs were also synthetized via the physical adsorption of the polyaniline (PANI), a conductive polymer, on the surface of the self-assembled peptide nanofibers by mixing the fiber dispersion with the polymerizing solution of aniline, without stirring [260]. Moreover, Sun *et al.* developed a biosensor for the electrochemical detection of tumor necrosis factor α(TNF-α) based on ferrocene carboxylic acid-functionalized peptide nanofibers. Such a sensor is able to detect TNF-α in a concentration range from 5 pg/mL to 10 ng/mL with a LOD of 2 pg/mL [261].

5. Protein- and Peptide-Based Nanomaterials in the Theranostic Outlook

One of the most exciting research fields in nanomedicine is represented by theranostic, a novel concept which involves the combination of diagnosis and therapy for potential personalized medicine in order to improve the accumulation and delivery of the active compounds at the diseased site, enhancing therapeutic efficacy and reducing the intensity of side effects on healthy tissues [72]. The so-called theranostic nanomedicine contains both a drug and an imaging agent within a multicomponent formulation, thus providing application in therapy and diagnosis, for instance in the recognition of specific targets and internalization through a specific mechanism, e.g., receptor-mediated endocytosis [262,263].

NMs such as metallic NPs, magnetic NPs or graphene-based nanostructures have intrinsic features for both diagnosis and therapy and can themselves act as theranostic platforms [263]; examples include the antiangiogenic nanogold, the antibacterial nanosilver and the reactive oxygen species (ROS) enhancer GO, respectively. Alternatively, they can be functionalized in multifaceted platforms for simultaneous therapy and diagnosis (see Figure 10), with several therapeutic and image contrast agents. The latter are sometimes introduced in the framework of a multiple imaging paradigm, e.g., with the NM functionalization of fluorophores for optical imaging and other contrast agents for X-ray, computed tomography, ultrasound and magnetic resonance imaging [264].

The drug delivery using theranostic NPs enables non-invasive *in vivo* imaging of the NP delivery process and may enable assessment of treatment responses at an early stage because they offer high capacity for drug loading as well as the ability to track and image the *in vivo* pathway of both the transporter and the drug in the body [265].

Over the past decade, more interests have been aroused in engineering protein-based nanoformulations for cancer treatment in a theranostic paradigm. A new generation of biocompatible endogenous protein-based nanoformulations is currently constructed through delivering cancer therapeutic and diagnostic agents simultaneously [266]. For this purpose, protein and peptide sequences can be incorporated with dyes, contrast agents, drug payloads and, possibly, nanomaterials, serving as imaging-guided combinatorial cancer therapeutics.

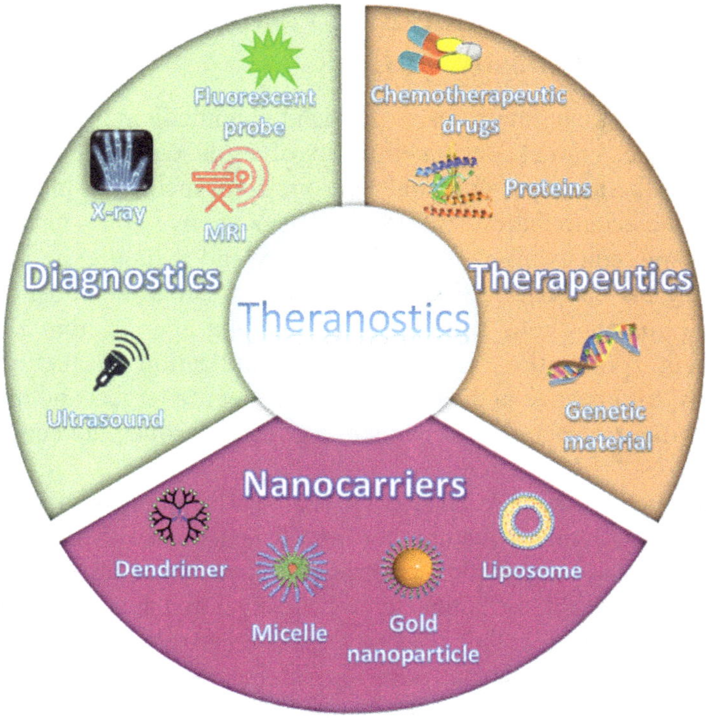

Fig. 10. Different classes of therapeutics, nanocarriers and diagnostic applications in theranostics.

Examples for protein-based cancer theranostics include the use of BSA [267], ferritin [268], transferrin [269], silk fibroin [270], lipoprotein [271] and lactoferrin [272].

Several studies on peptide-based theranostic platforms reported on tumor-targeting peptides to enable more precise diagnostic imaging for image-guided surgery, tumor-specific chemotherapeutic delivery and tumor-selective targeted radiotherapy [273]. Other examples include the self-assembly of peptide-photosensitizers and peptide-drugs as well as multicomponent cooperative self-assembly for the fabrication of nanotheranostics that integrate diagnosis and therapeutics for antitumor applications [274]. As an example, a dual-channel fluorescent cyclic RGD peptide was developed to track each of the *N*- and *C*-terminal fragments (with conjugated a fluorescent dye and a cisplatin prodrug on each terminus) separately during the tumor internalization process, for simultaneous cancer-targeted imaging and therapy [275].

In summary, nanomedicines hold a great promise for the diagnosis and treatment of human diseases. However, there are still questions not satisfactorily answered, such as: (i) the nanomaterial interaction with cells at the molecular level; (ii) the biodistribution and pharmacokinetics, which depend on the route of administration; (iii) the actual therapeutic efficacy. Another crucial subject is the mechanism of detoxification and clearance, since the accumulation of non-biodegradable NPs into biologically benign components, without an efficient clearance from the body, potentially amplifies their toxicity [22].

Theranostics have the potential to predict and evaluate therapy response, offering advantageous opportunities to control the treatments and to develop novel therapy even in a personalized manner. Protein- and peptide-based NMs have gained a lot of confidence in becoming important tools for a lot of medical applications due to their properties, which ensure better sensitivity and accuracy. These systems are currently studied and have proven effectiveness in targeting therapy and diagnosis by combining different imaging techniques with drug delivery strategies.

6. Conclusions

In this chapter, we introduced various types of bioengineered nanomaterials made of hybrid nanocomposites of peptide/protein and NMs. The latter include carbon-based nanostructures such as nanotubes and graphene, metal and metal oxide nanoparticles, inorganic oxides such as silica nanoparticles, organic polymers and macromolecules, including self-assembled peptide nanostructures.

Besides their easy fabrication, low-cost synthesis, and straightforward functionalization, NMs gained significance in technological applications due to their tunable physical, chemical and biological properties with enhanced performances over their bulk counterparts.

Due to recent advancements in nanoscience and nanotechnology, bioengineered nanomaterials are increasingly used for the fabrication of effective scaffolds for tissue engineering, biosensors and theranostic systems, contributing to outstanding advances in medicine, ranging from nano-pharmaceuticals to medical devices. Specifically, novel highly efficient delivery systems can be developed that are able to reduce drug toxicity and, meanwhile increase its solubility and bioavailability profile. Moreover, these multifunctional NMs provide innovative substrates for a highly sensitive analysis via signal amplification in analytical testing and chemical sensing. In this regard, we have discussed the fundamental differences of various types of biosensors, including magnetic, metallic nanoparticles and carbon-based devices as well as genosensors, immunosensors and enzymatic sensors used for the detection of active principles and based on different transduction approaches, such as electrochemistry, optic, and piezo-electric measurements.

Considering all these aspects, the hybrid peptide/protein nanomaterials provide new insights for a diversity of biomedical applications to fight against existing and novel diseases, thereby revolutionizing modern medicine.

List of Abbreviations

4-DPD	4,4-bipyridine
AgNP	silver nanoparticle
AuNP	gold nanoparticle
BBB	brain-blood barrier
BMP-2	bone morphogenic protein-2
BN	boron nitride nanosheet
BRCA1	breast cancer marker
BRET	bioluminescence resonance energy transfer
CBN	carbon-based nanomaterial
CCP	coiled-coil peptide
C-dot	carbon dot
CNT	carbon nanotube
DNA	desoxyribonucleic acid
DOX	doxorubicin
ECM	extracellular matrix
EDC	ethyl(dimethylaminopropyl)carbodiimide hydrochloride
ELP	elastin-like protein
FAD	flavin adenine dinucleotide
FAM	carboxyfluorescein
FQ	fluoroquinolone
FRET	fluorescence resonance energy transfer
GO	graphene oxide

HA	hydroxyapatite
hASC	human adipose stem cells
hBMP-2	bone morphogenetic protein-2
Hyp	4-hydroxyproline
LOD	limit of detection
LSPR	localized surface plasmon resonance
MRI	magnetic resonance imaging
NHS	*N*-hydroxysuccinimide
Nluc	nano luciferase
NM	nanomaterial
NP	nanoparticle
PANI	polyaniline
PCL	poly ε-caprolactone
PEG	polyethylene glycol
PHB	polyhydroxyl butyrate
PLA	polylactic acid
PLGA	polylactic-co-glycolic acid
PMMA	polymethylmethacrylate
PNIPAM	poly-*N*-isopropylacrylamide
P-NM	peptide/protein nanomaterial
Pro	proline
p-SC4	p-sufonatocalixarene
PU	polyurethane
PVP	polyvinylpyrrolidone
QD	quantum dot
rGO	reduced graphene oxide
Rluc	renilla luciferase
RNA	ribonucleic acid
ROS	reactive oxygen species
SAPN	self-assembled peptide nanostructure
SLN	solid lipid nanoparticle
SPR	surface plasmon resonance
TMD	transition metal dichalcogenide
TNF	tumor necrosis factor
VEGF	vascular endothelial growth factor
VIP	vasoactive intestinal peptide

References

1. Satriano, C., Munzone, A., Cucci, L. M., Giacomelli, C., Trincavelli, M. L., Martini, C., Rizzarelli, E. and La Mendola, D. (2018) Angiogenin-Mimetic Peptide Functionalised gold Nanoparticles for Cancer Therapy Applications. *Microchem. J.* 136, pp. 157–163.
2. Ventola, C. L. (2012) The Nanomedicine Revolution: Part 1: Emerging Concepts. *P T.* 37, pp. 512–525.
3. Bharali, D. J. and Mousa, S. A. (2010) Emerging Nanomedicines for Early Cancer Detection and Improved Treatment: Current Perspective and Future Promise. *Pharmacol. Therapeut.* 128, pp. 324–335.
4. Kim, J. K., Kim, H. J., Chung, J.-Y., Lee, J.-H., Young, S.-B. and Kim, Y.-H. (2013) Natural and Synthetic Biomaterials for Controlled Drug Delivery. *Arch. Pharm. Res.* 37, pp. 60–68.
5. Kundu, J., Chung, Y.-I., Kim, Y. H., Tae, G. and Kundu, S. C. (2010) Silk Fibroin Nanoparticles for Cellular Uptake and Control Release. *Int. J. Pharma.* 388, pp. 242–250.
6. Kim, B. Y. S., Rutka, J. T. and Chan, W. C. W. (2010) Nanomedicine. *N. Eng. J. Med.* 363, pp. 2434–2443.
7. Shaji, J. and Patole, V. (2008) Protein and Peptide Drug Delivery: Oral Approaches. *Ind. J. Pharm. Sci.* 70, pp. 269–277.
8. Lee, T., Yoo, S., Lee, K., Hwang, L. and Ryou. (2019) Self-Assembling Peptides and Their Application in the Treatment of Diseases. *Int. J. Mol. Sci.* 20, pp. 5850–5871.
9. Wang, H.-J., Di, L., Ren, Q.-S. and Wang, J.-Y. (2009) Applications and Degradation of Proteins Used as Tissue Engineering Materials. *Materials.* 2, pp. 613–635.
10. Liu, Q., Wang, J. and Boyd, B. J. (2015) Peptide-Based Biosensors. *Talanta.* 136, pp. 114–127.
11. Pokropivny, V. V. and Skorokhod, V. V. (2007) Classification of Nanostructures by Dimensionality and Concept of Surface Forms Engineering in Nanomaterial Science. *Mat. Sci. Eng: C.* 27, pp. 990–993.
12. Anilkumar, P., Lu, F., Cao, L., G. Luo, P., Liu, J. H., Sahu, S., N. Tackett Ii, K., Wang, Y. and Sun, Y. P. (2011) Fullerenes for Applications in Biology and Medicine. *Cur. Med. Chem.* 18, pp. 2045–2059.
13. Medintz, I. L. and Mattoussi, H. (2009) Quantum Dot-Based Resonance Energy Transfer and its Growing Application in Biology. *Phys. Chem. Chem. Phys.* 11, pp. 17–45.
14. Liu, T.-M., Conde, J., Lipiński, T., Bednarkiewicz, A. and Huang, C.-C. (2016b). Revisiting the Classification of NIR-Absorbing/Emitting Nanomaterials for *In vivo* Bioapplications. *NPG Asia Materials.* 8, pp. e295–e295.

15. Kawai, S., Saito, S., Osumi, S., Yamaguchi, S., Foster, A. S., Spijker, P. and Meyer, E. (2015) Atomically Controlled Substitutional Boron-Doping of Graphene Nanoribbons. *Nature Commun.* 6, pp. 1–6.
16. Tamanaha, C. R., Mulvaney, S. P., Rife, J. C. and Whitman, L. J. (2008) Magnetic Labeling, Detection, and System Integration. *Bios. Bioelectron.* 24, pp. 1–13.
17. Trapani, G., Linda Caruso, V. C., Cucci, L. M., Attanasio, F., Tabbi, G., Forte, G., La Mendola, D. and Satriano, C. (2020) Graphene Oxide Nanosheets Tailored With Aromatic Dipeptide Nanoassemblies for a Tuneable Interaction With Cell Membranes. *Front. Bioeng. Biotechnol.* 8, pp. 427.
18. Ganguly, A., Trovato, O., Duraisamy, S., Benson, J., Han, Y., Satriano, C. and Papakonstantinou, P. (2019) Organic Solvent Based Synthesis of Gold Nanoparticle–Semiconducting 2H-MoS2 Hybrid Nanosheets. *J. Phys. Chem. C.* 123, pp. 10646–10657.
19. Yang, G., Zhu, C., Du, D., Zhu, J. and Lin, Y. (2015) Graphene-Like Two-Dimensional Layered Nanomaterials: Applications in Biosensors and Nanomedicine. *Nanoscale.* 7, pp. 14217–14231.
20. Darweesh, H. H. M. (2018). Nanomaterials: Classification and Properties-Part I. *Journal of Nanoscience*, 1, pp. 1–11.
21. Hutter, E. and Fendler, J. H. (2004) Exploitation of Localized Surface Plasmon Resonance. *Adv. Mat.* 16, pp. 1685–1706.
22. Di Pietro, P., Strano, G., Zuccarello, L. and Satriano, C. (2016a) Gold and Silver Nanoparticles for Applications in Theranostics. *Curr. Top. Med. Chem.* 16, pp. 3069–3102.
23. Homberger, M. and Simon, U. (2010) On the Application Potential of Gold Nanoparticles in Nanoelectronics and Biomedicine. *Philos. Trans. Royal Soc. A: Mat. Phys. Engin. Sci.* 368, pp. 1405–1453.
24. Mineo, P., Abbadessa, A., Mazzaglia, A., Gulino, A., Villari, V., Micali, N., Millesi, S., Satriano, C. and Scamporrino, E. (2017) Gold Nanoparticles Functionalized with PEGylate Uncharged Porphyrins. *Dyes Pigm.* 141, pp. 225–234.
25. Forte, G., Travaglia, A., Magrì, A., Satriano, C. and La Mendola, D. (2014) Adsorption of NGF and BDNF Derived Peptides on Gold Surfaces. *Phys. Chem. Chem. Phys.* 16, pp. 1536–1544.
26. Cucci, L. M., Munzone, A., Naletova, I., Magrì, A., La Mendola, D. and Satriano, C. (2018) Gold Nanoparticles Functionalized with Angiogenin-Mimicking Peptides Modulate Cell Membrane Interactions. *Biointerphases* 13, p. 03C401.
27. Naletova, I., Cucci, L. M., D'angeli, F., Anfuso, C. M., Magrì, A., La Mendola, D., Lupo, G. and Satriano, C. (2019) A Tunable Nanoplatform of Nanogold Functionalised with Angiogenin Peptides for Anti-Angiogenic Therapy of Brain Tumours. *Cancers* 11, pp. 1322.

28. Abou El-Nour, K. M. M., Eftaiha, A. A., Al-Warthan, A. and Ammar, R. A. A. (2010) Synthesis and Applications of Silver Nanoparticles. *Arab. J. Chem.* 3, pp. 135–140.
29. Di Pietro, P., Zaccaro, L., Comegna, D., Del Gatto, A., Saviano, M., Snyders, R., Cossement, D., Satriano, C. and Rizzarelli, E. (2016b) Silver Nanoparticles Functionalized with a Fluorescent Cyclic RGD Peptide: A Versatile Integrin Targeting Platform for Cells and Bacteria. *RSC Adv.* 6, pp. 112381–112392.
30. Ramyadevi, J., Jeyasubramanian, K., Marikani, A., Rajakumar, G. and Rahuman, A. A. (2012) Synthesis and Antimicrobial Activity of Copper Nanoparticles. *Mat. Lett.* 71, pp. 114–116.
31. Mirsafaei, R., Heravi, M. M., Ahmadi, S., Moslemin, M. H. and Hosseinnejad, T. (2015) In Situ Prepared Copper Nanoparticles on Modified KIT-5 as an Efficient Recyclable Catalyst and its Applications in Click Reactions in Water. *J. Mol. Cat. A: Chem.* 402, pp. 100–108.
32. Tudisco, C., Cambria, M. T., Giuffrida, A. E., Sinatra, F., Anfuso, C. D., Lupo, G., Caporarello, N., Falanga, A., Galdiero, S., Oliveri, V., Satriano, C. and Condorelli, G. G. (2018) Comparison Between Folic Acid and gH625 Peptide-Based Functionalization of Fe3O4 Magnetic Nanoparticles for Enhanced Cell Internalization. *Nanoscale Res. Lett.* 13, p. 45.
33. Huber, D. L. (2005) Synthesis, Properties, and Applications of Iron Nanoparticles. *Small.* 1, pp. 482–501.
34. Bohara, R. A., Thorat, N. D. and Pawar, S. H. (2016) Role of Functionalization: Strategies to Explore Potential Nano-Bio Applications of Magnetic Nanoparticles. *RSC Adv.* 6, pp. 43989–44012.
35. Zhang, Y., Lv, Z., Zhou, J., Xin, F., Ma, J., Wu, H., Fang, Y., Jiang, M. and Dong, W. (2018) Application of Eukaryotic and Prokaryotic Laccases in Biosensor and Biofuel Cells: Recent Advances and Electrochemical Aspects. *Appl. Microbiol. Biotechnol.* 102, pp. 10409–10423.
36. Kuo, C.-L., Wang, C.-L., Ko, H.-H., Hwang, W.-S., Chang, K.-M., Li, W.-L., Huang, H.-H., Chang, Y.-H. and Wang, M.-C. (2010) Synthesis of Zinc Oxide Nanocrystalline Powders for Cosmetic Applications. *Ceram. Int.* 36, pp. 693–698.
37. Zou, Y., Huang, Z., Wang, Y., Liao, X., Yin, G. and Gu, J. (2013) Synthesis and Cellular Compatibility of Co-Doped ZnO Particles in Silk-Fibroin Peptides. *Colloids Surf. B: Biointerfaces.* 102, pp. 29–36.
38. Bai Aswathanarayan, J., Rai Vittal, R. and Muddegowda, U. (2017) Anticancer Activity of Metal Nanoparticles and Their Peptide Conjugates Against Human Colon Adenorectal Carcinoma Cells. *Artif. Cells Nanomed. Biotechnol.* 46, pp. 1444–1451.
39. Grigore, M., Biscu, E., Holban, A., Gestal, M. and Grumezescu, A. (2016) Methods of Synthesis, Properties and Biomedical Applications of CuO Nanoparticles. *Pharmaceuticals.* 9, p. 75.

40. Ishida, N., Hosokawa, Y., Imaeda, T. and Hatanaka, T. (2019) Reduction of the Cytotoxicity of Copper (II) Oxide Nanoparticles by Coating with a Surface-Binding Peptide. *Appl. Biochem. Biotechnol.* 190, pp. 645–659.
41. Dettin, M., Bagno, A., Gambaretto, R., Iucci, G., Conconi, M. T., Tuccitto, N., Menti, A. M., Grandi, C., Di Bello, C., Licciardello, A. and Polzonetti, G. (2009) Covalent Surface Modification of Titanium Oxide with Different Adhesive Peptides: Surface Characterization and Osteoblast-Like Cell Adhesion. *J. Biomed. Mat. Res. Part A.* 90A, pp. 35–45.
42. Fei Yin, Z., Wu, L., Gui Yang, H. and Hua Su, Y. (2013) Recent Progress in Biomedical Applications of Titanium Dioxide. *Phys. Chem. Chem. Phys.* 15, pp. 4844–4858.
43. Nelson, B., Johnson, M., Walker, M., Riley, K. and Sims, C. (2016) Antioxidant Cerium Oxide Nanoparticles in Biology and Medicine. *Antioxidants.* 5, pp. 15–35.
44. Cimini, A., D'angelo, B., Das, S., Gentile, R., Benedetti, E., Singh, V., Monaco, A. M., Santucci, S. and Seal, S. (2012) Antibody-Conjugated PEGylated Cerium Oxide Nanoparticles for Specific Targeting of Aβ Aggregates Modulate Neuronal Survival Pathways. *Acta Biomaterialia.* 8, pp. 2056–2067.
45. Wang, Y., Santos, A., Kaur, G., Evdokiou, A. and Losic, D. (2014) Structurally Engineered Anodic Alumina Nanotubes as Nano-Carriers for Delivery of Anticancer Therapeutics. *Biomaterials.* 35, pp. 5517–5526.
46. Athari, S. S., Pourpak, Z., Folkerts, G., Garssen, J., Moin, M., Adcock, I. M., Movassaghi, M., Ardestani, M. S., Moazzeni, S. M. and Mortaz, E. (2016) Conjugated Alpha-Alumina Nanoparticle with Vasoactive Intestinal Peptide as a Nano-Drug in Treatment of Allergic Asthma in Mice. *Eur. J. Pharmacol.* 791, pp. 811–820.
47. Rampazzo, E., Bonacchi, S., Genovese, D., Juris, R., Sgarzi, M., Montalti, M., Prodi, L., Zaccheroni, N., Tomaselli, G., Gentile, S., Satriano, C. and Rizzarelli, E. (2011) A Versatile Strategy for Signal Amplification Based on Core/Shell Silica Nanoparticles. *Chem. A Eur. J.* 17, pp. 13429–13432.
48. Zuccarello, L., Rampazzo, E., Petrizza, L., Prodi, L. and Satriano, C. (2016) The Influence of Fluorescent Silica Nanoparticle Surface Chemistry on the Energy Transfer Processes with Lipid Bilayers. *RSC Adv.* 6, pp. 52674–52682.
49. Palomba, F., Rampazzo, E., Zaccheroni, N., Malferrari, M., Rapino, S., Greco, V., Satriano, C., Genovese, D. and Prodi, L. (2020) Specific, Surface-Driven, and High-Affinity Interactions of Fluorescent Hyaluronan with PEGylated Nanomaterials. *ACS Appl. Mater. Interfaces.* 12, pp. 6806–6813.
50. Wei, Y., Gao, L., Wang, L., Shi, L., Wei, E., Zhou, B., Zhou, L. and Ge, B. (2017) Polydopamine and Peptide Decorated Doxorubicin-Loaded Mesoporous Silica Nanoparticles as a Targeted Drug Delivery System for Bladder Cancer Therapy. *Drug Delvi.* 24, pp. 681–691.

51. Slowing, I. I., Trewyn, B. G. and Lin, V. S. Y. (2007) Mesoporous Silica Nanoparticles for Intracellular Delivery of Membrane-Impermeable Proteins. *J. Am. Chem. Soc.* 129, pp. 8845–8849.
52. Liu, X., Chu, P. K. and Ding, C. (2010) Surface Nano-Functionalization of Biomaterials. *Mater. Sci. Eng.: R: Rep.* 70, pp. 275–302.
53. Dai, C., Guo, H., Lu, J., Shi, J., Wei, J. and Liu, C. (2011) Osteogenic Evaluation of Calcium/Magnesium-Doped Mesoporous Silica Scaffold with Incorporation of rhBMP-2 by Synchrotron Radiation-Based μCT. *Biomaterials.* 32, pp. 8506–8517.
54. Jun, S.-H., Lee, E.-J., Jang, T.-S., Kim, H.-E., Jang, J.-H. and Koh, Y.-H. (2013) Bone Morphogenic Protein-2 (BMP-2) Loaded Hybrid Coating on Porous Hydroxyapatite Scaffolds for Bone Tissue Engineering. *J. Mater. Sci: Mater. Med.* 24, pp. 773–782.
55. Song, Y., Ju, Y., Morita, Y., Xu, B. and Song, G. (2014) Surface Functionalization of Nanoporous Alumina with Bone Morphogenetic Protein 2 for Inducing Osteogenic Differentiation of Mesenchymal Stem Cells. *Mater. Sci. Eng: C.* 37, pp. 120–126.
56. Kojima, S., Nakamura, H., Lee, S., Nagata, F. and Kato, K. (2019) Hydroxyapatite Formation on Self-Assembling Peptides with Differing Secondary Structures and Their Selective Adsorption for Proteins. *Int. J. Mol. Sci.* 20, p. 4650.
57. Rivas, M., Del Valle, L., Alemán, C. and Puiggalí, J. (2019) Peptide Self-Assembly into Hydrogels for Biomedical Applications Related to Hydroxyapatite. *Gels* 5, p. 14.
58. Cha, C., Shin, S. R., Annabi, N., Dokmeci, M. R. and Khademhosseini, A. (2013) Carbon-Based Nanomaterials: Multifunctional Materials for Biomedical Engineering. *ACS Nano.* 7, pp. 2891–2897.
59. Simsikova, M. and Sikola, T. (2017) Interaction of Graphene Oxide with Proteins and Applications of their Conjugates. *J. Nanomed. Res.* 5, pp. 1–4.
60. Guo, C., Book-Newell, B. and Irudayaraj, J. (2011) Protein-Directed Reduction of Graphene Oxide and Intracellular Imaging. *Chem. Commun. (Camb).* 47, pp. 12658–12660.
61. Mahmoudi, M., Akhavan, O., Ghavami, M., Rezaee, F. and Ghiasi, S. M. A. (2012) Graphene Oxide Strongly Inhibits Amyloid Beta Fibrillation. *Nanoscale.* 4, pp. 7322–7325.
62. Li, M., Yang, X., Ren, J., Qu, K. and Qu, X. (2012) Using Graphene Oxide High Near-Infrared Absorbance for Photothermal Treatment of Alzheimer's Disease. *Adv. Mater.* 24, pp. 1722–1728.
63. Elhissi, A. M. A., Ahmed, W., Hassan, I. U., Dhanak, V. R. and D'emanuele, A. (2012) Carbon Nanotubes in Cancer Therapy and Drug Delivery. *J. Drug Delvi.* 2012, pp. 1–10.

64. Kotelnikova, R. A., Bogdanov, G. N., Frog, E. C., Kotelnikov, A. I., Shtolko, V. N., Romanova, V. S., Andreev, S. M., Kushch, A. A., Fedorova, N. E., Medzhidova, A. A. and Miller, G. G. (2003) Nanobionics of Pharmacologically Active Derivatives of Fullerene C60. *J. Nanoparticle Res.* 5, pp. 561–566.
65. Kalantar-Zadeh, K., Ou, J. Z., Daeneke, T., Strano, M. S., Pumera, M. and Gras, S. L. (2015) Two-Dimensional Transition Metal Dichalcogenides in Biosystems. *Adv. Funct. Mater.* 25, pp. 5086–5099.
66. Nicosia, A., Vento, F., Satriano, C., Villari, V., Micali, N., Cucci, L. M., Sanfilippo, V. and Mineo, P. G. (2020) Light-Triggered Polymeric Nanobombs for Targeted Cell Death. *ACS Appl. Nano Mater.* 3, pp. 1950–1960.
67. Ahmadi, M., Elmongy, H., Madrakian, T. and Abdel-Rehim, M. (2017) Nanomaterials as Sorbents for Sample Preparation in Bioanalysis: A Review. *Anal. Chimica Acta.* 958, pp. 1–21.
68. Han, J., Zhao, D., Li, D., Wang, X., Jin, Z. and Zhao, K. (2018) Polymer-Based Nanomaterials and Applications for Vaccines and Drugs. *Polymers* 10, pp. 31–44.
69. Venugopal, J. and Ramakrishna, S. (2005) Applications of Polymer Nanofibers in Biomedicine and Biotechnology. *Appl. Biochem. Biotechnol.* 125, pp. 147–158.
70. Sahoo, S. K., Parveen, S. and Panda, J. J. (2007) The Present and Future of Nanotechnology in Human Health Care. *Nanomed: Nanotechnol. Biol. Med.* 3, pp. 20–31.
71. Shi, J., Votruba, A. R., Farokhzad, O. C. and Langer, R. (2010) Nanotechnology in Drug Delivery and Tissue Engineering: From Discovery to Applications. *Nano Lett.* 10, pp. 3223–3230.
72. Onaciu, A., Jurj, A., Moldovan, C. and Berindan-Neagoe, I. (2019) Theranostic Nanoparticles and Their Spectrum in Cancer. *Silver Nanoparticles — Health and Safety [Working Title].*).
73. Consiglio, G., Di Pietro, P., D'urso, L., Forte, G., Grasso, G., Sgarlata, C., Cossement, D., Snyders, R. and Satriano, C. (2017) Surface Tailoring of Polyacrylate-Grafted Graphene Oxide for Controlled Interactions at the Biointerface. *J. Colloid Interface Sci.* 506, pp. 532–542.
74. Bamrungsap, S., Zhao, Z., Chen, T., Wang, L., Li, C., Fu, T. and Tan, W. (2012) Nanotechnology in Therapeutics: A Focus on Nanoparticles as a Drug Delivery System. *Nanomedicine.* 7, pp. 1253–1271.
75. Koutsopoulos, S. (2012) Molecular Fabrications of Smart Nanobiomaterials and Applications in Personalized Medicine. *Adv. Drug Del. Rev.* 64, pp. 1459–1476.
76. Seleci, M., Ag Seleci, D., Joncyzk, R., Stahl, F., Blume, C. and Scheper, T. (2016) Smart Multifunctional Nanoparticles in Nanomedicine. *BioNanoMater.* 17, pp. 31–41.

77. Lobatto, M. E., Fuster, V., Fayad, Z. A. and Mulder, W. J. M. (2011) Perspectives and Opportunities for Nanomedicine in the Management of Atherosclerosis. *Nat. Rev. Drug Discov.* 10, pp. 835–852.
78. Thiruppathi, R., Mishra, S., Ganapathy, M., Padmanabhan, P. and Gulyás, B. (2017) Nanoparticle Functionalization and Its Potentials for Molecular Imaging. *Adv. Sci.* 4, p. 1600279.
79. Elci, S. G., Jiang, Y., Yan, B., Kim, S. T., Saha, K., Moyano, D. F., Yesilbag Tonga, G., Jackson, L. C., Rotello, V. M. and Vachet, R. W. (2016) Surface Charge Controls the Suborgan Biodistributions of Gold Nanoparticles. *ACS Nano.* 10, pp. 5536–5542.
80. Arranja, A. G., Pathak, V., Lammers, T. and Shi, Y. (2017) Tumor-Targeted Nanomedicines for Cancer Theranostics. *Pharmacol. Res.* 115, pp. 87–95.
81. Soo Choi, H., Liu, W., Misra, P., Tanaka, E., Zimmer, J. P., Itty Ipe, B., Bawendi, M. G. and Frangioni, J. V. (2007) Renal Clearance of Quantum Dots. *Nat. Biotechnol.* 25, pp. 1165–1170.
82. Guo, Y., Wang, L., Lv, P. and Zhang, P. (2015) Transferrin-Conjugated Doxorubicin-Loaded Lipid-Coated Nanoparticles for the Targeting and Therapy of Lung Cancer. *Oncol. Lett.* 9, pp. 1065–1072.
83. Jin, Z., Lv, Y., Cao, H., Yao, J., Zhou, J., He, W. and Yin, L. (2016) Core-Shell Nanocarriers with High Paclitaxel Loading for Passive and Active Targeting. *Sci. Rep.* 6, p. 27559.
84. Park, D.-H., Cho, J., Kwon, O.-J., Yun, C.-O. and Choy, J.-H. (2016) Biodegradable Inorganic Nanovector: Passive versus Active Tumor Targeting in siRNA Transportation. *Angew. Chem. Int. Ed.* 55, pp. 4582–4586.
85. Tan, M. L., Choong, P. F. M. and Dass, C. R. (2010) Recent Developments in Liposomes, Microparticles and Nanoparticles for Protein and Peptide Drug Delivery. *Peptides.* 31, pp. 184–193.
86. Silva, R. F., Araújo, D. R., Silva, E. R., Ando, R. A. and Alves, W. A. (2013) l-Diphenylalanine Microtubes As a Potential Drug-Delivery System: Characterization, Release Kinetics, and Cytotoxicity. *Langmuir.* 29, pp. 10205–10212.
87. Liu, J., Liu, J., Chu, L., Zhang, Y., Xu, H., Kong, D., Yang, Z., Yang, C. and Ding, D. (2014) Self-Assembling Peptide of d-Amino Acids Boosts Selectivity and Antitumor Efficacy of 10-Hydroxycamptothecin. *ACS Appl. Mater. Interfaces.* 6, pp. 5558–5565.
88. Singh, D. P., Herrera, C. E., Singh, B., Singh, S., Singh, R. K. and Kumar, R. (2018) Graphene Oxide: An Efficient Material and Recent Approach for Biotechnological and Biomedical Applications. *Mater. Sci. Eng. C.* 86, pp. 173–197.
89. Atala, A., Kasper, F. K. and Mikos, A. G. (2012) Engineering Complex Tissues. *Sci. Translat. Med.* 4, pp. 160rv112–160rv112.

90. Hutmacher, D. W., Goh, J. C.-H. and Teoh, S. H. (2001) An Introduction to Biodegradable Materials for Tissue Engineering Applications. *Ann. Acad. Med. Singap*. 30, pp. 183–191.
91. Hosoyama, K., Lazurko, C., Muñoz, M., Mctiernan, C. D. and Alarcon, E. I. (2019) Peptide-Based Functional Biomaterials for Soft-Tissue Repair. *Front. Bioeng. Biotechnol.* 7, pp. 1–19.
92. Whitesides, G. M. (2002) Self-Assembly at All Scales. *Science.* 295, pp. 2418–2421.
93. Thadavirul, N., Pavasant, P. and Supaphol, P. (2014) Development of Polycaprolactone Porous Scaffolds by Combining Solvent Casting, Particulate Leaching, and Polymer Leaching Techniques for Bone Tissue Engineering. *J. Biomed. Mater. Res. Part A.* 102, pp. 3379–3392.
94. Nam, Y. S. and Park, T. G. (1999) Porous Biodegradable Polymeric Scaffolds Prepared by Thermally Induced Phase Separation. *J. Biomed. Mater. Res.* 47, pp. 8–17.
95. Kumbar, S. G., James, R., Nukavarapu, S. P. and Laurencin, C. T. (2008) Electrospun Nanofiber Scaffolds: Engineering Soft Tissues. *Biomed. Mater.* 3, pp. 1–15.
96. Jayawarna, V., Ali, M., Jowitt, T. A., Miller, A. F., Saiani, A., Gough, J. E. and Ulijn, R. V. (2006) Nanostructured Hydrogels for Three-Dimensional Cell Culture Through Self-Assembly of Fluorenylmethoxycarbonyl–Dipeptides. *Adv. Mater.* 18, pp. 611–614.
97. Wahid, F., Khan, T., Hussain, Z. and Ullah, H. (2018) Nanocomposite Scaffolds for Tissue Engineering; Properties, Preparation and Applications. *Appli. Nanocomposite Mater. Drug Delvi.* pp. 701–735.
98. Thevenot, D. R., Tóth, K., Durst, R. A. and Wilson, G. S. (1999) Electrochemical Biosensors: Recommended Definitions and Classification. *Pure Appl. Chem.* 71, pp. 2333–2348.
99. Gooding, J. J. (2018) Remembering Some of the Giants of Biosensing. *ACS Sens.* 3, pp. 2198–2199.
100. Wang, G., Han, R., Su, X., Li, Y., Xu, G. and Luo, X. (2017) Zwitterionic Peptide Anchored to Conducting Polymer PEDOT for the Development of Antifouling and Ultrasensitive Electrochemical DNA Sensor. *Biosens. Bioelectron.* 92, pp. 396–401.
101. Arya, S. K., Kongsuphol, P., Wong, C. C., Polla, L. J. and Park, M. K. (2014) Label Free Biosensor for Sensitive Human Influenza Virus Hemagglutinin Specific Antibody Detection Using Coiled-Coil Peptide Modified Microelectrode Array Based Platform. *Sens. Actuat. B Chem.* 194, pp. 127–133.
102. Panda, J. J. and Chauhan, V. S. (2014) Short Peptide Based Self-Assembled Nanostructures: Implications in Drug Delivery and Tissue Engineering. *Polym. Chem.* 5, pp. 4431–4449.

103. Shamsi, M. H., Kraatz, H. B. (2016) Scanning Electrochemical Microscopy: A Multiplexing Tool for Electrochemical DNA Biosensing. In: Aliofkhazraei, M., Makhlouf, A. (eds.), *Handbook of Nanoelectrochemistry*. Springer, Cham., pp. 1073–1094.

104. Shafiee, A., Ghadiri, E., Kassis, J., Pourhabibi Zarandi, N. and Atala, A. (2018) Biosensing Technologies for Medical Applications, Manufacturing, and Regenerative Medicine. *Curr. Stem Cell Rep.* 4, pp. 105–115.

105. Ngoepe, M., Choonara, Y., Tyagi, C., Tomar, L., Du Toit, L., Kumar, P., Ndesendo, V. and Pillay, V. (2013) Integration of Biosensors and Drug Delivery Technologies for Early Detection and Chronic Management of Illness. *Sensors.* 13, pp. 7680–7713.

106. Gao, X., Cui, Y., Levenson, R. M., Chung, L. W. K. and Nie, S. (2004) *In vivo* Cancer Targeting and Imaging with Semiconductor Quantum Dots. *Nat. Biotechnol.* 22, pp. 969–976.

107. Pickup, J. C., Hussain, F., Evans, N. D. and Sachedina, N. (2005) In Vivo Glucose Monitoring: The Clinical Reality and the Promise. *Biosens. Bioelectron.* 20, pp. 1897–1902.

108. Fagerstam, L. G., Frostell, A., Karlsson, R., Kullman, M., Larsson, A., Malmqvist, M. and Butt, H. (1990) Detection of Antigen-Antibody Interactions by Surface Plasmon Resonance. Application to Epitope Mapping. *J. Mol. Recognit.* 3, pp. 208–214.

109. Wang, J. (2002) Electrochemical Nucleic Acid Biosensors. *Anal. Chim. Acta* 469, pp. 63–71.

110. Alterman, M., Sjöbom, H., Säfsten, P., Markgren, P.-O., Danielson, U. H., Hämäläinen, M., Löfås, S., Hultén, J., Classon, B., Samuelsson, B. and Hallberg, A. (2001) P1/P1′ Modified HIV Protease Inhibitors as Tools in Two New Sensitive Surface Plasmon Resonance Biosensor Screening Assays. *Eur. J. Pharmaceut. Sci.* 13, pp. 203–212.

111. Zeng, Y., Zhu, Z., Du, D. and Lin, Y. (2016) Nanomaterial-Based Electrochemical Biosensors for Food Safety. *J. Electroanalyt. Chem.* 781, pp. 147–154.

112. Kerman, K., Saito, M., Tamiya, E., Yamamura, S. and Takamura, Y. (2008) Nanomaterial-Based Electrochemical Biosensors for Medical Applications. *TrAC Trends Analyt. Chem.* 27, pp. 585–592.

113. Maduraiveeran, G., Sasidharan, M. and Ganesan, V. (2018) Electrochemical Sensor and Biosensor Platforms Based on Advanced Nanomaterials for Biological and Biomedical Applications. *Biosens. Bioelectron.* 103, pp. 113–129.

114. Jianrong, C., Yuqing, M., Nongyue, H., Xiaohua, W. and Sijiao, L. (2004) Nanotechnology and Biosensors. *Biotechnol. Adv.* 22, pp. 505–518.

115. Awual, M. R., Khraisheh, M., Alharthi, N. H., Luqman, M., Islam, A., Rezaul Karim, M., Rahman, M. M. and Khaleque, M. A. (2018) Efficient

Detection and Adsorption of Cadmium(II) Ions Using Innovative Nano-Composite Materials. *Chem. Eng. J.* 343, pp. 118–127.

116. Awual, M. R., Hasan, M. M., Eldesoky, G. E., Khaleque, M. A., Rahman, M. M. and Naushad, M. (2016) Facile Mercury Detection and Removal from Aqueous Media Involving Ligand Impregnated Conjugate Nanomaterials. *Chem. Eng. J.* 290, pp. 243–251.
117. Hussain, M. M., Rahman, M. M., Arshad, M. N. and Asiri, A. M. (2017) Hg2+ Sensor Development Based on (E)-N′-Nitrobenzylidene-Benzenesulfonohydrazide (NBBSH) Derivatives Fabricated on a Glassy Carbon Electrode with a Nafion Matrix. *ACS Omega.* 2, pp. 420–431.
118. Wilchek, M. and Bayer, E. A. (1988) The Avidin-Biotin Complex in Bioanalytical Applications. *Analyt. Biochem.* 171, pp. 1–32.
119. Bruno, B. J., Miller, G. D. and Lim, C. S. (2013) Basics and Recent Advances in Peptide and Protein Drug Delivery. *Therapeutic Delvi.* 4, pp. 1443–1467.
120. Jain, A., Singh, S. K., Arya, S. K., Kundu, S. C. and Kapoor, S. (2018) Protein Nanoparticles: Promising Platforms for Drug Delivery Applications. *ACS Biomater. Sci. Eng.* 4, pp. 3939–3961.
121. Jones, O. G., Decker, E. A. and Mcclements, D. J. (2010) Comparison of Protein–Polysaccharide Nanoparticle Fabrication Methods: Impact of Biopolymer Complexation Before or After Particle Formation. *J. Coll. Interface Sci.* 344, pp. 21–29.
122. Kundu, J., Chung, Y.-I., Kim, Y. H., Tae, G. and Kundu, S. C. (2010) Silk Fibroin Nanoparticles for Cellular Uptake and Control Release. *Int. J. Pharm.* 388, pp. 242–250.
123. Yan, H.-B., Zhang, Y.-Q., Ma, Y.-L. and Zhou, L.-X. (2008) Biosynthesis of Insulin-Silk Fibroin Nanoparticles Conjugates and *In Vitro* Evaluation of a Drug Delivery System. *J. Nanoparticle Res.* 11, pp. 1937–1946.
124. Raza, F., Siyu, L., Zafar, H., Kamal, Z., Zheng, B., Su, J. and Qiu, M. (2022) Recent Advances in Gelatin-Based Nanomedicine for Targeted Delivery of Anti-Cancer Drugs. *Curr. Pharm. Des.* 28, pp. 380–394.
125. Coester, C., Nayyar, P. and Samuel, J. (2006) *In Vitro* Uptake of Gelatin Nanoparticles by Murine Dendritic Cells and Their Intracellular Localisation. *Eur. J. Pharm. Biopharm.* 62, pp. 306–314.
126. Coester, C. J., Langer, K., van Briesen, H. and Kreuter, J. (2008) Gelatin Nanoparticles by Two Step Desolvation a New Preparation Method, Surface Modifications and Cell Uptake. *J. Microencapsul.* 17, pp. 187–193.
127. Fan, T., Yu, X., Shen, B. and Sun, L. (2017) Peptide Self-Assembled Nanostructures for Drug Delivery Applications. *J. Nanomater.* 2017, pp. 1–16.
128. Habibi, N., Kamaly, N., Memic, A. and Shafiee, H. (2016) Self-Assembled Peptide-Based Nanostructures: Smart Nanomaterials Toward Targeted Drug Delivery. *Nano Today.* 11, pp. 41–60.

129. Saini, R. K., Bagri, L. P., Bajpai, A. K. and Mishra, A. (2018) Responsive Polymer Nanoparticles for Drug Delivery Applications. In: Makhlouf, A. S. H. and Abu-Thabit, N. H. (eds.), Stimuli Responsive Polymeric Nanocarriers for Drug Delivery Applications, Elsevier, Amsterdam, pp. 289–320.
130. Yishay-Safranchik, E., Golan, M. and David, A. (2014) Controlled Release of Doxorubicin and Smac-Derived Pro-Apoptotic Peptide from Self-Assembled KLD-Based Peptide Hydrogels. *Poly. Adv. Technol.* 25, pp. 539–544.
131. Deb, P. K., Al-Attraqchi, O., Chandrasekaran, B., Paradkar, A. and Tekade, R. K. (2019) Protein/Peptide Drug Delivery Systems: Practical Considerations in Pharmaceutical Product Development. In Tekade, R. K. (ed.), Basic Fundamentals of Drug Delivery. Elsevier, Amsterdam pp. 651–684.
132. Tesauro, D., Accardo, A., Diaferia, C., Milano, V., Guillon, J., Ronga, L. and Rossi, F. (2019) Peptide-Based Drug-Delivery Systems in Biotechnological Applications: Recent Advances and Perspectives. *Molecules.* 24, pp. 351–377.
133. Hamman, J. H., Enslin, G. M. and Kotz, A. F. (2005) Oral Delivery of Peptide Drugs. *BioDrugs.* 19, pp. 165–177.
134. Qiu, L., Zheng, C., Jin, Y. and Zhu, K. (2007) Polymeric Micelles as Nanocarriers for Drug Delivery. *Exp. Op. Therap. Pat.* 17, pp. 819–830.
135. Calvo, P., Remuñan-López, C., Vila-Jato, J. L. and Alonso, M. J. (1997) Chitosan and Chitosan/Ethylene Oxide-propylene Oxide Block Copolymer Nanoparticles as Novel Carriers for Proteins and Vaccines. *Pharm. Res.* 14, pp. 1431–1436.
136. Amidi, M., Romeijn, S. G., Borchard, G., Junginger, H. E., Hennink, W. E. and Jiskoot, W. (2006) Preparation and Characterization of Protein-Loaded *N*-Trimethyl Chitosan Nanoparticles as Nasal Delivery System. *J. Control. Release.* 111, pp. 107–116.
137. Agnihotri, S. A., Mallikarjuna, N. N. and Aminabhavi, T. M. (2004) Recent Advances on Chitosan-Based Micro- and Nanoparticles in Drug Delivery. *J. Control. Release.* 100, pp. 5–28.
138. Quiñones, J. P., Peniche, H. and Peniche, C. (2018) Chitosan Based Self-Assembled Nanoparticles in Drug Delivery. *Polymers.* 10, pp. 235–266.
139. Brown, S. D., Nativo, P., Smith, J.-A., Stirling, D., Edwards, P. R., Venugopal, B., Flint, D. J., Plumb, J. A., Graham, D. and Wheate, N. J. (2010) Gold Nanoparticles for the Improved Anticancer Drug Delivery of the Active Component of Oxaliplatin. *J. Am. Chem. Soc.* 132, pp. 4678–4684.
140. Satriano, C., Munzone, A., Cucci, L. M., Giacomelli, C., Trincavelli, M. L., Martini, C., Rizzarelli, E. and La Mendola, D. (2018) Angiogenin-Mimetic Peptide Functionalised Gold Nanoparticles for Cancer Therapy Applications. *Microchem. J.* 136, pp. 157–163.

141. Chin, J., Foyez Mahmud, K. A., Kim, S. E., Park, K. and Byun, Y. (2012) Insight of Current Technologies for Oral Delivery of Proteins and Peptides. *Drug Discov/Today Technol.* 9, e105–e112.
142. Yuan, H., Jiang, S.-P., Du, Y.-Z., Miao, J., Zhang, X.-G. and Hu, F.-Q. (2009) Strategic Approaches for Improving Entrapment of Hydrophilic Peptide Drugs by Lipid Nanoparticles. *Colloids Surf.: B Biointerfaces* 70, pp. 248–253.
143. Li, Z., Chen, J., Sun, W. and Xu, Y. (2010c). Investigation of Archaeosomes as Carriers for Oral Delivery of Peptides. *Biochem. Biophys. Res. Commun.* 394, pp. 412–417.
144. Wang, L.-Y., Gu, Y.-H., Su, Z.-G. and Ma, G.-H. (2006) Preparation and Improvement of Release Behavior of Chitosan Microspheres Containing Insulin. *Int. J. Pharm.* 311, pp. 187–195.
145. Shin, H., Jo, S. and Mikos, A. G. (2002) Modulation of Marrow Stromal Osteoblast Adhesion on Biomimetic Oligo[Poly(ethylene glycol) Fumarate] Hydrogels Modified with Arg-Gly-Asp Peptides and a Poly(ethylene glycol) Spacer. *J. Biomed. Mater. Res.* 61, pp. 169–179.
146. Panitch, A., Yamaoka, T., Fournier, M. J., Mason, T. L. and Tirrell, D. A. (1999) Design and Biosynthesis of Elastin-like Artificial Extracellular Matrix Proteins Containing Periodically Spaced Fibronectin CS5 Domains. *Macromolecules.* 32, pp. 1701–1703.
147. Rezania, A. and Healy, K. E. (1999) Biomimetic Peptide Surfaces That Regulate Adhesion, Spreading, Cytoskeletal Organization, and Mineralization of the Matrix Deposited by Osteoblast-like Cells. *Biotechnol. Prog.* 15, pp. 19–32.
148. West, J. L. and Hubbell, J. A. (1999) Polymeric Biomaterials with Degradation Sites for Proteases Involved in Cell Migration. *Macromolecules.* 32, pp. 241–244.
149. Mann, B. K., Gobin, A. S., Tsai, A. T., Schmedlen, R. H. and West, J. L. (2001) Smooth Muscle Cell Growth in Photopolymerized Hydrogels with Cell Adhesive and Proteolytically Degradable Domains: Synthetic ECM Analogs for Tissue Engineering. *Biomaterials.* 22, pp. 3045–3051.
150. Hofmann, S., Knecht, S., Langer, R., Kaplan, D. L., Vunjak-Novakovic, G., Merkle, H. P. and Meinel, L. (2006) Cartilage-Like Tissue Engineering Using Silk Scaffolds and Mesenchymal Stem Cells. *Tissue Eng.* 12, pp. 2729–2738.
151. Daamen, W., Veerkamp, J., Vanhest, J. and Vankuppevelt, T. (2007) Elastin as a Biomaterial for Tissue Engineering. *Biomaterials.* 28, pp. 4378–4398.
152. Cen, L., Liu, W., Cui, L., Zhang, W. and Cao, Y. (2008) Collagen Tissue Engineering: Development of Novel Biomaterials and Applications. *Pediatr. Res.* 63, pp. 492–496.

153. Meinel, A. J., Kubow, K. E., Klotzsch, E., Garcia-Fuentes, M., Smith, M. L., Vogel, V., Merkle, H. P. and Meinel, L. (2009) Optimization Strategies for Electrospun Silk Fibroin Tissue Engineering Scaffolds. *Biomaterials.* 30, pp. 3058–3067.
154. Amruthwar, S. S. and Janorkar, A. V. (2013) *In Vitro* Evaluation of Elastin-Like Polypeptide–Collagen Composite Scaffold for Bone Tissue Engineering. *Dental Mater,* 29, pp. 211–220.
155. Palumbo, F. S., Pitarresi, G., Fiorica, C., Rigogliuso, S., Ghersi, G. and Giammona, G. (2013) Chemical Hydrogels Based on a Hyaluronic Acid-Graft-α-Elastin Derivative as Potential Scaffolds for Tissue Engineering. *Mater. Sci. Eng C.* 33, pp. 2541–2549.
156. Avila Rodríguez, M. I., Rodríguez Barroso, L. G. and Sánchez, M. L. (2018) Collagen: A Review on Its Sources and Potential Cosmetic Applications. *J. Cosmet. Dermatol.* 17, pp. 20–26.
157. Kojima, S., Nakamura, H., Lee, S., Nagata, F. and Kato, K. (2019) Hydroxyapatite Formation on Self-Assembling Peptides with Differing Secondary Structures and Their Selective Adsorption for Proteins. *Int. J. Mol. Sci.* 20, pp. 4650–4662.
158. Zeeman, R., Dijkstra, P. J., Van Wachem, P. B., Van Luyn, M. J. A., Hendriks, M., Cahalan, P. T. and Feijen, J. (1999) Successive Epoxy and Carbodiimide Cross-Linking of Dermal Sheep Collagen. *Biomaterials.* 20, pp. 921–931.
159. Castaneda, L., Valle, J., Yang, N., Pluskat, S. and Slowinska, K. (2008) Collagen Cross-Linking with Au Nanoparticles. *Biomacromolecules.* 9, pp. 3383–3388.
160. Van Luyn, M. J. A., Van Wachem, P. B., Damink, L. H. H. O., Dijkstra, P. J., Feijen, J. and Nieuwenhuis, P. (1992) Secondary Cytotoxicity of Cross-Linked Dermal Sheep Collagens During Repeated Exposure to Human Fibroblasts. *Biomaterials.* 13, pp. 1017–1024.
161. Yoshioka, S. A. and Goissis, G. (2007) Thermal and Spectrophotometric Studies of New Crosslinking Method for Collagen Matrix with Glutaraldehyde Acetals. *J. Mater. Sci Mater. Med.* 19, pp. 1215–1223.
162. Davidenko, N., Bax, D. V., Schuster, C. F., Farndale, R. W., Hamaia, S. W., Best, S. M. and Cameron, R. E. (2015) Optimisation of UV Irradiation as a Binding Site Conserving Method for Crosslinking Collagen-Based Scaffolds. *J. Mater. Sci. Mater. Med.* 27, pp. 1–17.
163. Yung, C. W., Wu, L. Q., Tullman, J. A., Payne, G. F., Bentley, W. E. and Barbari, T. A. (2007) Transglutaminase Crosslinked Gelatin as a Tissue Engineering Scaffold. *J. Biomed. Mater. Res. Part A.* 83A, 1039–1046.
164. Li, N., Fan, X., Tang, K., Zheng, X., Liu, J. and Wang, B. (2016) Nanocomposite Scaffold with Enhanced Stability by Hydrogen Bonds Between Collagen, Polyvinyl Pyrrolidone and Titanium Dioxide. *Coll. Surf B Biointerfaces.* 140, pp. 287–296.

165. Muñoz-Ruíz, A., Escobar-García, D. M., Quintana, M., Pozos-Guillén, A. and Flores, H. (2019) Synthesis and Characterization of a New Collagen-Alginate Aerogel for Tissue Engineering. *J. Nanomater.* 2019, pp. 1–10.
166. Jha, B. S., Ayres, C. E., Bowman, J. R., Telemeco, T. A., Sell, S. A., Bowlin, G. L. and Simpson, D. G. (2011) Electrospun Collagen: A Tissue Engineering Scaffold with Unique Functional Properties in a Wide Variety of Applications. *J. Nanomater.* 2011, pp. 1–15.
167. J hill, M., Qi, B., Bayaniahangar, R., Araban, V., Bakhtiary, Z., Doschak, M. R., Goh, B. C., Shokouhimehr, M., Vali, H., Presley, J. F., Zadpoor, A. A., Harris, M. B., Abadi, P. P. and Mahmoudi, M. (2019) Nanomaterials for Bone Tissue Regeneration: Updates and Future Perspectives. *Nanomedicine.* 14, pp. 2987–3006.
168. Gong, T., Xie, J., Liao, J., Zhang, T., Lin, S. and Lin, Y. (2015) Nanomaterials and Bone Regeneration. *Bone Res.* 3, pp. 1–7.
169. Keeley, F. W., Bailey, A. J., Macmillan, J., Shrewry, P. R., Tatham, A. S., Bellingham, C. M. and Woodhouse, K. A. (2002) Elastin as a Self–Organizing Biomaterial: Use of Recombinantly Expressed Human Elastin Polypeptides as A Model for Investigations of Structure and Self–Assembly of Elastin. *Philos. Trans. Royal Soc. Lond. Series B Biol. Sci.* 357, pp. 185–189.
170. Daamen, W. F., Nillesen, S. T. M., Hafmans, T., Veerkamp, J. H., Van Luyn, M. J. A. and Van Kuppevelt, T. H. (2005) Tissue Response of Defined Collagen–Elastin Scaffolds in Young and Adult Rats with Special Attention to Calcification. *Biomaterials.* 26, pp. 81–92.
171. Palumbo, F. S., Pitarresi, G., Fiorica, C., Rigogliuso, S., Ghersi, G. and Giammona, G. (2013) Chemical Hydrogels Based on a Hyaluronic Acid-Graft-α-Elastin Derivative as Potential Scaffolds for Tissue Engineering. *Mater. Sci. Eng. C.* 33, pp. 2541–2549.
172. Pal, P., Nguyen, Q. C., Benton, A. H., Marquart, M. E. and Janorkar, A. V. (2019) Drug-Loaded Elastin-Like Polypeptide–Collagen Hydrogels with High Modulus for Bone Tissue Engineering. *Macromol. Biosci.* 19, 1900142.
173. Nicol, A., Gowda, C. and Urry, D. W. (1991) Elastic Protein-based Polymers as Cell Attachment Matrices. *J. Vasc. Surg.* 13, pp. 746–748.
174. González De Torre, I., Ibáñez-Fonseca, A., Quintanilla, L., Alonso, M. and Rodríguez-Cabello, J.-C. (2018) Random and Oriented Electrospun Fibers Based on a Multicomponent, In Situ Clickable Elastin-Like Recombinamer System for Dermal Tissue Engineering. *Acta Biomater.* 72, pp. 137–149.
175. Paiva Dos Santos, B., Garbay, B., Pasqua, M., Chevron, E., Chinoy, Z. S., Cullin, C., Bathany, K., Lecommandoux, S., Amédée, J., Oliveira, H. and Garanger, E. (2019) Production, Purification and Characterization of An Elastin-Like Polypeptide Containing the Ile-Lys-Val-Ala-Val (IKVAV) Peptide for Tissue Engineering Applications. *J. Biotechnol.* 298, pp. 35–44.

176. Mahara, A., Kiick, K. L. and Yamaoka, T. (2017) *In Vivo* Guided Vascular Regeneration with a Non-Porous Elastin-Like Polypeptide Hydrogel Tubular Scaffold. *J. Biomed. Mater. Res. Part A.* 105, pp. 1746–1755.
177. Altman, G. H., Diaz, F., Jakuba, C., Calabro, T., Horan, R. L., Chen, J., Lu, H., Richmond, J. and Kaplan, D. L. (2003) Silk-Based Biomaterials. *Biomaterials.* 24, pp. 401–416.
178. Jin, H.-J. and Kaplan, D. L. (2003) Mechanism of Silk Processing in Insects and Spiders. *Nature.* 424, pp. 1057–1061.
179. Bini, E., Knight, D. P. and Kaplan, D. L. J. J. O. M. B. (2004) Mapping Domain Structures in Silks from Insects and Spiders Related to Protein Assembly. *Journal of Molecular Biology.* 335, pp. 27–40.
180. Yao, Y., Masuda, H., Zhao, C. and Asakura, T. (2002) Artificial Spinning and Characterization of Silk Fiber from Bombyx mori Silk Fibroin in Hexafluoroacetone Hydrate. *Macromolecules* 35, pp. 6–9.
181. Jiao, Z., Song, Y., Jin, Y., Zhang, C., Peng, D., Chen, Z., Chang, P., Kundu, S. C., Wang, G., Wang, Z. and Wang, L. (2017) *In Vivo* Characterizations of the Immune Properties of Sericin: An Ancient Material with Emerging Value in Biomedical Applications. *Macromolecular Biosci.* 17, p. 1700229.
182. Ni, Y., Jiang, Y., Wang, K., Shao, Z., Chen, X., Sun, S., Yu, H. and Li, W. (2018) Chondrocytes Cultured in Silk-Based Biomaterials Maintain Function and Cell Morphology. *Int. J. Artif. Org.* 42, pp. 31–41.
183. Wang, J., Yang, Q., Cheng, N., Tao, X., Zhang, Z., Sun, X. and Zhang, Q. (2016) Collagen/Silk Fibroin Composite Scaffold Incorporated with PLGA Microsphere for Cartilage Repair. *Mater. Sci. Eng C.* 61, pp. 705–711.
184. Sofia, S., Mccarthy, M. B., Gronowicz, G. and Kaplan, D. L. (2001) Functionalized Silk-Based Biomaterials for Bone Formation. *J. Biomed. Mater. Res.* 54, pp. 139–148.
185. Wöltje, M., Brünler, R., Böbel, M., Ernst, S., Neuss, S., Aibibu, D. and Cherif, C. (2019) Functionalization of Silk Fibers by PDGF and Bioceramics for Bone Tissue Regeneration. *Coatings.* 10, pp. 8–25.
186. Li, N., Zhao, P. and Astruc, D. (2014) Anisotropic Gold Nanoparticles: Synthesis, Properties, Applications, and Toxicity. *Angew. Chem. Int. Ed. Engl.* 53, pp. 1756–1789.
187. Li, Y., Schluesener, H. J. and Xu, S. (2010b). Gold Nanoparticle-Based Biosensors. *Gold Bulletin.* 43, pp. 29–41.
188. Biju, V. (2014) Chemical Modifications and Bioconjugate Reactions of Nanomaterials for Sensing, Imaging, Drug Delivery and Therapy. *Chem. Soc. Rev.* 43, pp. 744–764.
189. Mulvaney, P. (1996) Surface Plasmon Spectroscopy of Nanosized Metal Particles. *Langmuir.* 12, pp. 788–800.
190. Kelly, K. L., Coronado, E., Zhao, L. L. and Schatz, G. C. (2003) The Optical Properties of Metal Nanoparticles: The Influence of Size, Shape, and Dielectric Environment. *J. Phys. Chem. B.* 107, pp. 668–677.

191. Reynolds, R. A., Mirkin, C. A. and Letsinger, R. L. (2000) Homogeneous, Nanoparticle-Based Quantitative Colorimetric Detection of Oligonucleotides. *J. Am. Chem. Soc.* 122, pp. 3795–3796.
192. Oldenburg, S. J., Genick, C. C., Clark, K. A. and Schultz, D. A. (2002) Base Pair Mismatch Recognition Using Plasmon Resonant Particle Labels. *Anal. Biochem.* 309, pp. 109–116.
193. Liu, J. and Lu, Y. (2004) Colorimetric Biosensors Based on DNAzyme-Assembled Gold Nanoparticles. *J. Fluor.* 14, pp. 343–354.
194. Wijaya, E., Lenaerts, C., Maricot, S., Hastanin, J., Habraken, S., Vilcot, J.-P., Boukherroub, R. and Szunerits, S. (2011) Surface Plasmon Resonance-Based Biosensors: From the Development of Different SPR Structures to Novel Surface Functionalization Strategies. *Curr. Opin. Solid State Mater. Sci.* 15, pp. 208–224.
195. Guo, X. (2012) Surface Plasmon Resonance Based Biosensor Technique: A Review. *J. Biophotonics.* 5, pp. 483–501.
196. Xu, Q., Mao, C., Liu, N.-N., Zhu, J.-J. and Sheng, J. (2006) Direct Electrochemistry of Horseradish Peroxidase Based on Biocompatible Carboxymethyl Chitosan–Gold Nanoparticle Nanocomposite. *Biosens. Bioelectron.* 22, pp. 768–773.
197. Xiao, Y. (2003) Plugging into Enzymes: Nanowiring of Redox Enzymes by a Gold Nanoparticle. *Science.* 299, pp. 1877–1881.
198. Li, M., Cushing, S. K., Liang, H., Suri, S., Ma, D. and Wu, N. (2013) Plasmonic Nanorice Antenna on Triangle Nanoarray for Surface-Enhanced Raman Scattering Detection of Hepatitis B Virus DNA. *Anal. Chem.* 85, pp. 2072–2078.
199. Haes, A. J. and Van Duyne, R. P. (2002) A Nanoscale Optical Biosensor: Sensitivity and Selectivity of an Approach Based on the Localized Surface Plasmon Resonance Spectroscopy of Triangular Silver Nanoparticles. *J. Am. Chem. Soc.* 124, pp. 10596–10604.
200. Hall, W. P., Ngatia, S. N. and Van Duyne, R. P. (2011) LSPR Biosensor Signal Enhancement Using Nanoparticle−Antibody Conjugates. *J. Phys. Chem. C.* 115, pp. 1410–1414.
201. Chen, J., Shi, S., Su, R., Qi, W., Huang, R., Wang, M., Wang, L. and He, Z. (2015) Optimization and Application of Reflective LSPR Optical Fiber Biosensors Based on Silver Nanoparticles. *Sensors.* 15, pp. 12205–12217.
202. Vilela, D., González, M. C. and Escarpa, A. (2012) Sensing Colorimetric Approaches Based on Gold and Silver Nanoparticles Aggregation: Chemical Creativity Behind the Assay. A Review. *Anal. Chim. Acta.* 751, pp. 24–43.
203. Li, H., Li, F., Han, C., Cui, Z., Xie, G. and Zhang, A. (2010a). Highly Sensitive and Selective Tryptophan Colorimetric Sensor Based on 4,4-Bipyridine-Functionalized Silver Nanoparticles. *Sens. Actu. B Chem.* 145, pp. 194–199.
204. Xiong, D., Chen, M. and Li, H. (2008) Synthesis of Para-Sulfonatocalix[4]arene-Modified Silver Nanoparticles as Colorimetric Histidine Probes. *Chem. Commun.* pp. 880–882.

205. Doria, G., Conde, J., Veigas, B., Giestas, L., Almeida, C., Assuncao, M., Rosa, J. and Baptista, P. V. (2012) Noble Metal Nanoparticles for Biosensing Applications. *Sensors (Basel).* 12, pp. 1657–1687.
206. Bishop, K. J. M., Wilmer, C. E., Soh, S. and Grzybowski, B. A. (2009) Nanoscale Forces and Their Uses in Self-Assembly. *Small.* 5, pp. 1600–1630.
207. Haun, J. B., Yoon, T.-J., Lee, H. and Weissleder, R. (2010) Magnetic Nanoparticle Biosensors. *Wiley Interdiscip. Rev. Nanomed. Nanobiotechnol.* 2, pp. 291–304.
208. Fischer, I., Hsu, C.-C., Gärtner, M., Müller, C., Overton, T. W., Thomas, O. R. T. and Franzreb, M. (2013) Continuous Protein Purification Using Functionalized Magnetic Nanoparticles in Aqueous Micellar Two-Phase Systems. *J. Chromatogr. A.* 1305, pp. 7–16.
209. Min, J. H., Woo, M.-K., Yoon, H. Y., Jang, J. W., Wu, J. H., Lim, C.-S. and Kim, Y. K. (2014) Isolation of DNA Using Magnetic Nanoparticles Coated with Dimercaptosuccinic Acid. *Anal. Biochem.* 447, pp. 114–118.
210. Templier, V., Roux, A., Roupioz, Y. and Livache, T. (2016) Ligands for Label-Free Detection of Whole Bacteria on Biosensors: A Review. *Trends Analyt. Chem.* 79, pp. 71–79.
211. Kamikawa, T. L., Mikolajczyk, M. G., Kennedy, M., Zhang, P., Wang, W., Scott, D. E. and Alocilja, E. C. (2010) Nanoparticle-Based Biosensor for the Detection of Emerging Pandemic Influenza Strains. *Biosens. Bioelectron.* 26, pp. 1346–1352.
212. Pal, S. and Alocilja, E. C. (2009) Electrically Active Polyaniline Coated Magnetic (EAPM) Nanoparticle as Novel Transducer in Biosensor for Detection of Bacillus Anthracis Spores in Food Samples. *Biosens Bioelectron.* 24, pp. 1437–1444.
213. Su, X., Chew, F. T. and Li, S. F. Y. (2000) Design and Application of Piezoelectric Quartz Crystal-based Immunoassay. *Analyt. Sci.* 16, pp. 107–114.
214. Murray, C. B., Norris, D. J. and Bawendi, M. G. (1993) Synthesis and Characterization of Nearly Monodisperse CdE (E = sulfur, selenium, tellurium) Semiconductor Nanocrystallites. *J. Am. Chem. Soc.* 115, pp. 8706–8715.
215. Park, J., Joo, J., Kwon, S. G., Jang, Y. and Hyeon, T. (2007) Synthesis of Monodisperse Spherical Nanocrystals. *Angew. Chemie Int. Ed.* 46, pp. 4630–4660.
216. Weller, H. (1993) Colloidal Semiconductor Q-Particles: Chemistry in the Transition Region Between Solid State and Molecules. *Angew. Chemie Int. Ed. Engl.* 32, pp. 41–53.
217. Petryayeva, E. and Algar, W. R. (2014) Multiplexed Homogeneous Assays of Proteolytic Activity Using a Smartphone and Quantum Dots. *Analyt. Chem.* 86, pp. 3195–3202.

218. Dabbousi, B. O., Rodriguez-Viejo, J., Mikulec, F. V., Heine, J. R., Mattoussi, H., Ober, R., Jensen, K. F. and Bawendi, M. G. (1997) (CdSe) ZnS Core–Shell Quantum Dots: Synthesis and Characterization of a Size Series of Highly Luminescent Nanocrystallites. *J. Phys. Chem. B.* 101, pp. 9463–9475.
219. Jaiswal, J. K., Mattoussi, H., Mauro, J. M. and Simon, S. M. (2002) Long-Term Multiple Color Imaging of Live Cells Using Quantum Dot Bioconjugates. *Nature Biotechnol.* 21, pp. 47–51.
220. Biju, V., Itoh, T. and Ishikawa, M. (2010) Delivering Quantum Dots to Cells: Bioconjugated Quantum Dots for Targeted and Nonspecific Extracellular and Intracellular Imaging. *Chem. Soc. Rev.* 39, pp. 3031–3056.
221. Boeneman, K., Delehanty, J.B., Susumu, K., Stewart, M. H., Deschamps, J. R., Medintz, I. L. (2012) Quantum Dots and Fluorescent Protein FRET-Based Biosensors. In: Zahavy, E., Ordentlich, A., Yitzhaki, S. and Shafferman, A. (eds.), Nano-Biotechnology for Biomedical and Diagnostic Research. Advances in Experimental Medicine and Biology, vol. 733. Springer, Dordrecht, pp. 63–74.
222. Medintz, I. L., Clapp, A. R., Brunel, F. M., Tiefenbrunn, T., Tetsuo Uyeda, H., Chang, E. L., Deschamps, J. R., Dawson, P. E. and Mattoussi, H. (2006) Proteolytic Activity Monitored by Fluorescence Resonance Energy Transfer Through Quantum-Dot–Peptide Conjugates. *Nat. Mater.* 5, pp. 581–589.
223. So, M.-K., Xu, C., Loening, A. M., Gambhir, S. S. and Rao, J. (2006) Self-Illuminating Quantum Dot Conjugates for *In Vivo* Imaging. *Nat. Biotechnol.* 24, pp. 339–343.
224. Frasco, M. and Chaniotakis, N. (2009) Semiconductor Quantum Dots in Chemical Sensors and Biosensors. *Sensors.* 9, pp. 7266–7286.
225. Kumar, M., Zhang, D., Broyles, D. and Deo, S. K. (2011) A Rapid, Sensitive, and Selective Bioluminescence Resonance Energy Transfer (BRET)-Based Nucleic Acid Sensing System. *Biosens. Bioelectron.* 30, pp. 133–139.
226. Yu, X., Wen, K., Wang, Z., Zhang, X., Li, C., Zhang, S. and Shen, J. (2016) General Bioluminescence Resonance Energy Transfer Homogeneous Immunoassay for Small Molecules Based on Quantum Dots. *Anal. Chem.* 88, pp. 3512–3520.
227. Kamkaew, A., Sun, H., England, C. G., Cheng, L., Liu, Z. and Cai, W. (2016) Quantum Dot–NanoLuc Bioluminescence Resonance Energy Transfer Enables Tumor Imaging and Lymph Node Mapping *In Vivo*. *Chem. Commun.* 52, pp. 6997–7000.
228. Vamvakaki, V. and Chaniotakis, N. (2007) Carbon Nanostructures as Transducers in Niosensors. *Sens. Actuators B Chem.* 126, pp. 193–197.

229. Cho, I. H., Lee, J., Kim, J., Kang, M. S., Paik, J. K., Ku, S., Cho, H. M., Irudayaraj, J. and Kim, D. H. (2018) Current Technologies of Electrochemical Immunosensors: Perspective on Signal Amplification. *Sensors (Basel).* 18, pp. 207–224.
230. Wang, J. (2005) Carbon-Nanotube Based Electrochemical Biosensors: A Review. *Electroanalysis.* 17, pp. 7–14.
231. Silveira, C. M., Baur, J., Holzinger, M., Moura, J. J. G., Cosnier, S. and Almeida, M. G. (2010) Enhanced Direct Electron Transfer of a Multihemic Nitrite Reductase on Single-walled Carbon Nanotube Modified Electrodes. *Electroanalysis.* 22, pp. 2973–2978.
232. Patolsky, F., Weizmann, Y. and Willner, I. (2004) Long-Range Electrical Contacting of Redox Enzymes by SWCNT Connectors. *Angew. Chemie Int. Ed.* 43, pp. 2113–2117.
233. Kucherenko, I. S., Soldatkin, O. O., Kucherenko, D. Y., Soldatkina, O. V. and Dzyadevych, S. V. (2019) Advances in Nanomaterial Application in Enzyme-Based Electrochemical Biosensors: A Review. *Nanoscale Adv.* 1, pp. 4560–4577.
234. Hassan, R. Y. A., Kamel, A. M., Hashem, M. S., Hassan, H. N. A. and Abd El-Ghaffar, M. A. (2018) A New Disposable Biosensor Platform: Carbon Nanotube/Poly(o-toluidine) Nanocomposite for Direct Biosensing of Urea. *J. Solid State Electrochem.* 22, pp. 1817–1823.
235. Zhang, Y., Lv, Z., Zhou, J., Xin, F., Ma, J., Wu, H., Fang, Y., Jiang, M. and Dong, W. (2018) Application of Eukaryotic and Prokaryotic Laccases in Biosensor and Biofuel Cells: Recent Advances and Electrochemical Aspects. *Appl. Microbiol. Biotechnol.* 102, pp. 10409–10423.
236. Kaçar, C., Erden, P. E. and Kılıç, E. (2017) Amperometric l-Lysine Biosensor Based on Carboxylated Multiwalled Carbon Nanotubes-SnO2 Nanoparticles-Graphene Composite. *Appl. Surf. Sci.* 419, pp. 916–923.
237. Tang, L., Wang, Y., Li, Y., Feng, H., Lu, J. and Li, J. (2009) Preparation, Structure and Electrochemical Properties of Reduced Graphene Sheet Films. *Adv. Funct. Mater.* 19, pp. 2782–2789.
238. Krishnan, S. K., Singh, E., Singh, P., Meyyappan, M. and Nalwa, H. S. (2019) A Review on Graphene-Based Nanocomposites for Electrochemical and Fluorescent Biosensors. *RSC Adv.* 9, pp. 8778–8881.
239. Smith, A. T., Lachance, A. M., Zeng, S., Liu, B. and Sun, L. (2019) Synthesis, Properties and Applications of Graphene Oxide/Reduced Graphene Oxide and Their Nanocomposites. *Nano Mater. Sci.* 1, pp. 31–47.
240. Hondred, J. A., Stromberg, L. R., Mosher, C. L. and Claussen, J. C. (2017) High-Resolution Graphene Films for Electrochemical Sensing via Inkjet Maskless Lithography. *ACS Nano.* 11, pp. 9836–9845.

241. Muñoz-Ruíz, A., Escobar-García, D. M., Quintana, M., Pozos-Guillén, A. and Flores, H. (2019) Synthesis and Characterization of a New Collagen-Alginate Aerogel for Tissue Engineering. *J. Nanomater.* 2019, pp. 1–10.
242. Ye, R., James, D. K. and Tour, J. M. (2018) Laser-Induced Graphene. *Acc. Chem. Res.* 51, pp. 1609–1620.
243. Wang, Y., Zhai, F., Hasebe, Y., Jia, H. and Zhang, Z. (2018) A Highly Sensitive Electrochemical Biosensor for Phenol Derivatives Using a Graphene Oxide-Modified Tyrosinase Electrode. *Bioelectrochem.* 122, pp. 174–182.
244. Chae, M.-S., Yoo, Y. K., Kim, J., Kim, T. G. and Hwang, K. S. (2018) Graphene-Based Enzyme-Modified Field-Effect Transistor Biosensor for Monitoring Drug Effects in Alzheimer's Disease Treatment. *Sens. Actuators B Chem.* 272, pp. 448–458.
245. Díaz Nieto, C. H., Granero, A. M., Lopez, J. C., Pierini, G. D., Levin, G. J., Fernández, H. and Zon, M. A. (2018) Development of a Third Generation Biosensor to Determine Hydrogen Peroxide Based on a Composite of Soybean Peroxidase/Chemically Reduced Graphene Oxide Deposited on Glassy Carbon electrodes. *Sens. Actuators B Chem.* 263, pp. 377–386.
246. Bhardwaj, S. K., Chauhan, R., Yadav, P., Ghosh, S., Mahapatro, A. K., Singh, J. and Basu, T. (2019) Bi-Enzyme Functionalized Electro-Chemically Reduced Transparent Graphene Oxide Platform for Triglyceride Detection. *Biomater. Sci.* 7, pp. 1598–1606.
247. Jiang, W.-S., Xin, W., Xun, S., Chen, S.-N., Gao, X.-G., Liu, Z.-B. and Tian, J.-G. (2017) Reduced Graphene Oxide-Based Optical Sensor for Detecting Specific Protein. *Sens. Actuators B Chem.* 249, pp. 142–148.
248. Ma, H., Wu, D., Cui, Z., Li, Y., Zhang, Y., Du, B. and Wei, Q. (2013) Graphene-Based Optical and Electrochemical Biosensors: A Review. *Analyt. Lett.* 46, pp. 1–17.
249. Shi, J., Guo, J., Bai, G., Chan, C., Liu, X., Ye, W., Hao, J., Chen, S. and Yang, M. (2015) A Graphene Oxide Based Fluorescence Resonance Energy Transfer (FRET) Biosensor for Ultrasensitive Detection of Botulinum Neurotoxin A (BoNT/A) Enzymatic Activity. *Biosens. Bioelectron.* 65, pp. 238–244.
250. Wang, H., Zhang, Q., Chu, X., Chen, T., Ge, J. and Yu, R. (2011) Graphene Oxide-Peptide Conjugate as an Intracellular Protease Sensor for Caspase-3 Activation Imaging in Live Cells. *Angew. Chemie Int. Ed.* 50, pp. 7065–7069.54
251. Yu, L., Banerjee, I. A., Gao, X., Nuraje, N. and Matsui, H. (2005) Fabrication and Application of Enzyme-Incorporated Peptide Nanotubes. *Bioconjugate Chem.* 16, pp. 1484–1487.

252. Ryu, J. and Park, C. B. (2010) High Stability of Self-Assembled Peptide Nanowires Against Thermal, Chemical, and Proteolytic Attacks. *Biotechnol. Bioeng.* 105, pp. 221–230.
253. De La Rica, R., Mendoza, E. and Matsui, H. (2010) Bioinspired Target-Specific Crystallization on Peptide Nanotubes for Ultrasensitive Pb Ion Detection. *Small.* 6, pp. 1753–1756.
254. Hartgerink, J. D., Granja, J. R., Milligan, R. A. and Ghadiri, M. R. (1996) Self-Assembling Peptide Nanotubes. *J. Am. Chem. Soc.* 118, pp. 43–50.
255. Reches, M. and Gazit, E. (2007) Biological and Chemical Decoration of Peptide Nanostructures via Biotin-Avidin Interactions. *J Nanosci. Nanotechnol.* 7, pp. 2239–2245.
256. Geroulanos, S., Oxelbark, S. and Turina, M. (1984) A Prospective, Randomized Comparative Study Between Cefazolin and Cefuroxime as Perioperative Antibiotic Prevention in Cardiovascular Surgery. *Schweiz. Med. Wochenschr.* 114, pp. 297–303.
257. Kartal, F., Kilinç, A. and Timur, S. (2007) Lipase Biosensor for Tributyrin and Pesticide Detection. *Int. J. Environ. Anal. Chem.* 87, pp. 715–722.
258. Yang, H., Fung, S. Y., Pritzker, M. and Chen, P. (2009) Ionic-Complementary Peptide Matrix for Enzyme Immobilization and Biomolecular Sensing. *Langmuir.* 25, pp. 7773–7777.
259. Castillo, J. J., Svendsen, W. E., Rozlosnik, N., Escobar, P., Martinez, F. and Castillo-Leon, J. (2013) Detection of Cancer Cells Using a Peptide Nanotube-Folic Acid Modified Graphene Electrode. *Analyst.* 138, pp. 1026–1031.
260. Ryu, J. and Park, C. B. (2009) Synthesis of Diphenylalanine/Polyaniline Core/Shell Conducting Nanowires by Peptide Self-Assembly. *Angew. Chemie Int. Ed.* 48, pp. 4820–4823.
261. Sun, Z., Deng, L., Gan, H., Shen, R., Yang, M. and Zhang, Y. (2013) Sensitive Immunosensor for Tumor Necrosis Factor α Based on Dual Signal Amplification of Ferrocene Modified Self-Assembled Peptide Nanowire and Glucose Oxidase Functionalized Gold Nanorod. *Biosens. Bioelectron.* 39, pp. 215–219.
262. Lammers, T., Aime, S., Hennink, W. E., Storm, G. and Kiessling, F. (2011) Theranostic Nanomedicine. *Acc. Chem. Res.* 44, pp. 1029–1038.
263. Muthu, M. S., Leong, D. T., Mei, L. and Feng, S.-S. (2014) Nanotheranostics - Application and Further Development of Nanomedicine Strategies for Advanced Theranostics. *Theranostics.* 4, pp. 660–677.
264. Singh, D., Dilnawaz, F. and Sahoo, S. K. (2020) Challenges of Moving Theranostic Nanomedicine into the Clinic. *Nanomedicine.* 15, pp. 111–114.
265. Pelaz, B., Alexiou, C., Alvarez-Puebla, R. A., Alves, F., Andrews, A. M., Ashraf, S., Balogh, L. P., Ballerini, L., Bestetti, A., Brendel, C., Bosi, S.,

Carril, M., Chan, W. C. W., Chen, C., Chen, X., Chen, X., Cheng, Z., Cui, D., Du, J., Dullin, C., Escudero, A., Feliu, N., Gao, M., George, M., Gogotsi, Y., Grünweller, A., Gu, Z., Halas, N. J., Hampp, N., Hartmann, R. K., Hersam, M. C., Hunziker, P., Jian, J., Jiang, X., Jungebluth, P., Kadhiresan, P., Kataoka, K., Khademhosseini, A., Kopeček, J., Kotov, N. A., Krug, H. F., Lee, D. S., Lehr, C.-M., Leong, K. W., Liang, X.-J., Ling Lim, M., Liz-Marzán, L. M., Ma, X., Macchiarini, P., Meng, H., Möhwald, H., Mulvaney, P., Nel, A. E., Nie, S., Nordlander, P., Okano, T., Oliveira, J., Park, T. H., Penner, R. M., Prato, M., Puntes, V., Rotello, V. M., Samarakoon, A., Schaak, R. E., Shen, Y., Sjöqvist, S., Skirtach, A. G., Soliman, M. G., Stevens, M. M., Sung, H.-W., Tang, B. Z., Tietze, R., Udugama, B. N., Vanepps, J. S., Weil, T., Weiss, P. S., Willner, I., Wu, Y., Yang, L., Yue, Z., Zhang, Q., Zhang, Q., Zhang, X.-E., Zhao, Y., Zhou, X. and Parak, W. J. (2017) Diverse Applications of Nanomedicine. *ACS Nano.* 11, pp. 2313–2381.

266. Gou, Y., Miao, D., Zhou, M., Wang, L., Zhou, H. and Su, G. (2018) Bio-Inspired Protein-Based Nanoformulations for Cancer Theranostics. *Front. Pharmacol.* 9, pp. 1–19.
267. Gao, F.-P., Lin, Y.-X., Li, L.-L., Liu, Y., Mayerhöffer, U., Spenst, P., Su, J.-G., Li, J.-Y., Würthner, F. and Wang, H. (2014) Supramolecular Adducts of Squaraine and Protein for Noninvasive Tumor Imaging and Photothermal Therapy In Vivo. *Biomaterials.* 35, pp. 1004–1014.
268. Turino, L. N., Ruggiero, M. R., Stefanìa, R., Cutrin, J. C., Aime, S. and Geninatti Crich, S. (2017) Ferritin Decorated PLGA/Paclitaxel Loaded Nanoparticles Endowed with an Enhanced Toxicity Toward MCF-7 Breast Tumor Cells. *Bioconjugate Chem.* 28, pp. 1283–1290.
269. Sonali, Singh, R. P., Singh, N., Sharma, G., Vijayakumar, M. R., Koch, B., Singh, S., Singh, U., Dash, D., Pandey, B. L. and Muthu, M. S. (2016) Transferrin Liposomes of Docetaxel for Brain-Targeted Cancer Applications: Formulation and Brain Theranostics. *Drug Deliv.* 23, pp. 1261–1271.
270. Liu, B., Wu, P., Sha, H., Qian, H., Wang, Q., Yang, Y., Yang, M., Bian, X. and Cheng, L. (2016). Anti-EGFR-iRGD Recombinant Protein Conjugated Silk Fibroin Nanoparticles for Enhanced Tumor Targeting and Antitumor Efficiency. *Onco Targets Ther.* 9, pp. 3153–3162.
271. Alberti, D., Protti, N., Toppino, A., Deagostino, A., Lanzardo, S., Bortolussi, S., Altieri, S., Voena, C., Chiarle, R., Geninatti Crich, S. and Aime, S. (2015) A Theranostic Approach Based on the Use of a Dual Boron/Gd Agent to Improve the Efficacy of Boron Neutron Capture Therapy in the Lung Cancer Treatment. *Nanomed. Nanotechnol. Biol. Med.* 11, pp. 741–750.
272. Kanwar, J. R., Kamalapuram, S. K., Krishnakumar, S. and Kanwar, R. K. (2016) Multimodal Iron Oxide (Fe3O4)-Saturated Lactoferrin Nanocapsules

as Nanotheranostics for Real-Time Imaging and Breast Cancer Therapy of Claudin-Low, Triple-Negative (ER-/PR-/HER2-). *Nanomedicine.* 11, pp. 249–268.

273. Wright, C. L., Pan, Q., Knopp, M. V. and Tweedle, M. F. (2016) Advancing Theranostics with Tumor-Targeting Peptides for Precision Otolaryngology. *World J. Otorhinolaryngol. Head Neck Surg.* 2, pp. 98–108.
274. Li, S., Zou, Q., Xing, R., Govindaraju, T., Fakhrullin, R. and Yan, X. (2019) Peptide-Modulated Self-Assembly as a Versatile Strategy for Tumor Supramolecular Nanotheranostics. *Theranostics.* 9, pp. 3249–3261.
275. Cho, H.-J., Park, S.-J., Lee, Y.-S. and Kim, S. (2019) Theranostic iRGD Peptide Containing Cisplatin Prodrug: Dual-Cargo Tumor Penetration for Improved Imaging and Therapy. *J. Control. Release.* 300, pp. 73–80.

https://doi.org/10.1142/9789811261664_0006

Chapter 6

Engineering Peptidyl and Protein Glutathione Peroxidase Mimics

Nicolas Delsuc

Laboratoire des biomolécules, LBM, Département de chimie, Ecole Normale Supérieure, PSL University, Sorbonne Université, Paris, France

nicolas.delsuc@ens.psl.eu

1. Introduction

Peptides are central in terms of size in the molecular continuum of pharmaceutical tools ranging from small molecules to proteins. However, their chemical and biochemical properties are very distinct from both classes of pharmaceutics. Until the end of the 20th century, examples of peptides on the market were very scarce, with insulin as the blockbuster [1,2]. This can be explained by the main drawbacks of peptides such as their poor stability in biological media, leading to suboptimal pharmacokinetics and their poor membrane permeability. However, since 2000, more and more peptides have entered clinical development and the number of approved peptides has increased gradually. The proteolytic instability and rapid clearance of peptides are nowadays seen as key advantages since peptides do not accumulate in tissues, are not metabolized in the liver avoiding drug–drug interactions and non-anticipated toxicology, contrarily to what happens with small molecules. In addition, their production is much easier than protein production and they present lower immunogenicity. The majority of peptidyl pharmaceutics are produced by chemical methods, using mainly solid-phase peptide synthesis, but some of them are produced using recombinant techniques. They have consequently benefited from the improvements in chemical and biological technologies for their production or delivery. Nowadays, approved peptides are used as drug-targeting proteins (mainly G-protein coupled receptors, GPCRs or other cell surface receptors) exploiting their recognition properties or means to deliver a cytotoxic payload or imaging agent. They are thus considered as "stoichiometric" drugs since one molecule reacts with one target (a protein for instance). On the contrary, a new class of drugs called catalytic drugs is emerging with promising applications [3,4]. Drugs based on catalysis afford potentially great advantages over stoichiometric drugs as they may allow decreasing the administrated doses and thus potential side effects. Catalytic drugs are mainly metal complexes inspired from metalloenzymes such as oxidoreductases, lyases, transferases, hydrolases, ligases and isomerases that catalyze elemental reactions very efficiently. Recently, five major groups of bioinspired catalytic drugs have been explored: photosensitizers used in photodynamic therapy to generate singlet oxygen [5], catalysts of transfer hydrogenation for the regeneration of NADH and NAD^+ [6], catalysts of peptide bonds or phospho-diester bond hydrolysis [3,7] used for hydrolytic cleavage of amyloids [8–10], HIV1 or hepatitis C RNA [12,13], thiol oxidants and in particular glutathione oxidants [14] and antioxidant enzymes mimics. The development of superoxide dismutase (SOD) [15–21] catalase (CAT) [21–24] and glutathione peroxidase (GPx) [23,25–29] mimics has attracted much attention as these enzymes play a central role in the redox homeostasis by controlling the levels of superoxide (SOD) and hydroperoxides (CAT and GPx) known as reactive oxygen species (ROS). SODs catalyze the dismutation of superoxide (O_2·-) into O_2 and H_2O_2, CAT the dismutation of H_2O_2 into O_2 and H_2O and GPx the reduction of ROOH into ROH. Among antioxidant enzyme mimics developed as catalytic drugs, several of them are peptides or involve a peptide as ligand of the metal cation bearing the redox properties essential for the catalysis. For example, peptidyl copper [30–35] or manganese [36,37] complexes have been developed as SOD mimics and CAT mimics. Concerning GPx, several strategies have been undertaken to develop selenium-containing GPx mimics and this will be the focus of this book chapter.

Glutathione peroxidase (GPx) is a family of enzymes that catalyze the reduction of hydroperoxides (ROOH) including hydrogen peroxide (H_2O_2) into their corresponding alcohols (ROH or H_2O for H_2O_2). Concomitantly thiols are oxidized into disulfide, with glutathione (GSH) as the mostly involved reductant [38]. Some GPx enzymes are selenoenzymes, meaning that they involve at their catalytic site a selenocysteine (Sec, U), often called the 21st amino acid [39]. Selenocysteine is an analog of the cysteine, the selenol group replacing the thiol group. Selenocysteine has a lower pKa (5.24–5.63) than cysteine's one (8.25), which suggests at physiological pH the Sec residue will be present predominantly in the reactive selenolate form [40]. In addition, it is a stronger nucleophile, a better leaving group and diselenides are more prone to nucleophilic attack than disulfides. Finally, Sec has also a lower reduction potential than Cys. Altogether, these properties make it very efficacious in proteins possessing antioxidant activities. The incorporation of the selenocysteine in GPx is not a post-translational modification but this amino acid is encoded by a UGA codon in messenger RNA, which is usually a STOP codon. In certain circumstances, that will not be discussed here, this STOP codon leads to the incorporation of selenocysteine [41].

Primarily, because of their ability to reduce hydroperoxides into less reactive species, GPxs were thought to detoxify organisms by preventing the formation of highly reactive radicals resulting from their degradation. GPx1 Knockout Mice ((−/−), mice with no GPx1) submitted to an oxidative stress induced by paraquat did not survive even if they were supplemented by selenium whereas selenium-supplemented wild type mice survived [42]. This clearly demonstrates that the mammalian GPx1 plays a crucial role as an antioxidant defense. However, later on, it has been shown that hydroperoxides are involved in various signaling pathways [43]. Consequently, the physiologic role of GPx is not restricted to antioxidant defense but to many other physiologic processes involving redox reactions. Brigelius-Flohé and Maiorino have recently reviewed the mammalian GPx functions thus giving an overview of their key regulating roles of multiple pathways that respond to hydroperoxides including H_2O_2 [44].

2. Mammalian GPx

2.1. *Mammalian isoforms: Localization and substrate specificities*

Mammalian GPx family is composed of eight different isoforms GPx1-8 (Table 1). Among these isoforms, GPx1-4 and GPx6 contain selenocysteine and are called SecGPxs whereas GPx5 and GPx7-8 possess a cysteine at their catalytic site (CysGPx) [45]. In addition to the composition of their active sites, these isoforms also differ from their location and thus from their substrates scope. GPx1 is found in the cytosol and reacts with soluble hydroperoxides such as H_2O_2, *t*-butyl hydroperoxide and hydroperoxide of simple lipids. GPx2, possessing a closely related structure, may possess the same substrates but has not been purified so far, thus preventing the study of its substrates scope. As GPx2 is mainly expressed in intestinal epithelium, it was suggested that its role was to reduce the toxicity of ingested lipid hydroperoxides [46]. GPx3 is also very similar to GPx1 but lacks an endoplasmic reticulum (ER) retention signal, which may be responsible for its release into the plasma where it reacts with soluble hydroperoxides as well. Three different isoforms of GPx4 have been described. They are located in the cytosol, mitochondria, nucleus or plasma membrane [47]. Very important features of GPx4 are that it is a monomeric protein, contrarily to the other Sec-containing GPx, and lacks the GSH-binding sequence. These specificities provide unique properties to GPx4: it is able to reduce, besides small hydroperoxides, hydroperoxides of complex lipids and of cholesterol and it can accommodate thiol proteins as reductant acting as thiol peroxidase. GPx5 is mainly secreted in the epididymis and is closely related to GPx3. GPx6 is homologous to GPx3 but very little is known about its reactivity. It is mainly located in the olfactory epithelium. GPx7 is the cysteine-containing counterpart of the GPx4 and is mainly located in the lumen of the ER. To finish, GPx8 is a membrane protein of the ER and the later detected member of the GPx family.

Since little is known about the catalytic cycle of the mammalian Cys-containing GPx, only SecGPxs that have been more deeply investigated will be discussed in the following.

2.2. *Catalytic activity of mammalian SecGPx*

The catalytic cycle of SecGPx comprises three steps (Figure 1(a)) [44,49]. The first step is the oxidation of the selenol under its selenolate

Table 1. Structural features, proven substrates and second-order kinetics constants of mammalian GPx. Adapted from references [44] and [48].

GPx type	Peroxidatic residue	Homo-tetramer	GSH-binding domain[a]	Reducing substrate	Location	Oxidizing substrate	Kinetic constants (M^{-1} s^{-1})
GPx1	Sec	Yes	R57, R103, R184, R185, K91′	GSH	Cytoplasm	H_2O_2, ROOH, soluble LOOH, ONOO–	k_{+1}: 4.1 10^7[b] k'_{+2}: 2.3 10^5[b]
GPx2	Sec	Yes	R57, R103, R184 conserved	n.d.	Gastro intestinal epithelium	n.d.	
GPx3	Sec	Yes	R103, R185 conserved	GSH, low rate with Trx and Grx	Plasma	H_2O_2, ROOH, soluble LOOH, PLOOH	k_{+1}: 4.0 10^7[b] k'_{+2}: 7.9 10^4[b]
GPx4	Sec	No	No	GSH, DTT, mercaptoethanol, protein thiols	Cytosol, mitochondria, nucleus	H_2O_2, ROOH, PLOOH, LOOH, ChOOH, $ONOO^-$, CEOOH	k_{+1}: 1.5 10^7[c] k'_{+2}: 5.7 10^4[c]
GPx5	Cys	Yes	R103, R185 conserved	n.d.	Epididymis	n.d.	
GPx6	Sec	Yes	n.d.	n.d.	Olfactory epithelium	n.d.	
GPx7	Cys	No	n.d.	GSH, PDI?	ER lumen	H_2O_2	
GPx8	Cys	No	n.d.	GSH, PDI?	ER membrane	H_2O_2	$k_{+1}{}^{a}$ 95[a] k'_{+2} n.d.

Notes-: [a] Bovine GPx numbering, [b] with H_2O_2, [c] with phosphatidylcholine hydroperoxide.
ChOOH, cholesterol hydroperoxide; CEOOH cholesterol ester hydroperoxide; DTT, dithiotreitol; Grx, glutaredoxin; LOOH, lipid (fatty acid) hydroperoxide; PLOOH, phospholipid hydroperoxide of different classes; ROOH, small synthetic hydroperoxides (e.g. cumene hydroperoxide and tert-butyl-hydroperoxide); Trx, thioredoxin; PDI, protein disulfide isomerase; n.d. not determined so far.

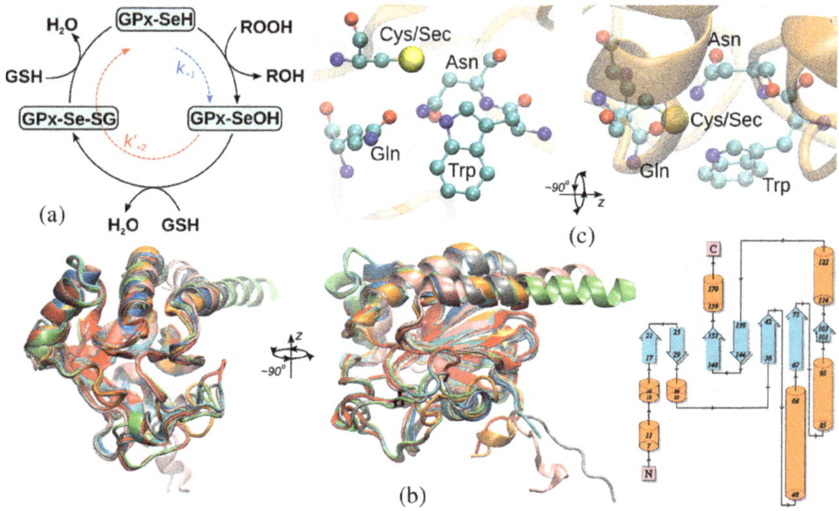

Fig. 1. Catalytic cycle and structural features of GPxs. (a) GPxs "canonical" catalytic cycle scheme. (b) Structure superimposition of several human GPx: GPx1, cyan (PDB 2F8A); GPx2, red (PDB 2HE3); GPx3, green (PDB 2R37); GPx4, orange (PDB 2OBI); GPx5, gray (PDB 2I3Y); GPx7, blue (PDB 2P31); GPx8, pink (PDB 3CYN). A topological diagram of GPx4 as a representative family member is also shown. (c) Catalytic tetrad of GPx: besides the reactive Cys/Sec residue, the conserved critical Gln, Trp, and Asn residues are highlighted. Copyright 2019, American Chemical Society [48].

(GPxSe$^-$) form of the GPxSeH Sec residue with hydroperoxide. This Sec residue and its Cys counterpart in Cys-containing GPx (CysGPx) are thus commonly called the peroxidatic residues. This oxidation leads presumably to the formation of a highly reactive selenenic acid (GPxSeOH) that has not been evidenced so far. In a second step, the selenenic acid is reduced with GSH to form water and a selenenylsulfide (GPxSeSG), which is then reduced in a final step by another GSH to produce GSSG on the one hand and to recover the GPxSeH on the other hand. The overall cycle is thus a three-substrate reaction following a non-sequential mechanism that in kinetics term is referred as a ping-pong mechanism [38]. The first step of the catalytic cycle, corresponding to the reaction with the hydroperoxide, is also called the peroxidatic part and the two last steps belong to the reductive part of the cycle as it includes two successive reductions. From this simplified two-part mechanism, two apparent second-order rate constants have been defined (k_{+1} and k'_{+2}) where k_{+1} describes the oxidation by hydroperoxide and k'_{+2} the sum of the rate constants for the two reductions. The overall rate is thus $v = [\text{GPx}]_0(k_{+1}[\text{ROOH}] + k'_{+2}[\text{GSH}])$. The relevant steady-state equation for the enzymatic peroxidase reaction following a ping-pong mechanism is written as follows:

$$\frac{v_0}{[\text{GP}X]_0} = \frac{k_{\text{max}}[\text{GSH}][\text{ROOH}]}{K_{m,ROOH}[\text{GSH}] + K_{m,GSH}[\text{ROOH}] + [\text{GSH}][\text{ROOH}]}$$

where k_{max} is a pseudo-first-order rate constant and $K_{\text{m,ROOH}}$ and $K_{\text{m,GSH}}$ are the Michaelis constants for the peroxide and thiol, respectively [50].

To determine the kinetics constants, the stopped flow techniques were indeed used to measure H_2O_2 concentrations [50]. An assay initially described by Wendel [51] and modified by Wilson *et al.* [52] was developed to measure in a more routine fashion the kinetics using a standard UV-vis spectrometer. This assay involves glutathione reductase (GR) with nicotinamide adenine dinucleotide phosphate (NADPH) to regenerate GSH from GSSG. In this situation, the GSH concentration remains essentially constant, leading to pseudo-zero order kinetics, and the decrease in NADPH can be continuously measured spectrophotometrically at 366 nm (Scheme 1). The decrease in NADPH concentration is directly related to the GPx activity. Nevertheless, the values obtained are still dependent on the GSH concentration during the cycle.

The catalytic site of GPx has first been described as a triad involving selenocysteine (Sec), glutamine (Gln) and tryptophan (Trp) [49]. It has been proposed that hydrogen bonds between the amido and imino groups of the Gln and Trp, respectively, with the Sec residue, activate the selenol to facilitate the nucleophilic attack on the hydroperoxide [54]. Following this attack, the selenolate is readily oxidized to the selenenic acid derivative. Later on, it has been shown by the evaluation of different GPx mutants of Drosophila melanogaster GPx (DmGPx), described as a paradigm of the GPx family, that an asparagine (Asn) plays also a pivotal role in the catalytic activity (Figures 1(b) and (c)) [55]. It has been emphasized that the contribution of the asparagine amido group for activation of the selenol (and the thiol for CysGPx) through hydrogen bonding is even more important than the glutamine and tryptophan contribution.

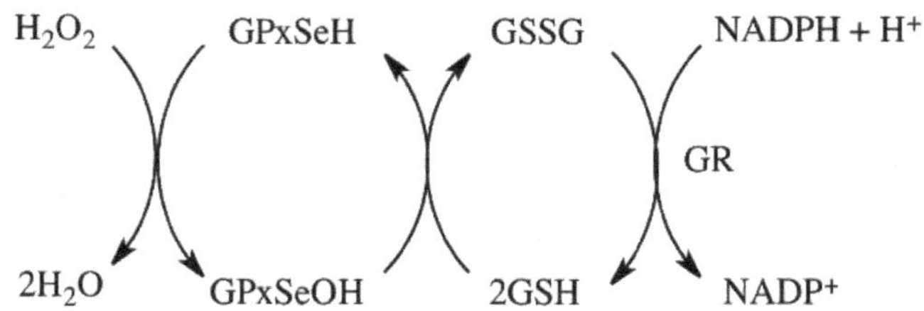

Scheme 1. Catalytic cycle of the GPx activity assay involving glutathione reductase (GR) and NADPH. Adapted from Ref. [53]. The resulting chemical equation is H^+ + NADPH + $H_2O_2 \rightarrow NADP^+ + 2H_2O$.

This tetrad is identical in all mammalian GPx active sites, except in GPx8 where the glutamine is replaced by a serine [56]. Another key feature of the GPx is their ability to interact or to direct the reductant to favor the reduction of the selenenic acid. The X-ray structure of the bovine GPx1 has shown that the catalytic site is surrounded by four arginines and one lysine that may interact with the negatively charged carboxylate groups of GSH [49]. Further investigations by molecular modeling have supported the importance of these residues for GSH binding [57].

Tremendous efforts have been devoted to the generation of GPx mimics to (i) better understand their catalytic activity and (ii) to develop efficient molecules able to supplement GPx when these enzymes are inactive or overwhelmed. Many small molecules containing selenium have been developed to mimic GPx with ebselen as the gold standard compound [58,59]. These organoselenium compounds have been extensively reviewed [25,28,29,60,61] and are not in the scope of this book chapter, which focuses on mimics involving proteins and peptides.

3. GPx Mimics

3.1. *Protein mimics of GPx*

3.1.1. *Engineering GPx by incorporating a selenocysteine into a protein scaffold*

In a pioneering work, Hilvert and coworkers have converted a serine of the active site of the serine protease subtilisin protein into a selenocysteine [62].

For this purpose, they have used two successive chemical reactions: a reaction with phenylmethanesulfonyl fluoride (PMSF) to generate a good leaving group followed by a nucleophilic substitution using hydrogen selenide (H_2Se) as nucleophile (Figure 2). They have then investigated in detail the GPx activity of this newly created selenosubtilisin (Table 2) [63–65]. In a similar way, Liu *et al.* converted a trypsin into a selenotrypsin that exhibited GPx-like activity (Table 2) [66]. Few years later, Branlant *et al.* converted the cysteine of the phosphorylating glyceraldehyde 3-phosphate dehydrogenase (GAPDH) active site into a selenocysteine [67]. This has been achieved by using the strategy developed by Böck *et al.* [68]. In brief, after having demonstrated that the cysteine can be replaced by the selenocysteine into the cysteine-specific tRNA by the cysteinyl-tRNA ligase, they produce the protein in bacteria under cysteine deprivation conditions and selenocysteine supplementation. This resulted in the incorporation of selenocysteine instead of cysteine. The produced selenoprotein (SeGAPDH) has shown similar second-order catalytic activity as selenosubtilisin but with optimum values for different hydroperoxides (Table 2). These modified proteins were all found much less efficacious than the native enzyme most probably because the active site of these mimics is buried inside the protein matrix whereas it is at the surface of native GPx enzyme and they do not possess a GSH-binding site.

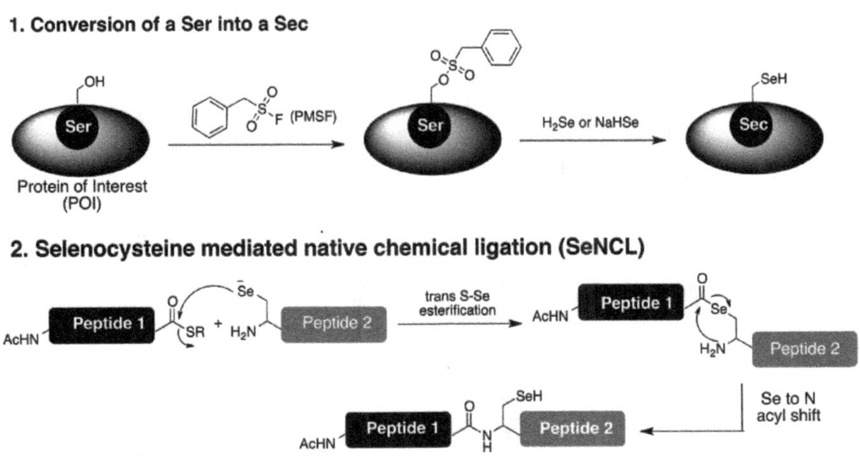

Fig. 2. Chemical strategies to incorporate a selenocysteine into a protein.

Table 2. Selected engineered GPx mimics and their kinetics parameters.

	Sec incorporation	ROOH	k_{cat} (app) min^{-1}	K_m, ROOH mM	$K_{m,thiol}$ μM	$k_{cat}/Km_{,ROOH}$ 10^6 M^{-1} min^{-1}	References
GPx1 (rabbit liver)[a]		H_2O_2	47200	0.0044		1000	[50,76,77]
Selenosubtilisin[b]	**Chemical conversion of Ser**	*t*-**BuOOH**	**2100 ± 200**	**530 ± 60**	**160 ± 20 (ArSH)**	**0.0039 ± 0.0002**	**[65]**
		CuOOH				**0.018 ± 0.001**	**[65]**
		H_2O_2	> 8000	> 0.3	> 400 (ArSH)	0.0137 ± 0.0008	[65]
Selenotrypsin[c]	Chemical conversion of Ser	H_2O_2	124 ± 4	1.25 ± 0.11	1310 ± 160	0.099	[66]
SeGAPDH[d]	Genetic incorporation	*t*-BuOOH	228	430	60 (ArSH)	0.00053	[67]
		CuOOH	14	2	140 (ArSH)	0.007	[67]
		H_2O_2	N.D.	N.D.	N.D.	0.023 ± 0.001	[67]
Se-4A4[a]	Chemical conversion of Ser	H_2O_2	619.5	0.09	270	6.86	[69,70]
Se-2F3[a]	Chemical conversion of Ser	H_2O_2	25400	1.19	20.4	21.1	[76]

Se-rGST T2-2[c]	Chemical conversion of Ser	H_2O_2	20000 ± 200	0.11 ± 0.02		180 ± 12	[75]
Se-GSTLu1-1[c]	Genetic incorporation	H_2O_2	2100 ± 30	0.21 ± 0.01	170	9.90 ± 0.28	[78]
Selenoglutaredoxin[e]	Sec Native chemical ligation	*t*-BuOOH	0.042				[79]
Biomprinted egg albumin[f]	Chemical conversion of Ser	H_2O_2	785				[80]
Bioimprinted selenosubtilisin[g]	Chemical conversion of Ser	H_2O_2	1170 ± 50	0.62 ± 0.08	300 ± 20	1.89 ± 0.05	[81]

Note: Reaction conditions: (a) [GSH] = 1 mM, [H_2O_2] = 0.5 mM, [NADPH] = 0.25 mM, [EDTA] = 0.1 mM, [GR] = 1 U and [NaN_3] = 1 mM in phosphate buffer (50 mM, pH 7) at 37°C. Reaction performed with the Wendel method.[51]. (b) [EDTA] = 1 mM, [$CaCl_2$] = 10 mM in buffer (citric acid 33 mM, HEPES 33 mM, MES 33 mM, pH 5.5) and 10% DMF at 25°C°. ArSH: 3-carboxy-4-nitrobenzenethiol. Reaction followed by stopped-flow spectroscopy. (c) [GSH] = 0.25 mM, [H_2O_2] = 0.5 mM, [NADPH] = 0.21 mM, [EDTA] = 1 mM, [GR] = 1 U, [NaN3] = 1 mM in phosphate buffer (50 mM, pH 7) at 37°C. Reaction performed with the Wendel method.[51]. (d) [ArSH] = 0.2 mM, [ROOH] = 10 mM, [EDTA] = 0.2 mM, ionic strength: 0.15 M in MES (100 mM, pH 5) at 25°C. ArSH: 4-nitrobenzenethiol. (e) [GSH] = 0.01-21 mM, [*t*-BuOOH] = 0.1 mM, [NADPH] = 0.21 mM, [EDTA] = 1 mM, [GR] = 5 U mL^{-1}, [NaCl] = 100 mM in phosphate buffer (50 mM, pH 7) at 25°C.[51] f) [GSH] = 1 mM, [H_2O_2] = 0.5 mM, [NADPH] = 0.25 mM, [GR] = 1 U in phosphate buffer (50 mM, pH 7) at 25°C. Reaction performed with the Wendel method.[51] g) [GSH] = 1 mM, [H2O2] = 0.5 mM, [NADPH] = 0.25 mM, [EDTA] = 1 mM, [GR] = 1 U, [$CaCl_2$] = 10 mM in PIPES buffer (50 mM, pH 7) at 37°C. Reaction performed with the Wilson method [52].

3.1.2. *Introducing GSH-binding properties into GPx mimics*

(a) Catalytic antibodies

In order to confer GSH-binding properties to such GPx mimics, Luo *et al.* have developed a selenium-containing monoclonal antibody with catalytic activity (abzyme) [69]. For this purpose, they have first produced a monoclonal antibody that selectively binds GSH with high affinity. Then, this antibody has been chemically modified following the 2-step procedure described by Hilvert [62] to substitute the hydroxyl group of serine residues of the monoclonal antibody L chain by selenol. In this construct (Se-4A4), both the GSH-binding domain and the active site were located on the variable part of the monoclonal antibody providing spatial proximity that conferred good catalytic activity (Table 2) [70]. A similarly prepared abzyme 4mG3 [71] has been investigated for its antioxidant properties on isolated myocardial mitochondria. It has been shown that 4mG3 was able to protect mitochondria submitted to a flow of reactive oxygen species produced by the enzymatic system xanthine oxidase/hypoxanthine [72]. Few years later, these abzymes were improved by modifying the preparation of the monoclonal antibodies and they ended up with GPx mimics whose second-order constant was only 2 orders of magnitude lower than native GPx one. In order to produce such mimics in high quantities, the variable region of the best monoclonal antibody (2F3) has been cloned and expressed as a single-chain fragment in different bacterial strains and then chemically modified to incorporate the reactive selenol (Se-2F3-scFv) [73]. Very interestingly, this new construct keeps the ability to reduce H_2O_2 and showed a very good activity (2840 U μmol^{-1}, which is 49% of that of the rabbit liver GPx: 5780 U μmol^{-1}) [74]. The antioxidant properties of Se-2F3-scFv were then investigated on a damaged-mitochondria model system and it showed the capacity to decrease mitochondrial swelling to inhibit lipid peroxidation and to maintain cytochrome c oxidase activity [74]. In addition, the antioxidant properties of this single-chain Fv on rat skin epidermal cells exposed to damaging UV-B were demonstrated: Se-2F3-scFv inhibited lipid peroxidation, preserved membrane integrity and increased cell viability [27].

(b) Engineering proteins that intrinsically possess affinity for glutathione

With the same goal of introducing GSH-binding properties to improve the efficacy of the GPx mimics, Luo *et al.* converted a glutathione *S*-transferase

(GST), which is modular, stable, easy to synthesize and more importantly already possesses a GSH-binding motif, into a GPx mimic. They have chemically converted the serine of the GST into a selenocysteine leading to a semi-synthetic GPx mimic called Se-rGST T2-2 with both high thiol selectivity and high catalytic efficiency (Table 2) [75]. However, using a chemical modification of serine residues lacks selectivity since several serines are present in GST.

To avoid that, they have used a GST mutant of the Australian sheep blowfly (*Lucilia cuprina*) LuGST1-1 where, first, the serine 9 (Ser9) of the catalytic site has been replaced by a cysteine and then the two cysteines (Cys86 and Cys200) were replaced by serine [78]. The authors argued that since these cysteines are apart from the active site and are not involved in a disulfide bridge, these substitutions did not impact the protein structure and catalytic activity. The LuGST1-1 mutant was converted into a selenoprotein (SeLuGST1-1) using the already described Böck *et al.* strategy [68] that relies on the fact that selenocysteine is charged on the cysteine-specific tRNA when the growth medium is depleted in cysteine and enriched in selenocysteine. SeLuGST1-1 appeared to be less efficient than Se-rGST T2-2 most probably because only a single residue has been converted into a selenocysteine in SeLuGST1-1 whereas several could have been introduced using the chemical strategy (Table 2). Hilvert *et al.* have also converted a mutant of *E. coli* glutaredoxin 1 (Grx1) into a GPx mimic using a three-fragment ligation strategy involving one conventional cysteine-based and one selenocysteine-based native chemical ligation step (SecNCL) (Figure 2) [79]. This semi-synthetic enzyme selenoglutaredoxin exhibited a low GPx-like activity, most probably because its monomeric structure does not prevent the formation of a diselenide dimer that competes with the formation of the required selenenylsufide intermediate (Table 2).

(c) Bio imprinted proteins

An alternative strategy that has been developed to produce protein-based GPx mimic with a GSH-binding domain relied on a combination of bioimprinting and chemical modification. This method requires a protein matrix and an imprinting molecule to generate a binding site. In brief, the bioimprinting relies on four steps: (i) protein unfolding, (ii) addition of the imprinting molecule to enable interactions between the molecule and the protein, (iii) crosslinking of the protein to block the conformation of the molecule-protein adduct, and (iv) removing of the imprinting molecule.

Finally, in the case of GPx mimics, serine residues were chemically converted into selenocysteines. Luo *et al.* used egg albumin as the protein matrix and a modified GSH as the imprinting molecule (*N*,*S*-bis(2,4-dinitrophenyl)glutathione, GSH-2DNP). Following this strategy, they produced an egg albumin imprinted GPx that was only seven times less active than the native GPx from rabbit liver (817 and 5780 U μmol^{-1} for the bio-imprinted protein and native GPx, respectively) [79]. To improve catalytic efficiency, another imprinted protein mimicking GPx has been produced starting from Hilvert's selenosubtilisin. The GSH-binding site was created through the crosslinking of the partially denaturated GSH-selenosubtilisin adduct using glutaraldehyde [81]. As expected, this bioimprinted selenosubtilisin reacted with GSH whereas selenosubtilisin did not and with second-order kinetics that are 2 orders of magnitude higher than selenosubtisilin.

3.2. *Peptides as GPx mimics*

As highlighted earlier, only a few of these semi-synthetic enzymes have been used in more biologically relevant conditions. As native proteins, semi-synthetic enzymes have poor pharmaceutical potentials since they have large molecular weight, can exhibit immunogenicity and membrane permeability issues. Consequently, smaller peptidyl mimics have been developed to overcome these shortcomings. They all include a selenocysteine residue as the peroxidatic residue which is oxidized into a diselenide to form dimers that are more stable than the monomers.

3.2.1. *Primary amino acid sequence models*

Yoshida *et al.* studied diselenide dimers of tri- and pentapeptides composed of the amino acids involved in the native primary sequence (residues 48 to 50 or 47 to 51) of the human GPx [53]. These peptides have been synthesized on solid support using a Fmoc strategy (Table 3, entries 1 and 2). Interestingly, they have shown that (H_2N-Leu-Sec-Gly OH)$_2$ and (H_2N-Ser-Leu-Sec-Gly-Thr-OH)$_2$ exhibited a GPx-like activity in the presence of GSH and that the longer peptide (H_2N-Ser-Leu-Sec-Gly-Thr-OH)$_2$ was less active than the shorter one (H_2N-Leu-Sec-Gly OH)$_2$. This thus suggested that the primary amino acid sequence around the GPx peroxidatic residue does not play a pivotal role for the antioxidant activity [26]. This was confirmed by Wehrle *et al.* who studied an

Table 3. Peptidyl SecGPx mimics and their GPx activity. The peroxidatic Sec residue is indicated in red, the residues involved in the catalytic tetrad in bold and residues that may confer GSH binding are in italic.

	Entry	Peptide sequence	*v*0 μM min^{-1}	GPx activity U μmol^{-1}	*k*cat/ Km,H_2O_2 M^{-1} min^{-1}	References
Primary sequence mimics	1	(H-Leu-**Sec**-Gly-OH)$_2$	44 ± 6[a]			[53]
	2	(H-Ser-Leu-**Sec**-Gly-Thr-OH)$_2$	39 ± 3[a]			[53]
	3	(H-**Sec**-Gly-Thr-Thr-Val-Arg-Asp-Tyr-Thr-Gln-OH)$_2$	18.0 ± 0.4[b]			[82]
	4	(H-(αMe)**Sec**-Gly-Thr-Thr-Val-Arg-Asp-Tyr-Thr-Gln-OH)$_2$	$_2$3.5 ± 1.9[b]			[82]
Catalytic triad mimics	5	(H-Gly-**Gln**-Ala-**Sec**-Ala-**Trp**-Gly-OH)$_2$	617 ± 50[a]			[83]
	6	(H-Gly-**Gln**-Ala-**Sec**-Ala-Ala-Gly-OH)$_2$	550 ± 83[a]			[83]
	7	(H-Gly-Ala-Ala-**Sec**-Ala-**Trp**-Gly-OH)$_2$	317 ± 17[a]			[83]
	8	(H-Gly-Ala-Ala-**Sec**-Ala-Ala-Gly-OH)$_2$	383 ± 33[a]			[83]
Catalytic tetrad mimics	9	(H-Lys-**Gln**-Gly-**Sec**-Gly-**Trp**-Gly-**Asn**-OH)$_2$	1167 ± 83[a]			[84]
	10	(H-Arg-**Gln**-Ala-**Sec**-Ala-**Trp**-**Asn**-Gly-OH)$_2$	783 ± 50[a]			[84]
	11	(H-Arg-**Gln**-Pro-**Sec**-Pro-**Trp**-**Asn**-Gly-OH)$_2$	833 ± 50[a]			[84]
	1$_2$	(c-Lys-**Gln**-Gly-**Sec**-Gly-**Trp**-Gly-**Asn**-)$_2$	1483 ± 133[a]			[84]
	13	(c-Lys-**Gln**-Gly-**Sec**-Gly-Ala-Gly-**Asn**-)$_2$	1400 ± 67[a]			[84]
	14	(c-Lys-**Gln**-Gly-**Sec**-Gly-**Trp**-Gly-Ala-)$_2$	1$_2$00 ± 50[a]			[84]
	15	(c-Lys-Ala-Gly-**Sec**-Gly-**Trp**-Gly-**Asn**-)$_2$	633 ± 67[a]			[84]

(*Continued*)

Table 3. (Continued)

	Entry	Peptide sequence	*v*0 μM min^{-1}	GPx activity U μmol^{-1}	*k*cat/ Km,H_2O_2 M^{-1} min^{-1}	References
GSH mimic	16	(H-γ-Glu-Sec-Gly-OH)$_2$	> $_2$10[a]			[53]
Mimic with GSH binding	17	(H-*Arg*-Gly-Sec-*Arg*-*Asn*-OH)$_2$		10.9	8.54 10^4 [c]	[85]
	18	(H-*Arg*- Sec-Gly-*Arg*-*Asn*-Ala-Gln-OH)$_2$		13[d]		[86]
15SeP$_1$	19	(H-Gly-Pro-Pro-Pro-Arg-His-Asn-Val-Tyr-Gly-Arg-Pro-Arg-Ala-Sec-OH)$_2$		190	3.07 10^7 [e]	[77]
15SeP	**20**	**(H-Trp-Pro-Phe-Leu-Arg-His-Asn-Val-Tyr-Gly-Arg-Pro-Arg-**Ala-Sec-OH)$_2$		**260**	**2.42 10^8 [e]** 6.60 10^2 [f]	**[77]** [87]
GPx (rabit liver)	21			5780	10^9	[34]

Note: Reaction conditions: (a) [GSH] = 4 mM, [H_2O_2] = 0.25 mM, [NADPH] = 0.3 mM, [GR] = 4 units mL^{-1} and [catalyst] = 50 μM in phosphate buffer (pH 7.4) at room temperature. (b) [GSH] = 0.1 mM, [NADPH] = 0.$_2$ mM, [EDTA] = 1 mM, [GR] = 4 unit/mL, [H_2O_2] = 0.2 mM, [catalyst] = 10 μM in potassium phosphate buffer (100 mM, pH 8) at $_2$5°C. (c) [GSH] = 0.5–3 mM, [H_2O_2] = 0.5-2 mM, [NADPH] = 0.25 mM, [EDTA] = 1 mM, [GR] = 1 unit, and [catalyst] = 5 μM in potassium phosphate buffer (50 mM, pH 7.4) at 37°C. (d) [GSH] = 1 mM, [H_2O_2] = 0.5 mM, [NADPH] = 0.25 mM, [EDTA] = 1 mM, [NaN3] = 1 mM, [GR] = 1 unit, and [catalyst] = 10-50 μM in sodium phosphate buffer (50 mM, pH 7) at 37°C. (e) [GSH] = 0.5–3 mM, [H_2O_2] = 0.2–2 mM, [EDTA] = 1 mM, [GR] = 1 unit, [NADPH] = 0.25 mM in potassium phosphate buffer (50 mM, pH 7). (f) [GSH] = 0.5–8 mM, [NADPH] = 0.25 mM, [EDTA] = 1 mM, [NaCl] = 100 mM, [NaN_3] = 1 mM, [GR] = 1 unit/mL, [catalyst] = 60 μM in potassium phosphate buffer (50 mM, pH 7) at 37°C.

extended primary sequence mimic of the human GPx (from residue 49 to 58) [82]. This peptide (Table 3, entry 3) exhibited a poor catalytic activity. However, by substituting the selenocysteine by α-methyl selenocysteine, they ended up with a more stable and active peptide (Table 3, entry 4). However, the initial rate was still low highlighting the fact that mimicking the primary sequence around the Sec residue is not a valuable strategy.

3.2.2. *Reproducing the catalytic triad using model peptides*

Through a Monte Carlo simulation, Iwaoka *et al.* determined amino acid sequences involving a selenocysteine that could be interesting to reproduce the catalytic triad of GPx [83]. A peptide possessing a GQAUAWG (Table 3, entry 5) sequence has emerged and has been studied as a diselenide dimer $(GQAUAWG)_2$ together with several variants lacking the glutamine or/and the tryptophan residues (Table 3, entries 5–8). All selenopeptides showed GPx-like activity higher than primary sequence mimics and the results supported a cooperative effect of the Gln and Trp residues on the activity. This highlights the importance of the catalytic triad. In addition, it has been proposed that Gln and Trp were involved in NH···Se hydrogen bonds in the selenolate form and that in the SeOH and SeSG forms, the amide of Gln was pushed away and the indole ring of the Trp was involved in a CH···Se hydrogen bond.

3.2.3. *Reproducing the catalytic tetrad using model peptides*

Later on, Iwaoka *et al.* introduced the 4th amino acid of the catalytic tetrad to improve the catalytic activity of the peptidyl mimics. An additional asparagine was added at C terminus either directly bound to the tryptophan (Table 3, entries 10 and 11) or with a glycine spacer (Table 3, entry 9) [84]. The incorporation of the glycine spacer appeared to be beneficial for the GPx-like activity. They have then head-to-tail cyclized these peptides using an N to S acyl migration followed by an intramolecular Sec-native chemical ligation (Sec-NCL) and oxidation (Scheme 2) to afford the corresponding dimeric cyclized peptides (Table 3, entries 12–15). Again, the cyclic peptide possessing the Gln, Sec, Trp and Asn separated by a single residue (Table 3, entry 12) exhibited the highest initial rate among the series. More importantly, the activity was also

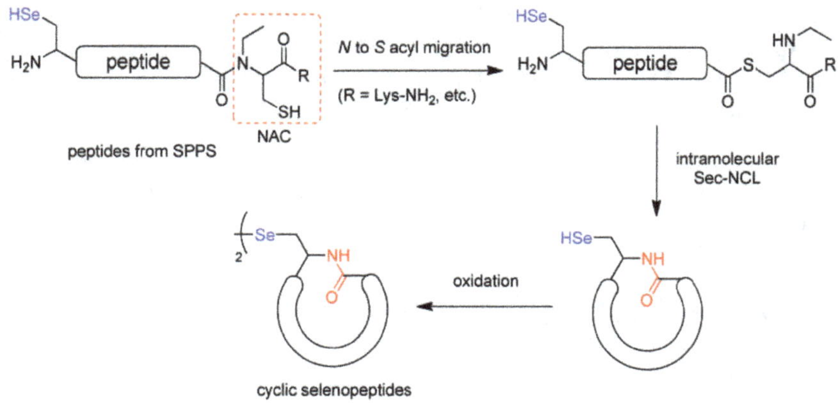

Scheme 2. Strategy for the synthesis of cyclic selenopeptides via tandem N-to-S acyl migration and intramolecular Sec-NCL. Reproduced by permission of The Royal Society of Chemistry [84].

higher than for the corresponding acyclic peptide suggesting that fixing the relative side-chain positions is beneficial. In addition, this study reveals that Gln (Table 3, entry 15 vs. 12) plays a crucial role whereas the substitution of the Trp by an Ala (Table 3, entry 13 vs. 12) or of the Asn for an Ala (Table 3, entry 14 vs. 12) did not impact the kinetics in a large extent.

3.2.4. *Glutathione mimic*

The diselenide dimer of selenoglutathione $(H_2N\text{-}\gamma\text{-Glu-Sec-Gly-OH})_2$ (GSeSeG) has been also investigated for its GPx-like activity (Table 3, entry 16) [53]. Interestingly, it showed remarkable antioxidant properties even in the absence of GSH. To explain such improved properties in comparison with primary sequence mimics that are of similar size (Table 3, entries 1–4), the authors have investigated in details the possible reactions that occurred during the assay (Scheme 3). They have shown that, among other explanations, the structural similarities of GSeSG with GSSH enable its direct reduction by glutathione reductase GR leading to the reactive GSeH intermediate. This was not the case with $(H_2N$-Leu-Sec-Gly

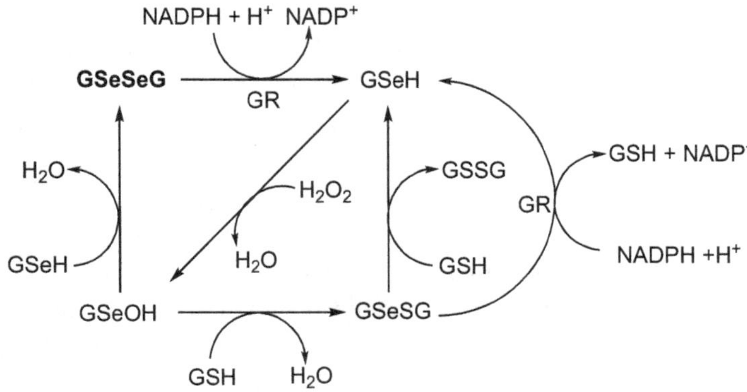

Scheme 3. Entire reaction mechanism for the antioxidative GPx activity of GSeSeG. Adapted from Ref. [53] .

OH)$_2$ and (H$_2$N-Ser-Leu-Sec-Gly-Thr-OH)$_2$ which suggests that the carboxylate of the γ-Glu residue is important for the regulation of the redox reactivity. Such effect has also been observed for small molecules reproducing GPx activity [88,89].

3.2.5. *Peptides with a GSH-binding site*

The measured catalytic activity of the above-mentioned peptides was always quite low and the residues surrounding the Sec amino acid have only a weak influence. These model peptides were poorly efficacious most probably because they lack a GSH-binding site. In the SecGPx structure published by Epp *et al.* [49], two arginines and a glutamine were presumably involved in the GSH binding through salt bridges and hydrogen bounds. This is why Yin *et al.* designed a peptide involving the Sec residue, an asparagine, replacing the glutamine and two arginine residues [85]. They have shown that this peptide ((H$_2$N-Arg-Gly-Sec-Arg-Asn-OH)$_2$) exhibited quite good catalytic activity through a ping-pong mechanism similar to those of GPx (Table 3, entry 17). This peptide has been assayed in cells and in mice as an anticancer agent. It showed promising properties but the link between its anticancer properties and its GPx-like activity has not been yet clearly established [85].

Inspired by this peptide, a longer sequence with an Ala-Gln dipeptide added at the *C*-terminus has been studied [86]. This dipeptide has been added since it has been shown to decrease ischemia-reperfusion (I-R) injuries in rats most probably by preserving GSH content [90]. GPx-like kinetics of this peptide have not been investigated in detail but it has shown a higher GPx-like activity than the shorter peptide (Table 3, entry 18 vs. 17). It has been investigated in a rat model of liver I-R and has exhibited a protective effect after an intravenous injection. In hepatic I-R, ROS produced during the reperfusion are indeed responsible for oxidative damages and are also involved in oxygen-radical-induced apoptosis [91]. Interestingly, this peptide was efficacious on both pathways, which opens up new therapeutic opportunities [86].

3.2.6. *Peptides selected from a phage display library*

To confer enhanced GSH-binding properties to the peptidyl mimics, Luo *et al.* created a 15-mer phage display library and selected the phages with high affinity for GSH [77]. The sequences of the selected peptides were then determined by DNA sequencing of the phages. The *C*-terminal serine of the peptide ($15P_1$) possessing the best association constant with GSH was then chemically modified into a selenocysteine leading to the selenopeptide $15SeP_1$ (Table 3, entry 19). This peptide exhibited a poor hydroperoxide affinity, consequently, the authors have mutated the first residues of the sequence with more hydrophobic residues that are often observed at the SecGPx catalytic site. The reported value of the second-order catalytic rate of the resulting peptide 15SeP is extremely high, only 1 order of magnitude weaker than the native GPx1 (Table 3, entry 20). However, this extremely high GPx-like activity has been questioned by Casi and Hilvert [87] that have published a much lower activity of the same peptide and no explanation was afforded to explain such discrepancies. Nevertheless, this peptide has been assayed for its antioxidant properties on rat epidermal cells submitted to a high H_2O_2 concentration. Luo *et al.* have shown that 15SeP significantly reduced lipid peroxidation, cell leakage and increased cell viability [77]. To note, this peptide is the only example of GPx mimic selected from a combinatorial library. Contrary to what has been done for the discovery of peptidyl SOD mimics and CAT mimics [35], no combinatorial library on solid support associated with GPx activity-based screening has been reported so far to develop peptidyl GPx mimics [33].

3.3. *GPx mimics with superoxide dismutase-like activity*

To ensure global protection from ROS in cells, antioxidant enzymes act cooperatively or synergistically: the balance between their antioxidant activities and their intracellular levels being very important. For example, a beneficial effect of a SOD-CAT conjugate has been described in a rat model of heart ischemia-reperfusion (I-R) injury whereas the SOD alone was found less efficacious or even detrimental at high doses [92]. Consequently, efforts have been devoted to the development of GPx mimics possessing also a SOD-like activity.

3.3.1. *Engineering proteins with a dual functionality*

A first example of a protein possessing such a dual activity has been reported by Luo *et al.* [93]. Serines of the pig blood Cu,ZnSOD have been chemically converted into selenocysteines by the already described 2-step procedure [62]. The resulting mutated SOD (Table 4) exhibited a low homogeneity as well as a low GPx activity. To circumvent this difficulty, Yu *et al.* combined the fusion protein technology with the production of a seleno semi-synthetic protein in bacteria supplemented in selenocysteine and deprived with cysteine [94]. They thus produced a Se-glutathione S-transferase (GST) fused with a SOD (Table 4). This construct showed both catalytic properties (SOD and GPx) and was able to reduce oxidation-induced damages in isolated mitochondria. However, the applications of such big macromolecules that are expressed in inclusion bodies are very limited.

3.3.2. *Miniaturization of dual functionality mimics*

In an attempt to decrease the size and the complexity of the resulting objects, an approach that has been undertaken consists of conserving key sequences of the Cu,ZnSOD3 (residues 96–138 and 161–167) and replacing the sequence in between (residues 139–160) that has a more variable composition among SODs [95] with the peptide 15SeP from Luo *et al.* possessing a GPx activity [77]. The resulting sequence has then been slightly modified according to molecular modeling studies [96]. Since Val2 and Phe33 were found close to the Sec58, these amino acids have been replaced by Gln2 and Trp33, respectively, to potentially reproduce the catalytic triad of the natural GPx. In addition, to produce this

Table 4. GPx mimics with an additional SOD-like activity

	Activity		Kinetics		
	SOD ($U\ \mu mol^{-1}$)	**GPx ($U\ \mu mol^{-1}$)**	**SOD (μmol^{-1})**	**k_{cat}/K_m,H_2O_2 ($10^6\ M^{-1}\ min^{-1}$)**	**References**
SOD[a]	6.94 10^5	0			[93]
Mutated SOD[a]	6.38 10^5	29			[93]
Se-GSTLu1-1-SOD[b]			12813	0.91	[94]
Se–CuZn-65P[c]	1254 U/mg	831		0.6	[96]
	1196 U/mg	112 U/mg			[97]
Se76P[a]	1278 U/mg	109 U/mg			[98]
SeCu32P[d]	164 ± 1.5 10^{-3}	146 ± 0.9		0.409	[99]
Se-SjGSTp35-Cu(II)[d]	1708 ± 21	2062 ± 22			[100]
GPx		5780		1000	[50,77]
SOD3	2970 U/mg				[101]

Note: Reaction conditions: (a) not reported. (b) [GSH] = 1 mM, [H_2O_2] = 0.5 mM, [NADPH] = 0.25 mM, [EDTA] = 1 mM, [GR] = 1 U and [NaN_3] = 1 mM in phosphate buffer (50 mM, pH 7) at 37°C. Reaction performed with the Wilson method [52]. (c) [GSH] = 1 mM, [H_2O_2] = 0.5 mM, [NADPH] = 0.25 mM, [GR] = 1 unit, and $m_{catalyst}$ = 0.5–2.5 μg in potassium phosphate buffer (50 mM, pH 7) at 37°C. Reaction performed with the Wilson method [52]. (d) [GSH] = 1 mM, [H_2O_2] = 0.5 mM, [NADPH] = 0.25 mM, [EDTA] = 1 mM, [NaN_3] = 1 mM, [GR] = 1 unit, and [catalyst] = 10–50 μM in PBS buffer (50 mM, pH 7) at 37°C. Reaction performed with the Wilson method [52].

construct, the Cys12 has been mutated by an alanine to enable the incorporation of the selenocysteine at the desired position (Cys58) through the utilization of a bacterial cysteine auxotrophic strain cultured in the absence of Cys in the growth medium and with a Sec supplementation. After peptide expression and cell lysis, $CuSO_4$ and $ZnSO_4$ were added into the cell-free extract to promote the metalation of the peptide. On the one hand, the resulting Se-CuZn-65P peptide exhibited a SOD activity that was unambiguously associated with the presence of a Cu cation (Table 4). On the other hand, the GPx activity required the presence of the Sec residue and was improved when the two residues of the catalytic triad (Gln2 and Trp33) were introduced. Se-CuZn-65P has shown a protective effect of mitochondria against oxidative damage on a free radical damage system. In addition, this selenopeptide protects hepatocytes against ethanol-induced cytotoxicity [97]. It has been demonstrated that this effect occurred through the diminution of mitochondrial oxidative damages but also through the prevention of the oxidation-mediated apoptosis.

The design of this peptide was further modified to improve its internalization in cells. TAT (YGRKKRRQRRR), a cell-penetrating peptide, has been added at the *N*-terminus of the Se–CuZn-65P leading to Se76P [98]. This modification did not impact both catalytic activities (Table 4) but its effect on cell penetration was not clearly evidenced.

To improve the pharmacological potential of such mimics, Zou *et al.* [99] attempted to reduce the size of the peptide by fusing the 15P peptide described by Sun *et al.* [77] with a peptidyl copper complex developed in Luo's group [102]. The 32-mer peptide was synthesized by solid phase peptide synthesis with a Ser residue instead of the Sec [99]. The Ser was converted after purification into a Sec using the Wu and Hilvert method [63] and the peptide was then metalated. The resulting SeCu32P selenopeptide (Table 4) exhibited poor catalytic activities. However, this difunctional peptide showed a better protective effect on Vero cells submitted to ROS damage than the two monofunctional peptides, highlighting the importance of the synergism between SOD and GPx activities. An analog of this dual activity peptide fused to a GST from Schistosoma japonicum GST (SjGST) has been expressed in *Escherichia coli* to generate a mimic with the three activities: SOD, GPx and GST [100]. After metalation and Sec introduction by the chemical modification of serines, the resulting Se-SjGSTp35-Cu(II) exhibited higher SOD and GPx activities than SeCu32P and an additional GST activity (2209 ± 23 U/μM of enzyme). This represents the first example of a trifunctional enzyme.

4. Conclusion

To catalytically reduce hydroperoxydes into their corresponding alcohols, three partners are involved: hydroperoxide, GPx and GSH. Efficacious catalysis by GPx thus requires that the GPx binds both ROOH and GSH with high affinity. That is why the development of GPx mimics reproducing such features is thus not very straightforward. This chapter has reviewed different strategies, ranging from protein engineering to small peptide design, that have been developed to mimic GPx, which already appeared as an appealing strategy to fight against oxidative stress in the early 90s. However, contrary to what has been done for SOD mimics, only a limited number of studies have been devoted to the utilization of GPx mimics in biologically relevant conditions, most probably because they lack stability and efficacy in intricate media such as cells or tissues. This highlights the urgent need to develop new strategies enabling the discovery of efficacious and stable GPx mimics.

List of Abbreviations

CAT	catalase
CEOOH	cholesterol ester hydroperoxide
ChOOH	cholesterol hydroperoxide
DTT	dithiotreitol
GPCR	G-protein coupled receptors
GPx	glutathione peroxidase
Grx	glutaredoxin;
GSH	glutathione
GSSG	glutathione disulfide
HIV	human immunodeficiency virus
LOOH	lipid (fatty acid) hydroperoxide
NAD^+	Nicotinamide adenine dinucleotide (oxidized form)
NADH	Nicotinamide adenine dinucleotide (reduced form)
PDI	protein disulfide isomerase
PLOOH	phospholipid hydroperoxide of different classes
PMSF	phenylmethanesulfonyl fluoride
RNA	ribonucleic acid
ROOH	small synthetic hydroperoxides
SOD	superoxide dismutase
Trx	thioredoxin

References

1. Henninot, A., Collins, J. C. and Nuss, J. M. (2018) The Current State of Peptide Drug Discovery: Back to the Future? *J. Med. Chem.*, 61(4), pp. 1382–1414.
2. Lau, J. L. and Dunn, M. K. (2018) Therapeutic Peptides: Historical Perspectives, Current Development Trends, and Future Directions. *Bioorg. Med. Chem.*, 26(10), pp. 2700–2707.

3. Suh, J. and Chei, W. S. (2008) Metal Complexes as Artificial Proteases: Toward Catalytic Drugs. *Curr. Opin. Chem. Biol.*, 12(2), pp. 207–213.
4. Soldevila-Barreda, J. J. and Sadler, P. J. (2015) Approaches to the Design of Catalytic Metallodrugs. *Curr. Opin. Chem. Biol.*, 25, pp. 172–183.
5. Josefsen, L. B. and Boyle, R. W. (2008) Photodynamic Therapy and the Development of Metal-Based Photosensitisers, Met-Based Drugs, 2008, p. 276109.
6. Liu, Z., Romero-Canelón, I., Qamar, B., Hearn, J. M., Habtemariam, A., Barry, N. P. E., Pizarro, A. M., Clarkson, G. J. and Sadler, P. J. (2014) The Potent Oxidant Anticancer Activity of Organoiridium Catalysts. *Angew. Chem. Int. Ed.*, 53(15), pp. 3941–3946.
7. Kim, H. M., Jang, B., Cheon, Y. E., Suh, M. P. and Suh, J. (2009) Proteolytic Activity of Co(III) Complex of 1-Oxa-4,7,10-Triazacyclododecane: A New Catalytic Center for Peptide-Cleavage Agents. *J. Biol. Inorg. Chem.*, 14(1), pp. 151–157.
8. Suh, J., Yoo, S. H., Kim, M. G., Jeong, K., Ahn, J. Y., Kim, M., Chae, P. S., Lee, T. Y., Lee, J., Lee, J., Jang, Y. A. and Ko, E. H., (2018) Cleavage Agents for Soluble Oligomers of Amyloid β Peptides. *Angew. Chem. Int. Ed.*, 46(37), pp. 7064–7067.
9. Chei, W. S., Lee, J.-W., Kim, J. B. and Suh, J. (2010) Cell-Penetration by Co(III)Cyclen-Based Peptide-Cleaving Catalysts Selective for Pathogenic Proteins of Amyloidoses. *Bioorg. Med. Chem.*, 18(14), pp. 5248–5253.
10. Chei, W. S., Ju, H. and Suh, J. (2011) New Chelating Ligands for Co(III)-Based Peptide-Cleaving Catalysts Selective for Pathogenic Proteins of Amyloidoses. *J. Biol. Inorg. Chem.*, 16(3), pp. 511–519.
11. Suh, J., Yoo, S. H., Kim, M. G., Jeong, K., Ahn, J. Y., Kim, M., Chae, P. S., Lee, T. Y., Lee, J., Lee, J., Jang, Y. A. and Ko, E. H. (2007) Cleavage Agents for Soluble Oligomers of Amyloid *β* Peptides. *Angew. Chem. Int. Ed.*, 46(37), pp. 7064–7067.
12. Bradford, S. S., Ross, M. J., Fidai, I. and Cowan, J. A. (2014) Insight into the Recognition, Binding, and Reactivity of Catalytic Metallodrugs Targeting Stem Loop IIb of Hepatitis C IRES RNA. *ChemMedChem*, 9(6), pp. 1275–1285.
13. Joyner, J. C., Keuper, K. D. and Cowan, J. A. (2013) Kinetics and Mechanisms of Oxidative Cleavage of HIV RRE RNA by Rev-Coupled Transition Metal–Chelates. *Chem. Sci.*, 4(4), p. 1707.
14. Dougan, S. J., Habtemariam, A., McHale, S. E., Parsons, S. and Sadler, P. J. (2008) Catalytic Organometallic Anticancer Complexes. *Proc. Natl. Acad. Sci.*, 105(33), pp. 11628–11633.
15. Salvemini, D., Muscoli, C., Riley, D. P. and Cuzzocrea, S. (2002) Superoxide Dismutase Mimetics. *Pulm. Pharmacol. Ther.*, 15(5), pp. 439–447.

16. Miriyala, S., Spasojevic, I., Tovmasyan, A., Salvemini, D., Vujaskovic, Z., St. Clair, D. and Batinic-Haberle, I. (2012) Manganese Superoxide Dismutase, MnSOD and Its Mimics. *Biochim. Biophys. Acta BBA — Mol. Basis Dis.*, 1822(5), pp. 794–814.
17. Batinić-Haberle, I., Rebouças, J. S. and Spasojević, I. (2010) Superoxide Dismutase Mimics: Chemistry, Pharmacology, and Therapeutic Potential. *Antioxid. Redox Signal.*, 13(6), pp. 877–918.
18. Iranzo, O. (2011) Manganese Complexes Displaying Superoxide Dismutase Activity: A Balance between Different Factors. *Bioorganic Chem.*, 39(2), pp. 73–87.
19. Batinic-Haberle, I. (2016) *Redox-Active Therapeutics*, Springer Science+Business Media, New York, NY.
20. Policar, C. (2016) Mimicking SODs, Why and How: Bio-Inspired Manganese Complexes as SOD Mimics. *Redox-Active Therapeutics*, Springer Science, New York, NY, pp. 125–164.
21. Signorella, S., Palopoli, C. and Ledesma, G. (2018) Rationally Designed Mimics of Antioxidant Manganoenzymes: Role of Structural Features in the Quest for Catalysts with Catalase and Superoxide Dismutase Activity. *Coord. Chem. Rev.*, 365, pp. 75–102.
22. Signorella, S. and Hureau, C. (2012) Bioinspired Functional Mimics of the Manganese Catalases. *Coord. Chem. Rev.*, 256(11–12), pp. 1229–1245.
23. Day, B. J. (2009) Catalase and Glutathione Peroxidase Mimics. *Biochem. Pharmacol.*, 77(3), pp. 285–296.
24. Tovmasyan, A., Maia, C. G. C., Weitner, T., Carballal, S., Sampaio, R. S., Lieb, D., Ghazaryan, R., Ivanovic-Burmazovic, I., Ferrer-Sueta, G., Radi, R., Reboucas, J. S., Spasojevic, I., Benov, L. and Batinic-Haberle, I. (2015) A Comprehensive Evaluation of Catalase-like Activity of Different Classes of Redox-Active Therapeutics. *Free Radic. Biol. Med.*, 86, pp. 308–321.
25. Huang, X., Liu, X., Luo, Q., Liu, J. and Shen, J. (2011) Artificial Selenoenzymes: Designed and Redesigned. *Chem. Soc. Rev.*, 40(3), pp. 1171–1184.
26. Iwoaka, M. (2013) Emulating Antioxidative Functions of Glutathione Peroxidase Using Selenopeptides. *Biochalcogen Chemistry: The Biological Chemistry of Sulfur, Selenium, and Tellurium*, C.A. Bayse, and J.L. Brumaghim, eds., American Chemical Society. Washington, DC, pp. 163–177.
27. Luo, G., Ren, X., Liu, J., Mu, Y. and Shen, J. (2003) Towards More Efficient Glutathione Peroxidase Mimics: Substrate Recognition and Catalytic Group Assembly. *Curr. Med. Chem.*, 10(13), pp. 1151–1183.
28. Mugesh, G. and Singh, H. B. (2000) Synthetic Organoselenium Compounds as Antioxidants: Glutathione Peroxidase Activity. *Chem. Soc. Rev.*, 29(5), pp. 347–357.

29. Mugesh, G., du Mont, W.-W. and Sies, H. (2001) Chemistry of Biologically Important Synthetic Organoselenium Compounds. *Chem. Rev.*, 101(7), pp. 2125–2180.
30. Corazza, A., Scarpa, M., Vianello, F., Zennaro, L., Gourova, N., Di Paolo, M. L., Signor, L., Marin, O. and Rigo, A. (1999) Enzyme Mimics Complexing Cu (II) Ion: Structure–Function Relationships. *Chem. Biol. Drug Des.*, 54(6), pp. 491–504.
31. Csire, G., Timári, S., Asztalos, J., Király, J. M., Kiss, M. and Várnagy, K. (2017) Coordination, Redox Properties and SOD Activity of Cu(II) Complexes of Multihistidine Peptides. J. *Inorg. Biochem.*, 177, pp. 198–210.
32. Csire, G., Turi, I., Sóvágó, I., Kárpáti, E. and Kállay, C. (2020) Complex Formation Processes and Metal Ion Catalyzed Oxidation of Model Peptides Related to the Metal Binding Site of the Human Prion Protein. *J. Inorg. Biochem.*, 203, p. 110927.
33. Vincent, A., Fores, J. R., Tauziet, E., Quévrain, E., Dancs, Á., Conte-Daban, A., Bernard, A.-S., Pelupessy, P., Coulibaly, K., Seksik, P., Hureau, C., Selmeczi, K., Policar, C. and Delsuc, N. (2020) An Easy-to-Implement Combinatorial Approach Involving an Activity-Based Assay for the Discovery of a Peptidyl Copper Complex Mimicking Superoxide Dismutase. *Chem. Commun.*, 56(3), pp. 399–402.
34. Mathieu, E., Tolbert, A. E., Koebke, K. J., Tard, C., Iranzo, O., Penner-Hahn, J. E., Policar, C. and Pecoraro, V. (2020) Rational De Novo Design of a Cu Metalloenzyme for Superoxide Dismutation. *Chem. - Eur. J.*, 26(1), pp. 249–258.
35. Coulibaly, K., Thauvin, M., Melenbacher, A., Testard, C., Trigoni, E., Vincent, A., Stillman, M. J., Vriz, S., Policar, C. and Delsuc, N. (2021) A di-Copper Peptidyl Complex Mimics the Activity of Catalase, A Key Antioxidant Metalloenzyme. *Inorg. Chem.*, 60(13), pp. 9309–9319.
36. Piacham, T., Isarankura-Na-Ayudhya, C., Nantasenamat, C., Yainoy, S., Ye, L., Bülow, L. and Prachayasittikul, V. (2006) Metalloantibiotic Mn(II)–Bacitracin Complex Mimicking Manganese Superoxide Dismutase. *Biochem. Biophys. Res. Commun.*, 341(4), pp. 925–930.
37. Singh, U. P., Singh, R. K., Isogai, Y. and Shiro, Y. (2006) Design and Synthesis of De Novo Peptide for Manganese Binding. *Int. J. Pept. Res. Ther.*, 12(4), pp. 379–385.
38. Ursini, F., Maiorino, M., Brigelius-Flohé, R., Aumann, K. D., Roveri, A., Schomburg, D. and Flohé, L. (1995) "[5] Diversity of Glutathione Peroxidases," *Methods in Enzymology*, Elsevier, pp. 38–53.
39. Soll, D. (2007) "The Genetic Code Revisited Four Decades after Francis Crick," *Nucleic Acids Symp. Ser.,* 51(1), pp. 13–14.

40. Muttenthaler, M. and Alewood, P. F. (2008) Selenopeptide Chemistry. *J. Pept. Sci.*, 14(12), pp. 1223–1239.
41. Baranov, P. V., Gesteland, R. F. and Atkins, J. F. (2002) Recoding: Translational Bifurcations in Gene Expression. *Gene*, 286(2), pp. 187–201.
42. Cheng, W.-H., Ho, Y.-S., Valentine, B. A., Ross, D. A., Combs, G. F. and Lei, X. G. (1998) Cellular Glutathione Peroxidase is the Mediator of Body Selenium to Protect against Paraquat Lethality in Transgenic Mice. *J. Nutr.*, 128(7), pp. 1070–1076.
43. Veal, E. A., Day, A. M. and Morgan, B. A. (2007) Hydrogen Peroxide Sensing and Signaling. *Mol. Cell*, 26(1), pp. 1–14.
44. Brigelius-Flohé, R. and Maiorino, M. (2013) Glutathione Peroxidases. *Biochim. Biophys. Acta BBA — Gen. Subj.*, 1830(5), pp. 3289–3303.
45. Kipp, A. P. (2017) Chapter Four — Selenium-Dependent Glutathione Peroxidases During Tumor Development. *Advances in Cancer Research*, K.D. Tew, and F. Galli, eds., Academic Press, pp. 109–138.
46. Chu, F. F., Doroshow, J. H. and Esworthy, R. S. (1993) Expression, Characterization, and Tissue Distribution of a New Cellular Selenium-Dependent Glutathione Peroxidase. GSHPx-GI., *J. Biol. Chem.*, 268(4), pp. 2571–2576.
47. Cardoso, B. R., Hare, D. J., Bush, A. I. and Roberts, B. R. (2017) Glutathione Peroxidase 4: A New Player in Neurodegeneration? *Mol. Psychiatry*, 22(3), pp. 328–335.
48. Zeida, A., Trujillo, M., Ferrer-Sueta, G., Denicola, A., Estrin, D. A. and Radi, R. (2019) Catalysis of Peroxide Reduction by Fast Reacting Protein Thiols. *Chem. Rev.*, 119(19), pp. 10829–10855.
49. Epp, O., Ladenstein, R. and Wendel, A. (1983) The Refined Structure of the Selenoenzyme Glutathione Peroxidase at 0.2-nm Resolution," *Eur. J. Biochem.*, 133(1), pp. 51–69.
50. Flohé, L., Loschen, G., Günzler, W. A. and Eichele, E. (1972) Glutathione Peroxidase, V. The Kinetic Mechanism, Hoppe-Seylers Z. *Physiol. Chem.*, 353, pp. 987–999.
51. Wendel, A. (1981) Glutathione Peroxidase. *Methods Enzymol.*, 77, pp. 325–333.
52. Wilson, S. R., Zucker, P. A., Huang, R. R. C. and Spector, A. (1989) Development of Synthetic Compounds with Glutathione Peroxidase Activity. *J. Am. Chem. Soc.*, 111(15), pp. 5936–5939.
53. Yoshida, S., Kumakura, F., Komatsu, I., Arai, K., Onuma, Y., Hojo, H., Singh, B. G., Priyadarsini, K. I. and Iwaoka, M. (2011) Antioxidative Glutathione Peroxidase Activity of Selenoglutathione. *Angew. Chem. Int. Ed.*, 50(9), pp. 2125–2128.
54. Maiorino, M., Aumann, K.-D., Brigelius-Flohé, R., Doria, D., van den Heuvel, J., McCarthy, J., Roveri, A., Ursini, F. and Flohé, L. (1995) Probing the Presumed Catalytic Triad of Selenium-Containing Peroxidases by

Mutational Analysis of Phospholipid Hydroperoxide Glutathione Peroxidase (PHGPx). *Biol. Chem. Hoppe. Seyler*, 376(11), pp. 651–660.

55. Tosatto, S. C. E., Bosello, V., Fogolari, F., Mauri, P., Roveri, A., Toppo, S., Flohé, L., Ursini, F. and Maiorino, M. (2008) The Catalytic Site of Glutathione Peroxidases. *Antioxid. Redox Signal.*, 10(9), pp. 1515–1526.
56. Toppo, S., Vanin, S., Bosello, V. and Tosatto, S. C. E. (2008) Evolutionary and Structural Insights Into the Multifaceted Glutathione Peroxidase (Gpx) Superfamily. *Antioxid. Redox Signal.*, 10(9), pp. 1501–1514.
57. Flohé, L., Toppo, S., Cozza, G. and Ursini, F. (2010) A Comparison of Thiol Peroxidase Mechanisms. *Antioxid. Redox Signal.*, 15(3), pp. 763–780.
58. Cadenas, E., Graf, P. and Sies, H. (1984) A Novel Biologically Active Seleno-Organic Coupound-I. *Biochem. Pharmacol.*, 33(20), pp. 3235–3239.
59. Wendel, A., Fausel, M., Safayhi, H., Tiegs, G. and Otter, R. (1984) A Novel Biologically Active Seleno-Organic Compound-II. *Biochem. Pharmacol.*, 33(20), pp. 3241–3245.
60. Nogueira, C. W., Zeni, G. and Rocha, J. B. T. (2004) Organoselenium and Organotellurium Compounds: Toxicology and Pharmacology. *Chem. Rev.*, 104(12), pp. 6255–6286.
61. Alberto, E. E., Soares, L. C., Sudati, J. H., Borges, A. C. A., Rocha, J. B. T. and Braga, A. L. (2009) Efficient Synthesis of Modular Amino Acid Derivatives Containing Selenium with Pronounced GPx-Like Activity. *Eur. J. Org. Chem.*, 2009(25), pp. 4211–4214.
62. Wu, Z. P. and Hilvert, D. (1989) Conversion of a Protease into an Acyl Transferase: Selenolsubtilisin. *J. Am. Chem. Soc.*, 111(12), pp. 4513–4514.
63. Wu, Z. P. and Hilvert, D. (1990) Selenosubtilisin as a Glutathione Peroxidase Mimic. *J. Am. Chem. Soc.*, 112(14), pp. 5647–5648.
64. Bell, I. M., Fisher, M. L., Wu, Z. P. and Hilvert, D. (1993) Kinetic Studies on the Peroxidase Activity of Selenosubtilisin. *Biochemistry*, 32(14), pp. 3754–3762.
65. Bell, I. M. and Hilvert, D. (1993) Peroxide Dependence of the Semisynthetic Enzyme Selenosubtilisin. *Biochemistry*, 32(50), pp. 13969–13973.
66. Liu, J.-Q., Jiang, M.-S., Luo, G.-M., Yan, G.-L. and Shen, J.-C. (1998) Conversion of Trypsin into a Selenium-Containing Enzyme by Using Chemical Mutation. *Biotechnol. Lett.*, 20(7), pp. 693–696.
67. Boschi-Muller, S., Muller, S., Dorsselaer, A. V., Böck, A. and Branlant, G. (1998) Substituting Selenocysteine for Active Site Cysteine 149 of Phosphorylating Glyceraldehyde 3-Phosphate Dehydrogenase Reveals a Peroxidase Activity. *FEBS Lett.*, 439(3), pp. 241–245.
68. Mueller, S., Senn, H., Gsell, B., Vetter, W., Baron, C. and Boeck, A. (1994) The Formation of Diselenide Bridges in Proteins by Incorporation of

Selenocysteine Residues: Biosynthesis and Characterization of (Se)2-Thioredoxin. *Biochemistry*, 33(11), pp. 3404–3412.

69. Luo, G. M., Zhu, Z. Q., Ding, L., Gao, G., Sun, Q. A., Liu, Z., Yang, T. S. and Shen, J. C. (1994) Generation of Selenium-Containing Abzyme by Using Chemical Mutation. *Biochem. Biophys. Res. Commun.*, 198(3), pp. 1240–1247.
70. Ding, L., Liu, Z., Zhu, Z., Luo, G., Zhao, D. and Ni, J. (1998) Biochemical Characterization of Selenium-Containing Catalytic Antibody as a Cytosolic Glutathione Peroxidase Mimic. *Biochem. J.*, 332(1), pp. 251–255.
71. Luo, G., Ding, L., Liu, Z., Yang, T. and Ni, J. (1998) A Selenium-Containing Abzyme, the Activity of Which Surpassed the Level of Native Glutathione Peroxidasea. *Ann. N. Y. Acad. Sci.*, 864(1), pp. 136–141.
72. Qi, D.-H., Luo, G.-M., Zhou, L. and Yang, T.-S. (1999) Protection of Myocardial Mitochondria Against Oxidative Damage by Selenium-Containing Abzyme M4G3. *Appl. Biochem. Biotechnol.*, 82(3), pp. 167–174.
73. Ren, X., Gao, S., You, D., Huang, H., Liu, Z., Mu, Y., Liu, J., Zhang, Y., Yan, G., Luo, G., Yang, T. and Shen, J. (2001) Cloning and Expression of a Single-Chain Catalytic Antibody that Acts as a Glutathione Peroxidase Mimic with High Catalytic Efficiency. *Biochem. J.*, 359(Pt 2), pp. 369–374.
74. You, D., Ren, X., Xue, Y., Luo, G., Yang, T. and Shen, J. (2003) A Selenium-Containing Single-Chain Abzyme with Potent Antioxidant Activity. *Eur. J. Biochem.*, 270(21), pp. 4326–4331.
75. Ren, X., Jemth, P., Board, P. G., Luo, G., Mannervik, B., Liu, J., Zhang, K. and Shen, J. (2002) A Semisynthetic Glutathione Peroxidase with High Catalytic Efficiency: Selenoglutathione Transferase. *Chem. Biol.*, 9(7), pp. 789–794.
76. Su, D., Ren, X., You, D., Li, D., Mu, Y., Yan, G., Zhang, Y., Luo, Y., Xue, Y., Shen, J., Liu, Z. and Luo, G. (2001) Generation of Three Selenium-Containing Catalytic Antibodies with High Catalytic Efficiency Using a Novel Hapten Design Method. *Arch. Biochem. Biophys.*, 395(2), pp. 177–184.
77. Sun, Y., Li, T., Chen, H., Zhang, K., Zheng, K., Mu, Y., Yan, G., Li, W., Shen, J. and Luo, G. (2004) Selenium-Containing 15-Mer Peptides with High Glutathione Peroxidase-like Activity. *J. Biol. Chem.*, 279(36), pp. 37235–37240.
78. Yu, H., Liu, J., Böck, A., Li, J., Luo, G. and Shen, J. (2005) Engineering Glutathione Transferase to a Novel Glutathione Peroxidase Mimic With High Catalytic Efficiency. *J. Biol. Chem.*, 280(12), pp. 11930–11935.
79. Casi, G., Roelfes, G. and Hilvert, D. (2008) Selenoglutaredoxin as a Glutathione Peroxidase Mimic. *ChemBioChem*, 9(10), pp. 1623–1631.
80. Liu, J., Luo, G., Gao, S., Zhang, K., Chen, X. and Shen, J. (1999) Generation of a Glutathione Peroxidase-like Mimic Using Bioimprinting and Chemical Mutation. *Chem. Commun.*, (2), pp. 199–200.

81. Liu, L., Mao, S., Liu, X., Huang, X., Xu, J., Liu, J., Luo, G. and Shen, J. (2008) Functional Mimicry of the Active Site of Glutathione Peroxidase by Glutathione Imprinted Selenium-Containing Protein. *Biomacromolecules*, 9(1), pp. 363–368.
82. Wehrle, R. J., Ste.Marie, E. J., Hondal, R. J. and Masterson, D. S. (2019) Synthesis of Alpha-Methyl Selenocysteine and Its Utilization as a Glutathione Peroxidase Mimic. *J. Pept. Sci.*, 25(6), p. e3173.
83. Takei, T., Urabe, Y., Asahina, Y., Hojo, H., Nomura, T., Dedachi, K., Arai, K. and Iwaoka, M. (2014) Model Study Using Designed Selenopeptides on the Importance of the Catalytic Triad for the Antioxidative Functions of Glutathione Peroxidase. *J. Phys. Chem. B*, 118(2), pp. 492–500.
84. Shimodaira, S., Takei, T., Hojo, H. and Iwaoka, M. (2018) Synthesis of Selenocysteine-Containing Cyclic Peptides via Tandem N-to-S Acyl Migration and Intramolecular Selenocysteine-Mediated Native Chemical Ligation. *Chem. Commun.*, 54(83), pp. 11737–11740.
85. Yin, J., Wang, B., Zhu, X., Qu, X., Huang, Y., Lv, S., Mu, Y. and Luo, G. (2017) The Small Glutathione Peroxidase Mimic 5P May Represent a New Strategy for the Treatment of Liver Cancer. *Molecules*, 22(9), p. 1495.
86. Jiang, Q., Pan, Y., Cheng, Y., Li, H. and Li, H. (2016) Protection of Rat Liver against Hepatic Ischemia-Reperfusion Injury by a Novel Selenocysteine-Containing 7-Mer Peptide. *Mol. Med. Rep.*, 14(3), pp. 2007–2015.
87. Casi, G. and Hilvert, D. (2007) Reinvestigation of a Selenopeptide with Purportedly High Glutathione Peroxidase Activity. *J. Biol. Chem.*, 282(42), pp. 30518–30522.
88. Sarma, B. K. and Mugesh, G. (2005) Glutathione Peroxidase (GPx)-like Antioxidant Activity of the Organoselenium Drug Ebselen: Unexpected Complications with Thiol Exchange Reactions. *J. Am. Chem. Soc.*, 127(32), pp. 11477–11485.
89. Bhabak, K. P. and Mugesh, G. (2009) Amide-Based Glutathione Peroxidase Mimics: Effect of Secondary and Tertiary Amide Substituents on Antioxidant Activity. *Chem. - Asian J.*, 4(6), pp. 974–983.
90. Jia, C.-J., Dai, C.-L., Zhang, X., Cui, K., Xu, F. and Xu, Y.-Q. (2006) Alanyl-Glutamine Dipeptide Inhibits Hepatic Ischemia-Reperfusion Injury in Rats. *World J. Gastroenterol.*, 12(9), pp. 1373–1378.
91. Yu, H.-C., Bai, L., Yue, S.-Q., Wang, D.-S., Wang, L., Han, H. and Dou, K.-F. (2013) Notch Signal Protects Non-Parenchymal Cells from Ischemia/Reperfusion Injury in Vitro by Repressing ROS. *Ann. Hepatol.*, 12(5), pp. 815–821.
92. Mao, G. D., Thomas, P. D., Lopaschuk, G. D. and Poznansky, M. J. (1993) Superoxide Dismutase (SOD)-Catalase Conjugates. Role of Hydrogen Peroxide and the Fenton Reaction in SOD Toxicity., *J. Biol. Chem.*, 268(1), pp. 416–420.

93. Luo, G., Liu, W., Sun, Q., Ding, L., Zhu, Z., Yan, G. and Yang, T. (1996) Preparation of Bifunctional Enzyme with Both Superoxide Dismutase and Glutathione Peroxidase Activities by Using Chemical Mutation. *Ann. N. Y. Acad. Sci.*, 799, pp. 50–55.
94. Yu, H., Ge, Y., Wang, Y., Lin, C.-T., Li, J., Liu, X., Zang, T., Xu, J., Liu, J., Luo, G. and Shen, J. (2007) A Fused Selenium-Containing Protein with Both GPx and SOD Activities. *Biochem. Biophys. Res. Commun.*, 358(3), pp. 873–878.
95. Antonyuk, S. V., Strange, R. W., Marklund, S. L. and Hasnain, S. S. (2009) The Structure of Human Extracellular Copper–Zinc Superoxide Dismutase at 1.7 Å Resolution: Insights into Heparin and Collagen Binding. *J. Mol. Biol.*, 388(2), pp. 310–326.
96. Yan, F., Yan, G., Lv, S., Shen, N., Mu, Y., Chen, T., Gong, P., Xu, Y., Lv, L., Liu, J., Shen, J. and Luo, G. (2011) A Novel 65-Mer Peptide Imitates the Synergism of Superoxide Dismutase and Glutathione Peroxidase. *Int. J. Biochem. Cell Biol.*, 43(12), pp. 1802–1811.
97. Cheng, W., Na, S., Gang-lin, Y., Chun-hong, S., Jian-jian, Z., Shao-wu, L., Gui-min, L. and Ying, M. (2014) The Protective Effect of a Metallic Selenopeptide with Superoxide Dismutase and Glutathione Peroxidase Activities Against Alcohol Induced Injury in Hepatic L02 Cells. *Int. J. Pept. Res. Ther.*, 20(3), pp. 307–324.
98. Xu, Y., Zhou, Y., Yin, R., Wang, C., Chu, H. and Wang, J. (2018) A Novel 76-Mer Peptide Mimic with the Synergism of Superoxide Dismutase and Glutathione Peroxidase. *Vitro Cell. Dev. Biol. — Anim.*, 54(5), pp. 335–345.
99. Zou, X., Ji, Y., Gao, G., Zhu, X., Lv, S., Yan, F., Han, S., Chen, X., Gao, C., Liu, J. and Luo, G. (2010) A Novel Selenium and Copper-Containing Peptide with Both Superoxide Dismutase and Glutathione Peroxidase Activities. *J. Microbiol. Biotechnol.*, 20(1), pp. 88–93.
100. Yan, F., Yang, W., Li, X., Lin, T., Lun, Y., Lin, F., Lv, S., Yan, G., Liu, J., Shen, J., Mu, Y. and Luo, G. (2008) A Trifunctional Enzyme with Glutathione S-Transferase, Glutathione Peroxidase and Superoxide Dismutase Activity. *Biochim. Biophys. Acta BBA — Gen. Subj.*, 1780(6), pp. 869–872.
101. Marklund, S. L. (1982) Human Copper-Containing Superoxide Dismutase of High Molecular Weight., *Proc. Natl. Acad. Sci.*, 79(24), pp. 7634–7638.
102. Luo, G.-M., Chen, H.-P. and Cheng, Y.-H. (1988) A New Metal-Peptide Complex Displays the Activity of Superoxide Dismutase. *Ann. N. Y. Acad. Sci.*, 542(1 Enzyme Engine), pp. 79–82.

https://doi.org/10.1142/9789811261664_0007

Chapter 7

DNA Recognition with Artificial Metallopeptides

Jacobo Gómez-González*, Ana Alcalde*, Miguel Vázquez López†, and M. Eugenio Vázquez‡

**Centro Singular de Investigación en Química Biolóxica e Materiais Moleculares (CiQUS), Departamento de Química Orgánica, Universidade de Santiago de Compostela, Santiago de Compostela, Spain*

†*Centro Singular de Investigacioìn en Quiìmica Bioloìxica e Materiais Moleculares (CiQUS), Departamento de Quiìmica Inorgaìnica, Universidade de Santiago de Compostela, Santiago de Compostela, Spain*

‡*eugenio.vazquez@usc.es*

1. Introduction

Chemists have been trying for many years to synthesize molecules that can specifically recognize DNA sequences, but regardless of the sustained efforts and progress in the area [1–7], specific targeting of DNA sites with small agents still represents a formidable and unmet challenge in Chemical Biology [8]. Despite the dominance of small organic molecules for the specific recognition of DNA sequences, over the past few decades, there has been an increased interest in the application of transition metal complexes for the development of DNA-based probes, reactive agents, and drugs, particularly since the successful application of cisplatin and its derivatives as anticancer agents [9–13]. However, severe side effects, such as nephrotoxicity, neurotoxicity, or drug-induced resistance, have hampered their clinical application, and fueled intense research efforts to develop safer alternatives with reduced side effects and improved DNA binding and therapeutic properties [14–16]; in this regard, peptides are highly versatile platforms that offer many advantages over the organic ligands traditionally used in coordination chemistry for the design of compounds with tailored properties. On the other hand, the developments experienced over the last 20 years in DNA nanotechnology [17–19] offer a new, and still unexplored, setting in which metal complexes will likely play a fundamental role.

There are many reviews that deal with the topic of DNA-binding metal complexes from different perspectives [20–24], but to our knowledge, regardless of the growing number of examples in the literature, the topic of DNA binding by metallopeptides has been largely overlooked so far [25].

Peptides are excellent supramolecular building blocks that encode in their amino acid sequence precise structural and functional information, and researchers have exploited this potential for engineering using a variety of peptide motifs, including coiled-coils, β-hairpins, amphipathic peptides, collagen triple helices, in combination with coordination chemistry to design complex supramolecular architectures [26–34]. Peptides are also ideal scaffolds that, by creating appropriate coordination environments, can easily interface metal ions with unique properties (e.g., luminescence, catalytic, magnetic, or photochemical properties) with biological systems [35–40]. The possibilities offered by the combination of these two highly versatile platforms have been exploited in the development of metallopeptide DNA-binding agents.

Although, in principle, both the metal complex and the peptide could simultaneously act as DNA-binding elements, most DNA-binding metallopeptides are designed so that the metal complex and the peptide domain have complementary roles. This modular configuration offers the greatest versatility and simplifies the design of the metallopeptides. Thus, a number of designs are based on known DNA-binding complexes, such as the intercalator $[Ru(bpy)_2(dppz)]^{2+}$, which are derivatized with peptide tags that endow the resulting conjugate with new and desirable properties (e.g., enhanced cellular internalization, or modulation of the target DNA sequence and affinity). A second class of DNA-binding metallopeptides is based on known DNA-binding peptides (typically, fragments of natural transcription factors), which are derivatized with metal-chelating units or metal complexes that complement the DNA-binding peptide with additional functionalities (e.g., nuclease activity, luminescence, dynamic conformational control). In some cases, the peptide tag and the metal complex do not have such clearly defined roles and act synergistically as a whole.

2. Natural DNA-Binding Peptides Modified with Metal Complexes

The regulation of gene transcription in eukaryotic cells relies on gene-specific transcription factors (TFs) that guide RNA polymerases to selected promoters [41]. These proteins are typically classified according to the structure of their specialized DNA-binding domains. Prominent among them is the family of *basic leucine zipper* (bZIP) transcription factors, which has become the preferred platform for researchers thanks to its structural simplicity, small size, and the wealth of functional, biophysical and structural information available.

GCN4 is a yeast transcription factor (TF) of the bZIP family that has been used as a model system for the development of many peptide-based DNA binders. A seminal paper by the group of P. S. Kim demonstrated in 1990 that the full leucine zipper region of the DNA-binding domain of GCN4 could be replaced by a disulfide bond. More specifically, the disulfide dimer of a 34-residue peptide comprising residues 222–253 of GCN4 plus a short *C*-terminal flexible linker (GGC) reproduced the DNA-binding properties of the natural GCN4 (nM affinity for the ATF/CREB site (5′-ATGAC GTCAT-3′) at 4°C). Not surprisingly, the monomeric peptide, resulting from reduction of the disulfide linker, did not show any measurable affinity under the same conditions [42]. Further studies defined the minimal GCN4 fragment that displays specific DNA binding as a disulfide dimer, corresponding to residues 226–248 of the basic region (AcDPAALKRARNTEAARRSRARKLQGGC-NH_2) [43].

Following Kim's work, the group of Prof. A. Schepartz reported in 1993 the dimerization of GCN4 peptides using a set of transition metal complexes (Figure 1). By exploiting the geometric constraints imposed by the coordination geometry they could explore the influence of the relative orientation of the attached basic regions on the recognition properties of the resulting GCN4 dimers. As expected, they found that only dimerizing

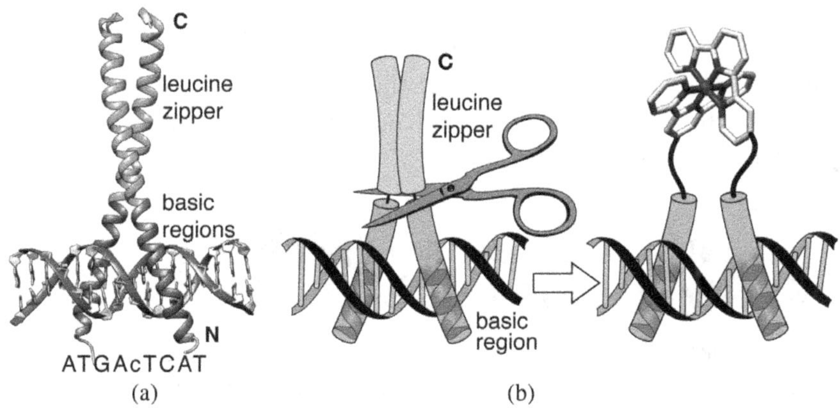

Fig. 1. (a) Structure of the DNA-binding domain of the GCN4 TF bound to the AP1/GCRE site; (b) schematic representation of the GCN4 dimers reported by Prof. A. Schepartz, showing metal complex that plays the role of the leucine zipper mediating the dimerization of the basic regions [44].

the minimal basic regions was not sufficient for DNA binding, but the geometry of the metal complexes had a strong effect on the binding affinity of the dimers, as well as in their sequence selectivity. Later, the authors thoroughly characterized the DNA binding of these and related bis(terpyridyl)iron(II) GCN4 metallopeptides [44,45] and found that, while the DNA-binding affinity of these complexes was close to that of the natural GCN4 DNA-binding domain for the ATF/CREB site (5′ATGAC GTCAT3'), they displayed enhanced sequence discrimination against the closely related AP1/GCRE (5′ATGA (c/g) TCAT3′) site.

The effect of the relative geometry of the GCN4 basic regions in DNA binding was also explored a few years later by the group of A. Peacock, who designed a GCN4 dimer in which the minimal GCN4 basic regions (**br**) were connected by a 2,2′:6′,2″-terpyridine linker. The peptide dimer was prepared by reaction of 6,6"-dibromomethyl-2,2′:6′,2″-terpyridine with a derivative of GCN4 basic region (residues 229–249) featuring an additional *C*-terminal GGCG-NH_2 sequence with a nucleophilic Cys. It was reasoned that the linker would experience a large *transoid* to *cisoid* conformational change upon metal ion coordination, which in turn would modify the relative orientation of the attached basic regions, and ultimately modulate its DNA-binding properties (Figure 2). Circular dichroism and UV/vis spectroscopy experiments demonstrated that coordination of this metal-chelating GCN4 linker to Cu(II) or Zn(II) ions promoted

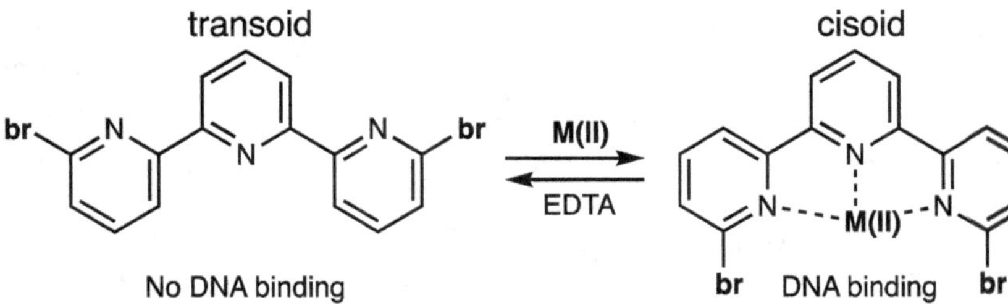

Fig. 2. Scheme of the metal-induced *transoid-cisoid* conformational change, and its effect in the relative geometry of the DNA-binding GCN4 basic region peptides (**br**). Only the *cisoid* conformation delivers the br peptide in an appropriate orientation that allows both of them to simultaneously interact with the DNA [46].

binding to its target sites ATF/CREB or AP1/GCRE. Interestingly, metal–ion coordination and DNA binding were fully reversible upon addition of excess EDTA, and a control dimer containing a 2,2′-bipyridine linker, which does not induce any geometric change in the relative orientation of the basic regions upon metal coordination, did not modify its DNA-binding properties in the presence of metal ions [46].

The folding of an α-helix from a random coil configuration is an entropically unfavorable process, indeed, peptides that form helices in solution are typically found as a complex mixture of all-helix, all-coil or, most frequently, central helices with frayed-coil ends. The conformational freedom of peptide chains can be reduced by introducing geometric constraints; the more extended strategy involves introducing bonds between distant side chains in the sequence (i.e., stapled peptides), using a variety of chemical modifications including triazole [47], hydrocarbons [48–51], lactams [52,53], as well as metal coordination, which was first demonstrated in 1990 by R. Ghadiri *et al.*, who introduced in a peptide sequence a pair of His residues at positions $(i,i+4)$. This arrangement places the imidazole groups at the appropriate distance to chelate transition metal ions, thereby locking the peptide backbone in a helical conformation. Furthermore, by replacing one of the His residues by a Cys, the authors could modify the coordination preferences of the peptide from Cu(II) to Cd(II) [54]. The same peptide was also stabilized using $[Ru(NH_3)_4]^{2+}$ showing good helical conformation [55].

Following this $(i,i+4)$ approach to stabilize the helical conformation, D. P. Fairlie and co-workers demonstrated that the pentapeptide $AcHAAAHNH_2$ adopted an α-helical conformation upon coordination of $[Pd(en)]^{2+}$ in water, and studied its folding by 2D NMR [56]. This system was also studied with $[Ru(NH_3)_4]^{2+}$ and showed a higher α-helical conformation than his analog of $[Pd(en)]^{2+}$ [57]. Importantly, these coordination staples can also stabilize longer peptides, such as fragments of the protein thermolysin [58].

Following this approach, we have recently used metal coordination to modulate the DNA-binding properties of a small fragment of the basic region of a bZIP transcription factor. The design is based on the GCN4 basic region peptide (**brHis$_2$**), which was modified to include two histidine residues at the designed $(i,i+4)$ position in its N-terminus. The resulting monomeric peptide is incapable of recognizing its consensus target DNA site due to the high entropic cost associated with its folding into the α-helical conformation, however, the addition of $[Pd(en)]^{2+}$ promotes a high-affinity interaction with excellent sequence selectivity. Furthermore, this interaction can be repeatedly switched on and off by the addition of a chelating agent such as diethyldithiocarbamate (DEDTC), or $[Pd(en)]^{2+}$, respectively. As expected, the control peptide featuring a single histidine residue (**brHis**) was not stabilized in the presence of $[Pd(en)]^{2+}$ and did not show DNA binding (Figure 3) [158].

DNA recognition is often a cooperative process involving the formation of multimeric complexes of TFs that cooperatively bind to specific sequences in the DNA [59]. This mechanism is the basis of the combinatorial targeting of a large number of sites using a relatively small set of

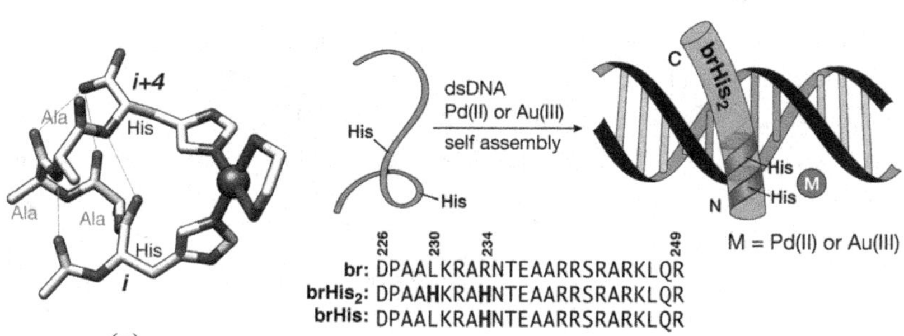

(a) (b)

Fig. 3. (a) Structure of the short α-helical peptide Ac-HAAAH-NH_2 coordinated with $[Pd(en)]^{+2}$, showing intrahelical hydrogen bonds and the coordination of the imidazole rings in the His side chains locking the α-helical conformation; (b) schematic representation of the unfolded peptide **brHis$_2$**, derived from the basic region of the GCN4 transcription factor, with two His residues at positions 230 and 234 $(i,i+4)$. The stabilized peptide binds to an ATF/CREB half-site (5′-GTCAT-3′) with good affinity thanks to this coordination staple.

transcription regulators (about 2,000 TFs in humans) [60,61]. For example, the members of bZIP family of TFs can form homodimers, or a variety of heterodimers with different partners that display different DNA-binding properties [62–64], integrating in this way multiple signaling pathways into complex networks of TFs [65,66]. Despite the advantages of combinatorial DNA binding, the challenges associated with its implementation have limited the development of artificial systems that display some level of cooperativity in their DNA recognition. In collaboration with Prof. J. L. Mascareñas, we showed in 2014 that the nickel-promoted assembly of the **brHis**$_2$ peptide derived from GCN4 TF and a bisbenzamidine equipped with a bipyridine unit allowed the specific recognition of composite sequences displaying a target AP1/GCRE (5′-ATGA-3′) half-site in tandem with an A/T-rich sequence (5′-AATTT-3′) targeted by the bisbenzamidine minor groove binder (Figure 4). Importantly, the Ni(II) ion not only mediates the formation of the heterodimeric complex, but also nucleates the **brHis**$_2$ α-helix, which otherwise would not fold and bind the DNA. The kinetic lability of the Ni(II) complex allows the disassembly of the supramolecular assembly by adding EDTA to sequester the nickel cation. This could be easily observed by the decrease in the intensity of the circular dichroism signal at 208/222 nm associated with the **brHis**$_2$ α-helix, as well as by electrophoretic mobility shift assay (EMSA) experiments in which the retarded band

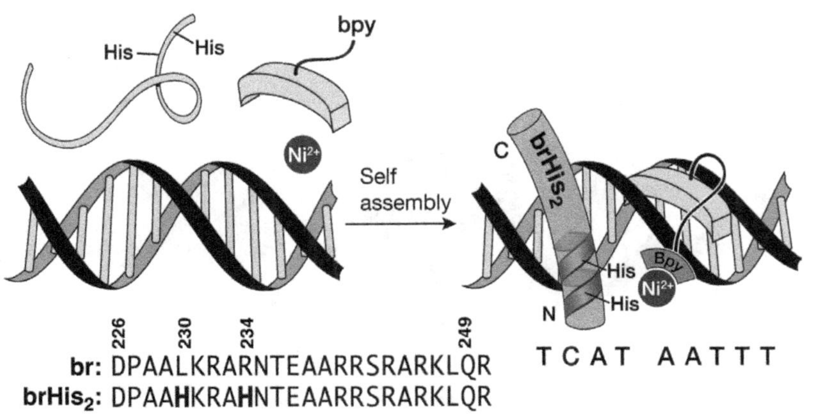

Fig. 4. Metal-induced cooperative assembly of multimeric DNA-binding metallopeptides. Schematic representation of the **brHis**$_2$ peptide in the presence of a bisbenzamidine-bipyridine DNA binder and Ni(II) self-assemble into a trimeric DNA-binding complex mediated by the Bpy ligand that links the bisbenzamidine and the peptide.

corresponding to the complex disappeared in the presence of 10 equiv of EDTA; this process was reversible, and addition of excess $Ni(ClO_4)_2$ reconstructed the supramolecular complex with the DNA [67]. A follow-up paper in 2016 applied this same strategy for the construction of a nickel-mediated trimeric DNA-binding metallopeptide composed of a basic region/AT-hook chimera equipped with a bipyridine ligand (**brHk**) and the **brHis$_2$** peptide. The metallopeptide complex assembled in the presence of Ni(II) salts was capable of self-assembling at specific DNA sequences of twelve base pairs [68]. Both systems exemplify the versatility of coordination chemistry to modulate the supramolecular assembly of stimuli-responsive DNA-binding metallopeptide complexes (Figure 5).

In 1987, the group of Prof. P. B. Dervan published a pioneering work describing, for the first time, the construction of a hybrid nuclease combining a sequence-specific DNA-binding peptide with a coordination complex. More specifically, they reported the synthesis of a 52-residue peptide corresponding to the helix-turn-helix DNA-binding domain of the Hin recombinase TF (residues 139–190), covalently modified on its N-terminus with an Fe(II)EDTA complex capable of producing oxidative cleavage of the DNA chain [69]. The synthesis of the hybrid was fairly straightforward and involved the on-resin modification of the Hin recombinase peptide with a protected EDTA derivative containing three of its carboxylates protected as benzyl esters (Figure 6(a)). The paper used Boc/Bzl solid-phase peptide synthesis protocols for the assembly of the

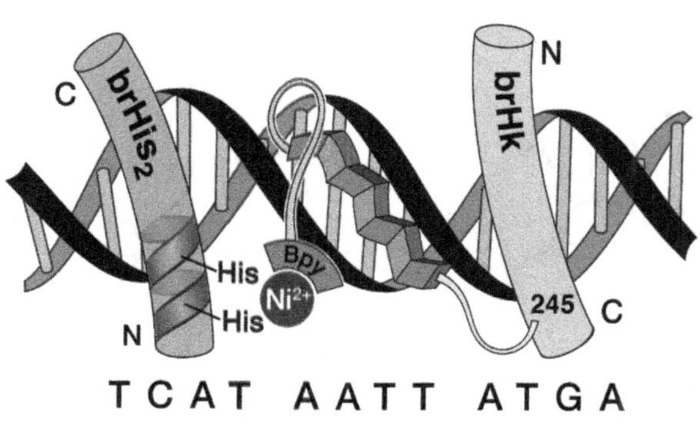

Fig. 5. Scheme of the multimeric DNA binding of a metal- trimeric DNA binding in which His^{230} and His^{234} residues in brHis$_2$ coordinate Ni(II) and connect this peptide with the GCN4br/AT-hook chimera (**brHk**).

peptide chain, which have been largely replaced by the safer and more convenient Fmoc/tBu protocols [70,71]. Upon incubation with a DNA oligonucleotide containing the Hin recombinase-binding site, the hybrid nuclease Fe(II)EDTA-Hin(139–190) was capable of producing specific cleavage pattern near the symmetry axis of the Hin recombination sites, which were consistent with specific recognition and delivery of the active complex to the vicinity of the DNA minor groove (Figure 6(a), bottom) [72].

The group of Prof. Steitz reported the semisynthesis of a DNA nuclease by selective modification of a single Cys residue present in the DNA-binding domain of the *E. coli* catabolite activator protein (CAP). Their elegant approach was possible thanks to the analysis of the atomic structure of the CAP-DNA complex (PDB ID 2CGP) [73] and highlights the benefits of having at hand such structural information during the design process. Thus, the inspection of the X-ray crystal structure showed that Cys^{178} is the solvent-accessible cysteine residue in the CAP helix-turn-helix DNA-binding domain, while the other two residues, Cys^{18} and Cys^{92}, are buried in the interior of the domain. On the other hand, the structure also confirmed that the modification of this residue would neither affect the structure of the CAP domain, nor hinder the CAP-DNA contacts mediating specific recognition. Thus, incubation of the expressed CAP DNA-binding domain with the electrophilic *N*-(iodoacetyl)-5-amino-1,10-phenanthroline afforded a single major product, which was purified by gel filtration (Figure 6(b)). The modified nuclease binds to a 22-base-pair DNA containing the CAP recognition site with near wilt-type affinity and, in the presence of Cu(II), cleaves the DNA at four adjacent nucleotides on each strand within the recognition site with high efficiency.

Following the same modular design that combines a sequence-specific DNA-binding domain with a catalytic metal complex, the group of Prof. Y. Sugiura reported in 2005 an engineered metalloprotein composed of fragments of the Cys_2-His_2 TFs Sp1 and GLI with the short peptide SP1 (DKDGDGYISAAE-NH_2) [74]. The SP1 peptide, which is derived from the calcium-binding loop III of calmodulin and binds Ce(IV) to give a metallopeptide with DNA hydrolytic activity [75], was introduced as a linker between the fingers two and three of Sp1 [76] Sp1(zf23), and the fingers four and five of GLI [77], GLI(zf45) to give the chimera Sp1(zf23)-P1-GLI(zf45), which in the presence of $(NH_4)Ce(NO_3)_6$ as a source of

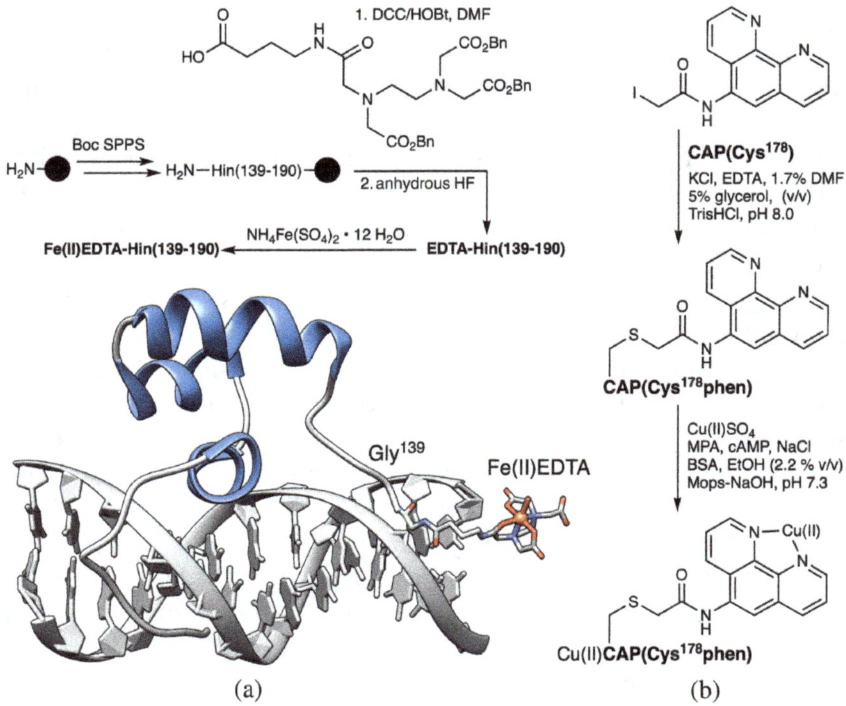

Fig. 6. (a) Top: Solid-phase peptide synthesis of the helix-turn-helix DNA-binding domain of Hin recombinase (residues 139–190) and modification with an EDTA derivative; deprotection and cleavage with anhydrous HF afforded the desired hybrid. Bottom: Model of the helix-turn-helix domain of Hin recombinase (PDB ID: 1HCR), [78] modified with the Fe(II)EDTA complex, showing the insertion of the N-terminal tail of Hin in the minor groove; (b) synthesis of the Cu(II)[(*N*-Acetl-5-amino-1,10-phenanthroline)-Cys^{178}]CAP complex by selective alkylation of the exposed Cys^{178} residue of the natural CAP protein.

Ce(IV) ions, showed a clear DNA cleavage pattern with enhanced hydrolysis in the region close to the SP1 linker, between the binding sites of Sp1(zf23), 5′-CCGCCC-3′, and GLI(zf45), 5′-TTGGGTGGTC-3′. The modular arrangement assigns distinct roles to the DNA-binding peptide domains, Sp1(zf23) and GLI(zf45), and the catalytic unit (Ce(IV)P1 complex), which facilitates the design of the nuclease.

In 2000, M. Y. Ogawa *et al.* reported a similar modification of a Cys residue engineered in the leucine zipper region of the GCN4 TF (Figure 7(b))

[79]. The authors replaced the natural Asp^{255} residue with a nucleophilic Cys that could be selectively alkylated in solution with a electrophilic complex $[Ru(bpy)_2(phen')]^{2+}$ (phen′ = *N*-(iodoacetyl)-5-amino-1,10-phenanthroline). The selection of position 255 for anchoring the metal complex ensured that the formation of the leucine zipper dimer would not be obstructed, and that that the photoactive $[Ru(bpy)_2(phen')]^{2+}$ complexes would be placed in close proximity to the DNA backbone upon specific binding of the dimer to the DNA (either ATF/CREB (5′-ATGAC GTCAT-3′), or AP1/GCRE (5′-ATGA (c/g) TCAT-3′sites). Gel mobility shift assays confirmed that the modification with the ruthenium(II) complex did not affect the DNA-binding properties of the GCN4-$[Ru(bpy)_2(phen')]^{2+}$ conjugate. Unfortunately, no photoinduced DNA damage was observed when the conjugate GCN4-$[Ru(bpy)_2(phen')]^{2+}$ was incubated with an oligonucleotide containing the ATF/CREB site, despite the conjugate binding to that sequence with wild-type affinity. The authors propose that the photoactive $[Ru(bpy)_2(phen')]^{2+}$ complex might be too far from the DNA (about 23 Å) for efficient diffusion of photogenerated $^1O_2$ to the nearest guanine site to induce DNA cleavage.

The calcium-binding loop has also been used in more challenging designs that integrate both the DNA targeting unit and the sequence with nuclease activity within the same peptidic domain. Thus, the group of Prof. S. J. Franklin reported in 2001 the design of a peptide chimera that combined helices $\alpha 2$ and $\alpha 3$ from the engrailed homeodomain DNA-binding domain with the consensus EF-hand calcium-binding loop (Figure 7(a)) [80]. The resulting peptide construct displayed high affinity for Eu(III) and Ce(IV) ions ($K_D = 4.7\ \mu$M and 3.8 μM, respectively), and binding to these metal ions induced significant folding of the peptide chain into an α-helical configuration required for DNA recognition. Furthermore, these metallopeptides displayed efficient nuclease activity, with modest sequence selectivity [81,82].

Recently, Tezcan and co-workers introduced coordinating groups at position $(i, i+7)$ with respect to a His residue, so that the α-helical conformation is induced by metal coordination. In their first report, they described different 8-hydroxiquinoline (Quin) derivatives attached to a Glu side chain; in this case, the helical conformation is induced in the presence of Zn(II), Cu(II), Co(II) and Ni(II) ions as a cross-linking agent. Moreover, the introduction of $Re(CO)_3$-Quin derivatives leads to luminescent peptides in the visible region, showing that these coordinating motifs can introduce structure and functionality in the engineered peptides in

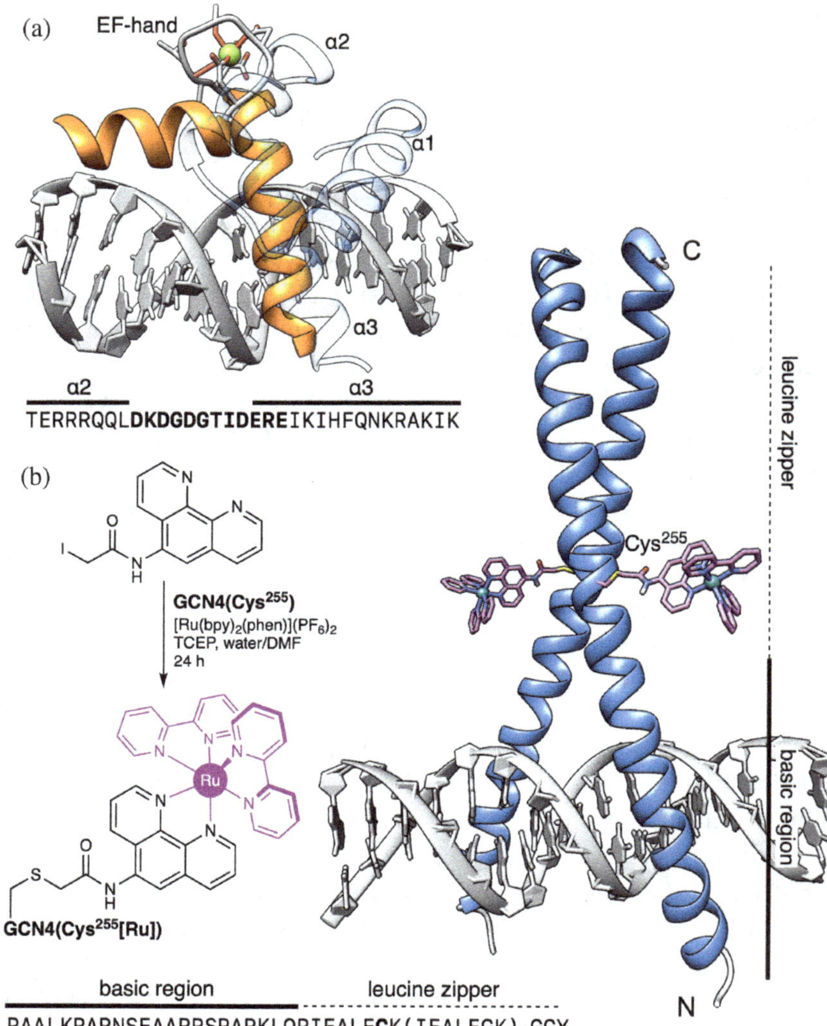

Fig. 7. (a) Structure of the EF-hand/homeodomain chimera (orange) superimposed to the engrailed homeodomain structure (PDB ID: 1EHN) shown in semi-transparent light-blue to show the match between $\alpha 2/\alpha 3$ and the EF-hand (PDB ID: 1OSA); sequence of the construct at the bottom, highlighting the $\alpha 2/\alpha 3$ and the sequence of the EF-hand (bold); (b) synthesis of the GCN4(Cys^{255})-$[Ru(bpy)_2(phen)]^{2+}$ metallopeptide by modification of the GCN4 Cys^{255} mutant in solution with the electrophilic *N*-iodoacetyl-5-amino-1,10-phenanthroline; structure of the DNA complex showing the metal complexes close to the DNA built from the reported GNC4/DNA complex (PDB ID: 1YSA).

order to study protein–protein interactions [83]. Following the same approach, they derivatized Cys side chain with a chelating phenanthroline group at (*i,i*+7), relative to the His residue. Coordination of Zn(II), Cu(II), Co(II) and Ni(II) promotes helical conformation of the basic region of a leucine zipper, showing that the coordination stabilizes the complex with the DNA [84].

3. DNA-Binding Metal Complexes Modified with Peptides

Cisplatin and its derivatives, carboplatin and oxaliplatin, are widely used chemotherapeutic drugs used to treat many types of cancers, including ovarian and testicular cancer, sarcoma, or lymphoma, among others. However, drug-induced resistance and severe side effects, particularly neurotoxicity, which can cause tinnitus, peripheral neuropathy, or partial hearing loss, have fueled intense research efforts to develop safer alternatives with reduced side effects and improved DNA binding and therapeutic properties [15,16,85]. In this context, in 2000, the group of J. Reedijk described the application of solid-phase synthesis methods for the assembly of a peptide-dichloroplatinum(II) conjugate [86]. The reported metallopeptide contained an ethylenediamine ligand attached to the *N*-terminus of a short Gly-Arg dipeptide tag. Interestingly, the Pt(II)-metallopeptide was completely assembled in the solid support, including the key platination step by treatment of the partially deprotected peptide ligand with 10 equiv of K_2PtCl_4 in a mixture of DMF/H_2O. Importantly, the final cleavage/deprotection of the metallopeptide required a modified cocktail lacking the commonly used triisopropylsilane scavenger (TFA/H_2O, 95/5, v/v) to avoid reduction of the coordinated Pt(II) (Figure 8). This breakthrough in solid-phase peptide synthesis of Pt(II) metallopeptides was soon followed by the application of this methodology for the automated parallel solid-phase synthesis of a small library of 36 Pt(II)-metallopeptide complexes, which was screened for *in vitro* anticancer activity against the A2780 cell line. Although the authors could not identify any compound with promising activity as cytotoxic agents, this study clearly demonstrated the potential of solid-phase peptide synthesis in the development of platinum drugs [87,88]. Additionally, the solid-phase peptide synthesis methodology could be extended for the synthesis of dinuclear peptide-like

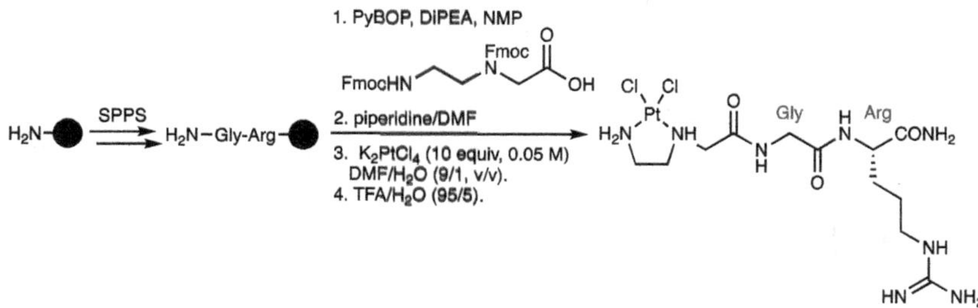

Fig. 8. Solid-phase peptide synthesis of peptide-dichloroplatinum(II) conjugates highlighting the key steps used to introduce the ethylenediamine chelator and the Pt(II) complex in the peptide while still attached to the resin. Adapted from Ref. [86]).

Pt(II) complexes with a bridging lysine linker, although in the initial report no significant activity was observed for the reported analogs [89].

The group of Prof. V. Marchán reported a number of cisplatin derivatives conjugated to peptides for improved targeting. In 2015, they described the synthesis of a cisplatin conjugate with a dicarba analog of the octreotide peptide, which is a stable cyclooctapeptide agonist that displays high affinity and specificity for the somatostatin sst_2 GPCR receptor subtype commonly overexpressed in tumoral cells (Figure 9(a)) [90,91].

The key step in the synthesis of the conjugate involved the coupling of the carba octreotide peptide attached to the resin with the (1-(carboxylic acid)-1,2-diaminoethane) platinum(II) complex activated with CIPC and *N*hydroxy succinimide as coupling reagents in DMF. The final peptide was deprotected/cleaved from the resin avoiding the use of triisopropylsilane as a scavenger as described by J. Reedijk; the product could be directly isolated from the reaction mixture by HPLC. *In vitro* studies showed that the conjugate retained the alkylating properties responsible for the cytotoxic activity of cisplatin drugs. Although no cytotoxicity studies were described in this initial report, these were included in a follow-up paper published in 2012 [92], in which they also report a set of new octreotide conjugates with ruthenium(II) and osmium(II) complexes (Figures 10(b) to 10(d)).

Of all the compounds, only the octreotide derivative of $[(\eta^6\text{-}p\text{-cym})RuCl\text{-}(imidazole\text{-}CO_2H)(PPh_3)]^+$, which was inert to ligand exchange, displayed antiproliferative activity against human tumor cell lines (e.g., $IC_{50}=63 \pm 2\ \mu M$ in MCF-7 cells), showing also active uptake and

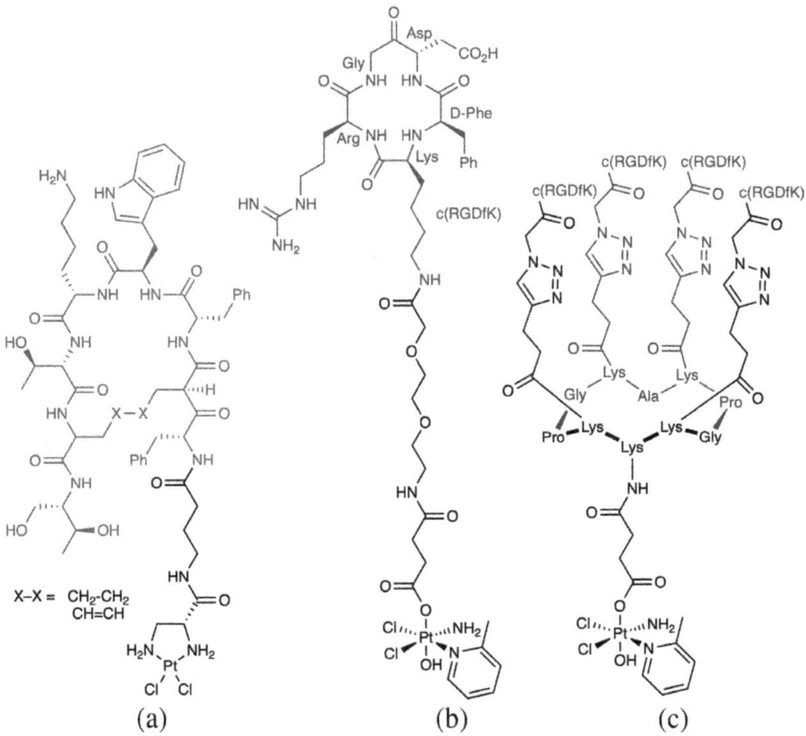

Fig. 9. Cisplatin derivatives conjugated to peptides for improved delivery: (a) carba octeotride-cisplatin conjugates; (b) monomeric picoplatin-*cyclo*-(RGDf) for integrin targeting; (c) multivalent picoplatin- *cyclo*-(RGDf)]$_4$.

participation of the somatostatin receptors targeted by the carboplatin octreotide peptide. Unfortunately, the parent complex by itself displayed even better IC_{50} in the same cell line (IC_{50}=3.32 ± 0.54 μM), comparable to that of cisplatin in the same conditions (IC_{50}=3.04 ± 0.25 μM), which clearly illustrates one of the greatest challenges in this field, which is that the peptide tags are not innocent bystanders, but could impact the activity of the metal complex warheads.

Following a similar approach, they also described the synthesis of a picoplatin attached to a *cyclo*-(RGDfK) peptide (Figure 9(b)) [93], which is known to target $\alpha_V\beta3$ and $\alpha_V\beta5$ integrin receptors overexpressed in some lung, breast, prostate, ovarian, or brain tumors [94,95]. The synthetic approach involved both solid phase and solution methods. The linear pentapeptide was

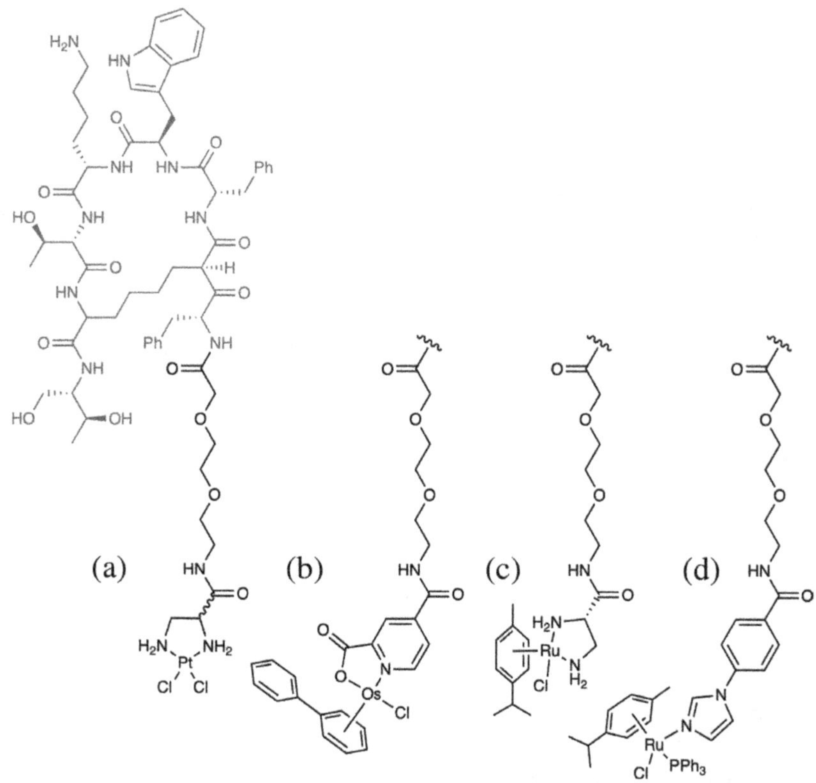

Fig. 10. Octreotide peptide (in light grey) conjugated to cytotoxic ruthenium(II) and osmium(II) complexes for targeted delivery to somatostatin receptors: (a) with $[PtCl_2(dap)]$ (dap = 1-(carboxylic acid)-1,2-diaminoethane); (b) $[(\eta^6\text{-bip})Os(4\text{-}CO_2\text{-pico})Cl]$ (bip = biphenyl, pico = picolinate); (c) $[(\eta^6\text{-}p\text{-cym})RuCl\text{-}(dap)]^+$ (*p*-cym = *p*-cymene); (d) $[(\eta^6\text{-}p\text{-cym})RuCl\text{-}(imidazole\text{-}CO_2H)(PPh_3)]^+$ [97].

assembled following standard solid-phase peptide synthesis methods on a 2-chlorotrityl chloride resin, which allowed its cleavage under mild conditions, while keeping the side-chain protecting groups in place; cyclization of the side-chain-protected peptide in solution afforded the peptide *cyclo*-[Arg(Pfb)GlyAsp(tBu)-(D)-Phe-Lys(alloc)], and selective cleavage of the alloc group in the Lys ε-NH_2 with $Pd(PPh_3)_4$, followed by a series of coupling and deprotection steps provided the desired picoplatin-*cyclo*-(RGDfK) conjugate [98]. A multivalent conjugate containing four targeting cyclopeptides attached to a regioselectively addressable functionalized template (RAFT) cyclodecapeptide scaffold was also synthesized following a related approach and click chemistry for the regioselective attachment of the *cyclo*-(RGDfK) units to the RAFT scaffold (Figure 9(c) [96]. Following the same strategy, they also developed an integrin-targeted photoactivatable Pt(IV) analog by combining a $[Pt(N_3)_2(OH)_2(py)_2]$ complex with the *cyclo*-(RGDfK) integrin ligand [97] (Figure 10).

Ruthenium(II) and rhodium(II) metallointercalators have been exhaustively studied over the years due to their stability and potential applications thanks to their unique redox and optical properties [10,22,98–100]. These complexes typically contain at least one large heteroaromatic ligand, such as dpq, dppz, or dppn (Figure 11), which intercalates between consecutive base pairs, usually through the major groove. Although the intercalation of these complexes does not provide much sequence specificity, these complexes offer extraordinary opportunities for the modulation of the DNA-binding properties, by taking advantage of ancillary ligands and stereochemical effects, not accessible with classic DNA-binding agents (e.g., early studies with $[Ru(phen)_3]^{2+}$ complex already identified the preference for intercalation of the Δ-isomers that match the symmetry of the B-DNA helix) [101,102]. In this context, peptides have been used to modulate the biological properties of these complexes, for example, facilitating cell internalization, or targeting intracellular compartments.

In 1994, the group of J. K. Barton reported the DNA-binding properties of a $[Rh(phi)_2(phen')]^{3+}$ (phen′=5-(amidoglutaryl)-1,10-phenanthroline) complex attached to the α_3-helix of the DNA-binding phage P_{22} c2 repressor to examine whether small peptides could enhance the

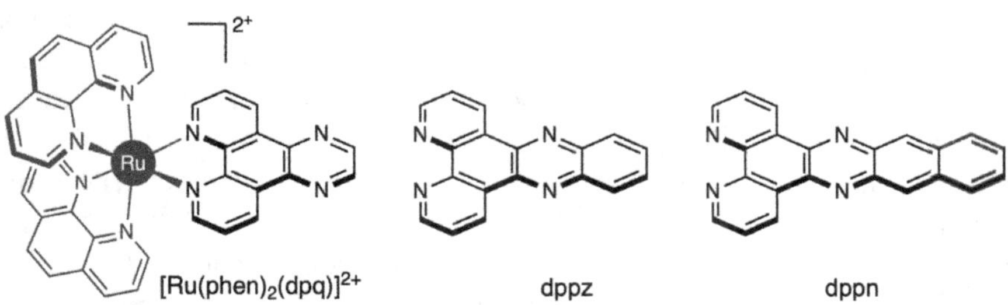

Fig. 11. Structures of the heteroaromatic ligand dpq (pyrazino[2,3-*f*][1,10]phenanthroline) as a ruthenium(II) metallointercalator, $[Ru(phen)_2(dppq)]^{2+}$, and the homologous ligands dppz (dipyrido[3,2-*a*:2′,3′-*c*]phenazine) and dppn (benzo [*i*]dipyrido[3,2-*a*:2′,3′-*c*] phenazine).

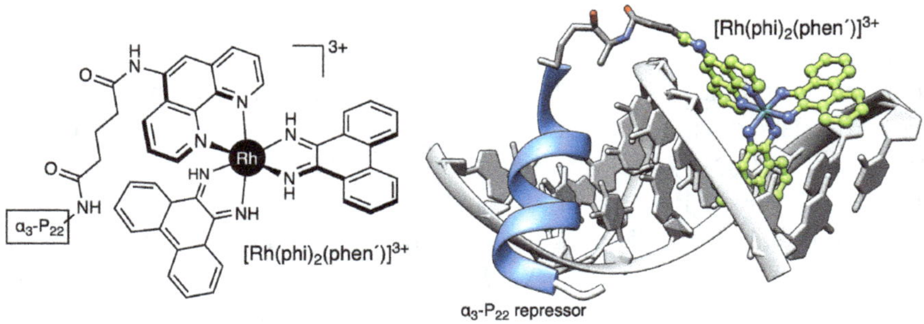

Fig. 12. Left: Structure of the $[Rh(phi)_2(phen')]^{3+}$-α_3-P22 conjugate. Right: Model of the interaction of the conjugate built from the X-ray crystal structure of the complex $[Ru(phen)_2(dppz)]^{2+}$ bound to d(TCGGTACCGA), PDB ID 4LY2, and the structure of the P_{22} c2 repressor bound to the operator sequence d(ATTTAAGATATCTTAAAT), PDB ID 2R1J [105]. The complex is shown in green, and the α_3-helix in blue. Adapted from Refs. [103 and 104].

DNA-binding properties of these metallointercalators [103,104]. The conjugate was assembled while the peptide was still attached to the solid phase by reaction of an *N*-terminal phen′ group, connected to the *N*-terminal en of the peptide through a succinic linker, with $[Rh(phi)_2(DMF)_2]^{3+}$; the metal-peptide conjugate was stable to standard cleavage/deprotection conditions. The results indicate that the nuclease activity of the complex is strongly dependent on the nature of the peptide tag, so that the Glu residue at position 10 of the short 13-residue peptide fragment (AANVAISQWERAA-NH_2) is required for strong sequence selectivity of the cleavage site at 5′-CC**A**-3′ (cleavage at the highlighted A base), while other mutations appear to affect the cleavage efficiency.

A few years later, the same group expanded this strategy reporting the synthesis of a synthetic DNA nuclease composed by a zinc-binding peptide attached to a rhodium(III) intercalator [106]. The design of this nuclease is similar to that of the P22 conjugate described previously, but in this case, the 16-residue α-helical peptide attached through its *N*-terminus to the rhodium intercalator was designed *de novo*, based on the sequences of metal-containing hydrolases. The sequence (DPDELE**H**AAK**H**EA-AAK-NH_2) contained two His residues at positions 7 and 11 (*i,i*+4, in bold), which created a zinc coordination site in the α-helix; the peptide also contained internal salt bridges (Glu-Lys) and Ala residues to stabilize the α-helical conformation. Importantly, the conjugate was able to induce efficient DNA cleavage in the presence of Zn(II) ions, while no nuclease activity was observed with a control peptide lacking the rhodium(III) complex, as well as in the absence of Zn(II), or in the presence of EDTA, indicating that the rhodium(III) metallointercalator delivers the reactive Zn(II) peptide nuclease to the major groove of the DNA double helix, thus allowing the stereospecific efficient cleavage to give 3′-hydroxyl DNA fragments at low micromolar concentrations. A few years later, the group applied the same principles for the design of a new nuclease containing a 22-residue long β-hairpin peptide derived from the *BamHI* restriction endonuclease (ADVYKEFIENSELKRVGAEFEA-NH_2) attached through its *N*-terminus to the metallointercalator $[Rh(phi)(bpy')]^{3+}$ (bpy′=4-(butyric acid)-4′-methyl-2,2′-bipyridine) [107]. As expected, conjugation of the *BamH1* peptide to the metallointercalator and the presence of Zn(II) ion in the reaction mixture were both essential for effective DNA cleavage.

A relatively recent example of these metallointercalator-peptide hybrids explored the effect of the peptide sequence in the internalization and cellular localization (Figure 13) [108]. In this study, the $[Ru(phen)(bpy')(dppz)]^{2+}$ complex (bpy′=4-(3-carboxypropyl)-4′-methyl-2,2′-bipyridine) was attached either to a well-known (*d*)-octaarginine (arg_8)

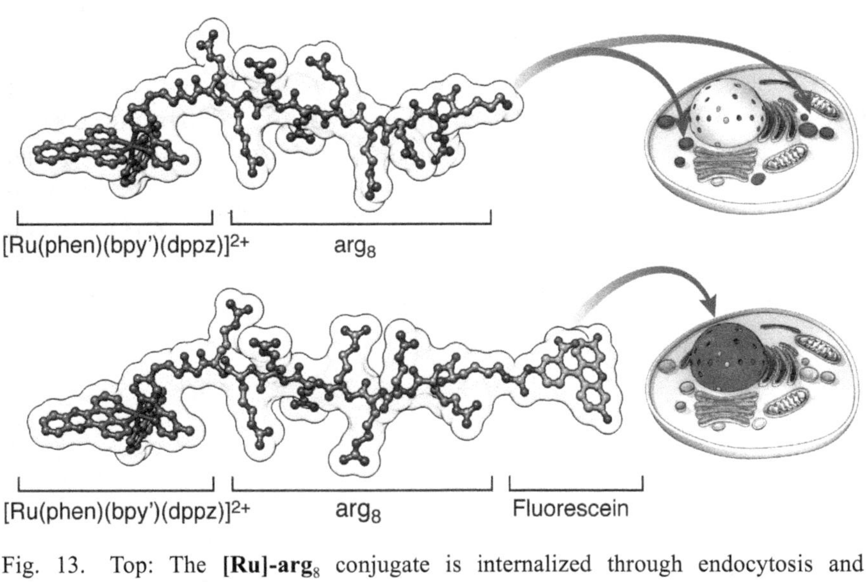

Fig. 13. Top: The **[Ru]-arg$_8$** conjugate is internalized through endocytosis and accumulates in vesicles in the cytoplasm; in contrast, the complex **[Ru]-arg$_8$-Flu** containing a fluorescein fluorophore attached to the same core structure is effectively delivered into the cell nucleus.

peptide transporter or to that same peptide modified with a fluorescein tag (**arg$_8$-Flu**). Interestingly, they found that, while the simple **[Ru]-arg$_8$** hybrid was readily internalized by endocytosis, and accumulated in endosomes in the cytoplasm, the **[Ru]-arg$_8$-Flu** derivative was readily internalized into the cell nucleus under the same conditions for which the complex without fluorescein was excluded. The observed difference in intracellular localization is consistent with other studies that demonstrate the role of charge and hydrophobicity compensation in peptide transporters [109]. This result demonstrates the potential role of the peptide appendages not only to modulate the DNA binding of metal complexes, but also for controlling their internalization properties as well as their intracellular delivery [110].

2,2′-Bipyridine (bpy) is one of the most widely used ligands in coordination chemistry; metal complexes derived from bpy usually present high association constants due to the chelating effect of the two nitrogen donors and the capacity of the bipyridine ligand to act as a π-acceptor. Due to the advantageous coordinative preferences of the bpy compared with natural amino acid side chains, bpy has been extensively used as ligand in artificial metallopeptides. The bpy unit can be functionalized in positions 4, 5 or 6 of the aromatic ring, so that it is possible to obtain amino acids equipped with the bpy group in their side chain (4bpa, 5bpa and 6bpa, respectively, Figure 14) [111,112].

However, the stereoselective synthesis of chiral bpy amino acids is far from straightforward, which led to the study of other bipyridine derivatives, such as 5′-amino-[2,2′-bipyridine]-5-carboxylic acid (5bpy). The 5bpy amino acid was first reported in 1996 by the Imperiali group, who used it for the development of peptide-based metal ion sensors [113]. A few years later, G. R. Newkome described a new synthetic route for the obtention of the 5bpy [114], which was modified in our group to access

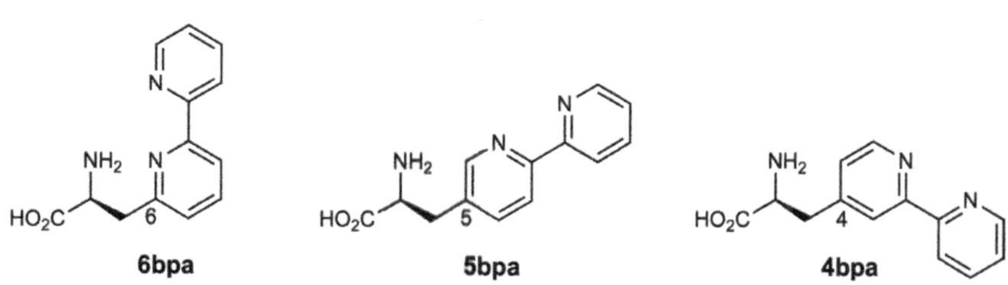

Fig. 14. Chiral amino acids equipped with chelating 2,2′-bpy units in their side chain.

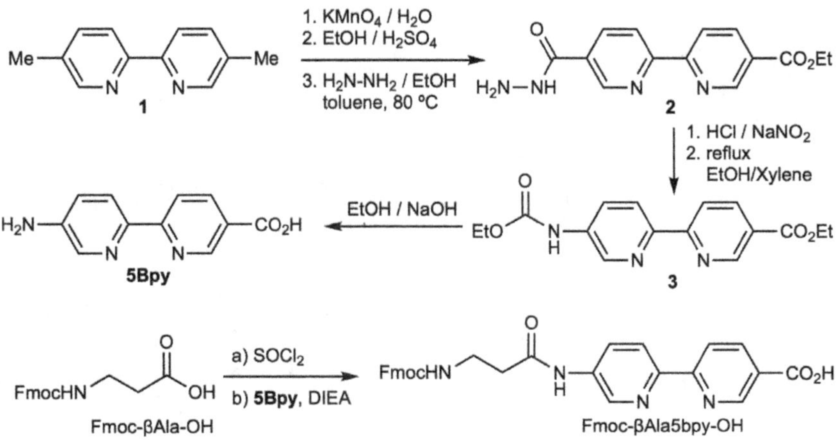

Fig. 15. Synthetic scheme for the synthesis of the Fmoc-βAla5bpy-OH building block for the solid-phase peptide synthesis of DNA-binding metallopeptides. Adapted from Ref. [120].

Fmoc-protected 5bpy derivatives suitable for solid-phase peptide in high yield [115].

Our group has extensively used the 5bpy building block during the past few years for the construction of DNA-binding peptides. Thus, in 2013, we reported the application of solid-phase peptide synthesis (SPPS) methodology to assemble linear peptide ligands containing two 5Bpy chelators; treatment of the peptide ligands while still attached to the solid support with the enantiopure Hua and von Zelewsky's Λ-*cis*-$[Ru(bpy)_2(py)_2]^{2+}$ or Δ-*cis*-$[Ru(bpy)_2(py)_2]^{2+}$ reagents (bpy = 2,2′-bipyridine, py = pyridine) [116,117], afforded the desired homochiral dinuclear Ru(II) complexes (e.g., $\Lambda\Lambda$-[Ac-(Ru(II)βAla5bpy)$_2$]) in good yields after cleavage/deprotection and purification [118]. The versatility of the solid-phase peptide synthesis methodology allowed us to easily synthesize derivatives tagged with an octaarginine domain, which has been shown to improve the internalization of molecular cargoes essentially in all types of cells (e.g., $\Lambda\Lambda$-[Ac-(Ru(II)βAla5bpy)$_2$]-Arg$_8$, Figure 16) [119] This methodology was later extended with the synthesis of a set of mono, di and trinuclear polypyridyl Ir(III) organometallopeptides as well as their octaarginine analogs, which displayed high DNA-binding affinity and sequence selectivity with preference for A/T-rich sequences. Moreover, the DNA affinity of the trinuclear Ac-(Ir(III)

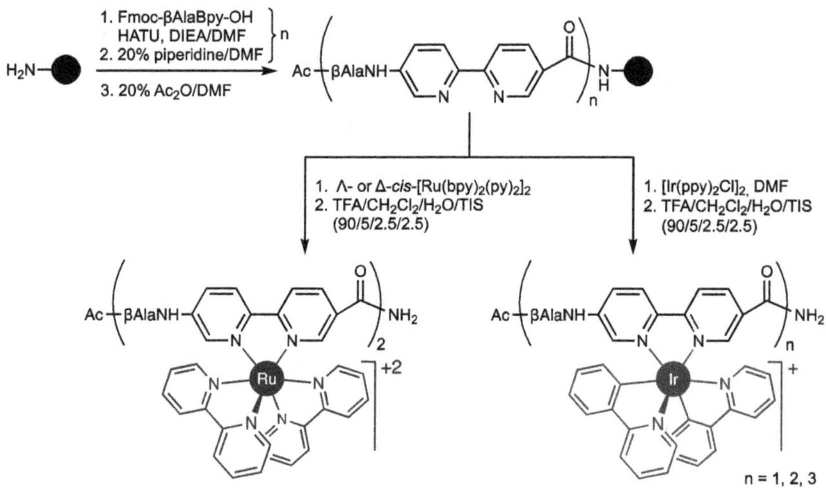

Fig. 16. Solid-phase peptide synthesis of the oligomeric metallopeptide ligands containing the *β*Ala5Bpy units. Metal coordination in the solid phase by reaction of the ligand with Hua and von Zelewsky's reagents affords the homochiral ΛΛ- or ΔΔRu(II) complexes; reaction with the iridium precursor affords, after cleavage/deprotection, the final complexes with one, two, and three cyclometallated Ir(III) units (n=1, 2, 3, respectively).

*β*Ala5bpy)$_2$–Arg$_8$ metallopeptide was in the order of the best-known organic DNA minor-groove binders [120]. This strategy was recently applied in our group for the synthesis of Ru(II) metallopeptides containing the dppz ligand and oligoarginine tails that displayed selective G-quadruplex binding [121].

Related dinuclear complexes attached to short peptide sequences (Gly$_3$, Gly$_2$-Lys, and Ahx-Lys) were recently described by the group of Prof. A. Garoufis in 2018 [122]. Their semi-synthetic approach involves the solid-phase derivatization of the peptide chains with the diruthenium oligopyridine Ru(II) complexes, which feature a carboxylate group for their attachment to the *N*-terminus of the sequence. Spectroscopic studies indicate that the complexes bind to the DNA minor groove and suggest that the attached peptides do not contribute to the observed DNA binding. This group has also described the application of similar methodologies for the assembly of mononuclear Ru(II) complexes to a short peptide derived from the sequence of the recognition loop of the *MunI* restriction enzyme (RGNAHER), which binds to the palindromic sequence 5′-C↓AATTG-3′

(cleavage site indicated by the downwards arrow) through the DNA major groove thanks to a combination of hydrogen bonds made by backbone and side chain atoms [123]. NMR studies in the presence of the oligonucleotide 5′-GCGCTTAAGCGC-3′ indicate the short peptide is not structured, and does not endow the complex with sequence selectivity, so that the metallopeptides (Λ- and Δ-isomers) bind to DNA via many different orientations [124]. In 2015, the group of Prof. U. Diederichsen reported a platinum metallopeptide chimera featuring a short cyclic peptide (*cyclo*-(XpGRNPKTGEDI); X=Dap, p=D-Pro) mimicking the minor groove-binding region of the IHF transcription factor, which would endow a platinum complex with DNA sequence selectivity, and an oligocationic lysine dendrimer, which would ideally complement such sequence-selective binding with complementary electrostatic interactions for increased affinity [125]. Unfortunately, EMSA assays showed that the platinum complex is the main contributor to DNA binding, and the IHF peptide does not endow the chimera with the desired sequence selectivity for targeting a particular DNA site. Indeed, the cyclic peptide by itself does not show significant DNA affinity and only the dendrimeric Lys unit appears to contribute to the overall binding through electrostatic interactions. These papers exemplify the complexities associated with the design of these bipartite systems, because the excision of the short peptide domains from their natural protein contexts usually results in loss of function, which might only be recovered by additional engineering of the natural sequences that stabilize the bioactive conformations [126–127].

4. Peptide Helicates

In 1995, Prof. J. M. Lehn described, for the first time, the DNA binding properties of a family of Cu(I) polynuclear complexes derived from Bpy, and suggested that the complex was inserted in the DNA major groove [129]. A few years later, the group of Prof. M. J. Hannon described the properties of a new bis iron *tris*-chelate helicate and its DNA binding through the major groove of the DNA, which caused a significant bend of the double helix [130,131]. Later work also demonstrated that the chirality of the helicate plays a key role in their binding so that the *M* isomer of the helicate binds preferably the major groove, whereas the *P* isomer appears to be inserted in the minor groove of the DNA [132]. In 2006, this group published the X-ray structure of the complex between the helicate and a three-way DNA junction, showing the insertion of the helicate cylinder in the hydrophobic cavity formed by the exposed surfaces of the base pairs at the center of the junction [133]. Subsequent studies related to this metallocylinder revealed its high activity against different cancer cell lines. The mechanism seems to be not genotoxic as in the case of cisplatin or other alkylating agents, but it acts reducing the mitochondrial activity, thus inhibiting the cellular growth [134].

In 2014, we described the application of solid-phase peptide synthesis methodology to assemble peptide ligands as precursor of metal helicates. In order to fully exploit the templating effect of the peptide scaffold, we designed a peptidic ligand capable of folding into a single-stranded dinuclear hairpin helicate [135]. The peptide sequence contains six 5Bpy units — to satisfy the coordination requirements of two octahedral metal centers — arranged in three strands, which are connected through two short loops (Figure 17). The loops are fundamental elements in the design because they include a short β-turn promoting sequence, -[(D/L)-Pro]-Gly- to preorganize the ligand, inducing its folding into a discrete complex, thus avoiding the formation of higher-order assemblies in the presence of metal ions. Moreover, the Pro residues are the only chiral residues in the sequence, and therefore the chirality of the resulting helicate would be defined by their chirality (D/L) [136,137]. Circular dichroism studies confirmed that upon incubation with Fe(II), the peptide precursors enantioselectively assembled into dimetallic helicates with ΛΛ- (for the L-Pro/L-Pro ligand) or ΔΔ- (for the D-Pro/D-Pro ligand) configurations. Fluorescence anisotropy titrations of rhodamine-labeled helicates confirmed that this complex displayed high affinity for three-way DNA junctions ($K_D \approx$ 3.5 μM for the ΛΛ- isomer, and 13.6 μM for the ΔΔ-helicate). In contrast, the binding of these species to double-stranded DNA was rather weak ($K_D \approx 40$ μM for A/T-rich oligonucleotides, and a $K_D \approx 100$ μM for G/C-rich oligos) [138].

We have recently shown that the trimeric bacteriophage T4 Fibritin foldon domain (T4Ff) can be engineered with metal-chelating 2,2′-bipyridine units on its *N*-terminus to yield a peptide ligand that stereoselectively assembles in the presence of Fe(II) ions into a parallel, three-stranded peptide helicate with *M* chirality. Inspection of the X-ray crystal structure of the T4Ff trimer (PDB IDs 4NCU or 1RFO) showed that the Gly residues at the *N*-terminus of the peptides are close to each other and could potentially accommodate an appended bpy unit without noticeable distortion of the T4Ff scaffold upon metal ion coordination (Figure 18).

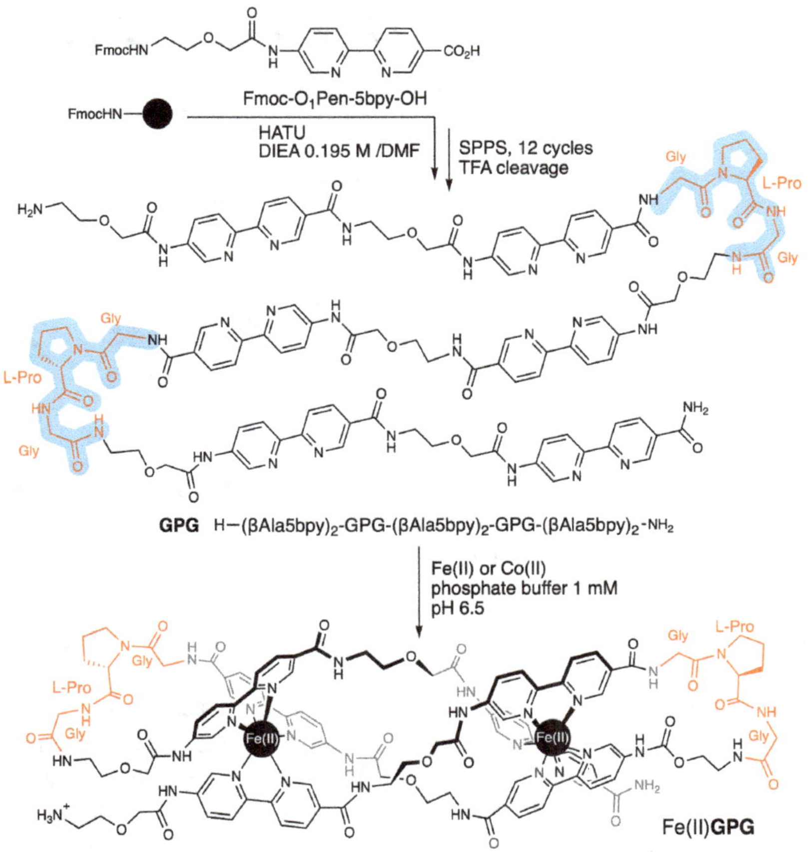

Fig. 17. Solid-phase peptide synthesis of a peptide helicate precursor. The Gly-Pro-Gly sequences induce the folding of the peptide chain and the formation of discrete, dinuclear helicates in the presence of Fe(II) ions.

Moreover, the natural orientation of the *N*-terminal polyproline helices in the folded T4Ff trimer templated the formation of a helicate complex with *M* helicity, which according to earlier studies was the preferred chirality for the efficient recognition of three-way junction DNA [138]. Indeed, the designed trimeric peptide helicate selectively recognizes three-way DNA junctions over double-stranded DNA with μM affinity, as shown by spectroscopic and gel shift mobility assays [139].

The group of Prof. M. Hannon reported in 2009 a three-stranded helicate complex featuring their classic bi-spyridylimine ligand derivatized with a

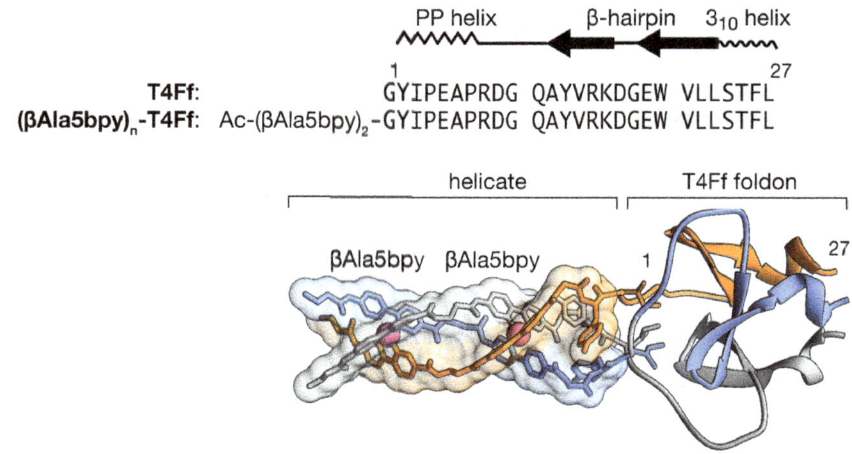

Fig. 18. Top: Sequence of the natural foldon (T4Ff) and sequence the peptide ligand containing the two 5Bpy units attached to the *N*-terminus of the natural foldon sequence. Bottom: the proposed structure for the $Fe(II)_2[5bpy5bpy\text{-}T4Ff]_3$ helicate. Adapted from Ref. [139].

short tripeptide sequence (GGS) [140]. The synthesis of this hybrid ligand involved the on-resin modification of the *N*-terminal amino group of the peptide sequence with 6-dimethoxymethyl-nicotinic acid; cleavage and deprotection under acidic conditions afforded a peptide-aldehyde intermediate, which then was reacted with 4,4′-methylenedianiline in the presence of $FeCl_2 \cdot 4H_2O$ to give the final three-stranded helicate (Figure 19). Alternatively, condensation of the peptide-aldehyde with 4,4′-methylenedianiline in the absence of metal salts produced the bis-imine ligand, which could coordinate various metal ions to give other types of helicates. Although the presence of the Ser residue in the sequence might induce a selective helical twist in the final helicate complexes, no spectroscopic evidence of such induction was found, suggesting that the remote Ser does not influence the helicity of the helicates. DNA binding and nuclease activity of these peptide derivatives were similar to those reported for the analogs lacking the peptide sequence.

5. Stimuli-Responsive Metallopeptides

Researchers have mainly focused their efforts on the design of static DNA-binding metallopeptides and although many of the systems discussed so far display some level of responsiveness, there are only a handful of purposely designed stimuli-responsive systems reported in the literature. Some of the

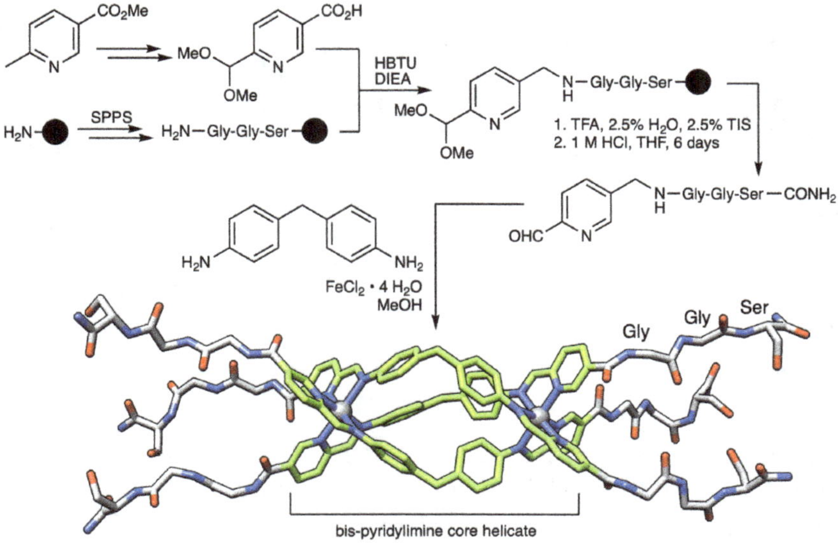

Fig. 19. Synthesis of the peptide-functionalized three-stranded helicates. The ligand was partially assembled in the solid phase and the reactive peptide-aldehyde intermediate was condensed with 4,4'-methylenedianiline in the presence of an Fe(II) salt to give the desired helicate. The core bis-imine helicate is highlighted in green in a model of the resulting peptide helicate.

earlier examples rely on the conformational control of a peptide domain that will only bind the DNA when folded into an α-helical conformation. A key development in that area was reported by the group of Y. Sugiura, who in 2004 demonstrated the effective conformational control of peptide helicity with metal ions [141]. Their approach involves the modification of the leucine zipper domain of a transcription factor called FOS to control its heterodimerization with its partner JUN. Thus, modification of a pair of Lys residues at positions *i* and *i+2* in the FOS leucine zipper region with metal-chelating iminodiacetic acid generates an artificial **FOS(KIda)**$_2$ analog featuring an artificial Fe(III) binding site; upon metal chelation, the Fe(III)**FOS(KIda)**$_2$ peptide is locked in a conformation that is incapable of folding its leucine zipper region into an α-helix, which is required for heterodimerization with JUN. In contrast, in the absence of Fe(III), the **FOS(KIda)**$_2$ analog is free to fold and form the coiled-coil structure with JUN, leading to the heterodimeric FOS/JUN bZIP complex (Figure 20).

This strategy to control the folding of a peptide α-helix was implemented in 2009 by the group of Futaki to develop a metal switch of the

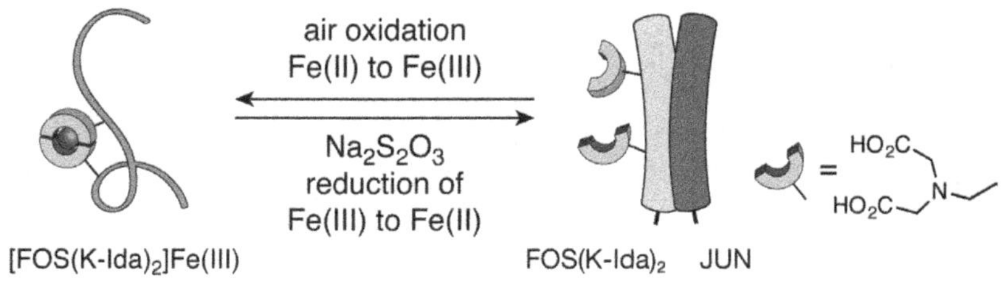

Fig. 20. Conformational control of α-helical peptide fragments modified with Ida chelators at positions i,i+2. The formation of the metal complex locks the peptide in a conformation that cannot dimerize with JUN.

DNA-binding domain of the GCN4 bZIP TF [142]. They introduced the Ida chelating units by modification of two pairs of Cys residues with *N*-(2-tosylthioethyl)iminodiacetic acid. The resulting pairs of chelating Cys derivatives, at position i,i+2 in the leucine zipper domain, controlled the folding of the GCN4 peptide, and through this, GCN4 homodimerization into the DNA-binding bZIP structure.

Thus, as described before for the **FOS(KIda)**$_2$ analog, incubation of **GCN4(CIda)**$_4$ with Co(II) impaired its dimerization and inhibited DNA binding (K_D > 1 μM), while in the absence of Co(II), the **GCN4(C-Ida)**$_4$ was capable of dimerizing and binding with high-affinity to the AP-1/GCRE site (K_D=22 ± 3.0 nM), being able to reproduce the recognition properties of the natural GCN4 dimer (K_D=15 nM). Remarkably, the addition of EDTA as a competitive chelator to a preformed Co(II)$_2$**GCN4(C-Ida)**$_2$ complex resulted in the recovery of the initial binding affinity in the absence of the metal ion (K_D=22 ± 1.1 nM), and addition to Co(II) to the complex of the **GCN4(CIda)**$_2$ with the DNA induced a large decrease in the α-helical content, which was consistent with structural alterations of the **GCN4(CIda)**$_2$ dimer that resulted in the disassembly of its complex with the DNA (Figure 21).

The formation of metal complexes has also been applied in combination with orthogonal stimuli, such as redox inputs, for the development of more sophisticated switches. Thus, in 2013, together with the group of Prof. J. L. Mascareñas, we described a DNA-binding peptide based on the GCN4 transcription factor that contained both a metal-chelating 5,5″-dimethyl-2,2′:6′,2″-terpyridine ligand attached to the side chain of a C-terminal Lys^{231} residue, and a redox-sensitive Cys residue on its

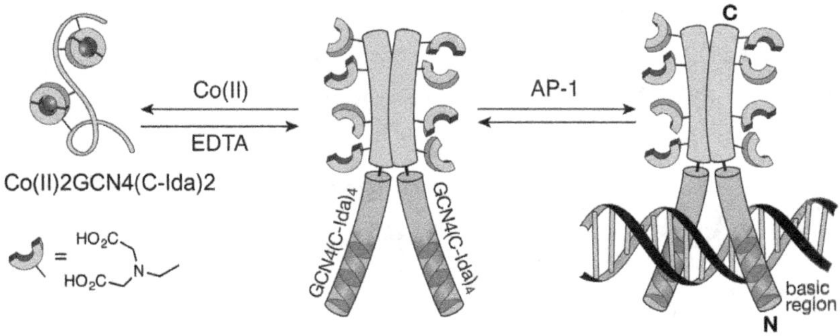

Fig. 21. Futaki's approach to metal-responsive DNA-binding peptides. The **GCN4(C-Ida)$_4$** peptide contains two metal-chelating *N*-(2-tosylthioethyl)iminodiacetic acid units in the leucine zipper region; in the absence of Co(II) ions, this peptide dimerizes (center) and binds to its target DNA (right); the addition of Co(II) induces a conformational change in the peptide that disrupts the leucine zipper helix and disassembles the dimer required for DNA binding (left) [142].

N-terminus **(Cys)GCN4(tpy)** that modified its DNA-binding profile — displaying different affinity and sequence selectivity — in response to specific chemical inputs [143]. Incubation of this bifunctional peptide with Ni(II) ions in the presence of the ATF/CREB site (5′ATGA cg TCAT3′) gave rise to a complex between the Ni(II)-mediated dimer of the GCN4 fragment Ni(II)[**(Cys)GCN4(tpy)**]$_2$ and the DNA, but under the same conditions, this peptide did not display significant affinity for the inverted sequence (5′TCAT cg ATGA3′). Remarkably, the sequence selectivity was reversed when the Cys residues were oxidized with DTNB, 5,5′-dithiobis-(2-nitrobenzoic acid), so that the disulfide dimer **(SS)[GCN4(tpy)]$_2$** preferentially bound to the inverted sequence (5′-TCAT cg ATGA-3′). Treatment of the **(SS)[GCN4(tpy)]$_2$**/DNA complex with tris(2-carboxyethyl) phosphine (TCEP) to reduce the disulfide bond resulted in the disassembly of the complex with the DNA (Figure 22).

Photolabile bisbipyridyl ruthenium(II) complexes have been described as effective caging groups characterized by high quantum yield and long wavelength of photolysis. We reported in 2014 the use of these types of complexes as a photocleavable dimerizer of TF fragments. More specifically, we reported the synthesis of a generally applicable Ru(II)[*cis*-bromoalkyl-(2,2′-bipyridine)] biselectrophilic reagent, which was used for the synthesis of homodimeric dimers of the GCN4 basic region, as

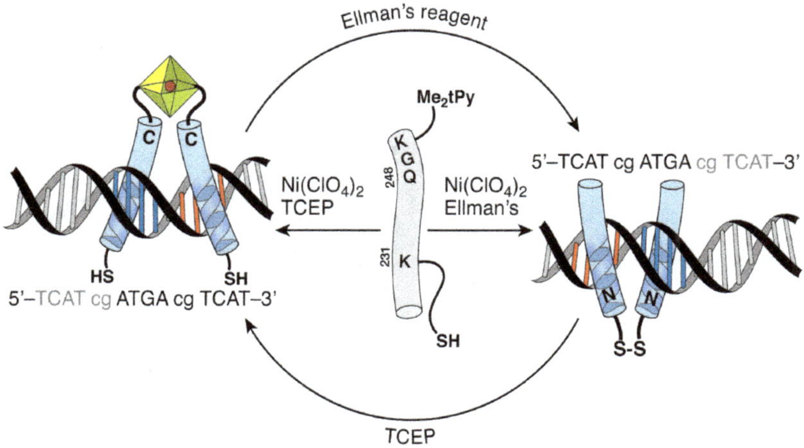

Fig. 22. Stimuli-responsive DNA binding with a GCN4 peptide fragment. The **(Cys) GCN4(tpy)** peptide (center) can be oxidized with Ellman's reagent to afford a disulfide-mediated dimer **(SS)[GCN4(tpy)]$_2$** (on the right-hand side of the image), which binds to the inverted sequence 5′-TCAT cg ATGA-3′ in the presence of Ni(II) ($K_D \approx 758$ nM); reduction of this peptide with TCEP yields an alternative dimer mediated by the terpyridine-nickel complex (Ni(II)[**(Cys)GCN4(tpy)**]$_2$, left) that binds with high affinity ($K_D \approx 670$ nM) to the consensus DNA (5′-ATGA cg TCAT-3′). The disulfide dimer can be recovered by oxidation with Ellman's reagent. Adapted from Ref. [143].

well as heterodimers of C/EBP and GCN4. In both cases, the dimeric constructs with the photolabile ruthenium(II) linker displayed good DNA-binding affinity and selectivity for their respective target sites. Furthermore, irradiation at 455 nm with a LED source caused the photolysis of the ruthenium(II) linker, and the disassembly of their complexes with the DNA (Figure 23) [144].

The amino terminal Cu(II)- and Ni(II)-binding sequence (ATCUN) is a classic tripeptide motif (Xaa-Xaa-His), first identified as a small metal-binding sequence in serum albumin, and then found at the *N*-terminus of many naturally occurring proteins, which has been studied for more than 50 years [145]. ATCUN peptides bind to both Cu(II) and Ni(II) ions with extremely high affinity ($K_D < 10^{-16}$ M), and their derived square-planar metal complexes show tight and sequence-selective DNA binding [146,147] through minor groove insertion. Importantly, Cu(II) and Ni(II) metallopeptides have also endonuclease activity in the presence of oxidizing agents [148–150], and have been extensively used as tags to

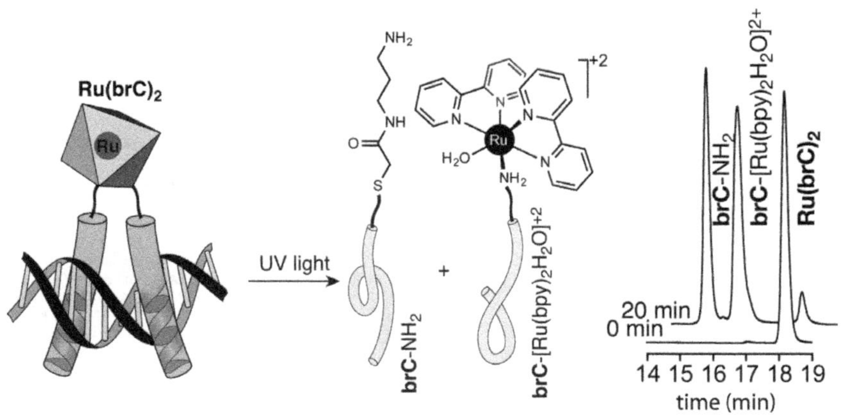

Fig. 23. Photocleavable (2,2′-bipyridyne)Ru(II) linkers in bZIP basic region dimers (either GCN4 homodimers or C/EBP-GCN4 heterodimers). The high-affinity, specific DNA complex can be disassembled by irradiation with long-wavelength light, and the different species resulting from the asymmetric photolysis of the ruthenium(II) linker can be identified by HPLC-MS (right).

endow nuclease activity to many DNA-binding systems [151,152]. In 2015, we reported the synthesis of a light-sensitive histidine building block for Fmoc/tBu solid-phase peptide synthesis in which the imidazole side chain was protected by a ruthenium(II) bisbipyridyl complex. This building block was used for the synthesis of a photoactivatable version of the ATCUN Arg-Gly-His (**RGH**) tripeptide (Figure 24). We demonstrated that the caged His residue could not coordinate Ni(II) ions but, upon irradiation at long wavelength (455 nm LED), the His residue was uncaged, therefore allowing Ni(II) coordination and formation of the square-planar complex Ni(II)**RGH**, which then could bind and cleave DNA *in vitro* [153].

A number of artificial nucleases containing the catalytic ATCUN tag attached to a DNA-binding module (either a peptide or a small molecule) have been reported. This design delivers the hydrolytic ATCUN complex in the vicinity of the DNA — ideally, with some degree of sequence selectivity — to induce its cleavage at particular sites. For example, in 2015, the group of Prof. J. A. Cowan described a Cu(II)GGHK-acridine conjugate (Figure 25) that selectively hydrolyzes a G-quadruplex DNA containing the human telomeric sequence (5′-AGGGTTA GGGTTAGGG

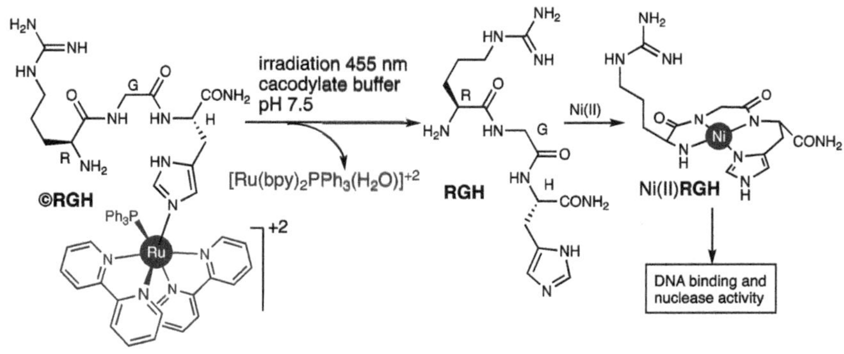

Fig. 24. Caged RGH peptide does not bind to Ni(II). Irradiation with red light at 455 nm releases the metal-chelating peptide, which folds and binds into the DNA minor groove, where it can exert its nuclease activity.

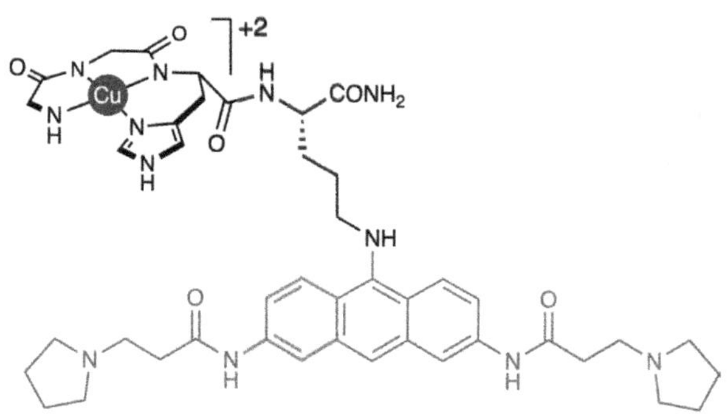

Fig. 25. Cu(II)GGHK-acridine conjugate. The acridine unit (red) targets the G4-DNA and delivers the active complex near the T5.A7 loop in the G-quadruplex.

TTAGGG-3′) [154]. The authors characterized the cleavage site, demonstrating the delivery of the ATCUN complex to the vicinity of the groove formed by the stacked G2-G4 trinucleotides and the T5-A7 loop, and demonstrated promising antitumoral activity against MCF7 breast carcinoma cells due to induced senescence. They have described a number of other nucleases [155], including RNA metallonucleases, that follow the same modular design in which a catalytic metal complex is attached to RNA targeting peptides [156,157].

6. Conclusions

As we have seen in this chapter, by exploiting this versatility, researchers have developed a number of metallopeptides capable of selectively recognizing the regular B-DNA through different binding modes (major or minor groove, intercalation, insertion), as well as other DNA secondary structures (three-way junctions, G-quadruplex). We have organized the DNA-binding metallopeptides according to whether the peptide fragment or the metal complex is mainly responsible for DNA recognition. Those examples in which the peptide has a significant contribution to the DNA recognition generally exploit small fragments of natural TFs to achieve high DNA sequence specificity, thanks to precise interactions between the amino acid side chains and the DNA bases and backbone; in these designs, the metal complex complements the DNA recognition of the peptide endowing it with additional properties, typically as switches, or nucleases. On the other hand, the examples in which the metal complexes take the burden of DNA recognition typically show less sequence specificity. The peptide tags in these designs are used to modulate the properties of the metal complex. Of course, those metallopeptides that combine both units, metal complex and peptide, in a synergistic fashion are the more interesting, but these are truly challenging systems and there are only a handful of examples in the literature. All these investigations have increased our knowledge about the nature of the interaction of metal complexes with DNA. Future developments will certainly exploit the unique properties of metal ions, and benefit from the progress in other areas of chemical biology, such as bioconjugation, (intra)cellular targeting and internalization, which still are in many ways unsolved obstacles for the development of these systems beyond the mere academic setting.

References

1. Roeland Boer, D., Canals, A. and Coll, M. (2008) DNA-Binding Drugs Caught in Action: The Latest 3D Pictures of Drug-DNA Complexes. *Dalton Trans*. 3, pp. 399–414.
2. Palchaudhuri, R. and Hergenrother, P. J. (2007) DNA as a Target for Anticancer Compounds: Methods to Determine the Mode of Binding and the Mechanism of Action. *Curr. Opin. Biotechnol*. 18, pp. 497–503.
3. Nelson. S. M., Ferguson. L. R. and Denny, W. A. (2007) Non-Covalent Ligand/DNA Interactions: Minor Groove Binding Agents. *Mutat. Res*. 623, pp. 24–40.

4. Tse, W. C. and Boger, D. L. (2004) Sequence-Selective DNA Recognition: Natural Products and Nature's Lessons. *Chem. Biol.* 11, pp. 1607–1617.
5. Kielkopf, C. L., White, S., Szewczyk, J. W., Turner, J. M., Baird, E. E., Dervan, P. B. and Rees, D. C. (1998) A Structural Basis for Recognition of A·T and T·A Base Pairs in the Minor Groove of B-DNA. *Science* 282, pp. 111–115.
6. Pazos, E., Mosquera, J., Vázquez, M. E. and Mascareñas, J. L. (2011) DNA Recognition by Synthetic Constructs. *ChemBioChem.* 12, pp. 1958–1973.
7. Boga, S., Bouzada, D., García Peña, D., Vázquez López, M. and Vázquez, M. E. (2018) Sequence-Specific DNA Recognition with Designed Peptides. *Eur. J. Org. Chem.* 2018, pp. 249–261.
8. Vázquez, M. E., Caamaño, A. M. and Mascareñas, J. L. (2003) From Transcription Factors to Designed Sequence-Specific DNA-Binding Peptides. *Chem. Soc. Rev.* 32, pp. 338–349.
9. Zeglis, B. M., Pierre, V. C. and Barton, J. K. (2007) Metallo-Intercalators and Metallo-Insertors. *Chem. Commun.* 44, pp. 4565–4579.
10. Haas, K. L. and Franz, K. J. (2009) Application of Metal Coordination Chemistry to Explore and Manipulate Cell Biology. *Chem. Rev.* 109, pp. 4921–4960.
11. Bruijnincx, P. C. A. and Sadler, P. J. (2008) New Trends for Metal Complexes with Anticancer Activity. *Curr. Opin. Chem. Biol.* 12, pp. 197–206.
12. Komor, A. C. and Barton, J. K. (2013) The Path for Metal Complexes to a DNA Target. *Chem. Commun.* 49, pp. 3617–3630.
13. Komeda, S. and Casini, A. (2012) Next-Generation Anticancer Metallodrugs. *Curr. Topics Med. Chem.* 12, pp. 219–235.
14. Reedijk, J. (2009) Platinum Anticancer Coordination Compounds: Study of DNA Binding Inspires New Drug Design. *Eur. J. Inorg. Chem.* 2009, pp. 1303–1312.
15. Kelland, L. (2007) The Resurgence of Platinum-Based Cancer Chemotherapy. *Nat. Rev. Cancer* 7, pp. 573–584.
16. Sun, R. W.-Y., Ma, D.-L., Wong, E. L.-M. and Che, C.-M. (2007) Some Uses of Transition Metal Complexes as Anti-Cancer and Anti-HIV Agents. *Dalton Trans.* 43, pp. 4884–4892.
17. Seeman, N. C. (2003) DNA in a Material World. *Nature* 421, pp. 427–431.
18. Chen, J. H. and Seeman, N. C. (1991) Synthesis from DNA of a Molecule with the Connectivity of a Cube. *Nature* 350, pp. 631–633.
19. Rothemund, P. W. K. (2006) Folding DNA to Create Nanoscale Shapes and Patterns. *Nature.* 440, pp. 297–302.
20. Smith, J. A., Keene, F. R., Li, F. and Collins, J. G. (2013) Noncovalent DNA Binding of Metal Complexes. In *Comprehensive Inorganic Chemistry II,* Reedijk, J. and Poeppelmeier, K., eds., 2nd edn., pp. 709–750. Amsterdam: Elsevier.

21. Zaki, M., Arjmand, F. and Tabassum, S. (2016) Current and Future Potential of Metallo Drugs: Revisiting DNA-Binding of Metal Containing Molecules and Their Diverse Mechanism of Action. *Inorg. Chim. Acta* 444, pp. 1–22.
22. Gill, M. R. and Thomas, J. A. (2012) Ruthenium(II) polypyridyl Complexes and DNA–From Structural Probes to Cellular Imaging and Therapeutics. *Chem. Soc. Rev.* 41, pp. 3179–3192.
23. Muhammad, N. and Guo, Z. (2014) Metal-Based Anticancer Chemotherapeutic Agents. *Curr. Opin. Chem. Biol.* 19, pp. 144–153.
24. Romero-Canelón, I. and Sadler, P. J. (2013) Next-Generation Metal Anticancer Complexes: Multitargeting via Redox Modulation. *Inorg. Chem.* 52, pp. 12276–12291.
25. Myari, A. and Hadjiliadis, N. (2009) DNA Recognition and Binding by Peptide–Metal Complex Conjugates. In *Metal Complex–DNA Interactions*, N. Hadjiliadis, N. and Sletten, E., eds., pp. 347–367. Chichester, UK: John Wiley & Sons, Ltd.
26. Yamagami, M., Sawada, T. and Fujita, M. (2018) Synthetic β-Barrel by Metal-Induced Folding and Assembly. *J. Am. Chem. Soc.* 140, pp. 8644–8647.
27. Scheib, K. A., Tavenor, N. A., Lawless, M. J., Saxena, S. and Horne, W. S. (2019) Understanding and Controlling the Metal-Directed Assembly of Terpyridine-Functionalized Coiled-Coil Peptides. *Chem. Commun.* 55, pp. 7752–7755.
28. Ghadiri, M. R., Soares, C. and Choi, C. (1992) Design of an Artificial Four-Helix Bundle Metalloprotein via A Novel Ruthenium(II)-Assisted Self-Assembly Process. *J. Am. Chem. Soc.* 114, pp. 4000–4002.
29. Leonard, J. P., Jensen, P., McCabe, T., O'Brien, J. E., Peacock, R. D., Kruger, P. E. and Gunnlaugsson, T. (2007) Self-Assembly of Chiral Luminescent Lanthanide Coordination Bundles. *J. Am. Chem. Soc.* 129, pp. 10986–10987.
30. Albrecht, M., Stortz, P. and Nolting, R. (2003) Peptide/Metal-Ligand Hybrids for the Metal-Assisted Stabilization of Peptide-Microstructures. *Synthesis* 2003, pp. 1307–1320.
31. Pires, M. M. and Chmielewski, J. (2009) Self-Assembly of Collagen Peptides into Microflorettes Via Metal Coordination. *J. Am. Chem. Soc.* 131, pp. 2706–2712.
32. Dublin, S. N. and Conticello, V. P. (2008) Design of a Selective Metal Ion Switch for Self-Assembly of Peptide-Based Fibrils. *J. Am. Chem. Soc.* 130, pp. 49–51.
33. Koebke, K. J. and Pecoraro, V. L. (2019) Noncoded Amino Acids in *de Novo* Metalloprotein Design: Controlling Coordination Number and Catalysis. *Acc. Chem. Res.* 52, pp. 1160–1116.

34. D'Souza, A., Mahajan, M. and Bhattacharjya, S. (2015) Designed Multi-Stranded Heme Binding β-Sheet Peptides in Membrane. *Chem. Sci.* 7, pp. 2563–2571.
35. Barthelmes, K., Reynolds, A. M., Peisach, E., Jonker, H. R. A., DeNunzio, N. J., Allen, K. N., Imperiali, B. and Schwalbe, H. (2011) Engineering Encodable Lanthanide-Binding Tags into Loop Regions of Proteins. *J. Am. Chem. Soc.* 133, pp. 808–819.
36. Franz, K. J., Nitz, M. and Imperiali, B. (2003) Lanthanide-Binding Tags as Versatile Protein Coexpression Probes. *Chem Bio Chem.* 4, pp. 265–271.
37. Uchinomiya, S., Ojida, A. and Hamachi, I. (2014) Peptide Tag/Probe Pairs Based on the Coordination Chemistry for Protein Labeling. *Inorg. Chem.* 53, pp. 1816–1823.
38. Pardoux, R., Sauge-Merle, S., Lemaire, D., Delangle, P., Guilloreau, L., Adriano, J.-M. and Berthomieu, C. (2012) Modulating Uranium Binding Affinity in Engineered Calmodulin EF-Hand Peptides: Effect of Phosphorylation. *PloS One* 7, pp. e41922.
39. Kochańczyk, T., Jakimowicz, P. and Krężel, A. (2012) Femtomolar Zn(II) Affinity of Minimal Zinc Hook Peptides — A Promising Small Tag for Protein Engineering. *Chem. Commun.* 49, pp. 1312–1314.
40. Daughtry, K. D., Martin, L. J., Sarraju, A., Imperiali, B. and Allen, K. N. (2012) Tailoring Encodable Lanthanide-Binding Tags as MRI Contrast Agents. *Chem Bio Chem.* 13, pp. 2567–2574.
41. Cramer, P. (2019) Eukaryotic Transcription Turns 50. *Cell* 179, pp. 808–812.
42. Talanian, R. V., McKnight, C. J. and Kim, P. S. (1990) Sequence-Specific DNA Binding by a Short Peptide Dimer. *Science* 249, pp. 769–771.
43. Talanian, R. V., McKnight, C. J., Rutkowski, R. and Kim, P. S. (1992) Minimum Length of a Sequence-Specific DNA Binding Peptide. *Biochemistry* 31, pp. 6871–6875.
44. Cuenoud, B. and Schepartz, A. (1993) Altered Specificity of DNA-Binding Proteins with Transition Metal Dimerization Domains. *Science* 259, pp. 510–513.
45. Palmer, C. R., Sloan, L. S., Adrian, J. C., Cuenoud, B., Paolella, D. N. and Schepartz, A. (1995) DNA Bending and Binding by Metallo–Zipper Models of bZIP Proteins. *J. Am. Chem. Soc.* 117, pp. 8899–8907.
46. Oheix, E. and Peacock, A. F. A. (2014) Metal-Ion-Regulated Miniature DNA-Binding Proteins Based on GCN4 and Non-Native Regulation Sites. *Chem. Eur. J.* 20, pp. 2829–2839.
47. Lau, Y. H., Wu, Y., de Andrade, P., Galloway, W. R. J. D. and Spring, D. R. (2015) A Two-Component "Double-Click" Approach to Peptide Stapling. *Nat. Prot.* 10, pp. 585–594.

48. Cromm, P. M., Spiegel, J. and Grossmann, T. N. (2015) Hydrocarbon Stapled Peptides as Modulators of Biological Function. *ACS Chem. Biol.* 10, pp. 1362–1375.
49. Kim, Y.-W., Grossmann, T. N. and Verdine, G. L. (2011) Synthesis of All-Hydrocarbon Stapled α-Helical Peptides by Ring-Closing Olefin Metathesis. *Nat. Prot.* 6, pp. 761–771.
50. Schafmeister, C. E., Po, J. and Verdine, G. L. (2000) An All-Hydrocarbon Cross-Linking System for Enhancing the Helicity and Metabolic Stability of Peptides. *J. Am. Chem. Soc.* 122, pp. 5891–5892.
51. Hilinski, G. J., Kim, Y.-W., Hong, J., Kutchukian, P. S., Crenshaw, C. M., Berkovitch, S. S., Chang, A., Ham, S. and Verdine, G. L. (2014) Stitched α-Helical Peptides via Bis Ring-Closing Metathesis. *J. Am. Chem. Soc.* 136, pp. 12314–12322.
52. Zhao, H., Liu, Q.-S., Geng, H., Tian, Y., Cheng, M., Jiang, Y.-H., Xie, M.-S., Niu, X.-G., Jiang, F., Zhang, Y.-O., Lao, Y.-Z., Wu, Y.-D., Xu, N.-H. and Li, Z.-G. (2016) Crosslinked Aspartic Acids as Helix-Nucleating Templates. *Angre. Chem. Int. Ed.* 55, pp. 12088–12093.
53. Bracken, C., Gulyas, J., Taylor, J. W. and Baum, J. (1994) Synthesis and Nuclear Magnetic Resonance Structure Determination of an α-Helical, Bicyclic, Lactam-Bridged Hexapeptide. *J. Am. Chem. Soc.* 116, pp. 6431–6432.
54. Ghadiri, M. R. and Choi, C. (1990) Secondary Structure Nucleation in Peptides. Transition Metal Ion Stabilized α-Helices. *J. Am. Chem. Soc.* 112, pp. 1630–1632.
55. Ghadiri, M. R. and Fernholz, A. K. (1990) Peptide Architecture. Design of Stable α-Helical Metallopeptides via A Novel Exchange-Inert Ruthenium(III) Complex. *J. Am. Chem. Soc.* 112, pp. 9633–9635.
56. Kelso, M. J., Hoang, H. N., Appleton, T. G. and Fairlie, D. P. (2000) The First Solution Structure of a Single α-Helical Turn. A Pentapeptide α-Helix Stabilized by a Metal Clip. *J. Am. Chem. Soc.* 122, pp. 10488–10489.
57. Ma, M. T., Hoang, H. N., Scully, C. C. G., Appleton, T. G. and Fairlie, D. P. (2009) Metal Clips that Induce Unstructured Pentapeptides to be α-Helical in Water. *J. Am. Chem. Soc.* 131, pp. 4505–4512.
58. Kelso, M. J., Hoang, H. N., Oliver, W., Sokolenko, N., March, D. R., Appleton, T. G. and Fairlie, D. P. (2003) A Cyclic Metallopeptide Induces α Helicity in Short Peptide Fragments of Thermolysin. *Angew. Chem. Int. Ed.* 42, pp. 421–424.
59. Chen, L. (1999) Combinatorial Gene Regulation by Eukaryotic Ttranscription Factors. *Curr. Opin. Struct. Biol.* 9, pp. 48–55.
60. Lambert, S. A., Jolma, A., Campitelli, L. F., Das, P. K., Yin, Y., Albu, M., Chen, X., Taipale, J., Hughes, T. R. and Weirauch, M. T. (2018) The Human Transcription Factors. *Cell* 172, pp. 650–665.

61. Reményi, A., Schöler, H. R. and Wilmanns, M. (2004) Combinatorial Control of Gene Expression. *Nat. Struct. Mol. Biol.* 11, pp. 812–815.
62. Garvie, C. W. and Wolberger, C. (2001) Recognition of Specific DNA Sequences. *Mol. Cell* 8, pp. 937–946.
63. Fujii, Y., Shimizu, T., Toda, T., Yanagida, M. and Hakoshima, T. (2000) Structural Basis for the Diversity of DNA Recognition by bZIP Transcription Factors. *Nat. Struct. Biol.* 7, pp. 889–893.
64. Baxevanis, A. D. and Vinson, C. R. (1993) Interactions of Coiled Coils in Transcription Factors: Where is the Specificity? *Curr. Opin. Gen. Dev.* 3, pp. 278–285.
65. Neph, S., Stergachis, A. B., Reynolds, A., Sandstrom, R., Borenstein, E. and Stamatoyannopoulos, J. A. (2012) Circuitry and Dynamics of Human Transcription Factor Regulatory Networks. *Cell* 150, pp. 1274–1286.
66. Ravasi, T., Suzuki, H., Cannistraci, C. V., Katayama, S., Bajic, V. B., Tan, K., Akalin, A., Schmeier, S., Kanamori-Katayama, M., Bertin, N., Carninci, P., Daub, C. O., Forrest, A. R. R., Gough, J., Grimmond, S., Han, J.-H., Hashimoto, T., Hide, W., Hofmann, O., Kamburov, A., Kaur, M., Kawaji, H., Kubosaki, A., Lassmann, T., van Nimwegen, E., MacPherson, C. R., Ogawa, C., Radovanovic, A., Schwartz, A., Teasdale, R. D., Tegnér, J., Lenhard, B., Teichmann, S. A., Arakawa, T., Ninomiya, N., Murakami, K., Tagami, M., Fukuda, S., Imamura, K., Kai, C., Ishihara, R., Kitazume, Y., Kawai, J., Hume, D. A., Ideker, T. and Hayashizaki, Y. (2010) An Atlas of Combinatorial Transcriptional Regulation in Mouse and Man. *Cell* 140, pp. 744–752
67. Sánchez, M. I., Mosquera, J., Vázquez, M. E. and Mascareñas, J. L. (2014) Reversible Supramolecular Assembly at Specific DNA Sites: Nickel-Promoted Bivalent DNA Binding with Designed Peptide and bipyridyl-bis(benzamidine) Components. *Angew. Chem. Int. Ed.* 53, pp. 9917–9921.
68. Rodríguez, J., Mosquera, J., Vázquez, M. E. and Mascareñas, J. L. (2016) Nickel-Promoted Recognition of Long DNA Sites by Designed Peptide Derivatives. *Chem. Eur. J.* 22, pp. 13474–13477.
69. Sluka, J. P., Horvath, S. J., Bruist, M. F., Simon, M. I. and Dervan, P. B. (1987) Synthesis of a Sequence-Specific DNA-Cleaving Peptide. *Science* 238, pp. 1129–1132.
70. Coin, I., Beyermann, M. and Bienert, M. (2007) Solid-Phase Peptide Synthesis: From Standard Procedures to the Synthesis of Difficult Sequences. *Nat. Prot.* 2, pp. 3247–3256.
71. Sluka, J. P., Griffin, J. H., Mack, D. P. and Dervan, P. B. (1990) Reagents and Methods for the Solid-Phase Synthesis of Protein-EDTA for use in Affinity Cleaving. *J. Am. Chem. Soc.* 112, pp. 6369–6374.
72. Sluka, J. P., Horvath, S. J., Glasgow, A. C., Simon, M. I. and Dervan, P. B. (1990) Importance of Minor-Groove Contacts for Recognition of DNA by the Binding Domain of Hin Recombinase. *Biochemistry*, 29, pp. 6551–6561.

73. Passner, J. M. and Steitz, T. A. (1997) The Structure of a CAP-DNA Complex Having Two cAMP Molecules Bound to Each Monomer. *Proc. Natl. Acad. Sci. USA* 94, pp. 2843–2847.
74. Nakatsukasa, T., Shiraishi, Y., Negi, S., Imanishi, M., Futaki, S. and Sugiura, Y. (2005) Site-Specific DNA Cleavage by Artificial Zinc Finger-Type Nuclease with Cerium-Binding Peptide. *Biochem. Bipohys. Res. Commun.* 330, pp. 247–252.
75. Wójcik, J., Góral, J., Pawłowski, K. and Bierzyński, A. (1997) Isolated Calcium-Binding Loops of EF-Hand Proteins can Dimerize to Form a Native-Like Structure. *Biochemistry* 36, pp. 680–687.
76. Yokono, M., Saegusa, N., Matsushita, K. and Sugiura, Y. (1998) Unique DNA Binding Mode of the N-Terminal Zinc Finger of Transcription Factor Sp1. *Biochemistry* 37, pp. 6824–6832.
77. Pavletich, N. P. and Pabo, C. O. (1993) Crystal Structure of a Five-Finger GLI-DNA Complex: New Perspectives on Zinc Fingers. *Science* 261, pp. 1701–1707.
78. Feng, J. A., Johnson, R. C. and Dickerson, R. E. (1994) Hin Recombinase Bound to DNA: The Origin of Specificity in Major and Minor Groove Interactions. *Science* 263, pp. 348–355.
79. Lasey, R. C., Banerji, S. S. and Ogawa, M. Y. (2000) Synthesis and Characterization of a Sequence-Specific DNA-Binding Protein that Contains Ruthenium Polypyridyl Centers. *Inorg. Chim. Acta* 300–302, pp. 822–828.
80. Kim, Y., Welch, J. T., Lindstrom, K. M. and Franklin, S. J. (2001) Chimeric HTH Motifs Based on EF-Hands. *J. Biol. Inorg. Chem.* 6, pp. 173–181.
81. Welch, J. T., Sirish, M., Lindstrom, K. M. and Franklin, S. J. (2001) De Novo Nucleases Based on HTH and EF-Hand Chimeras. *Inorg. Chem.* 40, pp. 1982–1984.
82. Kovacic, R. T., Welch, J. T. and Franklin, S. J. (2003) Sequence-Selective DNA Cleavage by a Chimeric Metallopeptide. *J. Am. Chem. Soc.* 125, pp. 6656–6662.
83. Smith, S. J., Du, K., Radford, R. J. and Tezcan, F. A. (2013) Functional, Metal-Based Crosslinkers for α-Helix Induction in Short Peptides. *Chem. Sci.* 4, pp. 3740–3747.
84. Smith, S. J., Radford, R. J., Subramanian, R. H., Barnett, B. R., Figueroa, J. S. and Tezcan, F. A. (2016) Tunable Helicity, Stability and DNA-Binding Properties of Short Peptides with Hybrid Metal Coordination Motifs. *Chem. Sci.* 7, pp. 5453–5461.
85. Wang, D. and Lippard, S. J. (2005) Cellular Processing of Platinum Anticancer Drugs. *Nat. Rev. Drug Discov.* 4, pp. 307–320.
86. Robillard, M. S., Valentijn, A. R., Meeuwenoord, N. J., van Der Marel G. A, van Boom J. H. and Reedijk, J. (2000) The First Solid-Phase Synthesis of a Peptide-Tethered Platinum(II) Complex. *Angew. Chem. Int. Ed.* 39, pp. 3096–3099.

87. Robillard, M. S., Bacac, M., van den Elst, H., Flamigni, A., van der Marel, G. A., van Boom, J. H. and Reedijk, J. (2003) Automated Parallel Solid-Phase Synthesis and Anticancer Screening of a Library of Peptide-Tethered Platinum(II) Complexes. *J. Comb. Chem.* 5, pp. 821–825.
88. Robillard, M. S., Davies, N. P., van der Marel, G. A., van Boom, J. H., Reedijk, J. and Murray, V. (2003) The Interaction of Peptide-Tethered Platinum(II) Complexes with DNA. *J. Inorg. Biochem.* 96, pp. 331–338.
89. van Zutphen, S., Robillard, M. S., van der Marel, G. A., Overkleeft, H. S., den Dulk, H., Brouwer, J. and Reedijk, J. (2003) Extending Solid-Phase Methods in Inorganic Synthesis: The First Dinuclear Platinum Complex Synthesised via The Solid Phase. *Chem. Commun.* 5, pp. 634–635.
90. Hannon, J. P., Nunn, C., Stolz, B., Bruns, C., Weckbecker, G., Lewis, I., Troxler, T., Hurth, K. and Hoyer, D. (2002) Drug Design at Peptide Receptors: Somatostatin Receptor Ligands. *J. Mol. Neurosci.* 18, pp. 15–27.
91. Di Cianni, A., Carotenuto, A., Brancaccio, D., Novellino, E., Reubi, J. C., Beetschen, K., Papini, A. M. and Ginanneschi, M. (2010) Novel Octreotide Dicarba-Analogues with High Affinity and Different Selectivity for Somatostatin Receptors. *J. Med. Chem.* 53, pp. 6188–6197.
92. Barragán, F., Carrion-Salip, D., Gómez-Pinto, I., González-Cantó, A., Sadler, P. J., de Llorens, R., Moreno, V., González, C., Massaguer, A. and Marchán, V. (2012) Somatostatin Subtype-2 Receptor-Targeted Metal-Based Anticancer Complexes. *Bioconjugate Chem.* 23(9), pp. 1838–1855.
93. Massaguer, A., González-Cantó, A., Escribano, E., Barrabés, S., Artigas, G., Moreno, V. and Marchán, V. (2015) Integrin-Targeted Delivery into Cancer Cells of a Pt(IV) Pro-Drug Through Conjugation to RGD-Containing Peptides. *Dalton Trans.* 44, pp. 202–212.
94. Kapp, T. G., Rechenmacher, F., Neubauer, S., Maltsev, O. V., Cavalcanti-Adam, E. A., Zarka, R., Reuning, U., Notni, J., Wester, H.-J., Mas-Moruno, C., Spatz, J., Geiger, B. and Kessler, H. (2017) A Comprehensive Evaluation of the Activity and Selectivity Profile of Ligands for RGD-binding Integrins. *Sci. Rep.* 7, pp. 39805.
95. Arosio, D. and Casagrande, C. (2016) Advancement in Integrin Facilitated Drug Delivery. *Adv. Drug. Del. Rev.*, 97, pp. 111–143.
96. Boturyn, D., Defrancq, E., Dolphin, G. T., Garcia, J., Labbe, P., Renaudet, O. and Dumy, P. (2008) RAFT Nano-Constructs: Surfing to Biological Applications. *J. Pept. Sci.* 14, pp. 224–240.
97. Gandioso, A., Shaili, E., Massaguer, A., Artigas, G., González-Cantó, A., Woods, J. A., Sadler, P. J. and Marchán, V. (2015) An Integrin-Targeted Photoactivatable Pt(IV) Complex as A Selective Anticancer Pro-Drug: Synthesis and Photoactivation Studies. *Chem. Commun.* 51, pp. 9169–9172.
98. Ali, A. and Bhattacharya, S. (2014) DNA Binders in Clinical Trials and Chemotherapy. *Bioorg. Med. Chem.* 22, pp. 4506–4521.

99. Komor, A. C. and Barton, J. K. (2013) The Path for Metal Complexes to a DNA Target. *Chem. Commun.* 49, pp. 3617–3630.
100. Zeglis, B. M., Pierre, V. C. and Barton, J. K. (2007) Metallo-Intercalators and Metallo-Insertors. *Chem. Commun.* 44, pp. 4565–4579.
101. Barton, J. K. (1986) Metals and DNA: Molecular Left-Handed Complements. *Science*. 233, pp. 727–734.
102. Barton, J. K., Danishefsky, A. and Goldberg, J. (1984) Tris(phenanthroline) Ruthenium(II): Stereoselectivity in Binding to DNA. *J. Am. Chem. Soc.* 106, pp. 2172–2176.
103. Sardesai, N. Y., Zimmermann, K. and Barton, J. K. (1994) DNA Recognition by Peptide Complexes of Rhodium(III): Example of a Glutamate Switch. *J. Am. Chem. Soc.* 116, pp. 7502–7508.
104. Sardesai, N. Y., Lin, S. C., Zimmerman, K. and Barton, J. K. (1995) Construction of Coordinatively Saturated Rhodium Complexes Containing Appended Peptides. *Bioconjugate Chem.* 6, pp. 302–312.
105. Watkins, D., Hsiao, C., Woods, K. K., Koudelka, G. B. and Williams, L. D. (2008) P22 c2 Repressor-Operator Complex: Mechanisms of Direct and Indirect Readout. *Biochemistry* 47, pp. 2325–2338.
106. Fitzsimons, M. P., and Barton, J. K. (1997) Design of a Synthetic Nuclease: DNA Hydrolysis by a Zinc-Binding Peptide Tethered to a Rhodium Intercalator. *J. Am. Chem. Soc.* 119, pp. 3379–3380.
107. Copeland, K. D., Fitzsimons, M. P., Houser, R. P. and Barton, J. K. (2002) DNA Hydrolysis and Oxidative Cleavage by Metal-Binding Peptides Tethered to Rhodium Intercalators. *Biochemistry* 41, pp. 343–356.
108. Puckett, C. A. and Barton, J. K. (2009) Fluorescein Redirects a Ruthenium-Octaarginine Conjugate to the Nucleus. *J. Am. Chem. Soc.* 131, pp. 8738–8739.
109. Carrigan, C. N. and Imperiali, B. (2005) The Engineering of Membrane-Permeable Peptides. *Anal. Biochem.* 341, pp. 290–298.
110. Puckett, C. A., Ernst, R. J. and Barton, J. K. (2010) Exploring the Cellular Accumulation of Metal Complexes. *Dalton Trans.* 39, pp. 1159–1170.
111. Imperiali, B., Prins, T. J. and Fisher, S. L. (1993) Chemoenzymic Synthesis of 2-Amino-3-(2,2′-bipyridinyl) Propanoic Acids. *J. Org. Chem.* 58, pp. 1613–1616.
112. Imperiali, B., Moats, R. A., Fisher, S. L. and Prins, T. J. (1992) A Conformational Study of Peptides with the General Structure Ac-L-Xaa-Pro-D-Xaa-L-Xaa-NH2: Spectroscopic Evidence for a Peptide with Significant β-Turn Character in Water and in Dimethyl Sulfoxide. *J. Am. Chem. Soc.* 114, pp. 3182–3188.
113. Torrado, A. and Imperiali, B. (1996) New Synthetic Amino Acids for the Design and Synthesis of Peptide-Based Metal Ion Sensors. *J. Org. Chem.* 61, pp. 8940–8948.

114. Newkome, G. R., Gross, J. and Patri, A. K. (1997) Synthesis of Unsymmetrical 5,5′-Disubstituted 2,2′-Bipyridines1. *J. Org Chem.* 62, pp. 3013–3014.
115. Rama, G., Ardá, A., Maréchal, J.-D., Gamba, I., Ishida, H., Jiménez-Barbero, J., Vázquez, M. E. and Vázquez López, M. (2012) Stereoselective Formation of Chiral Metallopeptides. *Chem. Eur. J.* 18, pp. 7030–7035.
116. Hayoz, P., Von Zelewsky, A. and Stoeckli-Evans, H. (1993) Stereoselective Synthesis of Octahedral Complexes with Predetermined Helical Chirality. *J. Am. Chem. Soc.* 115, pp. 5111–5114.
117. Hua, X. and von Zelewsky, A. (1995) Enantiomerically Pure Chiral RuII(LΛL)$_2$ Building Blocks for Coordination Compounds. *Inorg. Chem.* 34, pp. 5791–5797.
118. Gamba, I., Salvadó, I., Rama, G., Bertazzon, M., Sánchez, M. I., Sánchez-Pedregal, V. M., Martínez-Costas, J., Brissos, R. F., Gamez, P., Mascareñas, J. L., Vázquez López, M. and Vázquez, M. E. (2013) Custom-Fit Ruthenium(II) Metallopeptides: A New Twist to DNA Binding with Coordination Compounds. *Chem. Eur. J.* 19, pp. 13369–13375.
119. Goun, E. A., Pillow, T. H., Jones, L. R., Rothbard, J. B. and Wender, P. A. (2006) Molecular Transporters: Synthesis of Oligoguanidinium Transporters and Their Application to Drug Delivery and Real-Time Imaging. *ChemBioChem.* 7, pp. 1497–1515.
120. Gamba, I., Salvadó, I., Brissos, R. F., Gamez, P., Brea, J., Loza, M. I., Vázquez, M. E. and Vázquez López, M. (2016) High-Affinity Sequence-Selective DNA Binding by Iridium(III) Polypyridyl Organometallopeptides. *Chem. Commun.* 52, pp. 1234–1237.
121. Bouzada, D., Salvadó, I., Barka, G., Rama, G., Martínez-Costas, J., Lorca, R., Somoza, Á., Melle-Franco, M., Vázquez, M. E. and Vázquez López, M. (2018) Selective G-Quadruplex Binding by Oligoarginine-Ru(dppz) Metallopeptides. *Chem. Commun.* 54, pp. 658–661.
122. Ypsilantis, K., Plakatouras, J. C., Manos, M. J., Kourtellaris, A., Markopoulos, G., Kolettas, E. and Garoufis, A. (2018) Stepwise Synthesis, Characterization, DNA Binding Properties and Cytotoxicity of Diruthenium Oligopyridine Compounds Conjugated with Peptides. *Dalton Trans.* 47, pp. 3549–3567.
123. Deibert, M., Grazulis, S., Janulaitis, A., Siksnys, V. and Huber, R. (1999) Crystal Structure of MunI Restriction Endonuclease in Complex with Cognate DNA at 1.7 A Resolution. *EMBO J.* 18, pp. 5805–5816.
124. Myari, A., Hadjiliadis, N. and Garoufis, A. (2005) Synthesis and Characterization of the Diastereomers Lambda- and Delta-[Ru(bpy)2(m-bpy-L-Arg-Gly-L-Asn-L-Ala-L-His-L-Glu-L-Arg)]Cl2 1H NMR Studies on Their Interactions with the Deoxynucleotide Duplex d[(5'-GCGCTTAAGCGC-3')2] and d[(5'-CGCGATCGCG-3')2]. *J. Inorg. Biochem.* 99, pp. 616–626.

125. Rao, H., Damian, M. S., Alshiekh, A., Elmroth, S. K. C. and Diederichsen, U. (2015) Design, Synthesis and DNA Interactions of a Chimera Between a Platinum Complex and an IHF Mimicking Peptide. *Org. Biomol. Chem.* 13, pp. 11704–11713.
126. Pelay-Gimeno, M., Glas, A., Koch, O. and Grossmann, T. N. (2015) Structure-Based Design of Inhibitors of Protein-Protein Interactions: Mimicking Peptide Binding Epitopes. *Angew. Chem. Int. Ed.* 54, pp. 8896–8927.
127. Wójcik, P. and Berlicki, Ł. (2016) Peptide-Based Inhibitors of Protein-Protein Interactions. *Bioorg. Med. Chem. Lett.* 26, pp. 707–713.
128. Milroy, L.-G., Grossmann, T. N., Hennig, S., Brunsveld, L. and Ottmann, C. (2014) Modulators of Protein-Protein Interactions. *Chem. Rev.* 114, pp. 4695–4748.
129. Schoentjes, B. and Lehn, J.-M. (1995) Interaction of Double-Helical Polynuclear Copper(I) complexes with double-stranded DNA. *Helv. Chim. Acta* 78, pp. 1–12.
130. Hannon, M. J., Painting, C. L., Jackson, A., Hamblin, J. and Errington, W. (1997) An Inexpensive Approach to Supramolecular Architecture. *Chem. Commun.* 18, pp. 1807–1808.
131. Hannon, M. J., Moreno, V., Prieto, M. J., Moldrheim, E., Sletten, E., Meistermann, I., Isaac, C. J., Sanders, K. J. and Rodger, A. (2001) Intramolecular DNA Coiling Mediated by a Metallo-Supramolecular Cylinder. *Angew. Chem. Int. Ed Engl.* 40, pp. 879–884.
132. Meistermann, I., Moreno, V., Prieto, M. J. and Hannon, M. J. (2002) Intramolecular DNA coiling mediated by metallo-supramolecular cylinders: Differential binding of P and M helical enantiomers. *PNAS*, 99, pp. 5069–5074.
133. Oleksi, A., Blanco, A. G., Boer, R., Usón, I., Aymamí, J., Rodger, A., Hannon, M. J. and Coll, M. (2006) Molecular Recognition of a Three-Way DNA Junction by a Metallosupramolecular Helicate. *Angew. Chem. Int. Ed.* 45, pp. 1227–1231.
134. Hotze, A. C. G., Hodges, N. J., Hayden, R. E., Sanchez-Cano, C., Paines, C., Male, N., Tse, M.-K., Bunce, C. M., Chipman, J. K. and Hannon, M. J. (2008) Supramolecular Iron Cylinder with Unprecedented DNA Binding is a Potent Cytostatic and Apoptotic Agent Without Exhibiting Genotoxicity. *Chem. Biol.* 15, pp. 1258–1267.
135. Constable, E. C., Figgemeier, E., Hougen, I. A., Housecroft, C. E., Neuburger, M., Schaffner, S. and Whall, L. A. (2005) Hairpin Helicates: A Missing Link Between Double-Helicates and Trefoil Knots. *Dalton Trans.* 7, pp. 1168–1175.

136. Rama, G., Ardá, A., Maréchal, J.-D., Gamba, I., Ishida, H., Jiménez-Barbero, J., Vázquez, M. E. and Vázquez López, M. (2012) Stereoselective Formation of Chiral Metallopeptides. *Chem. Eur. J.* 18, pp. 7030–7035.
137. Gamba, I., Rama, G., Ortega-Carrasco, E., Berardozzi, R., Sánchez-Pedregal, V. M., Di Bari, L., Maréchal, J.-D., Vázquez, M. E. and Vázquez López, M. (2016) The Folding of a Metallopeptide. *Dalton Trans.* 45, pp. 881–885.
138. Gamba, I., Rama, G., Ortega-Carrasco, E., Maréchal, J.-D., Martínez-Costas, J., Vázquez, M. E. and Vázquez López, M. (2014) Programmed Stereoselective Assembly of DNA-Binding Helical Metallopeptides. *Chem. Commun.* 50, pp. 11097–11100.
139. Gómez-González, J., Peña, D. G., Barka, G., Sciortino, G., Maréchal, J.-D., Vázquez López, M. and Vázquez, M. E. (2018) Directed Self-Assembly of Trimeric DNA-Binding chiral Miniprotein Helicates. *Front. Chem.* 6, 520.
140. Cardo, L. and Hannon, M. J. (2009) Design and DNA-Binding of Metallo-Supramolecular Cylinders Conjugated to Peptides. *Inorg. Chim. Acta* 362, pp. 784–792.
141. Futaki, S., Kiwada, T. and Sugiura, Y. (2004) Control of Peptide Structure and Recognition by Fe(III)-Induced Helix Destabilization. *J. Am. Chem. Soc.* 126, pp. 15762–15769.
142. Azuma, Y., Imanishi, M., Yoshimura, T., Kawabata, T. and Futaki, S. (2009) Cobalt(II)-Responsive DNA Binding of a GCN4-bZIP Protein Containing Cysteine Residues Functionalized with Iminodiacetic Acid. *Angew. Chem. Int. Ed.* 48, pp. 6853–6856.
143. Mosquera, J., Jiménez-Balsa, A., Dodero, V. I., Vázquez, M. E. and Mascareñas, J. L. (2013) Stimuli-Responsive Selection of Target DNA Sequences by Synthetic bZIP Peptides. *Nat. Commun.* 4, 1874
144. Mosquera, J., Sánchez, M. I., Vázquez, M. E. and Mascareñas, J. L. (2014) Ruthenium Bipyridyl Complexes as Photocleavable Dimerizers: Deactivation of DNA-Binding Peptides Using Visible Light. *Chem. Commun.* 50, pp. 10975–10978.
145. Lau, S. J., Kruck, T. P. and Sarkar, B. (1974) A Peptide Molecule Mimicking the Copper(II) Transport Site of Human Serum Albumin. A Comparative Study Between the Synthetic Site and Albumin. *J. Biol. Chem.* 249, pp. 5878–5884.
146. Fang, Y.-Y., Ray, B. D., Claussen, C. A., Lipkowitz, K. B. and Long, E. C. (2004) Ni(II). Arg-Gly-His-DNA Interactions: Investigation into the Basis for Minor-Groove Binding and Recognition. *J. Am. Chem. Soc.* 126, pp. 5403–5412.
147. Harford, C. and Sarkar, B. (1997) Amino Terminal Cu(II)- and Ni(II)-Binding (ATCUN) Motif of Proteins and Peptides: Metal Binding, DNA Cleavage, and Other Properties. *Acc. Chem. Res.* 30, pp. 123–130.

148. Liang, Q., Eason, P. D. and Long, E. C. (1995) Metallopeptide-DNA Interactions: Site-Selectivity Based on Amino Acid Composition and Chirality. *J. Am. Chem. Soc.* 117, pp. 9625–9631.
149. Gonzalez, P., Bossak, K., Stefaniak, E., Hureau, C., Raibaut, L., Bal, W. and Faller, P. (2018) N-Terminal Cu-Binding Motifs (Xxx-Zzz-His, Xxx-His) and Their Derivatives: Chemistry, Biology and Medicinal Applications. *Chem. Eur. J.* 24, pp. 8029–8041.
150. Fang, Y.-Y., Claussen, C. A., Lipkowitz, K. B. and Long, E. C. (2006) Diastereoselective DNA Cleavage Recognition by Ni(II) x Gly-Gly-His-Derived Metallopeptides. *J. Am. Chem. Soc.* 128, pp. 3198–3207.
151. Agbale, C. M., Cardoso, M. H., Galyuon, I. K. and Franco, O. L. (2016) Designing Metallodrugs with Nuclease and Protease Activity. *Metallomics* 8, pp. 1159–1169.
152. Long, E. C. (1999) Ni(II)·Xaa-Xaa-His Metallopeptide–DNA/RNA Interactions. *Acc. Chem. Res.* 32, pp. 827–836.
153. Mosquera, J., Sánchez, M. I., Mascareñas, J. L. and Vázquez, M. E. (2015) Synthetic Peptides Caged on Histidine Residues with a Bisbipyridyl Ruthenium(II) Complex that can be Photolyzed by Visible Light. *Chem. Commun.* 51, pp. 5501–5504.
154. Yu, Z., Han, M. and Cowan, J. A. (2015) Toward the Design of a Catalytic Metallodrug: Selective Cleavage of G-Quadruplex Telomeric DNA by An Anticancer Copper-Acridine-ATCUN Complex. *Angew. Chem. Int. Ed.* 54, pp. 1901–1905.
155. Yu, Z. and Cowan, J. A. (2018) Metal Complexes Promoting Catalytic Cleavage of Nucleic Acids-Biochemical Tools and Therapeutics. *Curr. Opin. Chem. Biol.* 43, pp. 37–42.
156. Joyner, J. C. and Cowan, J. A. (2011) Targeted Cleavage of HIV RRE RNA by Rev-Coupled Transition Metal Chelates. *J. Am. Chem. Soc.* 133, pp. 9912–9922.
157. Bradford, S. and Cowan, J. A. (2012) Catalytic Metallodrugs Targeting HCV IRES RNA. *Chem. Commun.* 48, pp. 3118–3120.
158. Learte-Aymamí, S., Curado, N., Rodríguez, J., Vázquez, M. E. and Mascareñas, J. L. (2017) Metal-Dependent DNA Recognition and Cell Internalization of Designed, Basic Peptides. *J. Am. Chem. Soc.* 139, pp. 16188–16193.

https://doi.org/10.1142/9789811261664_0008

Chapter 8

Recombinant Production, Isotopic Labeling, Purification and NMR Characterization of Cysteine-rich Domains: The Case of the Death Receptors Involved in Cancer Treatment

Antoine Baudin[*], Anne Guichard[*,†], Lua Sobron[*], Gavin W. Collie[*,‡,§], Sabrina Rousseau[‡,¶], Gilles Guichard[*,‡], and Benoît Odaert[*,||]

[*]*Université de Bordeaux – CNRS – Bordeaux INP, Chimie et Biologie des Membranes et des Nano-objets (CBMN), Allée Geoffroy Saint Hilaire, Cedex, France*

[†]*Agenus UK Limited, Science Park, Milton Road, Cambridge, CB4 0WG, UK*

[‡]*Institut Européen de Chimie et Biologie, Univ. Bordeaux, Pessac France*

[§]*Discovery Sciences, IMED Biotech Unit, AstraZeneca, Cambridge, UK*

[¶]*Inserm U1212, ARNA Laboratory, Bordeaux, France*

[||]b.odaert@cbmn.u-bordeaux.fr

1. Biological Context

Tumor necrosis factor-a-Related Apoptosis-Inducing Ligand (TRAIL/Apo2L/TNFSF10) is a type II transmembrane trimeric protein that induces apoptosis of cancer cells while sparing normal ones [1]. Four membrane-bound TRAIL specific receptors have been described, comprising two Death Receptors (DR4/TNFRSF10A/TRAIL-R1 and DR5/TNFRSF10B/TRAIL-R2) that mediate the apoptogenic signal and two Decoy Receptors (DcR1/TNFRSF10C/TRAIL-R3 and DcR2/TNFRSF10D/TRAIL-R4) that bind the ligand but do not transduce the apoptogenic signal [2,3]. TRAIL binding induces receptor oligomerization [1], transduction of the apoptogenic signal to the intracellular death domain (DD) of the receptors and DISC formation. Autocleavage of the initiator caspases results in activation of the death-executing caspase cascade, leading to cell death [1,4,5,6]. Crystal structures of TRAIL complexed with the Extra Cellular Domain (residues 6–135 of our plasmid construct) of DR5 (DR5-ED) unravel the mechanism for receptor oligomerization ([7]: 1DOG.pdb; [8]: 1D4V.pdb; [9]: 1DU3.pdb): The elongated DR5 receptors snuggle into long crevices between pairs of monomers of the homotrimeric TRAIL ligand, but do not interact with each other. The TRAIL/DR5 interface is divided into two distinct patches, one near the bottom of the complex close to the membrane surface (90S loop of DR5) and one near the top (50S loop of DR5). The elongated structure of DR5-ED is arranged into three Cysteine-Rich Domains (CRD). CRD1 (32–48) adopts a beta hairpin conformation (B1B2) stabilized by the disulphide bridge 33–46 and is preceded by the N-terminal region in a disordered conformation. CRD2 (49–90) and CRD3 (91–135) possess two consecutive beta hairpins (B3-B6 and B7-B10, respectively) stabilized by three disulphide bridges (49–65, 68–81, 71–89 and 91–105, 108–122, 112–130, respectively). The 50S loop (residues S56–R67) and 90S loop (residues E99–R109) involved in TRAIL binding display similar conformations despite the absence of any sequence homology. The crystal structure of DR5-ED has also been solved in complex with the human glycoprotein UL141 ([10]: 4I9X.pdb) and with the Fab fragments of five anti-DR5 antibodies ([11]: 1ZA3.pdb; [12]: 2H9G.pdb; [13]: 4OD2.pdb; [14]: 4N90.pdb; [15]: 3X3F.pdb). No structural characterization of the isolated DR5-ED has yet been reported either by crystallography or NMR spectroscopy.

We report here for the first time the assignment of NMR resonances and the secondary structure determination of a TRAIL Death Receptor in solution, namely DR5/TRAIL-R2. Chemical shift assignment has been used to perform binding studies with TRAILmim peptidomimetics that bind to DR5 [16,17,18] and the results will be reported in a future publication. The assignment of resonances and secondary structure have been deposited to the BioMagResBank under the accession number 27400 [19].

2. Materials and Methods

2.1. *Production of the recombinant plasmid pETNusA-DR5(ED) by molecular cloning*

2.1.1. *Amplification of the DR5(ED) gene from the plasmid pET23m-DR5(ED) by using PCR*

For the Polymerase Chain Reaction (PCR) on the plasmid pET23m-DR5(ED) (Figure 1), two primers were used, the forward primer DR5-Fvs and the reverse primer DR5-Rvs:

DR5-Fvs: 5′-G**CCATGG**AGTCTGCTCTGATCACC-3′ Tm = 72.2°C
DR5-Rvs: 5′-C**GGATCC**TTATGATTCTTTGTGGACACATTCG-3′ Tm = 75.6°C

These primers contain respectively a NcoI and a BamHI restriction sites — as indicated in bold type — required for a later digestion. The PCR sample was prepared as per the New England BioLabs protocol of PCR Using Q5® HF DNA Polymerase, for a 50 μL reaction at a concentration of 100 ng.μL^{-1} and 10 μM for the plasmid and the primers, respectively. It was optimized with the component concentrations described in Table 1. These components were assembled on ice, before being heated in the thermocycler (Mastercycler® pro, Eppendorf) following the cycle described in Table 2. The PCR sample was analyzed on a 1.2% agarose gel prepared with 1.2 g of agarose dissolved in 100 mL of Tris Borate EDTA buffer (TBE) 1X. The gel was stained with SYBR® Safe 10,000X and Gel Loading Dye 6X (Blue) was added to the sample in order to visualize the DNA fragments. Around 30 μL of the sample were loaded on agarose gel, along with the 3 μL of molecular weight DNA ladder (1 kb Plus DNA Ladder). The migration was carried out at 110 V for 35–40 minutes and DNA bands were revealed with a UV light source. After gel analysis, the PCR product was excised and purified, following the protocol of ThermoScientific GeneJET Gel Extraction Kit, in 20 μL of elution buffer. DNA concentration was estimated by reading absorbance at 260 nm, using Beer–Lambert law (NanoDrop™ 2000c Spectrophotometer, ThermoScientific).

2.1.2. *Digestion of the DR5(ED) gene and the plasmid pETNusA using restriction enzymes*

As the NcoI and a BamHI restriction sites are also present into the plasmid pETNusA (Figure 2), a double digestion and a sequential digestion were

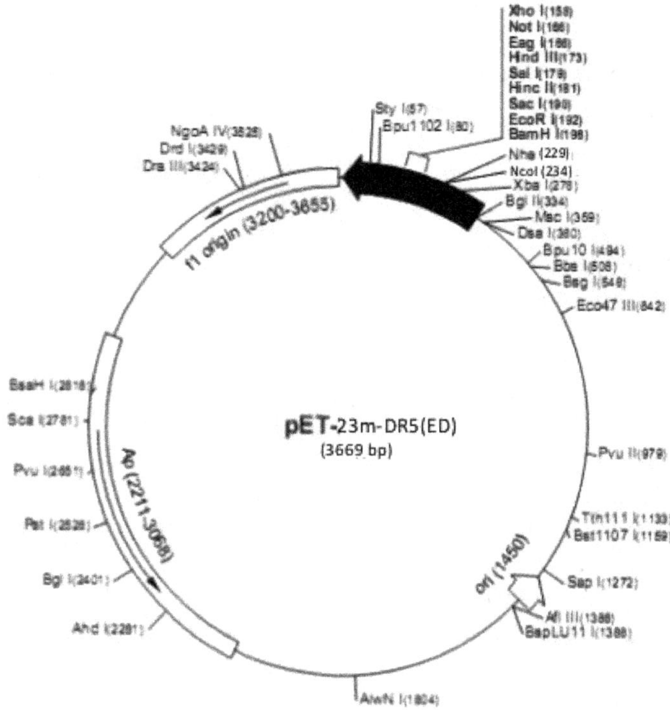

gatattaCC ATG GGG CAT CAT CAT CAT CAT CAT CCC GGG GCT AGC
NcoI 6 X His SmaI/XmaI NheI
gagtctgctctgatcacccaacaagacctagctccccagcagagagcggccccacaacaa
aagaggtccagcccctcagagggattgtgtccacctggacaccatatctcagaagacggt
agagattgcatctcctgcaaatatggacaggactatagcactcactggaatgacctcctt
ttctgcttgcgctgcaccaggtgtgattcaggtgaagtggagctaagtccctgcaccacg
accagaaacacagtgtgtcagtgcgaagaaggcaccttccgggaagaagattctcctgag
atgtgccggaagtgccgcacagggtgtcccagagggatggtcaaggtcggtgattgtaca
ccctggagtgacatcgaatgtgtccacaaagaatca
GGA TCC TAA
BamHI stop

Fig. 1. Restriction map of the plasmid pET23m-DR5(ED) and DR5(ED) gene DNA sequence.

performed, respectively, on the DR5(ED) gene and the plasmid pET-NusA, with the respective restriction enzymes in order to replace the GFP gene with the DR5(ED) gene.

Table 1. PCR amplification of the DR5(ED) gene from the plasmid pET23m-DR5(ED). For the Polymerase Chain Reaction (PCR) on the plasmid pET23m-DR5(ED) (100 ng.μL−1), two primers were used, the forward primer DR5-Fvs and the reverse primer DR5-Rvs (10 μM each), namely DR5-Fvs: 5′-GCCATGGAGTCTGCTCTGATCACC-3′ Tm = 72.2°C and DR5-Rvs: 5′-CGGATCCTTATGATTC-TTTGTGGA-CACATTCG-3′ Tm = 75.6°C. The PCR sample was prepared as per the New England BioLabs protocol of PCR Using Q5® HF DNA Polymerase, for a 50 μL reaction and was optimized with the above component concentrations.

Component	Final concentration
5X Q5 Reaction Buffer	1X
10 mM dNTPs	200 μM
10 μM DR5-Fvs	0.6 μM
10 μM DR5-Rvs	0.6 μM
Plasmid pET23m-DR5(ED)	200 ng
5X Q5 High GC Enhancer	1X
Q5 High-Fidelity DNA Polymerase	0.024 units/μL

Table 2. PCR amplification of the DR5(ED) gene from the plasmid pET23m-DR5(ED) The components of Table 1 were assembled on ice, before being heated in the thermocycler (Mastercycler® pro, Eppendorf) following the above cycle.

Step		Temperature/Time
Initial denaturation		98°C for 3 minutes
30 Cycles	Denaturation	94°C for 30 seconds
	Annealing	59°C for 30 seconds
	Extension	72°C for 45 seconds
Final extension		72°C for 5 minutes

Double digestion of the DR5(ED) gene obtained by PCR was realized in a 100 μL reaction volume. Around 550 ng of DR5(ED) gene was incubated at 37°C for 35 minutes (Fisher Scientific™ Dry Bath Incubator),

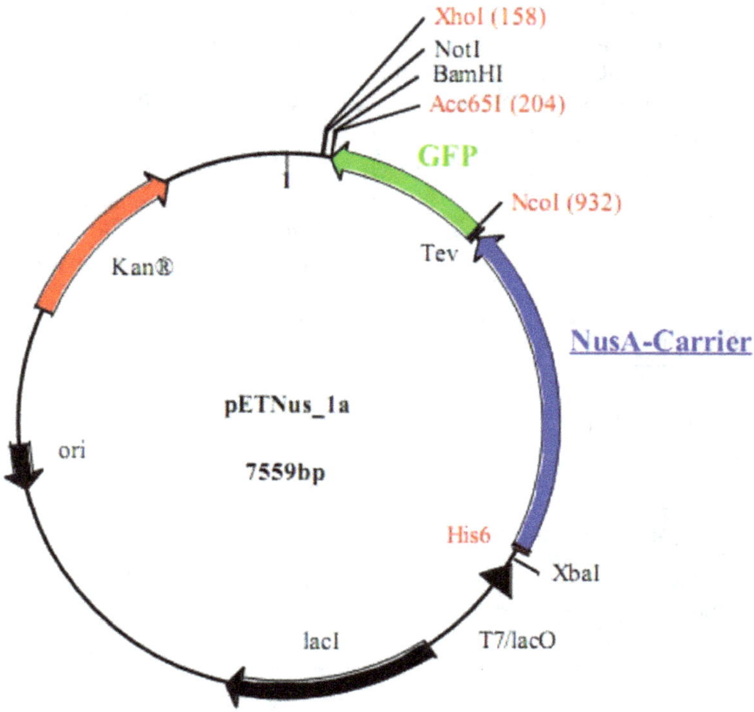

Fig. 2. Restriction map of the plasmid pETNusA coding for the His_6-NusA-GFP protein.

with 1 μL of each restriction enzyme — NcoI-HF and BamHI-HF — and 10 μL of CutSmart 10X. This cut DR5(ED) gene was then purified as per the Thermo Scientific GeneJET Gel Extraction Kit.

A sequential digest was performed on the plasmid pETNusA (207 ng·μL^{-1}). First, about 4 μg of plasmid vector was incubated at 37°C for 45 minutes (Fisher Scientific™ Dry Bath Incubator), in a 50 μL reaction, containing 1 μL of NcoI-HF enzyme and 5 μL of CutSmart 10X. The digest product was purified, following the protocol of ThermoScientific GeneJET Gel Extraction Kit. Once DNA was linearized, the plasmid was digested by the second restriction enzyme BamHI-HF. Approximatively 0.65 μg of this plasmid was incubated at 37°C for 1 hour (Fisher Scientific™ Dry Bath Incubator), with 1 μL of BamHI-HF enzyme and 2.2 μL of CutSmart 10X, in a 22.2 μL reaction. The cut plasmid pETNusA was purified according to the ThermoScientific GeneJET Gel Extraction Kit.

Samples from the digestion of the plasmid pETNusA were analyzed on 0.8% agarose gel prepared with 0.8 g of agarose dissolved in 100 mL of TBE 1X, along with the uncut plasmid as control. The DNA concentration of each digest product was calculated by OD measurement at 260 nm, using spectrophotometry (NanoDrop™ 2000c Spectrophotometer, ThermoScientific).

2.1.3. *Cohesive ends ligation*

The ligation of the DR5(ED) gene into the plasmid pETNusA was performed as per the New England BioLabs Quick Ligation™ Kit. Hence, around 50 ng of the cut plasmid pETNusA were added to a three-fold molar excess of cut insert, using a 5:1 insert:vector ratio. As the plasmid vector size is 6,822 bp and the insert size is 404 bp, the mass of the cut DR5(ED) gene needed was around 14.8 ng. The ligation mixture was incubated at room temperature for 10 minutes.

2.1.4. *Bacterial chemical transformation in DH5α cells*

The bacterial strain DH5*α* Competent *Escherichia coli* (*E. coli*) was used for the transformation of the recombinant plasmid pETNusA-DR5(ED) into *E. coli* cells, since it is optimized for the plasmid cloning. This strain is commonly used in biotechnology for bacterial transformation as it provides high transformation efficiency. Besides, DH5α strain has a recA1 mutation, which ensures higher insert stability, and endA1 mutation, which greatly increases recombinant plasmid yield and quality.

The bacterial transformation was realized as per the New England BioLabs Quick Ligation™ Kit. The heat shock was carried outputting samples successively at 4°C for 30 minutes, 42°C for 30 seconds and 4°C for 2 minutes. Then, the cells were incubated at 37°C under stirring (Infors HT® Ecotron) with 800 μL of Super Optimal broth with Catabolite repression (SOC) medium (2% peptone, 0.5% yeast extract, 10 mM NaCl, 2.5 mM KCl, 10 mM $MgCl_2$, 10 mM $MgSO_4$ and 20 mM Glucose). Kanamycin was added to Luria-Bertani (LB)-Agar medium, containing 15 g agar, 10 g tryptone, yeast extract 5 g and NaCl 5 g per liter — previously autoclaved at 120°C and 100 kPa for 20 minutes (ThermoScientific® Hearus oven) — to reach a concentration of 30 $\mu g \cdot mL^{-1}$. This medium was poured into Petri dishes and one plate was inoculated with 100 μL of transformed cells after 1 hour of incubation. Then, this cloning plate was incubated at 37°C overnight, lid downwards (Incu-Line® VWR). The strains resulting from this genetic transformation were named S1.

Two negative controls were performed to prove the efficiency of the cloning. One, named "0 DNA" control, was realized without DNA to confirm the DH5α cells cannot grow on Petri dishes without the plasmid that confers kanamycin resistance. For the second control, named ligation-transformation negative control, the ligation was carried out without insert to check that the plasmid used was totally cut by the two restriction enzymes.

Recovered colonies S1 were incubated with 10 mL of LB medium (10 g tryptone, yeast extract 5 g and NaCl 5 gL^{-1}) and Kanamycine (30 $\mu g.mL^{-1}$), at 37°C under stirring (Infors HT® Ecotron). After 24 hours of incubation, the samples were centrifuged at 6,800 g and 25°C, for 2 minutes (SIGMA® 4-16 KS centrifuge, rotor 12165H). Plasmids were recovered from the cell pellets through minipreparation, using the Thermo Scientific GeneJET Plasmid Miniprep Kit. The absorbance at 260 nm was measured by spectrophotometry (NanoDrop™ 2000c Spectrophotometer, ThermoScientific).

2.1.5. *Clone verifications*

To verify that the plasmids have the DR5(ED) gene, a PCR and a double digestion, with the restriction enzymes NcoI-HF and BamHI-HF, were performed on the plasmids pETNusA- DR5(ED) obtained by plasmid minipreparation. For these two controls, the conditions were the same as the ones mentioned previously, except that for the double digestion, around 3.5 μg of plasmid were used. Samples were then analyzed on a 1.2% agarose gel. Furthermore, a Sanger sequencing was carried out on these plasmids, using 5 μL of primer (5 μM) and 5 μL of plasmid with a concentration of 80 $ng \cdot \mu L^{-1}$ to 100 $ng \cdot \mu L^{-1}$.

2.2. *Production of DR5(ED) protein, using the recombinant plasmid pETNusA-DR5(ED)*

2.2.1. *Protein expression system*

The bacterial strain used for the production of the extracellular domain of the Death Receptor 5 was BL21(DE3) competent *E. coli*. This strain is commonly used in biotechnology for transformation — as it provides a great efficiency — and optimized for high protein expression yields.

Indeed, this strain contains the lDE3 prophage, in which there is a gene coding for the T7 RNA polymerase, which controls recombinant gene expression once induced with isopropyl β-D-1-thiogalactopyranoside (IPTG). Besides, the BL21(DE3) strain is deficient in proteases Lon and OmpT, which prevents the degradation of the over-expressed protein.

The expression vector used was the plasmid pETNusA (Figure 2), in which the GFP gene has been replaced by the DR5(ED) gene and enables its cytosolic expression, thanks to the T7 promoter recognized by the T7 RNA polymerase of the BL21(DE3) cells, upon induction with IPTG. This plasmid contains a kanamycin-resistance gene, essential for plasmid selection with BL21(DE3) cells. Furthermore, the plasmid pETNusA expresses an *E. coli* fusion carrier protein, named the *N*-utilizing substance A (NusA), which improves expression yield and solubility, and facilitates protein purification through affinity chromatography thanks to the 6His-Tag coding sequence at its *N*-terminus.

2.2.2. *Bacterial chemical transformation in BL21(DE3) cells*

The bacterial transformation was performed in the same way as for the transformation in DH5α cells, using around 220 ng of the recombinant plasmid pETNusA-DR5(ED) and 10 μL of BL21(DE3) cells. The strains resulting from this genetic transformation were named S2. A "0 DNA" control was realized to prove the efficiency of the transformation.

2.2.3. *Expression tests in LB medium*

To reduce the lag phase during the bacterial growth, a pre-culture was realized within 10 mL of LB medium, containing kanamycin (30 $\mu g \cdot mL^{-1}$), inoculated with a single colony S2. This pre-culture was incubated at 37°C, under stirring (Infors HT® Ecotron) until the absorbance at 600 nm reached 0.6. Afterwards, 250 mL of LB medium, in the presence of kanamycine (30 $\mu g \cdot mL^{-1}$), was inoculated with 9 mL of this pre-culture and incubated at 37°C, under stirring (MaxQ™ 600 incubator, ThermoScientific). When the OD measurement at 600 nm reached 0.6, corresponding to the exponential phase of the bacterial growth, IPTG was added to a final concentration of 0.5 mM (time t0). Culture medium of 1 mL was collected at 37°C at different times of induction — 5 minutes, 1 hour, 2 hours and

3 hours — and centrifuged 5 minutes (MiniSpin® Eppendorf) in order to recover the cell pellet, which was resuspended in an equivalent volume of SDS loading buffer. Samples were then heated at 95°C for 5 minutes and 10–20 μL of water was added to solubilize the solution, before being centrifuged for 5 minutes. Supernatants analyzed on SDS-PAGE gel were realized with a 15% polyacrylamide running gel with a 5% polyacrylamide stacking gel. About 15 μL of the samples was loaded on the gel, along with 5 μL of the molecular weight size marker (Color Prestained Protein Standard, Broad Range 11–245 kDa). The migration was carried out at 200 V for 55 minutes. Then, SDS-PAGE gel was stained with Coomassie blue G-250 and destained with the destain solution (20% acetic acid and 30% ethanol).

2.2.4. *Expression and production of DR5(ED) protein in LB medium*

A pre-culture was carried out with a single colony S2, in 20 mL of LB medium (tryptone 10g, yeast extract 5g, NaCl 5g per liter) supplemented with kanamycin (30 μg.mL^{-1}), and incubated at 37°C overnight, under stirring (Infors HT® Ecotron). This pre-culture, named P2, was then inoculated to 1L of LB medium, which was incubated at 37°C, under stirring (Excella® E25 New Brunswick Scientific). When the absorbance at 600 nm reached 0.6, IPTG was added to a final concentration of 0.5 mM. The protein induction was performed for 3 hours and 30 minutes at 37°C.

2.2.5. *Expression and production of DR5(ED) protein in M9 medium supplemented with 15NH4Cl*

The M9 medium has been designed to over-express and isotopically label proteins in order to perform structural studies by using heteronuclear Nuclear Magnetic Resonance (NMR). The only sources of nitrogen and carbon are provided by ^{15}N-labelled ammonium chloride and ^{13}C-labelled glucose, respectively. The medium was first prepared in its depleted form containing mineral salts (NaCl 0.5 g·L^{-1}, KH_2PO_4 3 g·L^{-1}, $Na_2HPO_4(2H_2O)$ 6 g·L^{-1}, pH 7.2) and was autoclaved at 120°C and 110 kPa for 20 minutes (ThermoScientific® Hearus oven). The medium is then cooled and completed by other salts ($MgSO_4$ 1 mM, $CaCl_2$ 0.4 mM, $FeCl_3$ 30 $\mu g \cdot mL^{-1}$), thiamine as vitamin (1 $\mu g \cdot mL^{-1}$) and kanamycin as antibiotics (30 $\mu g \cdot mL^{-1}$). The medium was then enriched by ^{15}N-labelled ammonium chloride (1 $g \cdot L^{-1}$) and ^{13}C-labelled or cold glucose (2 $g \cdot L^{-1}$).

Two percent of pre-culture P2 was centrifuged at 4,000 g for 6 minutes at a 4°C (SIGMA® 4-16 KS centrifuge, rotor 12165H). The cell pellet was resuspended in 1 mL and inoculated to 1L of the medium. The culture was performed at 37°C, under stirring (Excella® E25 New Brunswick Scientific), until the absorbance at 600 nm reached 0.6. Subsequently, IPTG was added to a final concentration of 0.5 mM and the temperature was decreased to 25°C. The protein induction was performed overnight for 18 hours. The reduction of the temperature slows down the general metabolism of the bacteria by limiting proteolysis and aggregation while favoring the proper folding of the over-expressed protein.

2.3. *Purification of DR5(ED) protein*

2.3.1. *Proteins recovery*

After protein induction (18 h in ^{15}N-M9 medium and 3 h30 in LB medium), cells were harvested by centrifugation at 4,500 rpm and 4°C for 20 minutes (Avanti® J-26 XP Beckman Coulter, rotor JLA 9.1000) and stored at −80°C.

Cell pellets were thawed and resuspended in 20 ml of high salt lysis buffer for the first purification protocol (50 mM Tris pH 7.5, 500 mM NaCl, 5 mM imidazole) or low salt lysis buffer for the second protocole (50 mM Tris pH 8, 0.5 mM NaCl, 20 mM imidazole), in the presence of phenylmethylsulfonyl fluoride (PMSF) at 1 mM as a serine protease inhibitor. Cell lysis was performed by sonication (Branson Digital Sonifier 150) at an amplitude of 40% for 5 minutes with pulsations and intervals of 30 seconds. Membranes and cell debris were eliminated through the centrifugation of the cell lysate at 50,000 rpm at 4°C for 30 minutes (Avanti™ J-30I, Beckman Coulter, rotor JA 30.50). The supernatant, containing soluble proteins, was supplemented by the Complete Protease Inhibitor Cocktail tablet (Roche) and a pinch of DNAse I (Sigma-Aldrich), and was filtered using 0.22 mm membranes. All purification steps were carried out with Fast Protein Liquid Chromatography (FPLC) on an AKTA Purifier system (GE Healthcare) and controlled by following the UV absorbance of aromatic residues at 280 nm. Fractions obtained after each purification step were analyzed by SDS-PAGE 15%.

2.3.2. *Protein purification by affinity chromatography on Ni-NTA resin*

The Immobilized Metal ions Affinity Chromatography (IMAC) was realized with a Ni-NTA HisTrap™ HP column (GE Healthcare), of which the stationary phase is composed by an NTA (NitriloTriacetic Acid)-agarose resin, chelated with immobilized nickel ions (Ni^{2+}). Histidine residues present in the His-Tag sequences of proteins bind with high specificity and affinity to the nickel ions, resulting in their retention. As imidazole has a similar structure to histidine residues, his-tagged proteins are eluted by competition with imidazole.

The protein samples, incubated or not with the TEV protease, were loaded into the Ni-NTA column previously equilibrated with the adequate lysis buffer. His-tagged proteins, such as NusA-DR5(ED) and TEV, bind to the column, while DR5(ED) is recovered in the flow-through. The resin was then washed with 10 column volumes (1 CV = 5 mL) of the adequate lysis buffer at a low concentration of imidazole (20 mM) in order to remove non-specific binding, and the protein of interest was eluted with the lysis buffer at a high concentration of imidazole (300 mM). The flow rate was set-up between 2 and 5 $mL{\cdot}min^{-1}$.

2.3.3. *TEV cleavage*

The recombinant plasmid pETNusA-DR5(ED) contains a cleavage site sequence (**E**NL**YFQ**-**G**AM) recognized by the protease of the Tobacco Etch Virus (TEV) and located between the His_6-NusA and the DR5(ED) genes. The protein of interest consists of 135 residues by including 3 N-ter residues (GAM) remaining from the TEV cleavage site.

In order to have a complete cleavage, it is essential to remove any trace of imidazole by exchanging the buffer in 50 mM Tris-HCl at basic pH (7,5–8) with PD-10 desalting column (GE Healthcare Life Sciences). TEV protease cleavage was then carried out overnight at 4°C or for 90 minutes at 30°C, at a TEV:NusA-DR5 mass ratio of 1:100.

2.3.4. *Purification of DR5(ED) by anion exchange chromatography (AIEX)*

The DR5(ED) protein may be recovered in the flow-through of a second IMAC or be purified by Anion Exchange Chromatography. The sample was then loaded on an HiTrap™ Q HP 5 mL column (GE Healthcare), pre-equilibrated with the appropriate buffer (20 mM Tris 50 mM NaCl pH 7.8). DR5(ED) is eluted at a NaCl concentration of 280 mM, while His_6-NusA is eluted at a NaCl concentration of 380 mM. The flow rate was 5 mL·min^{-1}.

2.3.5. *Protein purification by size exclusion chromatography (SEC)*

The purity of the sample, prior or not to the TEV cleavage, was enhanced by a step of size exclusion chromatography.

In the first purification protocol, the samples issued from IMAC before TEV cleavage were purified by SEC to separate the monomeric form (72 kDa) of the NusA-DR5(ED) from unwanted oligomeric forms as well as lower molecular weight compounds which may interfere with the further purification process of the momomeric form (15 kDa) of DR5(ED). The samples were therefore loaded on a HiLoad™ 16/600 Superdex 200 prep grade column (GE Healthcare), previously equilibrated with the appropriate buffer 20 mM Tris pH 50 mM NaCl pH 7.8. The column has a separation range for molecules with molecular weights between 10 and 600 kDa. The flow rate was comprised between 0.8 and 1 mL·min^{-1}.

In the second purification protocol, the samples issued from the second IMAC after TEV cleavage were purified by SEC to separate the monomeric form (15 kDa) of the DR5(ED) from oligomeric forms and remaining traces of NusA (57 kDa) or other contaminants. The samples were therefore loaded on a Superdex™ 75 10/300 GL column (GE Healthcare), previously equilibrated with the buffer 20 mM Tris pH 50 mM NaCl pH 7.8. The column has a separation range for molecules with molecular weights between 3 and 70 kDa. The flow rate was 1 mL·min^{-1}.

2.4. *NMR sample preparation*

Once the purity of the DR5(ED) proteins has been found satisfactory by analysis on SDS-PAGE 15%, the NMR samples coming from the production in LB (unlabeled protein) and M9 media (uniformly ^{15}N or $^{15}N^{13}C$ labelled protein) were buffer exchanged with 20 mM Na_2HPO_4 50 mM NaCl pH 6.3 in 10% or 100% D_2O using PD-10 columns (GE Healthcare). The NMR samples were concentrated in two steps with 3 kDa molecular weight cutoff filters, by using both Amicon Tube (Amicon® Ultra-15 3kDa Merck Millipore) by centrifugation at 5,000 g and 4°C for 30 minutes (SIGMA® 2-16 K centrifuge, rotor 12151) and Amicon Eppendorf (Amicon® Ultra-0.5 mL 3K, Merck Millipore) by centrifugation at 14,000 g and 4°C for 15 minutes (Centrifuge 5427R eppendorf). TriMethylSilylPropionate (TMSP) was added to NMR samples at 10 to 50 mM concentration to be used as an internal reference or has been used as an external reference. $^{13}C^{15}N$-DR5 sample concentration was made to 300 μM for assignment.

2.5. *Mass spectroscopy*

The average mass of intact DR5 was measured on a MALDI-TOFTOF mass spectrometer (Ultraflex III, Bruker) used in linear mode with sinapinic acid (Sigma-Aldrich) as a matrix [10 mg/mL solution in 50% acetonitrile in 0.1% aqueous trifluoroacetic acid (TFA)]. The dried droplet method was used for sample loading on a stainless steel target. The instrument was calibrated using an external calibration with a mixture of four standard proteins: Insulin ($[M+H]^+_{average}$= 5,734.51), Ubiquitin ($[M+H]^+_{average}$= 8,565.76), Cytochrom C ($[M+H]^+_{average}$= 12,360.97), Myoglobin ($[M+H]^+_{average}$= 16,952.30) (Bruker). Mass spectrometry (MS) study was performed to measure the average mass of the produced DR5 in order to assess its integrity. This analysis demonstrated the presence of one major form corresponding to an average mass M = 14,998 Da (mean of four individual analyzes). The mass difference between the theoretical mass of the recombinant protein calculated from the sequence (15,020.34 Da, taking into account all disulfide bonds in oxydized form) and the experimental mass is in accordance with the mass tolerance accepted for this measurement.

2.6. *NMR spectroscopy*

Spectra were acquired at 303 K on a Bruker Avance III 700 MHz and 800 MHz spectrometers, equipped with a TXI triple resonance probe and cryoprobe, respectively. All data were processed using NMRPipe (Delaglio *et al.*, 1995) and analyzed by using CCPNMR analysis 2.4 software [20]. Chemical shifts were referenced to TriMethylSilylPropanoic acid (TMSP) inside the samples [21]. The ^{1}H, ^{1}Hα, ^{13}Cα, ^{1}Hβ, ^{13}Cβ and ^{15}N backbone resonances of DR5-ED were derived by sequence-specific triple resonance 3D NMR spectra, namely HNCO, HN(CA)CO, HNCA, HN(CO)CA, HNCACB, CBCA(CO)NH, HNHA and HBHA(CO)NH. Side-chain resonance assignment was partially achieved by 3D NMR spectra, namely HC(C)H-TOCSY, (H)CCH-TOCSY, H(C)CH-COSY, ^{15}N-HSQC-NOESY (120 ms mixing time) and ^{15}N-HSQC-TOCSY (60 ms mixing time), as well as by 2D NMR spectra in 100% D_2O, namely aliphatic and aromatic ^{1}H^{13}C-HSQC, CBHD, CBHE, ^{1}H^{1}H-TOCSY and ^{1}H^{1}H-NOESY ([22] Sattler *et al.*, 1999).

3. Results and Discussion

3.1. *Production of the recombinant plasmid pETNusA-DR5(ED) by molecular cloning*

To produce the plasmid pETNusA-DR5(ED), the DR5(ED) gene was copied using PCR and excised out of the source DNA — the commercial plasmid pET23m-DR5(ED) — using restriction enzymes. Then, it was ligated to the plasmid vector pETNusA, which was prepared in a linear form using restriction enzymes.

3.1.1. *Amplification of the DR5(ED) gene from the plasmid pET23m-DR5(ED) by using PCR*

The PCR on the plasmid pET23m-DR5(ED) was performed with the forward primer DR5-Fvs: 5′-GCCATGGAGTCTGCTCTGATCACC-3′, which contains the ATG initiation codon, required for the expression of the DR5(ED) protein. The reverse primer used for this PCR was the DR5-Rvs: 5′-CGGATCCTTATGATTCTTTGTGGACACATTCG-3′, which contains a TAA stop codon, signaling the termination of translation. These two primers recognize specific sequences of the plasmid pET23m-DR5(ED), of about 20 nucleotides, resulting in the amplification of a 412 bp DNA segment — the DR5(ED) gene. Besides, their GC-contents are, respectively, 58% and 44% and thus, amplification of the DR5(ED) gene was improved by the addition of 1X Q5 High GC Enhancer.

PCR product was loaded on a 1.2% agarose gel (Figure 3), which revealed a unique band between 400 and 500 bp, which seems to correspond to the size of the DR5(ED) gene (412 bp). This band was then extracted and purified in order to obtain the DR5(ED) genes highly pure. Furthermore, the DNA assay indicated that the PCR product concentration was 30.4 ng·μL^{-1}, which was sufficient for cloning.

3.1.2. *Digestion of the DR5(ED) gene and the plasmid pETNusA, using restriction enzymes*

In order to insert the DR5(ED) gene into the plasmid pETNusA, we had to cut it with the same restriction enzymes as for the plasmid. As mentioned

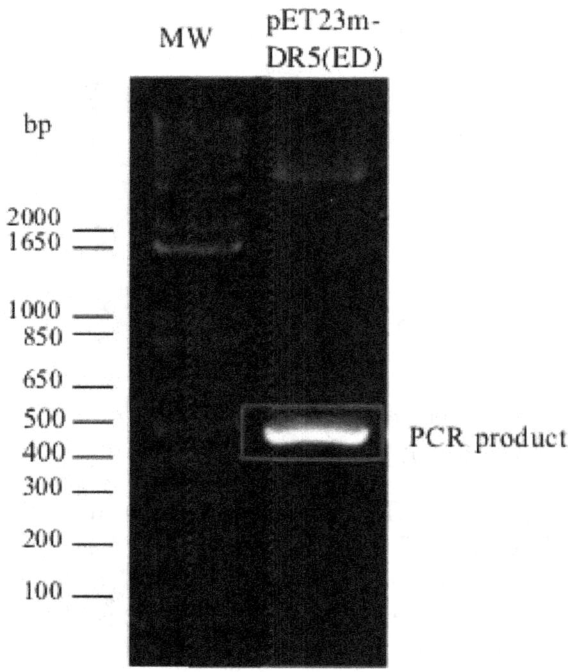

Fig. 3. Amplification by PCR of the DR5(ED) gene from the plasmid pET23m-DR5(ED). For PCR, the plasmid pET23m- DR5(ED) was incubated with the primer pair: DR5-Fvs 5′-GCCATGGAGTCTGCTCTGATCACC-3′ and DR5-Rvs 5′-CGGATCCTTATGATT-CTTTGTGGACACATTCG-3′, and subjected to a PCR reaction for 30 cycles (94°C–30 sec, 59°C–30 sec, 72°C–45 sec). The PCR product was then separated on 1.2% agarose gel, stained with SYBR® Safe 10,000X. MW: molecular weight.

earlier, the primers were designed to insert NcoI and BamHI restriction sites to the 5′ and 3′ extremities of the gene, respectively. This allowed us to treat the gene with both of these enzymes, as well as for the plasmid, which also has these restriction sites. These two enzymes — NcoI-HF and BamHI-HF — recognize very similar sequences and thus, produce compatible cohesive ends, required for the ligation of the insert with the vector.

The digestion of the plasmid pETNusA was performed in two steps in order to optimize the yield of fully cut plasmid. Samples from this digestion were separated on a 0.8% agarose gel (Figure 4). Compared to the plasmid uncut (Lane 2), on which there are two forms of the original plasmid — the "nicked circle" form and the supercoiled form — we can assume that the plasmid pETNusA was successfully cut by the NcoI restriction enzyme. This plasmid was then purified and 47.2 ng·μL^{-1} of DNA was retrieved and used for the second digestion with the BamHI

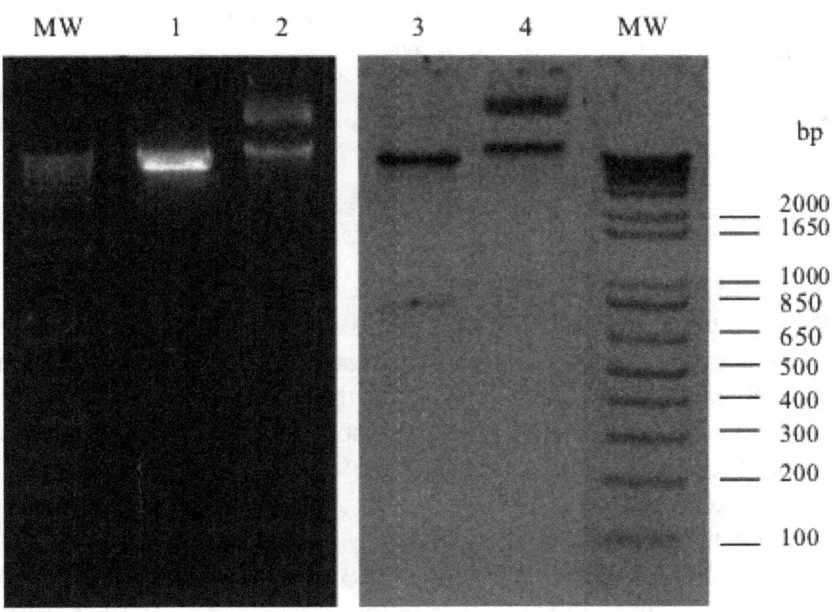

Fig. 4. Digestion of the plasmid pETNusA by the restriction enzymes NcoI and BamHI. Digest products were separated on 0.8% agarose gel, stained with SYBR® Safe. Controls with the original plasmid enable the checking of the digestion of the plasmid. MW: molecular weight; Lane 1: pETNusA cut by NcoI-HF; Lanes 2 and 4: pETNusA uncut; Lane 3: pETNusA cut by NcoI-HF and BamHI-HF.

enzyme. Digest product was analyzed on agarose gel (lane 3), on which we could observe a band between 650 bp and 850 bp, which seems to correspond to the size of the insert from the plasmid pETNusA cut (737 bp). Hence, the top band observed on lane 3 corresponded to the cut plasmid and was extracted from the gel. The OD measurement at 260 nm reveals that 13.6 ng·μL^{-1} of cut plasmid pETNusA were purified.

The DR5(ED) gene was digested by a double digest with the restriction enzymes NcoI-HF and BamHI-HF; and purified, resulting in the obtaining of 15.7 ng·μL^{-1} of cut DR5(ED) gene.

3.1.3. *Cohesive ends ligation*

The ligation procedure was realized with the Quick T4 DNA ligase, which provides fast and efficient DNA ligation of phosphorylated double-strand DNA fragments. The overall concentration of insert and vector should be between 1 ng·μL^{-1} and 10 ng·μL^{-1} for efficient ligation. As 54.4 ng of cut plasmid pETNusA and 15 ng of cut DR5(ED) gene were used, there was 3.47 ng·μL^{-1} of DNA, in the 20 μL reaction.

Besides, the insert:vector ratio was 5:1, which is optimal for single insertion. This ligation procedure enabled obtaining the recombinant plasmid pETNusA-DR5(ED).

3.1.4. *Bacterial transformation in DH5α cells*

DH5α cells were transformed with the recombinant plasmid pETNusA-DR5(ED), which contains a kanamycin-resistance gene. The cells were then plated on a Petri dish, containing kanamycin for bacteria selection. After 24 hours of incubation at 37°C, there were 19 CFU (Colony-Forming Units) on the plate, which corresponds to a transformation efficiency of 270 CFU·μg^{-1} of DNA. This transformation efficiency was sufficient to inoculate pre-cultures.

In order to check the cloning efficiency, two negative control transformations were performed, one with no DNA, the other one with a ligation mixture that did not contain the insert, in order to check that the plasmid used was cut. We did not observe any colony from those controls, which showed us that the cloning was efficient. Afterwards, four S1 colonies were selected to test whether each contained the recombinant plasmid.

The S1 colonies were recovered from the cloning plate to realize pre-cultures so as to be able to retrieve the recombinant plasmids. The recombinant plasmids pETNusA-DR5(ED) were obtained from the cell pellet of the culture medium by plasmid minipreparation. Hence, 221 ng·μL^{-1} of these plasmids were recovered as indicated by OD measurement at 260 nm.

3.1.5. *Clone verifications*

To check the validity of the cloning, three verifications were carried out on the recombinant plasmid pETNusA-DR5(ED): A DNA sequencing, a PCR with both primers DR5-Fvs and DR5- Rvs, and a double digestion with the restriction enzymes NcoI-HF and BamHI-HF.

Samples from the PCR and the double digestion were separated on 1.2% agarose gel (Figure 5) in order to prove the DR5(ED) gene was

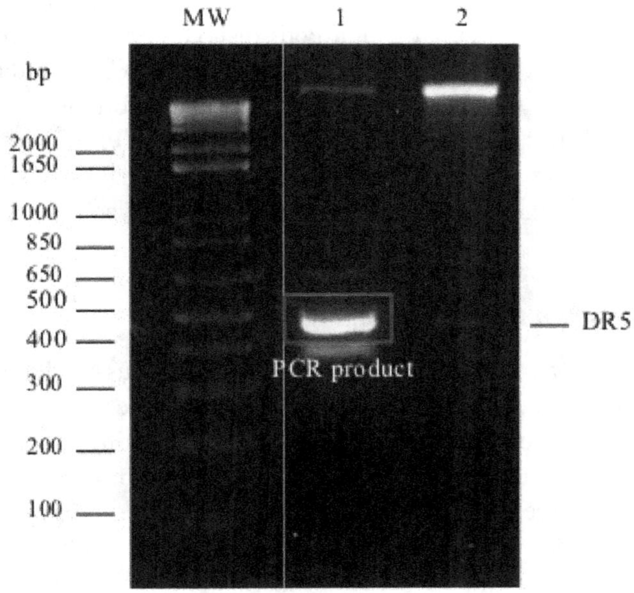

Fig. 5. Clone verifications. The recombinant plasmid pETNusA- DR5(ED) was amplified by PCR (Lane 1) and digested by the restriction enzymes NcoI-HF and BamHI-HF (Lane 2). For the PCR, the primer pair used is DR5-Fvs: 5′-GCCATGGAGTCTGCTCTGATCACC-3′ and DR5- Rvs: 5′-CGGATCCTTATGATTCTTTGTGGACACATTCG-3′, and the sample was subjected to a PCR reaction for 30 cycles (94°C–30 sec, 59°C–30 sec, 72°C–45 sec). PCR and digest products were separated on 1.2% agarose gel, stained with SYBR® Safe. MW: molecular weight.

isolated from the recombinant plasmid. On both lanes, we could observe one band between 400 and 500 bp, which should correspond to the size of the DR5(ED) gene (412 bp). Hence, the recombinant plasmid pETNusA-DR5(ED) carried the DR5(ED) gene, as expected.

DNA sequencing allowed to confirm these results, as it showed a similitude of 381 bp between the sequences of the DR5(ED) gene and the recombinant plasmid. Therefore, it may be possible to produce and purify the DR5(ED) protein from the plasmid pETNusA- DR5(ED).

3.2. *Production of DR5(ED) protein, using the recombinant plasmid pETNusA-DR5(ED)*

3.2.1. *Bacterial transformation*

BL21(DE3) cells were transformed with the recombinant plasmid pET-NusA-DR5(ED) and inoculated on a Petri dish containing kanamycin for plasmid selection. After 24 hours of incubation at 37°C, more than 1,000 CFU were tallied on the plate, corresponding to a transformation efficiency of 4.5.103 CFU$\cdot\mu g^{-1}$ of DNA. Thus, the transformation efficiency was sufficient for a further inoculation of pre-cultures. This genetic transformation was confirmed by the "0 DNA" control, which did not contain any CFU.

3.2.2. *Expression tests in LB and M9 media*

Expression tests were carried out to check that the NusA-DR5(ED) protein can be produced with the expression system described in Materials and Methods. The cell culture was carried out at 37°C in LB medium and at 25°C in M9 medium, under stirring to increase the oxygene (O_2) available required for the cell growth. The protein expression was induced by 0.5 mM IPTG, added during the exponential phase (OD600 nm = 0.6).

Samples of each time of induction in LB medium were analyzed on SDS-PAGE gel (Figure 6). On lanes 3 to 5, there was a large band between 58 kDa and 80 kDa, which corresponds to the DR5(ED) protein (15 kDa) fused to the His-tagged NusA protein (57 kDa). Besides, the intensity of the band grew larger with the induction time. This indicated to us that the fusion protein was successfully over-expressed in BL21(DE3) cells transformed with the recombinant plasmid. In rich medium (LB), there was no lag phase and only a short-acceleration phase during the bacterial growth,

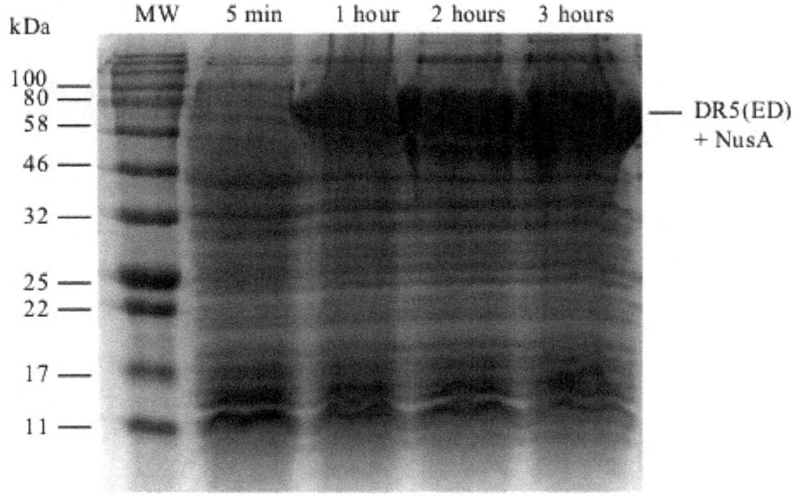

Fig. 6. Expression in BL21(DE3) cells transformed with pETNusA-DR5(ED) in LB medium. After 5 min, 1 hour, 2 hours and 3 hours of induction with IPTG (Lanes 2–5), samples were retrieved and separated on SDS-PAGE gel 15%, stained with Instant Blue.

in contrast to what was observed in the M9 medium (Figure 7). Therefore, the protein induction in the minimum medium was performed overnight, but at a reduced temperature (25°C) in order to increase the production of correctly folded and soluble proteins versus misfolded or aggregated proteins in inclusion bodies. Nevertheless, the expression yield is two to three times lower in the mimimum than in the rich medium, as the cell densities reached at the end of the culture (M9 medium: OD600 nm = 1.2–1.4; LB medium: OD600 nm = 2–3) strongly depend on the amount of source of energy, which is limited in M9 medium to 2 $g{\cdot}L^{-1}$ of ^{13}C-labelled glucose due to its expensiveness.

3.3. *Extents of assignments and data deposition*

Analysis of the 3D sequential NMR experiments allowed us to assign 111 out of the 125 expected ^{15}N and ^{1}H backbone resonances (135 residues less 9 prolines and the N-terminal glycine). The backbone assignment is nearly complete (89%), except for 14 residues (A2, Q11, S40, D54, D61, C68, V76, T87, V88, C91, F96, R97, R106, K107). Ten peaks

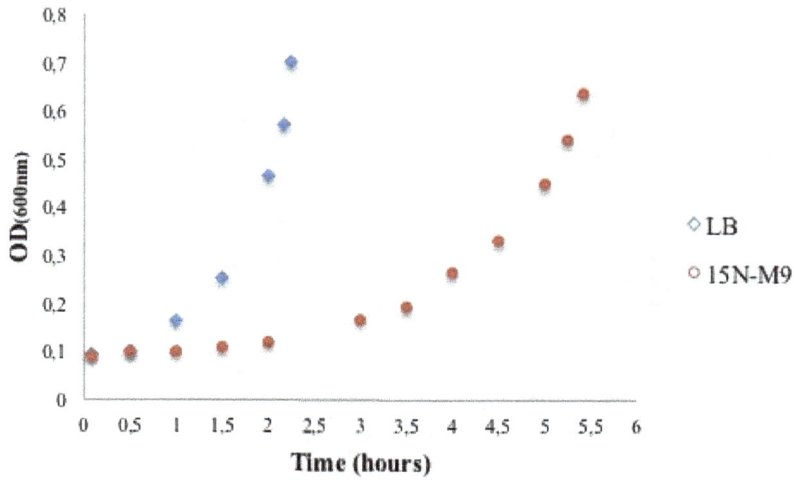

Fig. 7. Cell growth of BL21(DE3) cells transformed with pETNusA-DR5(ED). Comparison of the OD measurements at 600 nm (OD600 nm) as a function of time, in rich medium (LB) and in M9 minimum medium isotopically labeled with nitrogen ^{15}N (^{15}N-M9).

of the $^{1}H^{15}N$ HSQC spectrum, however, remain unassigned (Figure 8). The presence of additional peaks corresponding to a minor conformation was observed for residues located in the *N*-terminal flexible region (S5, L7, I8, T9, D12, A14, A20, K24, S26, S27, S29) and for the tryptophan residue W125. Such minor conformations probably result from the surrounding proline residues in a *cis* conformation (P15, P21, P28 and P124). Slow conformational exchange has also been observed in the loop of the first beta hairpin (residues 41–44) and may arise from conformational heterogeneity of the disulphide bridge 33–46 or protein oligomerization. We were able to extend the assignment up to 94%, 93% and 87% for the CO, Cα and Cβ chemical shifts, respectively. Hα, Cα, Cβ and CO chemical shift values allowed us to assess the secondary structure of the protein in solution by using random coil values [23] and TALOS-N software [24]. We found 8 of the 10 expected strands from crystal structures of DR5 complexes and one additional strand at the *N*-terminus (Figure 9), namely b0[residues 32:33], b1[37:39], b2[46:48], b3[54:55], b4[69:70], b5[75:79], b6[86:91], b9[116:120] and b10[129:132].

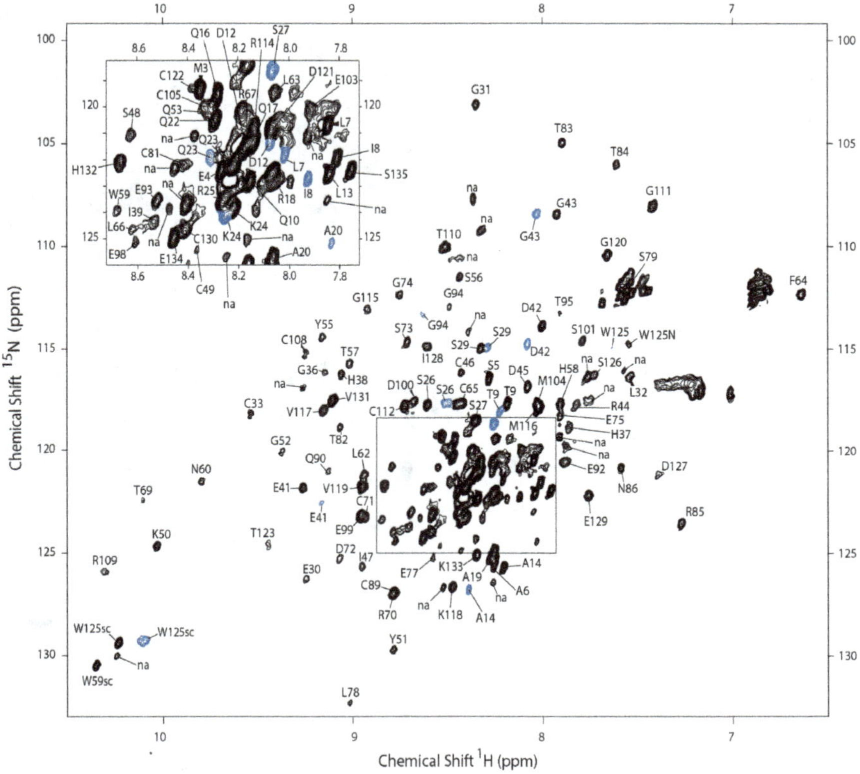

Fig. 8. Annotated ^{1}H-^{15}N HSQC spectrum of DR5-ED. The spectrum was acquired at 303K on a Bruker Avance III 800 MHz spectrometer equipped with a 5 mm TXI ^{1}H/^{13}C/^{15}N/^{2}H cryoprobe. The ^{15}N^{13}C labelled protein was at a concentration of 300 mM in 20 mM Na_2HPO_4 pH 6.3 50 mM NaCl in a mixture of 90% H_2O/ 10% D_2O. The assignment of the peaks is indicated with the amino acid letter followed by the residue number. For clarity, a more detailed view of the central region is displayed separately in the top left corner of the spectrum. Unassigned peaks are labeled by the letters na. Assigned peaks corresponding to the major (65%) and minor (35%) conformations for the same residue are, respectively, colored in black and cyan.

An excellent agreement (Figure 10) has been found for the protein in solution with the X-ray structures of DR5-ED bound to TRAIL (1DOG.pdb, 1DU3.pdb and 1D4V.pdb), to FAB fragments (1ZA3, 2H9G, 3X3F, 4OD2 and 4N90) and to the glycoprotein UL141 (4I9X.pdb). Most of the resonances for the residues of the third expected b-hairpin

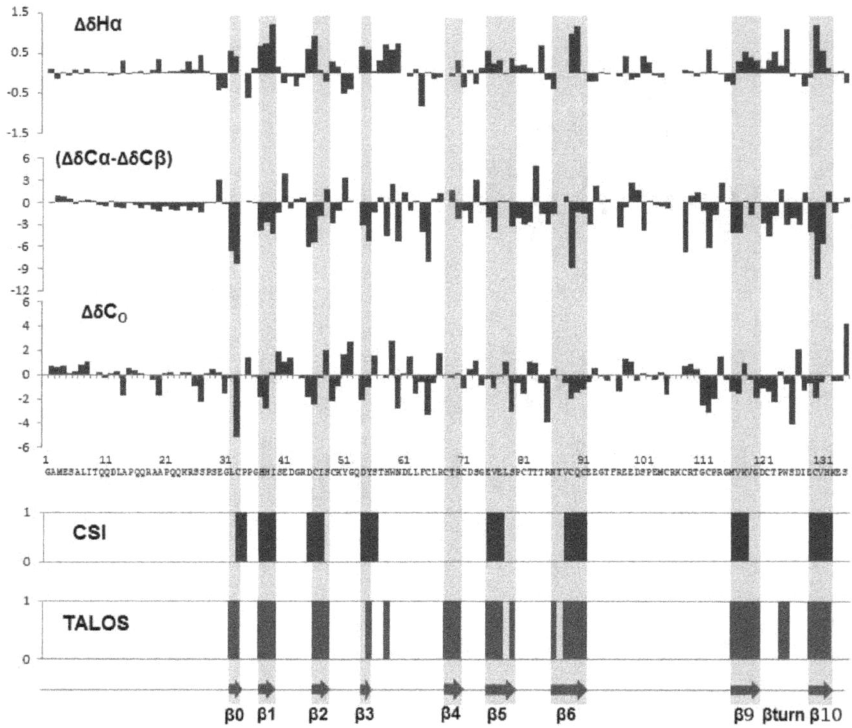

Fig. 9. Secondary structure of DR5-ED in solution. Assignment of secondary structure results from the TALOS prediction based on the backbone resonance values. Chemical Shift Indexes (CSI) are calculated with chemical shift values of ^{13}Ca, ^{13}Cb, ^{13}CO and ^{1}Ha resonances. The ten strands of the consecutive five beta hairpins are sequentially annotated by the letter beta followed by the corresponding number.

b7[94:96]-b8[104:106] were not found in the 3D NMR spectra. All the unassigned residues seem to be clustered in the vicinity of the beta sheets (b1: residue S40; b3: D54; b4: C68; b5: V76, b6: T87 and V88, b7: F96 and R97; b8: R106 and K107). These residues have not yet been assigned because peaks are missing or are too weak in intensity, probably arising from an excessive linebroadening beyond detection due to the presence of a conformational exchange on the intermediate millisecond timescale. The backbone and side-chain ^{1}H, ^{13}C and ^{15}N chemical shift values of DR5-ED have been deposited at BioMagResBank under the accession number 27400.

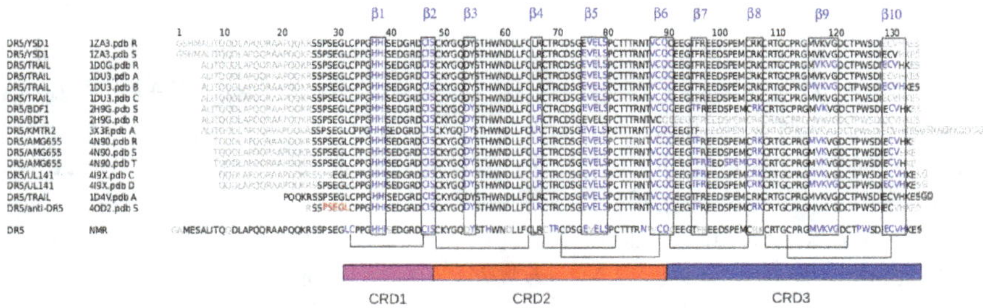

Fig. 10. Comparison of DR5-ED secondary structures in crystals and in solution. Alignment of the DR5-ED protein sequences used in crystallography and NMR spectroscopy. Crystal structures of the DR5 bound to TRAIL or Fab fragments of anti-DR5 antibodies are indicated on the left of the figure with the pdb code and the subunit. Visible and missing residues are, respectively, in black and grey. Residues in the beta conformation are in blue. Disulphide bridges are indicated. The three Cysteine Rich Domains (CRD) are represented schematically by rectangles in different colors.

Acknowledgments

We thank the structural biology platform at the Institut Européen de Chimie et Biologie (UMS 3033) for access to NMR spectrometers and technical assistance. Antoine Baudin was supported by a French Ph.D. fellowship afforded to the University of Bordeaux by the Ministère de la Recherche (MNERT) and a fourth- year Ph.D. extension by the Ligue Nationale Contre le Cancer (LCC). The project was funded by the Ligue Contre le Cancer de la Gironde. We thank Dr. Yong-Sung Kim from the Ajou University of the Republic of Korea for providing us the plasmid containing the gene coding for DR5-ED.

List of Abbreviations

DR5	Death Receptor 5
ED	Extra Cellular Domain
HSQC	Heteronuclear Single Quantum Coherence transfer
TRAIL	Tumor necrosis factor-a-Related Apoptosis-Inducing Ligand

References

1. Ashkenazi, A. and Dixit, V. M. (1998). Death Receptors: Signaling and Modulation. *Science* 281(5381), pp. 1305–1308.

2. MacFarlane, M., Ahmad, M., Srinivasula, S. M., Fernandes-Alnemri, T., Cohen, G. M. and Alnemri, E. S. (1997) Identification and Molecular Cloning of Two Novel Receptors for the Cytotoxic Ligand TRAIL. *J. Biol. Chem.* 272(41), pp. 25417–25420.
3. Walczak, H., Degli-Esposti, M. A., Johnson, R. S., Smolak, P. J., Waugh, J. Y., Boiani, N., Timour, M. S., Gerhart, M. J., Schooley, K. A., Smith, C. A., Goodwin, R. G. and Rauch, C. T. (1997) TRAIL-R2: A Novel Apoptosis-Mediating Receptor for TRAIL. *EMBO J.* 16(17), pp. 5386–5387.
4. Newsom-Davis, T., Prieske, S. and Walczak, H. (2009) Is TRAIL The Holy Grail of Cancer Therapy? *Apoptosis* 14(4), pp. 607–623.
5. Takeda, K., Stagg, J., Yagita, H., Okumura, K. and Smyth, M. J. (2007) Targeting Death-Inducing Receptors in Cancer Therapy. *Oncogene.* 26(25), pp. 3745–3757.
6. Mérino, D., Lalaoui, N., Morizot, A., Solary, E. and Micheau, O. (2007) TRAIL in Cancer Therapy: Present and Future Challenges. *Expert Opin. Ther. Targets.* 11(10), pp. 1299–1234.
7. Hymowitz, S. G., Christinger, H. W., Fuh, G., Ultsch, M., O'Connell, M., Kelley, R. F., Ashkenazi, A. and de Vos, A. M. (1999) Triggering Cell Death: The Crystal Structure of Apo2L/TRAIL in a Complex with Death Receptor 5. *Mol. Cell* 4(4), pp. 563–571.
8. Mongkolsapaya, J., Grimes, J. M., Chen, N., Xu, X. N., Stuart, D. I., Jones, E. Y. and Screaton, G. R. (1999) Structure of the TRAIL-DR5 Complex Reveals Mechanisms Conferring Specificity in Apoptotic Initiation. *Nat. Struct. Biol.* 6(11), pp. 1048–1053.
9. Cha, S. S., Sung, B. J., Kim, Y. A., Song, Y. L, Kim, H. J., Kim, S., Lee, M. S. and Oh, B. H. (2000) Crystal Structure of TRAIL-DR5 Complex Identifies a Critical Role of the Unique Frame Insertion in Conferring Recognition Specificity. *J. Biol. Chem.* 275(40), pp. 31171–31177.
10. Nemčovičová, I., Benedict, C. A. and Zajonc, D. M. (2013) Structure of Human Cytomegalovirus UL141 Binding to TRAIL-R2 Reveals Novel, Non-Canonical Death Receptor Interactions. *PloS Pathog.* 9(3), pp. e1003224.
11. Fellouse, F. A., Li, B., Compaan, D. M., Peden, A. A., Hymowitz, S. G. and Sidhu, S. S. (2005) Molecular Recognition by a Binary Code. *J. Mol. Biol.* 348(5), pp. 1153–1162.
12. Li, B., Russell, S. J., Compaan, D. M., Totpal, K., Marsters, S. A., Ashkenazi, A., Cochran, A. G., Hymowitz, S. G., Sidhu, S. S. (2006) Activation of the Proapoptotic Death Receptor DR5 by Oligomeric Peptide and Antiobody Agonists. *J. Mol. Biol.* 361(3), pp. 522–536.
13. Adams, C., Totpal, K., Lawrence, D., Marsters, S., Pitti, R., Yee, S., Ross, S., Deforge, L., Koeppen, H., Sagolla, M., Compaan, D., Lowman, H., Hymowitz, S. and Ashkenazi, A. (2008) Structural and Functional Analysis

of the Interaction Between the Agonistic Monoclonal Antibody Apomab and the Proapoptotic Receptor DR5. *Cell Death Differ.* 15(5), pp. 751–761.
14. Graves, J. D., Kordich J. J., Huang, T. H., Piasecki, J., Bush, T. L., Sullivan, T., Foltz, I. N., Chang, W., Douangpanya, H., Dang, T., O'Neill, J. W., Mallari, R., Zhao, X., Branstetter, D. G., Rossi, J. M., Long, A. M., Huang X. and Holland, P. M. (2014) Apo2L/TRAIL and the Death Receptor 5 Agonist Antibody AMG 655 Cooperate to Promote Receptor Clustering and Antitumor Activity. *Cancer Cell* 26(2), pp. 177–189.
15. Tamada, T., Shinmi, D., Ikeda, M., Yonezawa, Y., Kataoka, S., Kuroki, R., Mori, E. and Motoki, K. (2015) TRAIL-R2 Superoligomerization Induced by Human Monoclobal Agonistic Antibody KMTR2. *Sci Rep.* 5, pp. 17936.
16. Pavet, V., Beyrath, J., Pardin, C., Morizot, A., Lechner, M. C., Briand, J. P., Wendland, M., Maison, W., Fournel, S., Micheau, O., Guichard, G. and Gronemeyer, H. (2010) Multivalent DR5 Peptides Activate the TRAIL Death Pathway and Exert Tumoricidal Activity. *Cancer Res.* 70(3), pp. 1101–1110.
17. Pulka-Ziach, K., Pavet, V., Chekkat, N., Estieu-Gionnet, K., Rohac, R., Lechner, M. C., Smulski, C. R., Zeder-Lutz, G., Altschuh, D., Gronemeyer, H., Fournel, S., Odaert, B. and Guichard, G. (2015) Thioether Analogues of Disulfide-Bridged Cyclic Peptides Targeting Death Receptor 5: Conformational Analysis, Dimerisation and Consequences for Receptor Activation. *Chembiochem* 16(2), pp. 293–301.
18. Beyrath, J., Chekkat, N., Smulski, C. R., Lombardo, C. M., Lechner, M. C., Seguin, C., Decossas, M., Spanedda, M. V, Frisch, B., Guichard, G. and Fournel, S. (2016) Synthetic Ligands of Death Receptor 5 Display a Cell-Selective Agonistic Effect at Different Oligomerization Levels. *Oncotarget.* 7(40), pp. 64942–64956.
19. Baudin, A., Guichard, A., Collie, G. W., Rousseau, S., Chaignepain, S., Hocquellet, A., Berbon, M., Loquet, A., Mackereth, C., Guichard, G. and Odaert B. (2018) 1H, 13C, 15N NMR Resonance Assignments and Secondary Structure Determination of the Extra-Cellular Domain from the Human Proapoptotic TRAIL-R2 Death Receptor 5 (DR5-ED). *Biomol. NMR Assignment* 12(2), pp. 309–314.
20. Skinner, S. P., Fogh, R. H., Boucher, W., Ragan, T. J., Mureddu, L. G., Vuister, G. W. (2016) CcpNmr Analysis Assign: A Flexible Platform for Integrated NMR Analysis. *J. Biomol. NMR.* 66, pp. 111–124.
21. Wishart, D. S., Bigam, C. G., Yao, J., Abildgaard, F., Dyson, H. J., Oldfield, E., Markley, J. L. and Sykes, B. D. (1995) 1H, 13C and 15N Chemical Shift Referencing in Biomolecular NMR. *J. Biomol. NMR* 6, pp. 135–140.
22. Sattler, M., Schleucher, J. and Griesinger, C. (1999) Heteronuclear Multidimensional NMR Experiments for the Structure Determination of Proteins in Solution Employing Pulsed Field Gradients. *Prog. NMR Spectr.* 34, pp. 93–158

23. Wang, Y. and Jardetzky, O. (2002) Probability-Based Protein Secondary Structure Identification Using Combined NMR Chemical-Shift Data. *Protein Sci.* 11(4), pp. 852–61.
24. Yang, S. and Bax, A. (2013) TALOS-N: Protein Backbone and Sidechain Torsion Angles Predicted from NMR Chemical Shifts Using Artificial Neural Networks. *J. Biomol. NMR* 56, pp. 227–241.

https://doi.org/10.1142/9789811261664_0009

Chapter 9

Substrate Binding Free Energy Profiles: Probing Enzyme–Substrate Interactions by Molecular Dynamics Simulations

Juergen Pleiss and Henrique Carvalho*

Institute of Biochemistry and Technical Biochemistry, University of Stuttgart, Stuttgart, Germany

**henrique.carvalho@itb.uni-stuttgart.de*

1. Introduction

Enzymes are promising catalysts for a greener chemistry due to their sustainable production, high catalytic activity, and selectivity. Understanding the molecular basis of enzyme–substrate interactions is a prerequisite for engineering variants with a broadened substrate scope, increased selectivity for biocatalytic applications, or for finding novel enzymes in genomic or metagenomic sequence libraries for the synthesis of desired products.

The interactions of a substrate molecule with the active site of an enzyme have been studied by three different methods: molecular docking [1], molecular dynamics simulation of the substrate in a productive orientation in the active site [2], and quantum chemical calculations of the reaction path [3]. Functionally relevant residues were identified with these methods, which stabilize the substrate in its productive orientation, as well as positions which prevent the productive orientation of a substrate or mediate its binding in a non-productive orientation [4], thus being promising candidates for mutation. These modeling approaches have been successful, if the chemical step represents the kinetic bottleneck of the catalytic cycle. However, there is growing evidence that substrate access or product exit might be the rate-limiting steps [5] or might contribute to selectivity [6]. Due to the rapidly increasing availability of computational resources, unbiased simulations of protein–ligand interactions have become feasible to study the binding of multiple ligand molecules in solution [7]. First reports also demonstrate the feasibility of this approach to study enzyme–substrate interactions [4,8,9].

For enzyme-catalyzed reactions, the dependency of the initial reaction rate on the concentration of the substrate and product is indicative of the enzyme mechanism [10]. Kinetic parameters derived by fitting of experimental data are a prerequisite to process design [11]. However, it is desirable to model the concentration effects from first principles, because understanding the kinetics and thermodynamics of substrate binding on an atomic level will enable the identification and removal of kinetic bottlenecks by protein engineering. Here, we report how to apply unbiased molecular dynamics simulations to address such effects, where the protein is embedded in a water box with an increasing substrate concentration. Two enzymes are compared: lipase B of *Candida antarctica* (CALB), which acts on a wide range of fatty acid esters [12], and the thioesterase of *Escherichia coli* (TAP), which catalyzes hydrolysis of long-chain fatty acid esters [13]. We use methanol as a model substrate, since it is accepted by CALB as a substrate in alcoholysis reactions [12]. On the other hand, TAP is not known to accept methanol as a substrate, and alcoholysis activity has not been described. The enzymes are modeled as acyl-enzyme intermediate (details of the catalytic mechanism are given below).

CALB and TAP are of high industrial interest. CALB is widely used due to its broad substrate range, high stereoselectivity, activity, and robustness [14]. TAP is a multifunctional lysophospholipase and acyl-CoA thioesterase. Because it also acts as thioesterase, arylesterase, and protease, it also has high industrial potential [15,16]. CALB and TAP share the Ser-His-Asp catalytic triad in their active sites, but have a different fold. CALB has 316 residues and belongs to the α/β hydrolase family [17], while TAP has 190 and belongs to the SGNH-hydrolase family. As in all lipases, the active site of CALB is located at the bottom of a hydrophobic binding pocket [18] (Scheme 1(a)). The active site of TAP is located in a cleft at the protein surface [16] (Scheme 1(b)).

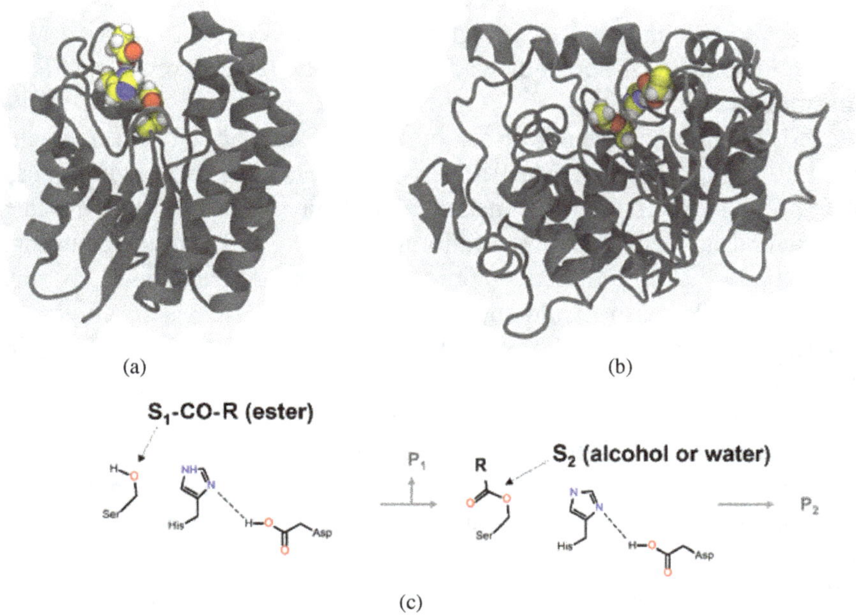

Scheme 1. Crystal structure of CALB (a) and TAP (b), with catalytic triad Ser/His/Asp residues shown in yellow vdW and protein backbone shown in cartoon. The Ping-Pong Bi-Bi mechanism (c). The first (thio)ester substrate (S_1-CO-R) donates an acyl moiety (R) to a catalytic Ser residue, leading to the formation of the first product (P_1) and an acyl-intermediate Ser residue. The reaction proceeds by a second substrate (S_2), which can be either an alcohol (in esterases) or water (in hydrolases), which accepts the acyl moiety leading to the formation of the second product (P_2-CO-R), which can be either an ester (in esterases) or acid (in hydrolases), and the regeneration of the free form of the enzyme. In this work, only the interaction of an S_2 substrate with the acyl-intermediate form of the enzyme is considered.

2. Unbiased Molecular Dynamics Simulations

2.1. *Simulation settings*

MD simulations of a molecular system containing a protein, substrate molecules, and solvent can be used to investigate the driving forces and the molecular details of binding of a substrate molecule in its productive conformation close to the active site [4,8]. By simulating multiple substrate molecules in an aqueous solvent, experimental reaction conditions are reproduced, such as substrate concentration, temperature, and the type of solvent. The approach is straightforward and relies on unbiased MD simulation methods, and thus can be widely applied to other enzyme–substrate systems.

MD simulations are performed by the MD simulation software package GROMACS version 5 [19]. The NPT ensemble is used, with a constant pressure of 1 bar and a constant temperature of 294 K. The v-rescale and Berendsen algorithms are used for temperature and pressure coupling, respectively [20,21]. Electrostatic interactions are calculated by the smooth particle-mesh Ewald summation [22]. A single protein molecule (CALB, PDB ID: 5A71 [23], or TAP, PDB ID: 1U8U [16]) is placed in the center of a cubic box, and methanol molecules are inserted randomly into the box. The box size and the number of methanol molecules are chosen to approximate the experimental substrate concentrations of interest: the box volume varied between 513 and 1659 nm^3, and the number of substrate molecules between 45 and 2500. The simulation boxes containing the protein and substrate molecules are then solvated with SPC/E water molecules [24,25]. For each concentration, 10 independent MD simulation replicates are performed to improve the statistics of binding events. Each system is first minimized for a maximum of 10000 steps using a steepest descent algorithm, followed by 1000 steps using a conjugate gradient algorithm. The system is then equilibrated for 105 ns, with positions restraints applied during the initial 5 ns to all substrate atoms as well as to the protein heavy atoms (force constant: 1000 $kJ \cdot mol^{-1} \cdot nm^{-2}$). After equilibration, the system is simulated for 100 ns, and trajectory frames are saved each 5 ps.

2.2. *Force field*

The all-atom force field OPLS-AA (Optimized Potentials for Liquid Simulations) is widely applied for simulations of small molecules and proteins [26]. We use a variant of OPLS-AA with optimized parameters for the hydroxyl group of methanol which reproduces its experimentally derived self-diffusion coefficient [27]. Protein force field definitions are obtained using the tool pdb2gmx of GROMACS 5. For both proteins, a pH of 7.0 is assumed, therefore the side chains of Asp/Glu and Lys/Arg are negatively and positively charged, respectively, except for Asp134 of CALB and Asp154 of TAP, which are considered as protonated (neutral) [28].

The catalytic histidine (His224 of CALB, His157 of TAP) is modeled with a single hydrogen on the δ-nitrogen, whereas all histidines in TAP are modeled with a hydrogen on the ε-nitrogen, in both cases with neutral net charge. The *N*- and *C*-termini are charged positively and negatively, respectively. The acyl-enzyme intermediate is generated by modeling the catalytic residues Ser105 (CALB) and Ser10 (TAP) as ^{acyl}Ser with an acetyl moiety covalently linked to the oxygen of the serine side chain. The model is based on the crystal structure of *Mycobacterium smegmatis* acyltransferase (PDB ID: 2q0s [29]), where the serine is covalently linked to the inhibitor 4-nitrophenyl *n*-hexylcarbamate. The OPLS-AA force field parameters for the Ac- ^{acyl}Ser-NH_2 amino acid are obtained from the LigParGen server using the 1.14*CM1A-LBCC charge model [30–32]. The Ac and NH_2 groups are removed and the partial charges of the side chain atoms are slightly adjusted to achieve a total charge of 0 for the ^{acyl}Ser residue.

3. Binding Free Energy Profile of Methanol

3.1. *Distance of near attack conformation*

The reaction mechanism of enzymes containing the Ser-His-Asp catalytic triad, such as CALB and TAP, has been described as a Ping-Pong Bi-Bi mechanism [28]. The reaction proceeds when an ester or thioester binds into the active site, followed by a nucleophilic attack of the catalytic serine, the formation of an acyl-enzyme intermediate, and the release of the alcohol product (Scheme 1(c)). [33] Subsequently, either water or alcohol acts as a second substrate (hydrolysis or alcoholysis, respectively) by a nucleophilic attack to the acyl-enzyme intermediate, resulting in the release of the final product (acid or ester, respectively). While MD simulations do not allow one to model the breaking or forming of bonds, the method is applied to study the access of a substrate molecule from the bulk to the active site and the productive binding. The productive binding of methanol to acylated CALB and TAP is described by near attack conformations (NAC), *i.e.*, non-covalent productive binding poses of the substrate which resemble the transition state and which can be accessed by MD simulations [33].

For each of the protein–substrate systems, the occurrence of NAC is measured by analyzing a set of relevant distances (Scheme 2): between

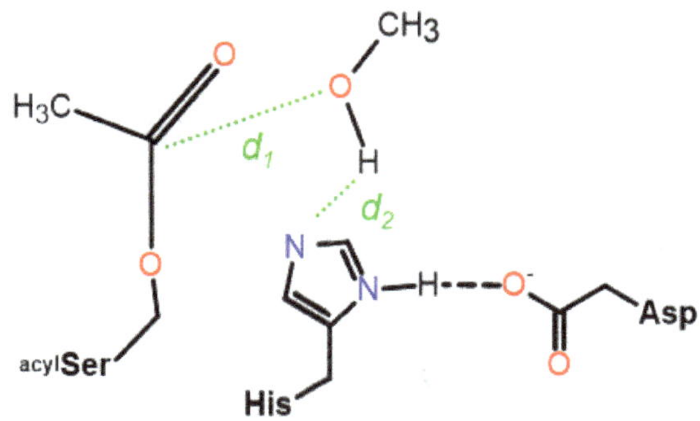

Scheme 2. Catalytic Ser/His/Asp triad of CALB and TAP. Distances used for d_{NAC} calculation shown in green.

the hydroxyl oxygen of methanol and the carbonyl carbon of the ^{acyl}Ser (d_1) and the distance between the hydroxyl hydrogen of methanol and the nitrogen of catalytic histidine (d_2). The reaction coordinate d_{NAC} is calculated as the root mean square of the two distances:

$$d_{NAC} = \sqrt{\frac{d_1^2 + d_2^2}{2}} \tag{1}$$

The lower bound of d_{NAC} (2.25 Å) is due to vdW repulsive terms defined in the OPLS-AA force field, while the upper bound is limited by the size of the simulation box (variable, from 9 to 12 Å). The d_{NAC} is calculated for all substrate molecules in each individual simulation at intervals of 5 ps.

3.2. *Binding free energy profiles*

The binding free energy profile describes the effect of the protein on the distribution of substrate molecules in a simulation box at a given concentration [4]. It reflects how the substrate molecules interact with the protein and how these interactions depend on the substrate concentration. It is obtained by calculating the ratio of the sampled distribution of substrate molecules in a box containing the protein, N_{enzyme}, and a reference distribution at the same bulk concentration, but in the absence of the protein, $N_{\mathrm{reference}}$. Assuming thermal equilibrium and thus a Boltzmann distribution [34], the free energy difference $\Delta G(i)$ is calculated from the ratio between $N(i)_{\text{enzyme}}$ and $N(i)_{\text{reference}}$ as follows:

$$\frac{\Delta G(i)}{k_B T} = -\ln \frac{N(i)_{\text{enzyme}}}{N(i)_{\text{reference}}} \tag{2}$$

where $k_B = 1.38 \cdot 10^{-23}$ J/K is the Boltzmann constant and T the temperature (in K). Therefore, this method is considered as a "direct counting" approach to obtain the free energy and thus a qualitative and quantitative description of enzyme–substrate interactions. N_{enzyme} is calculated as a function of d_{NAC} by counting the number of methanol molecules in each ith spherical shell by the following:

$$N(i)_{\text{enzyme}} = \frac{\bar{N}}{N_T} \tag{3}$$

where $\bar{N}$ represents the number of methanol molecules N at a distance between d_{NAC} and $d_{\text{NAC}}+\delta$, where the shell thickness δ is set to 0.5 Å, averaged over 10 simulation replicates, and N_T is the total number of sampled conformers (20000 per simulation replicate). The standard errors of N are calculated and used to obtain the corresponding standard errors of ΔG. The reference number of methanol molecules $N_{\text{reference}}$ for each ith spherical shell at a given bulk concentration *[methanol]* is calculated by the following:

$$N(i)_{\text{reference}} = 3\left(\frac{4}{3}\pi\left(d_{NAC} + \delta\right)^3 - d_{NAC}{}^3\right)\left[methanol\right]N_0\right) \tag{4}$$

where d_{NAC} and δ are in Å, [*methanol*] in M and N_0 is the Avogadro constant, and the pre-factor 3 is used to account for the distribution of molecules in 3D Cartesian space. The bulk concentration after equilibration is obtained by least square fitting of $N_{\text{reference}}$ to N_{enzyme} in the region 30 Å < $d_{\text{NAC}} \leq 40$ Å, where no protein effects occur (Figure 1). Therefore, ΔG equals 0 in this region. The distribution of d_{NAC} values is obtained by standard analysis tools of MD simulation software packages or by dedicated Python libraries such as MDAnalysis [35,36], and a histogram of N_{enzyme} is generated. For d_{NAC} regions occupied by the protein, ΔG tends to be positive, since the substrate cannot occupy the same volume

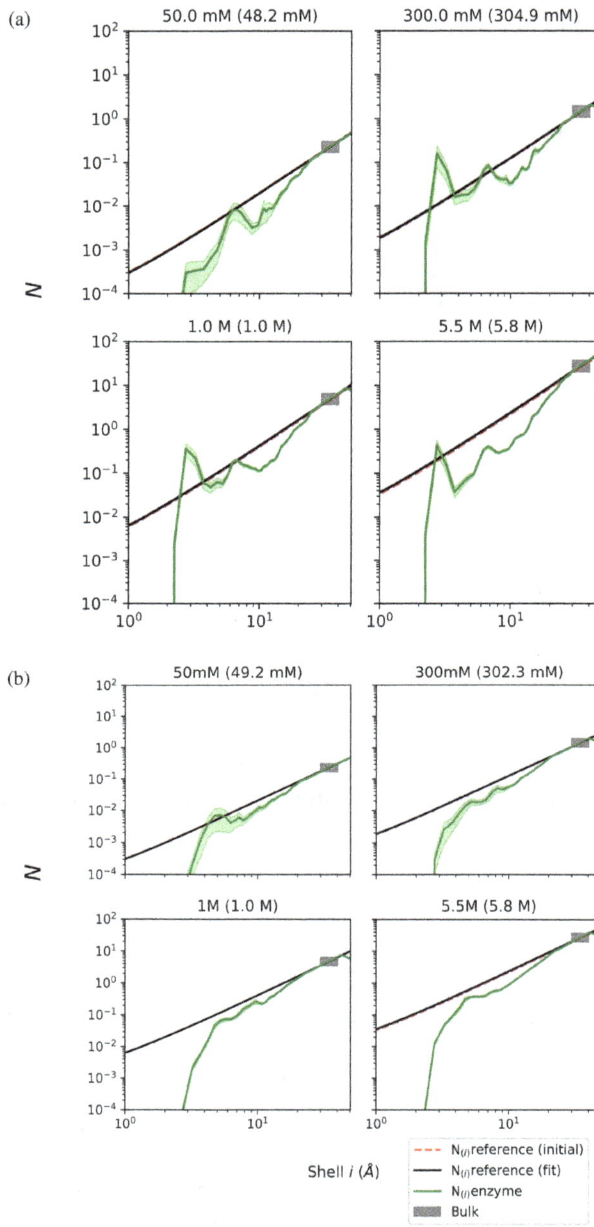

Fig. 1. Determination of the bulk concentration of methanol for (a) CALB and (b) TAP. Values of the methanol concentration in the bulk were obtained by least square fitting shown in the plot titles. Region used for fitting of $N_{\text{reference}}$ to N_{enzyme} represented in gray boxes.

as the protein. In both TAP and CALB, this occurs at $d_{NAC} < 25$ Å. Regions with negative ΔG values indicate accumulation of the substrate, and therefore correspond to regions with an attractive interaction with the substrate.

3.3. *Binding free energy profile of CALB*

For all methanol concentrations, the binding free energy profiles of the CALB-methanol systems have two minima, which correspond to two methanol binding sites within the CALB protein (Figure 2). The global minimum at d_{NAC} = 2.75 Å corresponds to the productive binding of the substrate in close proximity to the catalytic ^{acyl}Ser105 and His224. Below this value, the interactions between CALB and methanol become

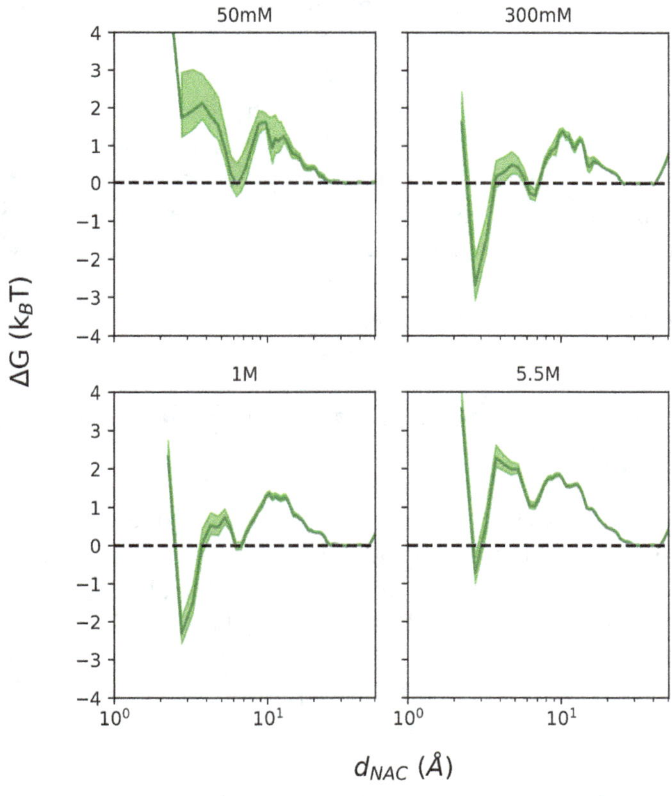

Fig. 2. Binding free energy profile (ΔG in k_BT units) of the CALB-methanol system as a function of d_{NAC}. Solid line and shaded regions correspond to mean value and standard error from 10 simulation replicas, respectively.

increasingly unfavorable due to steric repulsion, and no methanol molecule was found at $d_{NAC} < 2.25$ Å. The local minimum at $d_{NAC} = 6$ Å corresponds to a second binding site within the binding pocket of CALB and depends on the methanol concentration. At increasing methanol concentrations, the binding energy profiles gradually shift to higher values, indicating a gradual saturation especially at the two minima.

3.4. *Binding free energy profile of TAP*

For the TAP-methanol system, the ΔG values gradually increase below $d_{NAC} < 25$ Å, except for a shallow local free energy minimum at $d_{NAC} \approx 6$ Å (Figure 3). This minimum is far from the productive binding site close to ^{acyl}Ser10 and His174 ($d_{NAC} = 2.75$ Å), where ΔG is positive (up to 5 k_BT), thus indicating an unfavorable interaction. The binding free energy profiles are similar for different substrate concentrations, indicating the absence of saturation. Thus, the ability to interact with methanol as a substrate in a productive orientation is exclusively found in CALB. The binding free energy profiles at different substrate concentrations act as a fingerprint of the interactions between enzymes and substrates. However, at lower concentrations such as 50 mM, the errors in the binding free energy profile increase, in particular at low d_{NAC} values, due to insufficient sampling because the number of substrate molecules and thus the frequency of binding events decrease.

4. Structural Analysis of Enzyme–Substrate Interactions

The binding free energy minima are preferred binding sites of the substrate methanol, and the corresponding frames with d_{NAC} value of interest are retrieved from the simulation trajectory and analyzed, thus selecting the few relevant frames out of the 10^5 frames of the set of simulations. The structural analysis of frames corresponding to productive binding ($d_{NAC} = 2.75 \pm 0.05$ Å) at 1 M for CALB and TAP shows major differences in how methanol and the acetyl moiety of the ^{acyl}Ser intermediate are positioned in the active sites of the two enzymes (Figure 4). In CALB, the methanol molecule is buried within the active site, with the hydroxyl group oriented toward the carbonyl carbon of the ^{acyl}Ser105 and the ε-nitrogen of His224;

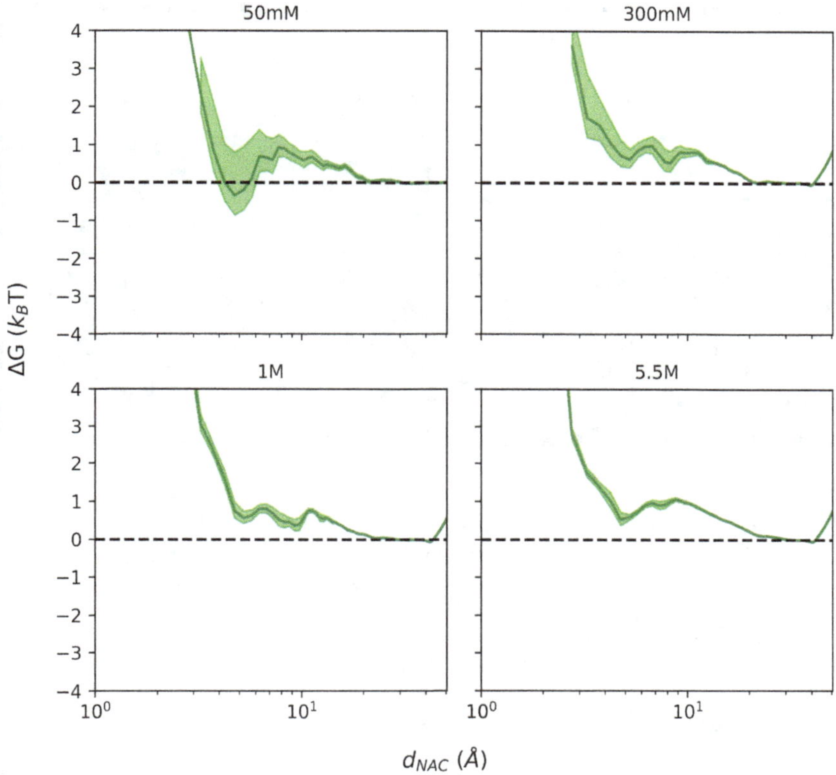

Fig. 3. Binding free energy profile (ΔG in k_BT units) of the TAP-methanol system as a function of d_{NAC}. Solid line and shaded regions correspond to mean value and standard error from 10 simulation replicas, respectively.

its methyl group is bound in the stereoselectivity pocket formed by ^{acyl}Ser105 and Trp104, and the carbonyl oxygen of ^{acyl}Ser105 points toward the oxyanion hole. In TAP, the hydroxyl moiety of methanol has a similar orientation as in CALB, but the methyl moiety is exposed toward the bulk, and the carbonyl oxygen of ^{acyl}Ser10 fails to be bound in the oxyanion hole. The unproductive binding of the acyl moiety in TAP might be caused by the short-chain acyl moiety, in accordance with the preference of TAP for long-chain fatty acid esters. For longer acyl chains, a stabilization of ^{acyl}Ser10 intermediate might occur by additional interactions along the fatty acid binding site, which might mediate the productive orientation of the carbonyl in the oxyanion hole.

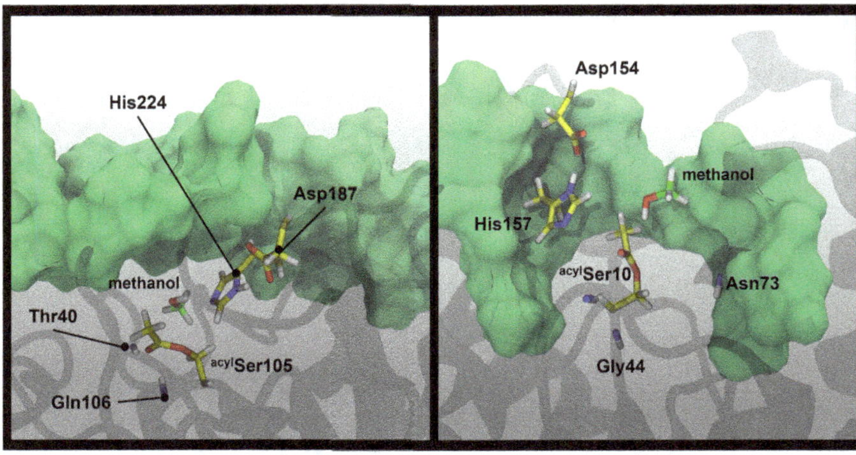

(a) (b)

Fig. 4. Details of the interactions between methanol and (a) CALB and (b) TAP. The protein backbone is shown in transparent gray cartoon, the protein surrounding the active site in green surface. Catalytic ^{acyl}Ser, His, and Asp residues are shown yellow and methanol in green licorice.

5. Methanol Binding Affinity

The binding affinity of CALB and TAP toward methanol at increasing methanol concentrations is determined by counting the number of molecules N_{mol} present in each spherical shell at d_{NAC} with a width of 1 Å. N_{mol} is obtained for each replicate and used to calculate the mean number of bound methanol molecules $\bar{N}$ and the corresponding standard deviations. The Langmuir adsorption model is used to derive the corresponding dissociation constant (K_D in M) and maximum number of absorbed molecules N_{max} [37] as follows:

$$N_{mol} = \frac{N_{max} \cdot [methanol]}{K_D + [methanol]} \tag{5}$$

Spherical shells with standard errors higher than 50% for K_D are discarded, and the values of K_D and N_{max} are plotted as a function of d_{NAC}.

The comparison of CALB and TAP reveals fundamental differences in the affinity of the two proteins toward methanol (Figure 5). CALB exhibits tight methanol binding at the active site (2 Å < d_{NAC} ≤ 3 Å) with

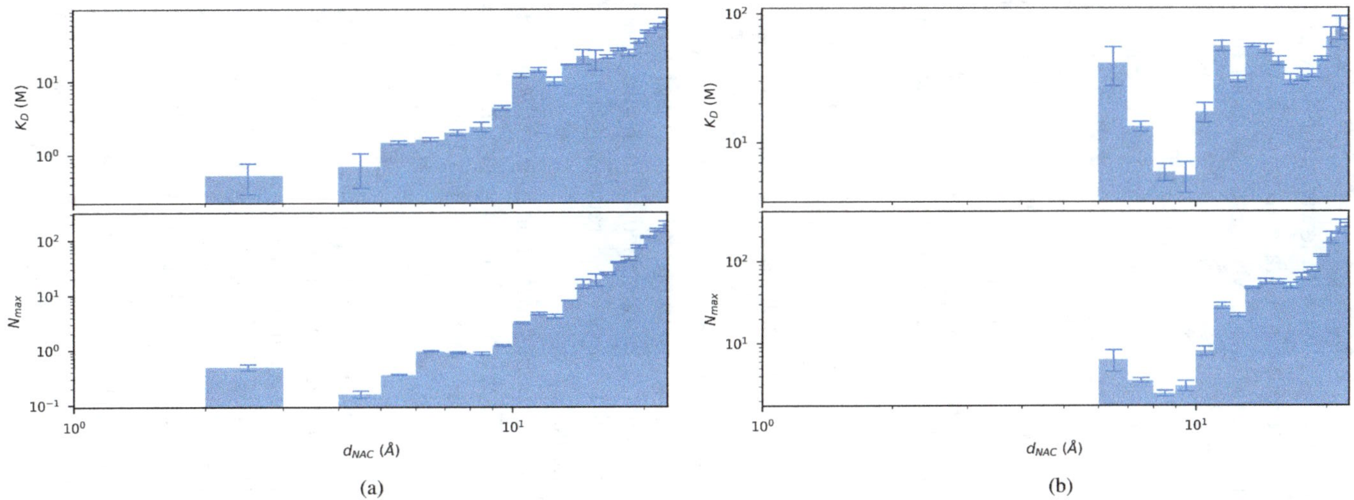

Fig. 5. Fitting of d_{NAC} values within the protein region to a Langmuir adsorption model for (a) CALB and (b) TAP. Fitted parameters K_{D} (top panel) and $N_{\max}$ (bottom panel) obtained from bins of 1 Å d_{NAC} values, error bars correspond standard errors.

submolar affinity (K_D = 0.5 ± 0.2 M, N_{max} = 0.5 ± 0.1) and binds to the binding pocket (6 Å < d_{NAC} ≤ 7 Å) with lower affinity (K_D = 1.6 ± 0.1 M, N_{max} = 0.9 ± 0.1). On the protein surface (d_{NAC} > 7 Å), the affinity for methanol is further reduced (K_D > 2 M) and the number of bound methanol molecules is increased (N_{max} > 0.9), due to the increasing binding area, which can accommodate a higher number of methanol molecules as compared to the narrow active site and binding pocket. In contrast, methanol binding to the active site cleft (d_{NAC} ≤ 6 Å) and surface (d_{NAC} > 7 Å) of TAP does not follow the Langmuir adsorption model (K_D > 10 M, except for a binding patch (8 Å < d_{NAC} ≤ 9 Å) with a low affinity (K_D = 2.4 ± 0.2 M, N_{max} = 6 ± 0.9). The absence of a measurable binding affinity toward methanol at the active site agrees with the absence of stabilizing interactions at the active site and adjacent regions, as shown above.

6. Methanol Interaction Hotspots

The identification of local minima in the binding free energy profiles provides valuable information to identify which regions of the protein interact with the substrate. By focused analysis of the trajectory frames corresponding to these energy minima, interaction hotspots are located, and structural determinants are identified, which are specific to each enzyme. These interaction hotspots also represent major targets for the design of protein variants.

For both enzymes, the frames corresponding to the global free energy minima (CALB: d_{NAC} = 2.75 ± 0.5 Å, TAP: d_{NAC} = 5 ± 0.5 Å) are extracted, superposed, and the three-dimensional density of methanol is calculated by using the density map tool MDAnalysis. The simulation box is considered as a cubic grid with a spacing of 1 Å, and the average number of molecules within each volume cell is calculated, resulting in a three-dimensional density map of methanol (in M). To ensure sufficient sampling (number of frames > 30), an isosurface at 1 M is calculated, which results from the analysis of 33726 frames for CALB and 14027 frames for TAP (Figure 6). CALB exhibits a methanol patch in the active site as well as within the substrate access channel (Trp104, Gly39, Gly41, Thr42), and TAP in the active site cleft. For both CALB and TAP, the remaining protein surface contains several interaction hotspots, indicating that, when methanol is bound at the site, concurrent binding events also take place away from the active site. For CALB, the occurrence of hotspots along the

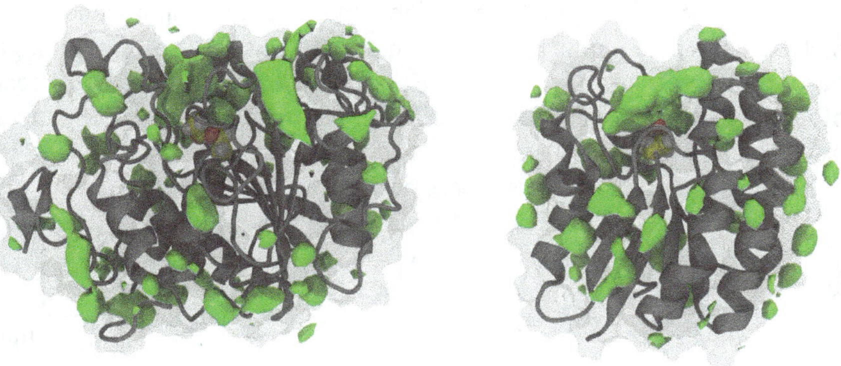

(a) (b)

Fig. 6. Interactions of methanol with (a) CALB and (b) TAP. Left panel: density map of methanol in isolated frames (CALB: $d_{NAC} = 2.75 \pm 0.05$ Å, TAP: $d_{NAC} = 5 \pm 0.05$ Å), with ^{acyl}Ser represented in yellow vdW representation, and methanol isosurface (22 M) in green.

substrate access channel favors the accumulation of methanol in this region, which causes inhibition of the enzyme at high concentrations of methanol [9].

7. Concluding Remarks

By examining the methanol concentration dependency of the binding profiles of CALB and TAP, specific features of the two enzymes are identified, providing a bridge between the microscopic properties of the modeled systems and the macroscopic properties of the enzymes. The calculated K_D of methanol in different regions of CALB and TAP surfaces allowed to distinguish between esterase-specific binding at the active site and substrate acces channel of CALB (esterase), but not in TAP (hydrolase). In CALB, methanol binding at the active site is stabilized by additional interactions with residues forming the substrate access channel, as well as oxyanion hole stabilization. On the other hand, in TAP, such stabilizing interactions do not occur as the active site cleft is small and exposed to the solvent, and therefore methanol is less prone to act as a substrate for the alcoholysis reaction.

The comparison of binding free energy profiles at different substrate concentrations is a valuable tool to develop a comprehensive understanding of enzymatic reactions by modeling approaches. The method has broad applicability. It cannot only be used for the investigation of different enzyme–substrate pairs but also for studying the effects of co-solvents, detergents, additives, or inhibitors. Concentration studies by molecular dynamics simulations are a valuable predictive tool for enzyme engineering and bioprocess design.

References

1. Hermann, J. C. *et al.* (2006). Predicting Substrates by Docking High-Energy Intermediates to Enzyme Structures. *J. Am. Chem. Soc.* 128, pp. 15882–15891.
2. Zhang, Y., Kua, J. and McCammon, J. A. (2003). Influence of Structural Fluctuation on Enzyme Reaction Energy Barriers in Combined Quantum Mechanical/Molecular Mechanical Studies. *J. Phys. Chem. B* 107, pp. 4459–4463.
3. Lodola, A. *et al.* (2010). Structural Fluctuations in Enzyme-Catalyzed Reactions: Determinants of Reactivity in Fatty Acid Amide Hydrolase from Multivariate Statistical Analysis of Quantum Mechanics/Molecular Mechanics Paths. *J. Chem. Theory Comput.* 6, pp. 2948–2960.
4. Ferrario, V., Fischer, M., Zhu, Y. and Pleiss, J. (2019). Modelling of Substrate Access and Substrate Binding to Cephalosporin Acylases. *Sci. Rep.* 9, pp. 1–13.
5. Fierke, C. A., Johnson, K. A. and Benkovic, S. J. (1987) Construction and Evaluation of the Kinetic Scheme Associated with Dihydrofolate Reductase from *Escherichia coli. Biochemistry* 26, pp. 4085–4092.
6. Lafaquière, V. *et al.* (2009) Control of Lipase Enantioselectivity by Engineering the Substrate Binding Site and Access Channel. *ChemBioChem* 10, pp. 2760–2771.
7. Pan, A. C., Xu, H., Palpant, T. and Shaw, D. E. (2017) Quantitative Characterization of the Binding and Unbinding of Millimolar Drug Fragments with Molecular Dynamics Simulations. *J. Chem. Theory Comput.* 13, pp. 3372–3377.
8. Ferrario, V. and Pleiss, J. (2019) Molecular Simulations of Enzymes under Non-natural Conditions. *Eur. Phys. J. Spec. Top.* 227, pp. 1631–1638.
9. Carvalho, H. F., Ferrario, V. and Pleiss, J. (2021) Molecular Mechanism of Methanol Inhibition in CALB-Catalyzed Alcoholysis: Analyzing Molecular Dynamics Simulations by a Markov State Model. *J. Chem. Theory Comput.* pp. acs.jctc.1c00559.
10. Bisswanger, H. (Wiley-VCH Verlag GmbH & Co. KGaA, 2017). *Enzyme Kinetics*.

11. Fedosov, S. N. *et al.* (2013) Kinetic Model of Biodiesel Production using Immobilized Lipase Candida Antarctica Lipase B. *J. Mol. Catal. B Enzym.* 85–86, pp. 156–168.
12. Lotti, M., Pleiss, J., Valero, F. and Ferrer, P. (2018) Enzymatic Production of Biodiesel: Strategies to Overcome Methanol Inactivation. *Biotechnol. J.* 13, pp. 1700155.
13. Grisewood, M. J. *et al.* (2017) Computational Redesign of Acyl-ACP Thioesterase with Improved Selectivity toward Medium-Chain-Length Fatty Acids. *ACS Catal.* 7, pp. 3837–3849.
14. Ortiz, C. *et al.* (2019) Novozym 435: The "perfect" Lipase Immobilized Biocatalyst? *Catal. Sci. Technol.* 9, pp. 2380–2420.
15. Grisewood, M. J. *et al.* (2017) Computational Redesign of Acyl-ACP Thioesterase with Improved Selectivity towards Medium-Chain Fatty Acids. *ACS Catal.* pp. acscatal.7b00408.
16. Lo, Y. C., Lin, S. C., Shaw, J. F. and Liaw, Y. C. (2003) Crystal Structure of Escherichia Coli Thioesterase I/protease I/lysophospholipase L1: Consensus Sequence Blocks Constitute the Catalytic Center of SGNH-hydrolases through a Conserved Hydrogen Bond Network. *J. Mol. Biol.* 330, pp. 539–551.
17. Fischer, M. and Pleiss, J. (2003) The Lipase Engineering Database: A Navigation and Analysis Tool for Protein Families. *Nucleic Acids Res.* 31, pp. 319–321.
18. Pleiss, J., Fischer, M. and Schmid, R. D. (1998) Anatomy of Lipase Binding Sites: The Scissile Fatty Acid Binding Site. *Chem. Phys. Lipids* 93, pp. 67–80.
19. Abraham, M. J. *et al.* (2015) GROMACS: High Performance Molecular Simulations through Multi-level Parallelism from Laptops to Super-computers. *SoftwareX* 1–2, pp. 19–25.
20. Bussi, G. *et al.* (2007) Canonical Sampling Through Velocity Rescaling. *J. Chem. Phys.* 126, pp. 014101.
21. Parrinello, M. and Rahman, A. (1981) Polymorphic transitions in single crystals: A New Molecular Dynamics Method. in *J. Appl. Phys.* 52, pp. 7182–7190.
22. Essmann, U. *et al.* (1995) A Smooth Particle Mesh Ewald Method. *J. Chem. Phys.* 103, pp. 8577–8593.
23. Stauch, B., Fisher, S. J. and Cianci, M. (2015) Open and Closed States of Candida Antarctica Lipase B: Protonation and the Mechanism of Interfacial Activation. *J. Lipid Res.* 56, pp. 2348–2358.
24. Berendsen, H. J. C., Grigera, J. R. and Straatsma, T. P. (1987) The Missing Term in Effective Pair Potentials. *J. Phys. Chem.* 91, pp. 6269–6271.
25. Ferrario, V. and Pleiss, J. (2018) Simulation of Protein Diffusion: A Sensitive Probe of Protein-Solvent Interactions. *J. Biomol. Struct. Dyn.* 37(6), pp. 1534–1544.

26. Jorgensen, W. L. and Tirado-rives, J. (1988) The OPLS Potential Functions for Proteins. Energy Minimizations for Crystals of Cyclic Peptides and Crambin. *J. Am. Chem. Soc.* 110, pp. 1657–1666.
27. Kulschewski, T. and Pleiss, J. (2013) A Molecular Dynamics Study of Liquid Aliphatic Alcohols: Simulation of Density and Self-diffusion Coefficient Using a Modified OPLS Force Field. *Mol. Simul.* 39, pp. 754–767.
28. Escorcia, A. M., Sen, K., Daza, M. C., Doerr, M. and Thiel, W. (2017) Quantum Mechanics/Molecular Mechanics Insights into the Enantio-selectivity of the O-Acetylation of (R,S)-Propranolol Catalyzed by Candida Antarctica Lipase B. *ACS Catal.* 7, pp. 115–127.
29. Mathews, I. *et al.* (2007) Structure of a Novel Enzyme that Catalyzes Acyl Transfer to Alcohols in Aqueous Conditions. *Biochemistry* 46, pp. 8969–8979.
30. Dodda, L. S., Vilseck, J. Z., Tirado-Rives, J. and Jorgensen, W. L. (2017) 1.14*CM1A-LBCC: Localized Bond-Charge Corrected CM1A Charges for Condensed-Phase Simulations. *J. Phys. Chem. B* 121, pp. 3864–3870.
31. Dodda, L. S., Cabeza de Vaca, I., Tirado-Rives, J. and Jorgensen, W. L. (2017) LigParGen Web Server: An Automatic OPLS-AA Parameter Generator for Organic Ligands. *Nucleic Acids Res.* 45, pp. W331–W336.
32. Jorgensen, W. L. and Tirado-Rives, J. (2005) Potential Energy Functions for Atomic-level Simulations of Water and Organic and Biomolecular Systems. *Proc. Natl. Acad. Sci.* 102, pp. 6665–6670.
33. Bruice, T. C. and Lightstone, F. C. (1999) Ground State and Transition State Contributions to the Rates of Intramolecular and Enzymatic Reactions. *Acc. Chem. Res.* 32, pp. 127–136.
34. Ankins, P. W. and DePaula, J. (2011). *Physical Chemistry for the Life Sciences*. W. H. Freeman and Company, New York.
35. Gowers, R. *et al.* (2016). MDAnalysis: A Python Package for the Rapid Analysis of Molecular Dynamics Simulations. *J. Comput. Chem.* 32, pp. 98–105.
36. Michaud-Agrawal, N., Denning, E. J., Woolf, T. B. and Beckstein, O. (2011) MDAnalysis: A Toolkit for the Analysis of Molecular Dynamics Simulations. *J. Comput. Chem.* 32, pp. 2319–2327.
37. Markham, E. C. and Benton, A. F. (1931) The Adsorption of Gas Mixtures by Silica. *J. Am. Chem. Soc.* 53, pp. 497–507.

https://doi.org/10.1142/9789811261664_0010

Chapter 10

Peptide-based Artificial Metalloenzymes by Design

Ornella Maglio[†], Marco Chino[*], Daniele D'Alonzo[*], Linda Leone[*], Flavia Nastri[*], and Angela Lombardi[*,‡]

[*]Department of Chemical Sciences, University of Napoli Federico II, Napoli, Italy
[†]IBB, National Research Council, Napoli, Italy

[‡]alombard@unina.it

1. Introduction

Metalloproteins are involved in a variety of functions crucial for life, such as electron transfer, dioxygen binding, storage and activation, and energy production [1]. In contrast, the number of utilized metal-based prosthetic groups is relatively small, and similar metal cofactors are able to perform different functions [2,3]. Metalloprotein activity arises from a strong partnership between the protein matrix and the metal cofactor: the metal ion endows protein with an array of chemical properties, while the protein stabilizes it in solution and directs its reactivity toward a unique and distinct path. Indeed, through specific interactions, ranging from coordinate and hydrogen bond, to hydrophobic and ionic interactions, the protein matrix finely tunes the metal cofactor properties, such as the ability of switching among various redox and coordination states, thus producing different chemistries and functions [2]. The way this occurs at the molecular level is very fascinating and, in some cases, still unclear [4].

The development of metalloenzyme mimics has emerged as a significant approach to shed light on this phenomenon and to obtain artificial biocatalysts with improved or new functions with respect to their natural counterparts [5–21]. Small molecule-based synthetic mimics have been and still represent a benchmark for understanding structure–function relationship in metalloproteins [22–32]. They are quite accurate in reproducing the metal ion first coordination sphere and its spectroscopic behaviors, by mimicking those ligands directly interacting with the central metal ion. However, similar success has not been achieved with functionality. The results on these mimics clearly demonstrated that reproducing metalloenzyme performance requires ligands with increasing levels of complexity around the metal site, able to generate second sphere interactions, often crucial in assisting catalysis. One of the most feasible solutions to this multifaceted problem is to use peptide-based ligands, as they seem good candidates to mimic the behaviors of the natural metal ion environment.

This chapter, by reviewing the published literature in the last two decades, illustrates the efforts made for reproducing metalloenzyme activities in artificial systems, by using peptide-based scaffolds. We first discuss the advantages of using peptides and small proteins to capture metalloenzymes behaviors. Then we highlight the power of peptides for metalloenzyme design, relatively to both synthetic and structural facets. Finally, we analyze several case studies, organized according to the peptide scaffolds that house different metal ion coordination environments, such as hemes and/or metalloporphyrins, mononuclear and dinuclear metal-binding sites. The power of the selected examples in reproducing key biological functions of native metalloenzymes, or even in catalyzing reactions still unknown to nature, is highlighted.

2. Capturing Metalloprotein Behaviors in Artificial Molecules: The Option of Peptide Scaffolds

Efforts to capture metalloenzyme behaviors into artificial molecules have been undertaken with the aim of providing insights for structure–activity relationships and understanding the minimal requirements for function. Starting from the construction of simple structural mimics, the use of peptide-based scaffolds and the insertion of further levels of complexity around the metal ion site have enabled the development of artificial metalloenzymes with fine-tuned and broad activities.

Why peptides-based scaffolds are good candidates for developing metalloprotein mimics? Peptides offer numerous advantages, by combining the simplicity of small molecules and the complexity of protein structures. They simultaneously have sufficient size and chemical diversity to allow the construction of catalytic and functional metal-sites, thus recreating the natural metal cofactor environment. Further, they can be routinely, reliably and quickly prepared with good yields, through automated-chemical synthesis and/or recombinant methods [33–39].

Peptide fragments can be designed with defined structures. Recent design strategies [7–9,40–43] and computational tools [44–50] allow obtaining peptide-based molecules with precise three-dimensional folds and are often able to tolerate substantial changes in the sequence. Thus, peptides can be very useful in reproducing the geometrical arrangements of the ligands in the metal-binding site. In this respect, some metal-binding sites are rather easy to mimic. For instance, in heme enzymes, where the metal ion is firmly held in the porphyrin ring, the designed peptide should embrace the macrocycle, granting the active site with additional first and second coordination sphere ligands, thus fine-tuning its catalytic and redox behaviors [7,51–53]. In more elaborate active sites, such as in metalloenzymes containing dinuclear metal-binding sites with bridging ligands, the structural preferences of the designed peptides should assure geometrically specific metal binding and activity [8,54]. In this respect, to obtain a functional metalloenzyme mimic, many variables should be simultaneously considered and satisfied: (i) the correct fold of the peptide chain; and (ii) the coordination requirements of the metal ion. Thus, the full control over the structure of both the peptide-based scaffold and the metal site is required to introduce functionality into an artificial molecule. Further, one of the most difficult conditions to reproduce is the delicate balance between protein conformational stability and metal ion site flexibility [54]. These demanding tasks can be achieved by using designed peptides.

2.1. *Peptides as scaffolds for artificial metalloenzyme design: Synthesis, structural properties and design strategies*

Over the last decades, the field of peptide chemistry has been significantly revitalized by virtue of several technological improvements. The growing knowledge in peptide chemistry enables us to address many relevant tasks. It is now possible to construct peptide-based molecules that

(i) self-assemble in a defined and programmable manner, giving rise to targeted three-dimensional structures; (ii) accommodate recognition and catalytic sites in their structure, thus recapitulating the key features of naturally evolved enzymes; and (iii) fulfill a definite function.

Advances in peptide chemical synthesis [33–36] and recombinant methods [37–39] allow for peptides and small proteins to be generated with a variety of chemical modifications, including the incorporation of non-proteinogenic amino acids (NPAAs) (Figure 1), as well as modifications of the peptide backbone (acetylation [55], phosphorylation [56], methylation [57], glycosylation [58,59]). Recent efforts in orthogonal translation system improvement, combined with the application of genetically recoded organisms, have enabled the production of recombinant proteins with single or multiple site-specifically incorporated NPAAs [39,60,61]. However, the repertoire of NPAAs that can be incorporated in proteins through recombinant techniques is still limited, and chemical synthesis can offer a valuable alternative solution [35,36]. The introduction of NPAAs into peptides may be particularly useful for boosting the properties of the final molecule [62].

For instance, D-amino acids and/or β- and γ-amino acids (Figure 1(a)) can have a substantial effect on the half-life of peptides, decreasing the binding affinity of proteolytic enzymes and increasing peptide stability [63,64]. C$\alpha\alpha$-alkylated amino acids in peptides, such as α-amino isobutyric acid (Aib) (Figure 1(b)), significantly reduce the flexibility of the backbone and can act as a promoter and stabilizer of helical structures [65,66], thus influencing the three-dimensional structure of the molecule, and consequently its function [67]. Finally, the incorporation of NPAAs has revealed a valuable approach for the design of functional metal-binding sites (Figure 1(c)). Several laboratories have explored their use in metalloprotein design and have shown their utility to tune metal-binding properties [68–73]. The use of NPAAs is devised to (i) probe the effect of individual amino acids on the protein structure and function; (ii) help in understanding the protein structure-function relationships [72,73]; (iii) add novel chemical functional groups in proteins, thus generating molecules with new properties [72]; and (iv) offer new solutions for the design of high-affinity metal-binding sites by substituting flexible side-chain ligands with unnatural chelating side chains [69].

Chemical modifications of the peptide sequence, besides influencing the chemical stability and expanding the sets of ligands for the design of metal-binding sites, can significantly modify the conformational

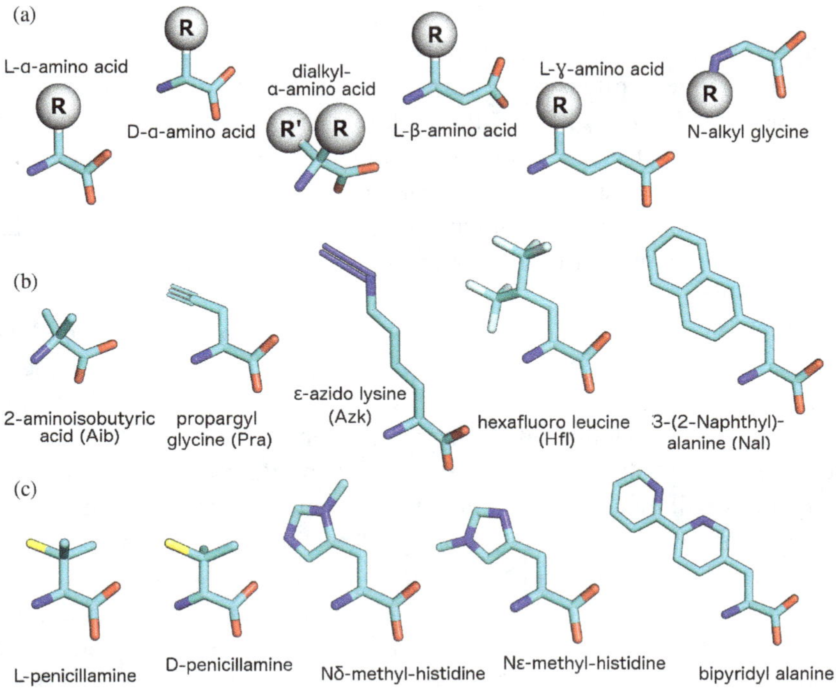

Fig. 1. Non-proteinogenic amino acids (NPAAs) in peptides. (a) Main chain structures of selected amino acids, as building blocks in peptides. (b) Structure-inducing NPAAs, useful for driving specific main-chain conformation, structure-tethering/stapling by click chemistry and enhancing hydrophobic or π stacking interactions. (c) Metal-binding NPAAs. The structures were generated with PyMOL (PyMOL Molecular Graphics System, version 1.7.4; Schrödinger).

properties of the molecule. This is an important aspect for the development of functional molecules. The propensity of a peptide to adopt a precise secondary structure, such as α-helix, β-strand and/or turn, as well as a defined tertiary structure, is ultimately dictated by its amino acid sequence. Thus, the accurate selection of amino acids can drive toward a desired 'structural element'.

Nowadays, for some structural elements, we have good "rules" that relate primary sequence and conformation, and this finding allows constructing complex peptide structures [40,44–46,74,75]. By replicating and recombining in precise patterns a set of these small stable structural elements, well-defined folding and structural motifs can be achieved [40,76].

Further, the self-assembly of these building blocks can generate more complex molecular architectures [47].

Tailor-made peptides offer great potential for the design of artificial functional metalloenzymes, as they allow a high level of structural and functional control over a metal-binding site. Several strategies and approaches allow shaping peptide structure and flexibility to tune reactivity. Indeed, subtle conformational changes may be necessary for metal ions to cycle among various oxidation states and for functional groups to assist catalysis.

Functional artificial metalloenzymes can be rationally designed taking inspiration from natural protein of known structure. In this respect, miniaturization is a suitable strategy to build the minimal peptide sequence, which contains sufficient information for proper folding and for an accurate reconstruction of the active site structure [77,78]. Using this approach, small metalloporphyrin-peptide conjugates have been designed and demonstrated to possess a variety of catalytic properties, including peroxidase [71], peroxygenase [79] or hydrogen evolution activities [80,81]. Further, this strategy was revealed to be valuable for developing biomimetic structures resembling iron-sulfur centers [77]. Functional peptides and small proteins have been successfully developed through *de novo* design [8–12,82,83]. In its purest and most challenging form, *de novo* design involves the construction of a polypeptide sequence, which is not directly related to any natural protein, intended to fold into a well-defined three-dimensional structure and to incorporate a metal cofactor into a precise geometry. The power of this approach is that the structure can be systematically varied and screened for different functions. Further, it allows inserting metal-binding sites into protein scaffolds, which are completely unrelated to the natural ones [82,84–89].

As an alternative approach, the functional properties of natural metalloproteins can be repurposed or enhanced by rational redesign [5,15,90,91]. This approach entails a careful choice of the scaffold, which should tolerate the mutations required for the construction of the desired metal-binding site. This strategy has been also used to insert catalytically competent metal-cofactors into native protein scaffolds, thus obtaining hybrid catalysts [20,92]. Finally, peptide fragments or small proteins can be designed to interact, thus affording supramolecular assembly [47]. This approach has been revealed to be very powerful for the development of artificial metalloenzymes endowed with functional complexity. All these strategies take advantages of computational algorithms and directed evolution approaches to introduce mutations and generate variants to be screened for activity [40,44–49,93].

3. Peptide Scaffolds Housing Hemes and Metalloporphyrins

A considerable amount of work in the design of artificial metalloenzymes has been devoted to the construction of peptide-based systems resembling structure and function of heme-enzymes [5,6,52,53].

These enzymes are a fascinating example of the effect of the protein matrix in tuning the chemistry of a single cofactor, the heme, to access a wide range of reactivity [1,6,52,53]. For example, in peroxidases and catalases, the protein matrix modulates the heme ability to process H_2O_2 in either selective substrate oxidation or in hydrogen peroxide dismutation, respectively. Efforts have been initially aimed at identifying the key factors allowing heme to selectively perform one process over the other, by designing small peptide sequences embracing the macrocycle and providing first and second coordination sphere interactions. Subsequently, more sophisticated properly folded peptide scaffolds have been conceived to improve and even expand the catalytic properties of heme-peroxidases.

Umezawa and coworkers prepared synthetic peptide-porphyrin conjugates, made up of small amino acid sequences covalently linked to the porphyrin ring, to probe the effect of charged residues on pathway selectivity, between catalase and peroxidase-like reactions [94]. Covalent linkage between metalloporphyrin and peptides was achieved by Cu-catalyzed click coupling between 5-azido-3-pyridyl groups, located at the meso positions of the porphyrin, and several propiolic acid N-capped peptides. Upon selecting scrambled sequences of Gly, Lys, Glu, His, or Cit (Citrulline), the peptide-Mn-porphyrin conjugates were assayed as artificial catalase and/or peroxidase mimics. Interestingly, a suitable choice of the amino acid residues moved the catalytic activity from catalase to peroxidase. In particular, Glu or His residues favored peroxidase activity, whereas the positively charged Lys-Gly-Cit-NH_2 sequence drove toward catalase activity.

The role of peptide sequences in providing several key interactions for heme peroxidase-like activity has been deeply investigated by the use of Microperoxidases (MPs). MPs derive from the proteolytic digestion of cytochrome *c*, in which the heme is covalently linked to the peptide chain through two thioether bonds [95]. MPs can be considered simplified peroxidase models, as they hold a His residue acting as the iron proximal ligand and an open catalytic site, freely accessible to both hydrogen peroxide (the natural oxidant in peroxidases) and organic substrates. However, they lack a distal site that is known to assist H_2O_2 activation during catalysis. In order to study the role of second-coordination sphere interactions in the catalytic properties of these heme-peptide conjugates, Monzani and coworkers studied a series of synthetic derivatives of MPs [96], by covalently elongating the N-terminal amino group of MP8 with one or two proline residues [97]. These derivatives exhibited a greatly enhanced catalytic activity in the H_2O_2-mediated oxidation of *p*-cresol, estimated by comparing the second-order rate constants k_1 (e.g., pH 9, MP8: k_1 13,300 $M^{-1}s^{-1}$; Pro-MP8, k_1 13,500 $M^{-1}s^{-1}$; Pro_2-MP8: k_1 17,500 $M^{-1}s^{-1}$). This suggested a marked contribution of positively charged Pro N-terminus in assisting H_2O_2-mediated catalysis, e.g., promoting the cleavage of hydrogen peroxide. As negative control, Pro-MP8 protected as Fmoc carbamate exhibited a reduced catalytic activity (Fmoc-Pro-MP8, k_1 5,300 $M^{-1}s^{-1}$). In a subsequent work, the oxidation of 4-(2-aminoethyl)-phenol (tyramine) and 3-(4-hydroxyphenyl)propionic acid (HPA) was performed by a number of MPs, obtained either by tryptic digestion or by chemical synthesis [98]. Comparative data indicated that protection of terminal functionalities of MP8 with aromatic Fmoc and Mtr groups enhanced the affinity in substrate binding, leading to lower K_m values; however, the same groups contributed in reducing the k_{cat} of the reactions.

A longstanding approach developed by our research group relies on the design of miniaturized heme-enzymes, named Mimochromes (MCs, Figure 2) [5–7,52,53]. As summarized in the previous paragraph, miniaturization is a structure-guided design of artificial enzymes, which own the minimal peptide sequence necessary for reproducing the activity of the parent native enzymes [77,78].

Based on a detailed analysis of the structure of the β-chain F helix fragment of human deoxyhemoglobin [99], MCs were conceived as composed of two small α-helical peptide chains, covalently bound to a deuteroporphyrin through its propionic acid functionalities [100]. The coordination of one or two His axial ligands to the metal center and the presence of ion-pair interchain interactions were devised to stabilize a sandwich structure containing a helix–heme–helix motif [5,6,52,53]. Starting from bis-His hexacoordinated, structurally defined but

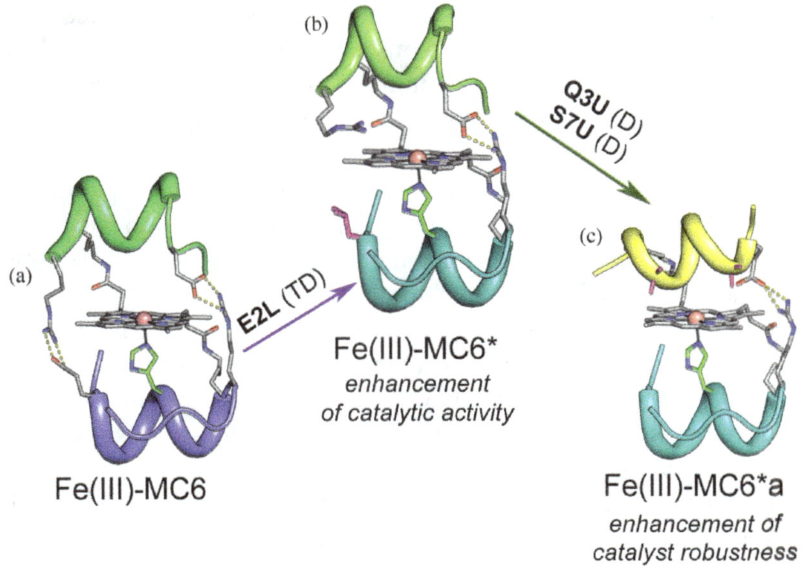

Fig. 2. Miniaturized heme-enzymes: Mimochromes. (a) Computational model of MC6, showing the tetradecapeptide (TD) that bears the His axial ligand, and the decapeptide (D) that lacks metal-coordinating residues. (b) Computational model of MC6*. The E2L mutation in the TD chain of MC6 is illustrated. (c) Computational model of MC6*a, showing the two Aib residues inserted into the D chain. (Adapted with permission from Ref. [5]. Copyright 2019 Elsevier. The structures were generated using PyMOL (PyMOL Molecular Graphics System, version 1.7.4; Schrödinger).

catalytically inactive prototype molecules [101–104], subsequent rounds of design were aimed at engineering functionality in the optimized scaffold. The first round of redesign afforded Mimochrome VI (MC6, Figure 2(a)), which mimics the asymmetry of natural proteins in both primary and secondary coordination spheres [105]. MC6 was characterized by a tetradecapeptide (*TD*) chain, bearing the His axial ligand, while a second decapeptide (*D*) chain lacks the coordinating residue, thereby creating a substrate-binding pocket on the heme distal side. Differently from its predecessors, MC6 demonstrated the ability to activate H_2O_2, thus catalyzing the oxidation of ABTS (2,2′-azino-bis(3-ethylbenzothiazoline-6-sulfonic acid)) as substrate. Despite the relative structural simplicity of the peptide scaffold, the catalytic efficiency of MC6 is comparable (k_{cat}/K_m 4.4 × 10^6 $M^{-1}s^{-1}$) to that of the natural peroxidase HRP (Horseradish peroxidase: k_{cat}/K_m 3.8 ×

10^6 $M^{-1}s^{-1}$) [105]. In subsequent studies, mutations were introduced in the MC6 scaffold to explore the effects of second-shell interactions [106] and of conformational constraints [71] in tuning catalysis. A E2L mutation in the TD chain afforded Mimochrome VI* (MC6*, Figure 2(b)), whose Fe(III) derivative displayed a four-fold enhancement in the catalytic efficiency of ABTS oxidation with respect to MC6 (k_{cat}/K_m 1.6×10^7 $M^{-1}s^{-1}$) [106]. The further incorporation of two non-proteinogenic, helix-inducing Aib residues in the D chain of MC6* produced an even more robust and active scaffold, Mimochrome VI*a [71] (MC6*a, Figure 2(c)). Indeed, Fe(III)-MC6*a displays a 20-fold higher catalytic efficiency than natural HRP in the same model reaction (k_{cat}/K_m 6.4×10^7 M^{-1} s^{-1}). Very recently, the FeMC6*a proficiency in catalyzing the luminol oxidation and further light emission was employed to develop a batch assay for H_2O_2 determination [107].

MC6*a resulted in a versatile scaffold toward metal replacement [53]. By swapping iron to cobalt, an electrocatalyst for hydrogen-evolution reactions in water was obtained [80,81] capable of catalyzing the reaction with a turnover number (TON) exceeding 230,000. Replacement of iron with manganese afforded Mn(III)-MC6*a, which exhibits an interesting catalytic activity through a direct oxygen-transfer pathway, in the oxidation of a variety of aryl thioethers [79]. Furthermore, Mn(III)-MC6*a promotes the selective oxidation of indole at its C3 position, leading to a 3-oxindole derivative (2-TFE-3-oxindole) with unprecedented product selectivity (86% at pH 8.5) compared to native or artificial heme-enzymes [108].

Finally, Fe(III)-MCs have been successfully conjugated to gold nanoparticles (AuNPs) and/or immobilized onto electrode surfaces, with redox properties and peroxidase activity being preserved upon conjugation [109–112]. All these results demonstrate the power of structurally defined minimal peptide sequences in tuning metalloporphyrin activity, thus resembling the role of native protein scaffolds.

Subsequently, Venanzi and coworkers exploited conformationally constrained peptides for developing hemeprotein mimics. Following a similar Mimochrome design approach, a biomimetic peroxidase ($FemP(10N)_2$) was obtained by conjugation of a Fe(III)-mesoporphyrin with two α-helical decapeptides [113]. In this case, the presence of six Aib residues in each peptide sequence was conceived to provide high helical propensity of the chains, while coordinating Glu residues replaced proximal His of native heme-enzymes. $FemP(10N)_2$ was able to promote the oxidation of both D- and L-DOPA to dopaquinone, with a weak stereoselectivity for the L-isomer and a moderate catalytic efficiency (k_{cat}/K_m up to 5.31×10^5 $M^{-1}s^{-1}$).

Increasing the complexity of the peptide moieties around the porphyrin enables the insertion of additional interactions that may affect activity. To this end, *de novo* design has been successfully used for the construction of heme-enzyme models. In most cases, α-helical coiled coils, and especially four-helix bundles, have been identified as suitable peptide scaffolds, for the incorporation of heme or, generally, metalloporphyrins [6,7]. As an example, our group exploited this structural motif in the design of MiniPeroxidase 3 (MP3) (Figure 3) [114].

Inspired by the heme-binding motif of bacterioferritin (BFR), this new hemeprotein model was developed by covalently linking deuteroporphyrin to two different peptide chains, to obtain an asymmetric helix-loop-helix/heme/helix-loop-helix (α2-heme-α2) sandwich arrangement. Similar to globins and peroxidases, the Fe(III) ion in MP3 is penta-coordinated with a His residue on one chain acting as an axial ligand. A distal

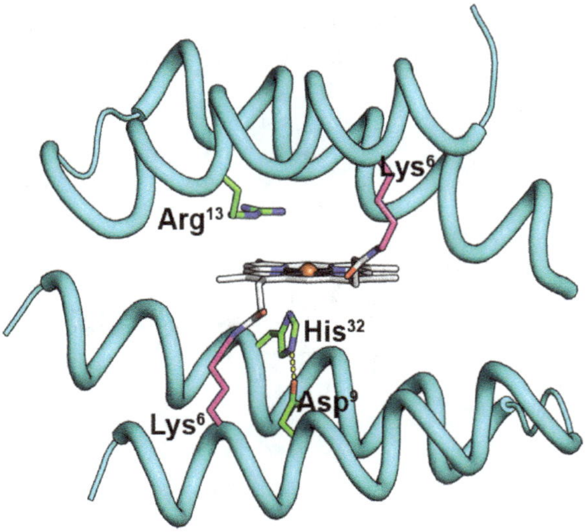

Fig. 3. Molecular model of Fe(III)-MP3 with key residues depicted as sticks: the His[32]–coordinating residue and the hydrogen-bonded Asp[9] residue on the proximal site, the catalytic Arg[13] residue on the distal site and the heme group, which is covalently linked to the peptide chains through the side chain of two lysine residues. The structures were generated using PyMOL (PyMOL Molecular Graphics System, version 1.7.4; Schrödinger).

site, designed to accommodate exogenous ligands or substrates, holds an Arg residue, which may assist the activation of hydrogen peroxide as in HRP [115]. When evaluated in the H_2O_2-mediated oxidation of ABTS, Fe(III)-MP3 showed a catalytic efficiency (k_{cat}/K_m 1.57 × 10^6 $M^{-1}s^{-1}$), comparable to that of polyhistidine-tagged recombinant R38A-HRP (k_{cat}/K_m 1.65 × 10^6 $M^{-1}s^{-1}$), while it was lower with respect to the native enzyme [114].

Recently, Anderson and coworkers used the four-helix bundle motif to develop heme-binding protein based on artificial maquettes [12]. Maquettes (French word for scale model) are four-helix bundles, first designed by Dutton and coworkers, which were demonstrated to function as electron-transfer or oxygen carrier proteins, upon insertion of heme and/or other types of redox-active cofactors [116,117]. Remarkably, Anderson's group established that maquettes can be recognized and modified by the post-translational cytochrome *c* maturation system of *E. coli* for covalent incorporation of the heme cofactor *in vivo*, affording the "*c*-type cytochrome maquettes" (CTMs) [118] (Figure 4). Starting from a non-catalytic CTM, a mono-histidine peroxidase-like heme active site was introduced through a simple design process, based on three amino acid mutations, which were conceived to restrict conformational flexibility, improve the hydrophobic core packing and remove one heme ligand [119]. The resulting enzyme,

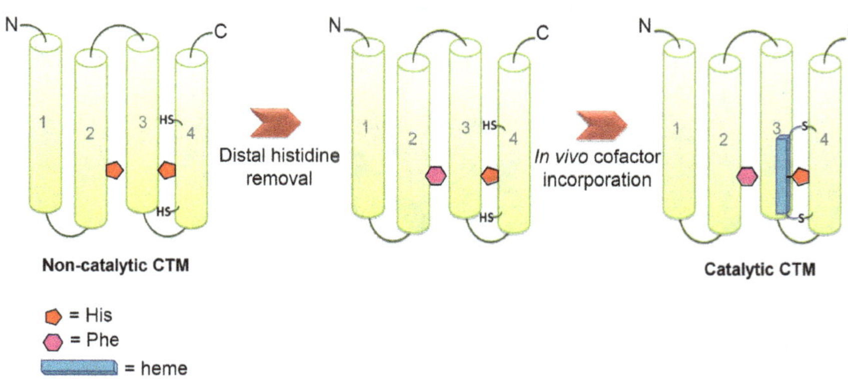

Fig. 4. Schematic representation of design strategy for *c*-type cytochrome maquettes (CTMs). Starting from a non-catalytic CTM, the mutation of the distal heme *c*-ligating His ligand results in the mono-His ligated C45. The corresponding *in vivo* incorporation of the cofactor yielded the corresponding heme protein, endowed with catalytic properties. Reprinted with permission from Ref. [6]. Copyright 2018 Wiley Periodicals, Inc.

named C45, displays peroxidase-like activity in ABTS oxidation (k_{cat}/K_m 3.2×10^6 $M^{-1}s^{-1}$). In addition, C45 is stable at high temperatures, in the presence of organic solvents, and retains its catalytic activity at 70°C close to its denaturation temperature (86°C). C45 also catalyzes the oxidation of a variety of other substrates, including guaiacol, luminol, *o*-phenylenediamine, *p*-anisidine, 5-aminosalycilic acid, 2,4,6-trichlorophenol and its brominated and fluorinated analogs, as resulting from the lack of a rationally designed substrate recognition site [119].

In a recent excellent work, the catalytic activity of C45 has been extended to abiotic transformations, including the stereoselective transfer of carbenes to olefins, aldehydes and amines, as well as the use of carbene-based catalysis for ring-expansion of pyrroles, even in whole cells [120] (Figure 5). Despite the growing number of artificial metalloenzymes involved in non-natural catalysis, especially acting as carbene transferases [20], C45 represents the earliest example of a *de novo* protein catalyzing abiotic reactions. Interestingly, the capability of this artificial metalloenzyme

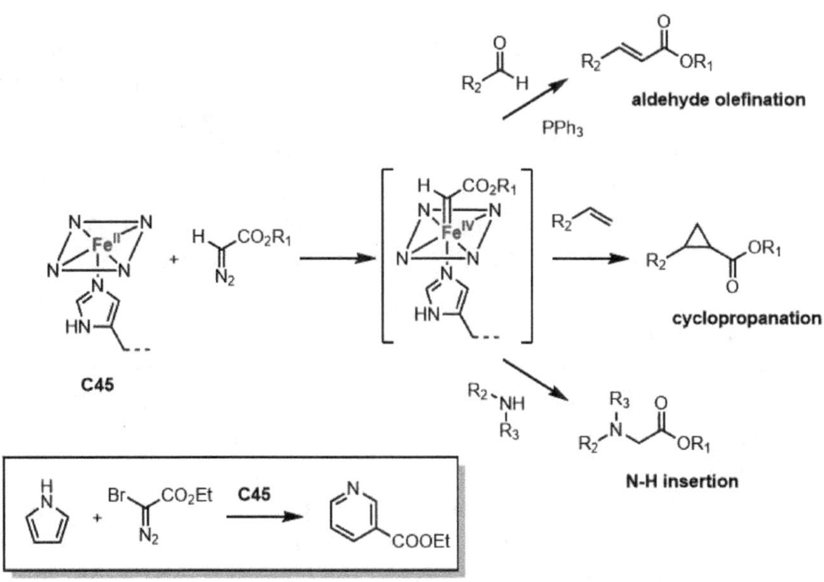

Fig. 5. Abiotic catalysis promoted by C45, including aldehyde olefination, olefin cyclopropanation and amine N–H insertion reactions. The common heme-based metallocarbenoid intermediate is reported in square brackets. The pyrrole ring-expansion reaction is highlighted.

to function *in vivo* has important perspectives in the development of engineered biosynthetic pathways within living organisms.

In the area of *de novo* proteins with a four-helix bundle fold, Hecht and coworkers developed a different approach, identifying catalytically active *de novo* proteins from a combinatorial library. In particular, they exploited the binary patterning of polar and non-polar amino acids, to drive peptide sequences to fold into four-helix bundles [83].

The majority of the *de novo* binary-patterned proteins was found to bind the heme cofactor, and a substantial amount of the resulting heme-containing proteins displayed peroxidase-like activity in ABTS oxidation, albeit with limited efficiency [121,122]. When exposed to immobilized heme on gold electrode surface, the peroxidase activity of one protein approached that of HRP [123]. In addition, such *de novo* heme-enzymes were used as starting materials for laboratory-based evolution [124]. Random mutagenesis experiments, followed by color-based screening of a relatively small number (hundreds or thousands) of variants, yielded novel sequences with improved peroxidase activity (3-fold enhancement compared to the parental sequence).

While *de novo* design of heme-proteins using α-helical structures has been highly successful, the use of β-sheets or β-strands as peptide scaffolds has been long overlooked, as the chemical stability of these structures may often be affected by heterogeneous aggregation or amyloid formation processes [125–127]. However, the development of model systems containing β-sheet structures has considerably increased our understanding of the design rules for making stable, well-folded and soluble β-sheet systems [128,129], thus drawing increasing interest in view of potential applications in metalloprotein design. In this context, Bhattacharjya and coworkers succeeded in designing membrane- and water-soluble peptides adopting defined β-hairpin or β-sheet structures, which were able to efficiently bind heme [130–134]. In early studies, the structural and functional characterizations of designed β-hairpin octapeptides (IV8 and IV8FA) were described in dodecylphosphocholine (DPC) detergent micelles [130] . Both peptides contained a ^{D}Pro-Gly segment for the nucleation of type I′ or type II′ β-turn. Studies revealed that the β-turn of the hairpin was located in proximity to the micelle head groups, whereas the residues at the β-strands were positioned into the hydrophobic milieu of the micelles. The interfacial localization of the β-turn residues was suggested to be responsible for the facile His-heme coordination and thereby for peroxidase activity toward tetramethylbenzidine (TMB), which was comparable to that of more complex designed proteins [135].

In subsequent studies, slightly longer peptides (19–26 residues) were employed, adopting four- or six-stranded β-sheet topologies, and ligating up to two hemes through *bis*-His coordination between adjacent antiparallel β-strands (Figure 6).

All the designed peptides contained ω-amino acids, for optimizing a high-affinity heme-binding pocket in the adjacent β-strands. The four-stranded peptides were found to bind a single heme inside a hydrophobic binding pocket in an aqueous environment, with a binding affinity comparable to that of naturally occurring heme proteins (K_D values down to pM range) [133]. Recently, the same authors designed and characterized water-soluble mini-proteins (<40 amino acids). These proteins were able to fold into multi-stranded antiparallel β-sheet structures, and coordinate multiple hemes either by stacking or sideways, thus mimicking naturally occurring multi-heme protein conduits [131]. The designed proteins displayed peroxidase activity in ABTS oxidation, with catalytic efficiencies (k_{cat}/K_m values up to 4.35×10^7 $M^{-1}s^{-1}$) inversely correlating with the binding affinity [132].

In the last decade, the application of peptides in materials science has been also explored [136]. In this respect, the engineering of

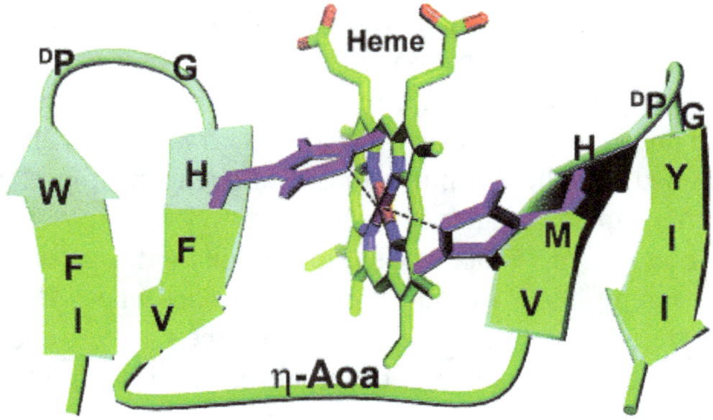

Fig. 6. Model structure of a *de novo* designed β-sheet mini-protein binding heme with peroxidase-like activity. The side chains of the two axial ligands coordinating heme are shown as sticks. Reprinted with permission from Ref. [132]. Published by The Royal Society of Chemistry.

peptide-based biomaterials endowed with functionality is a very demanding task. Along these lines, Fry and coworkers attempted to merge the utility of peptide-based biomaterials with the reactivity of the heme group for the development of functional materials [137]. By starting on self-assembling amphiphile peptides, mutations into the sequences allowed the authors to obtain different coordination environments around the heme. A strong relation between morphology and coordination of non-covalently linked heme *b* was found, the latter spanning from low-spin, *bis*-histidine ligation in micelles up to high-spin, single-histidine coordination in fibers. Further, the heme-containing peptide assemblies were shown to bind carbon monoxide and catalyze peroxidase-like reactions. Finally, the peroxidase activity was strongly influenced by the supramolecular morphology of the assemblies, where micelles exhibited enhanced catalytic activity over fibers. This work demonstrates that the design of conformational changes in small peptide sequences may afford controlled biomaterials.

More recently, Zozulia and Korendovych exploited short peptides capable of self-assembly into amyloid structures for creating functional materials [138]. They used very short peptides adopting β-sheet conformation to accommodate hemin in a functional manner. The spectroscopic characterization confirmed the β-sheet conformation of the peptides and the hemin binding. Furthermore, the circular dichroism (CD) analysis indicated that the amyloid structure provided a chiral environment around the porphyrin ring.

Indeed, the resulting assemblies were found capable of promoting enantioselective cyclopropanation of aromatic styrene derivatives with efficiencies comparable to engineered proteins. Interestingly, methylated peptides did not adopt β-sheet structures. Furthermore, no enantioselectivity was obtained with these peptides thus confirming the importance of the higher-ordered supramolecular structure for activity.

The selected examples above described point out the power of peptide scaffolds in tuning heme and metalloporphyrin activities. Thanks to the possibility offered by peptides to easily modify the structure and composition of the cofactor environment, different reactivities can be implanted into the artificial molecule. By increasing the complexity of the scaffold, it is possible to span from structure–activity relationship studies to the development of catalysts and/or biomaterials endowed with a variety of key reactivities.

4. Peptide Scaffolds Housing Mononuclear Metal Sites

Outstanding examples of designed metalloproteins containing mononuclear metal-binding sites have appeared in the literature over the years, and many strategies have been used to include and alter the metal surroundings in order to obtain functional metalloproteins.

In this respect, impressive contributions have been reported by Pecoraro and coworkers, who implanted catalytic and structural mononuclear sites into a *de novo* designed three-helix bundle [10,11,88,89,139–141]. Specifically, these researchers incorporated into the TRI family of peptides two spatially-separated metal-binding sites, endowed with different functions: a Zn(II)His_3OH tetrahedral coordination site, tucked within the protein's hydrophobic core, mimicking the active site of the natural enzyme carbonic anhydrase (CA), and a Hg(II)Cys_3 site for structure stabilization. The TRI peptides [142,143] (Table 1), based on the heptad sequence LKALEEK [144,145], form a parallel three-stranded coiled-coil (3SCC) with a hydrophobic interior that adopts a native fold in aqueous solution. The peptides were chemically synthesized, and this allowed simple incorporation of NPAAs, in either the primary or secondary coordination spheres, thus tuning coordination environment and catalytic efficiency [73]. The mutation of Leu residues, whose side chains are oriented towards the hydrophobic core (*a* and *d* positions of the heptad repeats), to Cys and His residues, near the N-terminus and the C-terminus respectively, determined the creation of the two different metal-binding sites within the interior of the bundle [146,147] (Figure 7).

The artificial metalloenzyme ($[Hg(II)]_S[Zn(II)(H_2O/OH^-)]_N(TRI\ L9CL23H)_3^{n+}$) is the first example of peptide-based metalloprotein model containing two different metals in two different coordination environments, endowed with distinct functions (catalytic and structural). Most remarkably, it represents an artificial hydrolytic metalloenzyme with unprecedented catalytic efficiency, approaching at pH 9.5 that of the natural counterpart. Indeed, the metalloenzyme was capable of catalyzing the *p*-nitrophenyl acetate (*p*NPA) hydrolysis with efficiency only ~100-fold less than that of CA-II (the fastest α-CA isozyme) and at least 550-fold better than small molecule mimics [146,147]. The artificial enzyme was also remarkably active in CO_2 hydration, the native reaction catalyzed by

Table 1. Peptide sequences of the TRI family and derivatives.

Peptide		Sequences[a]				
		2	9 12	16	23	30
		a b c d e f g	a b c d e f g	a b c d e f g	a b c d e f g	a b c d e f g
CoilSer (CS)	Ac-E	W E A L E E K	L K A L E S K	L Q A L E K K	L E A L E H G	$-NH_2$
CSL9CL23H	Ac-E	W E A L E E K	***C*** K A L E S K	L Q A L E K K	L E A L E H G	$-NH_2$
CSL9XL23H	Ac-E	W E A L E K K	***X*** A A L E S K	L Q A L E K K	***H*** E A L E H G	$-NH_2$
TRI	Ac-G	L K A L E E K	L K A L E E K	L K A L E E K	L K A L E E K	$G-NH_2$
TRIL9C	Ac-G	L K A L E E K	***C*** K A L E E K	L K A L E E K	L K A L E E K	$G-NH_2$
TRIL12C	Ac-G	L K A L E E K	L K A ***C*** E E K	L K A L E E K	L K A L E E K	$G-NH_2$
TRIL16C	Ac-G	L K A L E E K	L K A L E E K	***C*** K A L E E K	L K A L E E K	$G-NH_2$
TRIL19C	Ac-G	L K A L E E K	L K A L E E K	L K A ***C*** E E K	L K A L E E K	$G-NH_2$
TRIL9CL19C	Ac-G	L K A L E E K	***C*** K A L E E K	L K A ***C*** E E K	L K A L E E K	$G-NH_2$
TRIL12AL16C	Ac-G	L K A L E E K	L K A ***A*** E E K	***C*** K A L E E K	L K A L E E K	$G-NH_2$
TRIL16X	Ac-G	L K A L E E K	L K A L E E K	***X*** K A L E E K	L K A L E E K	$G-NH_2$
TRIL12L_DL16C	Ac-G	L K A L E E K	L K A ***L_D*** E E K	***C*** K A L E E K	L K A L E E K	$G-NH_2$
TRI-L23H	Ac-G	L K A L E E K	L K A L E E K	L K A L E E K	***H*** K A L E E K	$G-NH_2$
TRIL9CL23H	Ac-G	L K A L E E K	***C*** K A L E E K	L K A L E E K	***H*** K A L E E K	$G-NH_2$
Protein	loop	a b c d e f g	a b c d e f g	a b c d e f g	l o o p	
	MGS	W A E F K Q R	L A A I K T R	L Q A L	G G S	
α_3D	EAE	L A A F E K E	I A A F E S E	L Q A Y	K G K G	
	NPE	V E A L R K E	A A A I R D E	L Q A Y R H N		
	MGS	W A E F K Q R	L A A I K T R	***H*** Q A L	G G S	
α_3DH_3[b]	EAE	***H*** A A F E K E	I A A F E S E	L Q A Y	K G K G	
	NPE	V E A L R K E	A A A I R D E	***H*** Q A Y R ***V*** N		***GSGA***

[a]*X* = Penicillamine. L_D = D-leucine. Residues in bold and italics indicate substitutions.

[b]Mutations with respect to *α_3*D are in bold and italics.

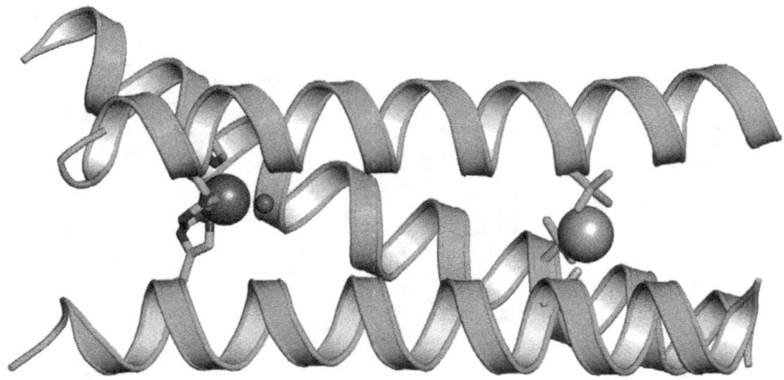

Fig. 7. Crystal structure of $[Hg(II)]_S[Zn(II)(H_2O/OH^-)]_N(CS\ L9PenL23H)_3^{n+}$ (PDB code 3PBJ), a structural analogue of $[Hg(II)]_S[Zn(II)(H_2O/OH^-)]_N(TRI\ L9CL23H)_3^{n+}$. The structural Hg(II)$Cys_3$ site (right) and the catalytic Zn(II)$(His)_3(H_2O/OH^-)$ site (left) are depicted.

CA, with a catalytic efficiency ~100-fold higher than previously reported models, and within ~500-fold of CA-II.

The designed peptide-based scaffold demonstrated to be well suited to accommodate the threefold symmetric histidine binding site of CA, thus allowing the authors to reproduce the core elements necessary for function into a completely different scaffold, with respect to the native enzyme (α-helices in the TRI construct versus β-sheets in CA) [146,147].

The TRI peptide was also used to incorporate the type 2 copper center of nitrite reductase (CuNiR) (Figure 8). CuNiR is an enzyme that converts NO_2 to NO, and this conversion is achieved by coupling the redox-active type 1 copper center to the catalytic type 2 copper center $Cu(His_3)(H_2O)$. The catalytic center shows a distorted-tetrahedral environment, intermediate between the standard preferences of Cu(I) and Cu(II). This enables nitrite to bind to the oxidized type 2 copper center before the electron is transferred from the type 1 copper center. Cu ion was incorporated into the hydrophobic core of a simplified scaffold $(TRI\ L23H)_3$ containing three histidine residues. These residues provided a layer of three nitrogen donors, thus mimicking the type 2 catalytic site of NiR [148,149]. The substitution of Zn(II) with Cu(II) in the CA mimic produced a highly stable catalyst able to generate nitric oxide from nitrite using ascorbate as a sacrificial electron donor [148,149].

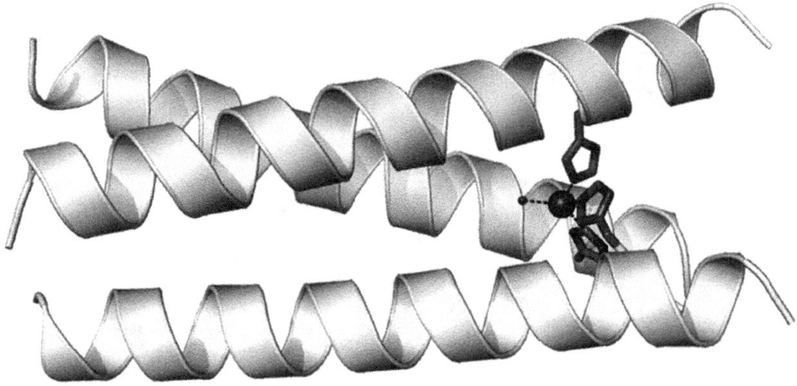

Fig. 8. Molecular model of Cu(I/II)(TRI L23H)$_3^{+/2+}$ based on the crystal structure of [Hg(II)]$_S$[Zn(II)(H$_2$O)]$_N$(CS L9CL23H)$_3^+$ (PDF code 3PBJ). The copper-binding site is highlighted. Reprinted with permission from Ref. [148]. Copyright 2012 National Academy of Sciences, USA.

Several rounds of redesign provided a series of TRI peptide analogs, and amino acids mutations in the second coordination sphere of the copper center allowed to increase the nitrite reductase activity up to 75-fold, thus producing a CuNiR catalyst with the highest catalytic efficiency and turnovers for artificial catalysts in aqueous media (TON > 1,000, k_{cat}/K_m up to 1.0 $M^{-1}s^{-1}$) [85]. These results highlight the versatility of the coiled-coil scaffolds, which can also incorporate 'rare earths' metal ions without any related biological counterparts [150]. Further, these peptide scaffolds allow reactivity modulation by the simple incorporation of different residues, including NPAAs.

In an effort to overcome the symmetry limitations imposed by the homo-trimeric TRI scaffolds, the same authors used α_3D, a single-stranded antiparallel three-helix bundle, previously developed in the DeGrado lab [151] to create a new CA catalytic site [152]. Three core leucine residues towards the C-terminal region of the α_3D protein were mutated to histidines (see Table 1) and the new metalloenzyme, namely Zn(II)-α_3DH$_3$, was found to catalyze the CO_2 hydration with a catalytic efficiency 14-fold faster than the best small molecule model, but slightly less efficient, compared to that of the TRI-based compounds. Compared with the native enzyme, Zn(II)-α_3DH$_3$ is 1,400-fold slower than the fastest isoform CA-II. Nevertheless, α_3D with its single peptide chain that enables key mutations to protein sequence, represents a useful scaffold for catalysis. In a more recent report, an elongated version of α_3D, GRα_3D, was designed for obtaining functional superoxide dismutase (SOD) mimics [89]. Four constructs were prepared with different binding sites: H3 (His3), H4 (His4), H2DH (His3Asp with two His and one Asp in the same plane), and H3D (His3Asp with three His in the same plane).

The analysis carried out on the Cu(II) complexes demonstrated that all the resulting models were good structural mimics of Cu-only SODs and exhibited SOD activity, albeit much slower than the native enzyme. Furthermore, this study showed that all four His residues from the native active site are not required for SOD activity within a *de novo* designed construct and highlighted again the usefulness of these stable scaffolds for the design of functional metalloenzymes.

Peptide-based artificial metalloenzymes with hydrolytic activity were also developed by Kuhlman's group. They designed MID1 [153], a homodimeric peptide, containing two interfacial Zn(II)His_3 sites. MID1 derived from a monomeric, 46 residues helix-turn-helix motif, capable of self-assembling in the presence of zinc ions. The designed model featured two zinc-binding sites, each consisting of four tetrahedrally arranged histidines, two His residues from one monomer and two from the other one. The crystal structure of MID1 unexpectedly revealed two ZnHis_3 sites at the interface. A tartrate molecule from the crystallization buffer occupied the fourth coordination position (Figure 9).

The absence of the fourth histidine ligand into the metal site created a small hydrophobic binding pocket, thus favoring the formation of a $(His)_3O$ zinc-binding site, a common catalytic motif for zinc hydrolases. MID1-zinc was demonstrated to catalyze carboxyester and phosphoester hydrolysis. It successfully catalyzed the hydrolysis of *p*NPA with a TON > 50 and a k_{cat}/K_m of 470 $M^{-1}s^{-1}$ at pH = 8.5.

In an elegant contribution, Hilvert and coworkers described the evolution of MID1 [154]. They transformed the zinc-binding peptide MID1 into a single-chain protein, MID1sc, obtaining a globular enzyme capable of accelerating ester cleavage with high enantiospecificity and catalytic efficiency. MID1sc10, the product of several rounds of directed evolution and site-directed mutagenesis, was found to catalyze the hydrolysis of *p*NPA, with enhanced activity (10,000 fold) with respect to MID1sc. Notably, MID1sc10 exhibits high efficiency ($k_{cat}/K_m \sim 10^6$ $M^{-1}s^{-1}$), outperforming

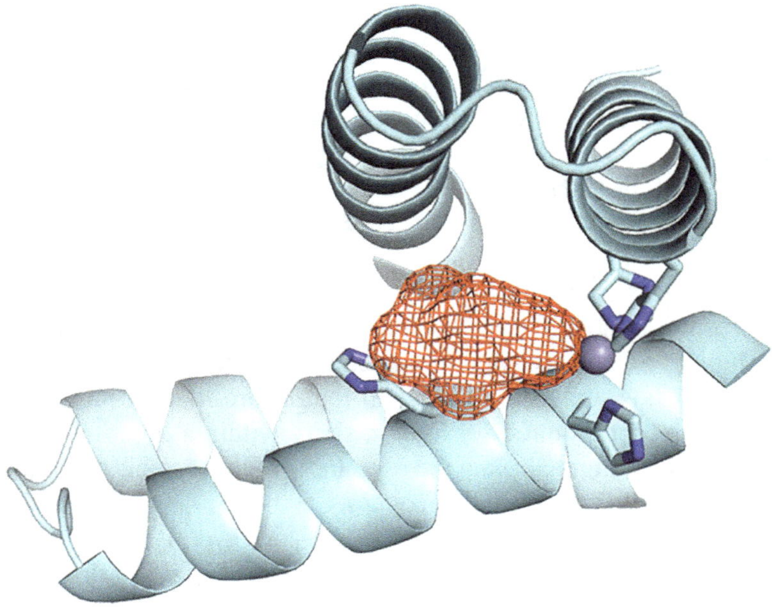

Fig. 9. X-ray structure of MID1-zinc (PDB code 3V1C). The mesh represents a cleft above the open zinc coordination site. The His residues are depicted as sticks, and the Zn(II) ion as a ball. Reprinted with permission from Ref. [153]. Copyright 2012 American Chemical Society.

several artificial esterases and CA, when assayed in the same reaction. More recently, they applied specific mutations to MID1sc protein and generated a highly active and stereoselective catalyst for an abiological hetero-Dies-Alder reaction [155]. The artificial enzyme displays a catalytic proficiency that exceeds all previously characterized Diels-Alderases.

These works prove that coupled biological and computational methods lead to structure optimization in a simple peptide-based scaffold, dramatically increasing the activity of the artificial metalloenzyme. These studies have also contributed to a deeper understanding of the structural features crucial for hydrolytic activity. Further, they highlighted the possibility to recapitulate native metalloprotein functions into protein architectures that are different from the natural ones.

Design approaches have been also applied to convert proteins that are not catalytically active, such as zinc fingers, into hydrolytic enzymes. Sugiura and coworkers, inspired by the Cys_2His_2-type zinc finger motif

(Figure 10(a), (b)), synthesized a series of zinc finger mutants, in which one coordinating residue was replaced to convert the tetracoordinate-zinc site into a tri-coordinate-zinc site [156,157].

All the synthesized peptides retained the ability of binding one equivalent of zinc ion and folding into compact structures, like the wild-type zinc finger peptide, despite their tridentate coordination. The resulting complexes contained at least one water molecule bound to the zinc ion and were capable to catalyze the hydrolysis of *p*NPA as well as the hydrolysis of amino acid esters with considerable enantioselectivity. Similarly, Durani and coworkers reprogrammed, by a computational approach, a zinc finger protein ($\alpha\beta\beta$ fold) to function as a hydrolase enzyme [158,159].

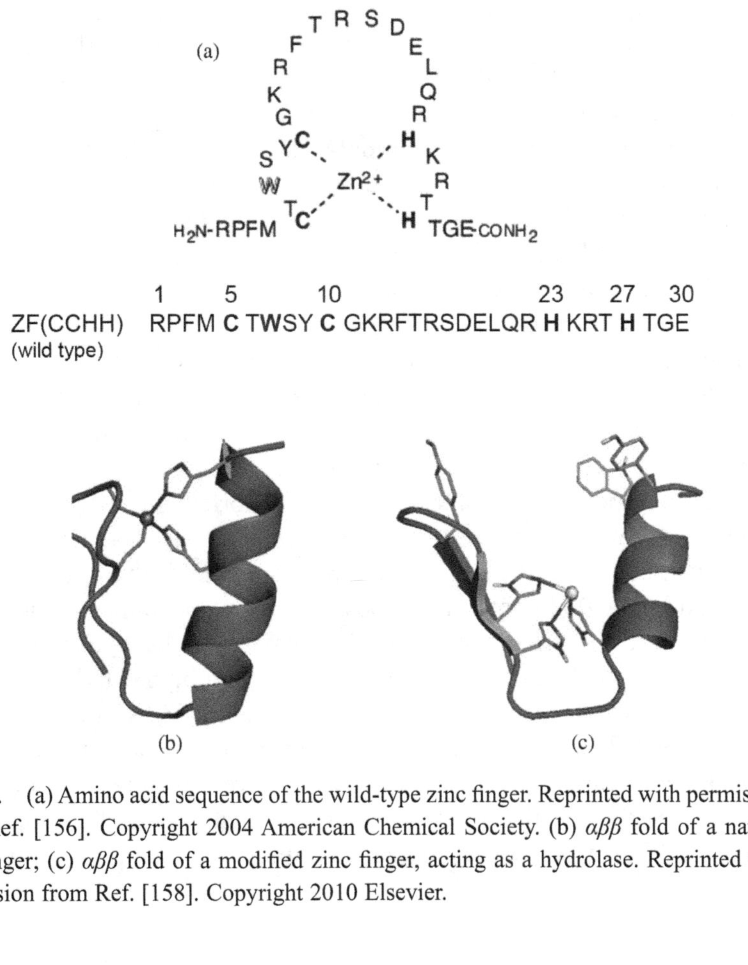

Fig. 10. (a) Amino acid sequence of the wild-type zinc finger. Reprinted with permission from Ref. [156]. Copyright 2004 American Chemical Society. (b) $\alpha\beta\beta$ fold of a natural zinc finger; (c) $\alpha\beta\beta$ fold of a modified zinc finger, acting as a hydrolase. Reprinted with permission from Ref. [158]. Copyright 2010 Elsevier.

First, they designed a 21-residue $\alpha\beta\beta$ protein with a tri-coordinate zinc-binding site ($ZnHis_3$) to mimic CA. (Figure 10(c)). The coordination and activation of zinc as a hydrolase catalyst were achieved successfully but not the binding of the substrate and its enzyme-like hydrolysis.

The activity was then repurposed through a precise redesign process. The resulting peptides were found to strongly bind Zn(II) and their Zn(II)-complexes catalyzed the hydrolysis of *p*NPA, as a surrogate ester substrate for CO_2, with an efficiency many-fold superior than other reported small molecule CA mimics, albeit lower than the natural enzyme.

Computational methods have significantly contributed to artificial metalloenzyme development by assisting the redesign of metal centers in native proteins or by *de novo* design of non-native scaffolds.

Recently, Iranzo and coworkers, using a computational multi-state design (MSD) approach, developed new artificial zinc hydrolases based on small protein scaffolds [160]. They explored two different routes (Figure 11). In the first, they redesigned the zinc site of a native zinc-finger metallopeptide, Sp1f2 (Figure 11(a)). In the second, a native scaffold, the villin headpiece C-terminal subdomain HP35, was *de novo* designed for zinc-binding and catalytic activity (Figure 11(b)). Both metallopeptides (RD01 and RD02, respectively) fold upon metal binding and are capable of catalyzing the *p*NPA hydrolysis, even though the catalytic efficiencies of the designed hydrolases are still far from those of native systems, such as CA-II.

The development of functional metalloenzymes by computational methods represents not only a valuable strategy for incorporating a metal-binding site into natural proteins or non-native scaffolds but also offers a useful approach to explore new reactivities.

In this respect, Baker and coworkers reported milestone results in redesigning native metalloenzymes that catalyze noncognate chemical transformations [161,162]. An organophosphate hydrolytic activity was implanted into a zinc-containing mouse adenosine deaminase. The resulting artificial organophosphate hydrolase catalyzes the hydrolysis of an organophosphate substrate, diethyl 7-hydroxycoumarinyl phosphate (DECP), with a catalytic efficiency (k_{cat}/K_m) of $\sim 10^4$ $M^{-1}s^{-1}$ (a net increase in activity $\sim 10^7$-fold higher than the native adenosine deaminase) [163].

In recent years, Tezcan and coworkers have developed an attractive and powerful design strategy that allows the construction of complex protein assemblies with sophisticated structures, by using small natural

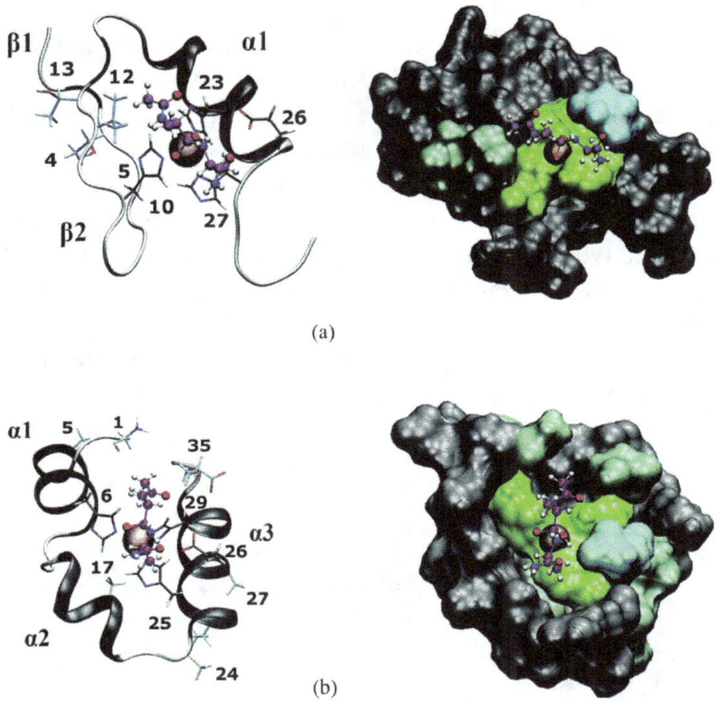

Fig. 11. (a) RD01 model based on the Sp1f2 scaffold. (b) RD02 model (F6H variant) based on the HP35 scaffold. Adapted with permission from Ref. [160]. Published by the Royal Society of Chemistry.

proteins as synthetic building blocks [47,164–168]. This approach utilizes folded monomeric proteins, as the heme protein cytochrome cb_{562} (Cyt), for building highly ordered supramolecular complexes through metal-mediated self-assembly (MDPSA, Metal-Directed Protein Self-Assembly) [47,164]. These supramolecular structures can be further modified by proper engineering of the interacting interfaces (MeTIR, Metal Templated Interface Redesign) via covalent, non-covalent or further metal-coordination interactions, thus affording versatile metalloprotein scaffolds provided with allostery [47,169], reversible redox activity, and small-molecule binding [170].

For example, by using these strategies, cytochrome cb_{562} was converted into a tetrameric assembly housing two structural zinc sites (three His and one Asp) and two catalytic zinc sites (two His, one Glu and one H_2O)

within the interfaces (Figure 12). The artificial proteins (namely, Zn_8:AB3_4 and Zn_8:AB5_4) show hydrolase activity toward *p*NPA and the β-lactam antibiotic ampicillin [47,167,168].

Impressively, these proteins were the first reported examples of artificial proteins displaying β-lactamase activity *in vivo*, thus endowing *E. coli* with antibiotic resistance. Subsequent optimization of the Zn_8:AB5_4 using rational design and directed evolution did not lead to significant improvement in the catalytic efficiency, possibly because of the local protein rigidity surrounding the Zn centers and the lack of mutable loops close to the active sites.

More recently, the same group applied the MeTIR strategy to modify Cyt surface-exposed hydrophobic residues with the aim of directing its self-assembly toward lower oligomerization states. By this approach, they

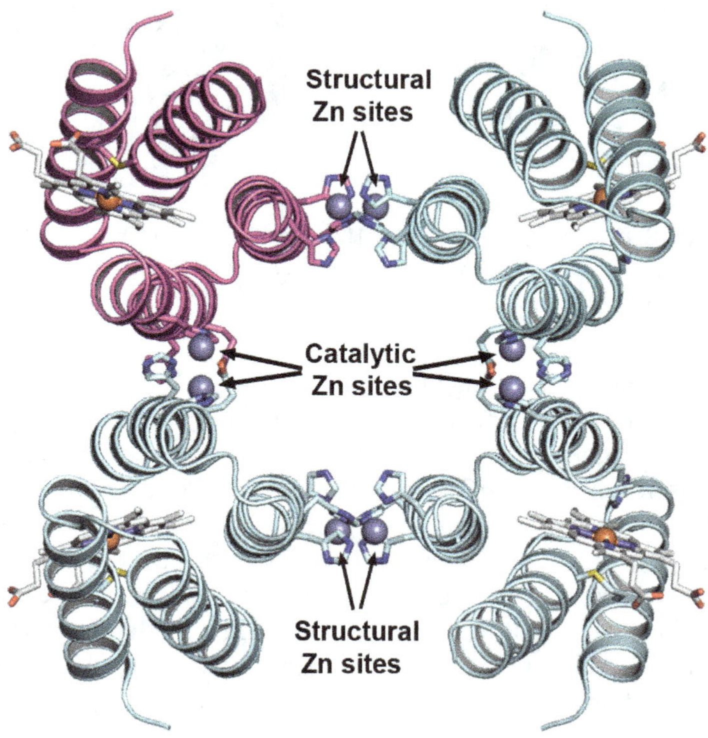

Fig. 12. Crystal structure of Zn_8:AB3_4 (PDB ID: 4U9E) [167] with structural and catalytic zinc sites depicted. A monomeric heme protein self-assembles into an oligomeric complex upon Zn(II) binding, thus acting as a multi-component hydrolase.

obtained the TriCyt1 monomer that, in the presence of a variety of metal ions such Mn(II), Fe(II), Co(II), Ni(II), Cu(II) and Zn(II), forms trimeric structural arrangements $(TriCyt1)_3$ featuring an His_6 coordination site, rarely observed in nature [171]. Interface redesign on $(TriCyt1)_3$ gave new variants $(TriCyt2)_3$ and $(TriCyt3)_3$, characterized by an increased structural stability with respect to the parent $(TriCyt1)_3$, and still housing a preorganized His_6 metal-binding site that is able to bind all mid-to-late first-row transition-metal ions with high affinity.

5. Peptide Scaffolds Housing Dinuclear Metal Sites

Many natural metalloenzymes use multi-metal ions as catalytic sites, as well as electron- or proton-delivery systems [1,15]. Examples of naturally occurring dinuclear metal cofactors involve the diiron, dimanganese, dicopper, dinickel, and dizinc sites, which are found in important classes of enzymes, such as monoxygenases, desaturases, oxidases, hydroxylases, and hydrolases [1]. Several dinuclear metal sites are housed within a conserved four-helix bundle. This motif is found in many structural contexts and in proteins that are functionally diverse [172] and is characterized by four α-helices packed against each other. It is compact, thermodynamically stable and able to tolerate residue substitutions, deletions and insertions without perturbing the global three-dimensional fold. As a consequence, the four-helix bundle scaffold is ideal as a template for *de novo* protein design and for developing novel artificial metalloenzymes [8,54,173].

A premier example of functional *de novo* designed metalloproteins containing a dinuclear site at the heart of a four-helix bundle is "Due Ferri" (two-irons; DF) family, developed by DeGrado's and our groups. DF design was aimed at reproducing in minimal peptide-based four-helix bundles the properties of the more complex natural diiron-oxo proteins, such as the alternative oxidases and methane monooxygenases. Such proteins catalyze a variety of O_2-dependent reactions and cycle between the diferrous and the diferric forms [8,54].

Starting from the first principles, we developed a family of antiparallel four-helix bundles, made up of two non-covalently associated helix-loop-helix (α2) motifs, four disconnected helices or a single chain (Table 2, Figure 13). All designed proteins were initially programmed to catalyze the O_2-dependent two-electron oxidation of phenols. Their activity was then repurposed through a precise redesign process [8,54].

The first member, DF1, was developed using a mathematical parameterization of the backbone [8,174]. We designed an $\alpha2$ peptide motif containing 48 amino acid residues, able to specifically self-assemble into an antiparallel dimeric four-helix bundle and to bind the dimetal cofactor near the center of the structure. Each helix-loop-helix peptide motif contains a Glu-Xxx-Xxx-His sequence in the helix 2, which serves a His side chain as well as a bridging Glu carboxylate to the site. A second Glu carboxylate ligand on helix 1 provides a fourth protein ligand per metal ion (Table 2, Figure 13).

Although DF1 behaved as a native-like protein and was able to bind the metal ions as predicted, unfortunately, it was not able to support any function because the access to its active site was hampered by a pair of hydrophobic leucine residues [174]. Adding functionality in this stable, uniquely folded DF1 protein thus required expansion of the active site to accommodate substrates.

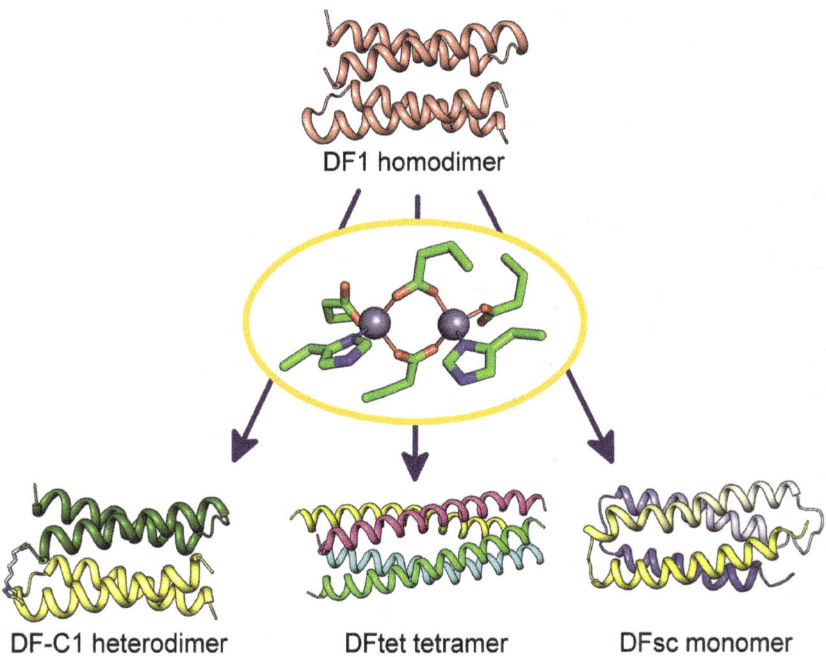

Fig. 13. Different DF protein constructs were derived from the DF1 homodimeric precursor. The highlighted His2Glu4 dimetal-binding site can be implanted in each of the different scaffolds, resulting in specific modulation of function. Side chains are represented as sticks, metal ions as spheres.

Table 2. Peptide sequence of the DF family. Coordinating residues and active-site access residues are in bold.

Sequences[a]										
Homodimers										
DF1	Ace	DY-----	LRELLK**L**	**E**LQ**L**IKQ	YREALEYV--KL	-----PV	LAKILED	**E**EK**H**IEW	LETILG	NH_2
DF3	Ace	DY-----	LRELLK**G**	**E**LQ**G**IKQ	YREALEYT--HN	-----PV	LAKILED	**E**EK**H**IEW	LETILG	NH_2
Heterodimer (two peptide chains covalently linked)										
DF-C1 ChainZ	aha	DY-----	LRELLK**F**	**E**LQ**G**IKQ	LREALEYT--HN	-----PV	QAKILED	**E**EK**H**IEW	LETILG	NH_2
DF-C1 ChainK	Ace	DY-----	LRELLK**G**	**E**LQ**T**AKL	FREALEXT--HN	-----PV	LAKIQED	**E**EK**H**IEW	NETILG	NH_2
Monomer (one single peptide chain)										
DFsc(1-29)	M	DE-----	LRELLK**A**	**E**QQAIKI	YKEVLKKA--KE	-----GD				
(30-60)		EQELARL	IQEIVK**A**	**E**KQAVKV	YKEAAE----KA	-----RN				
(61-89)		PEKRQV-	IDKILED	**E**EK**H**IEW	LKAASK-----Q	-----GN				
(90-115)		AEQFASL	VQQILQD	**E**QR**H**VEE	IEKKN					
3H-DFsc(1-30)	M	DE-----	LRELLK**G**	**E**QQGIKI	LKEVLKKA--KE	-----GD				
(31-60)		EQELARL	NQEIVK**G**	**E**KQGVKV	YKEAAE----KA	-----RN				
(61-89)		PEKRQV-	IDKILED	**E**EK**H**IEW	HKAASK-----Q	-----GN				
(90-115)		AEQFASL	VQQ**H**LQD	**E**QR**H**VEE	IEKKN					
Tetramer (four peptide chains)										
DFtet										
A	K	LKELKSK	LKELLK**L**	**E**LQ**A**IKQ	YKELKAE	LKEL				
Aa	E	LKELKSE	LKELLK**L**	**E**LQ**A**IKQ	FKELKAE	LKEL				
Ab	K	LKKLKSR	LKKLLKL	ELQAIHQ	YKKLKAR	LKKL				
B	E	LEELESE	LEKILED	**E**ER**H**IEW	LEKLEAK	LKEL				

Note: [a]X stands for propargyl glycine and **aha** stands for 6-azidohexanoic acid.

A detailed analysis of the energetic and structural consequences associated with the replacement of the bulky leucine residues lining the access site with smaller alanine and/or glycine residues was performed on DF1 variants [175–179]. In parallel, the effects of these substitutions on the catalytic activity were explored in a combinatorial manner with DFtet [8,54] peptides, by analyzing the O_2-dependent oxidation of 4-aminophenol (4AP) to 4-benzoquinine monoimine (4BQM).

Gaining catalytic activity required the substitution of all the four buried Leu with helix-breaking Gly residues. It was therefore necessary to redesign the $\alpha 2$ loop in DF1 to compensate for these highly destabilizing changes. The resulting protein, DF3, was revealed to be an artificial phenol oxidase, whose structure was confirmed by solution NMR [180,181]. DF3 was indeed capable of catalyzing the oxidation of 4AP. Further, as intended in the design, the active site cleft in DF3 could also accommodate a larger substrate, such as 3,5-di-*tert*-butylcatechol (DTBC). Indeed, di-Fe(III)-DF3 catalyzed the oxidation of this catechol derivative to the corresponding quinone (DTBQ), with a 5-fold higher value of k_{cat}/K_m than that for 4AP, reflecting an increase in k_{cat}.

In order to get a fine-tuning of the active site reactivity and specificity, further design on the $\alpha 2$ scaffold was aimed at engineering second-shell active site interactions. To this end, a careful observation of natural monooxygenase structures, such as methane and toluene monooxygenases, revealed that symmetry is broken in the proximity of the active site [28]. Starting from this observation, the design strategy was implemented in order to obtain an asymmetric DF scaffold, derived by the covalent ligation of two functionalized $\alpha 2$ peptides through click chemistry [182].

One of the major advantages of the click chemistry-based methodology relies on its orthogonality to solid-phase peptide synthesis. Once selected the binding positions, the peptides to be ligated could be easily functionalized during the synthetic step, by introducing in their sequences two NPAAs bearing the azide and alkyne moieties. Using a recently developed computational method [183], we designed DF-C1 [72], an asymmetric version of DF3 with an active site modeled after toluene monooxygenase (TOMO). Indeed, DF-C1 second-shell ligands were changed to those in TOMO, and a single Thr and Phe were introduced into the inner and outer regions of the substrate access site, respectively. The two $\alpha 2$ motifs (K and Z chains) were obtained by solid-phase peptide synthesis and comprised propargyl glycine (Pra) (see Figure 1(b)), and 6-azidohexanoic acid (6aha) as the alkyne and the azide moiety respectively, for the click reaction. DF-C1 not only oxidizes 4AP to 4BQM, but it is also able to further promote its oxidative dimerization and store the reactive oxidation intermediate in the purposely designed binding pocket, thus avoiding its diffusion in solution. Thus, DF-C1 mimics natural proteins that guide substrates through reactive species to create stable products without releasing any highly reactive or toxic species. Altogether, this work clearly demonstrates the advantage of incorporating NPAAs for stabilizing desired peptide tertiary structures.

As outlined above, an alternative approach to evaluate how systematic changes to the structure of DFs scaffold would affect its metal binding, substrate binding and catalytic properties was based on a series of heterotetrameric four-helix bundles, comprising four disconnected helical peptides (DFtet) (Figure 13) [184–186]. DFtet helical peptides were chemically synthesized and comprised 33 amino acid residues to guarantee, through an extended hydrophobic interface, the tetramer stability. One of the resulting heterotetramers, G4-DFtet, with all Gly residues in the proximity of the metal site, exhibited the most rapid rate of iron oxidation, with no detectable intermediates. G4-DFtet showed also the greatest binding ability toward phenol, which binds to the diferric site. Again, G4-DFtet was able to perform the rapid two-electron oxidation of 4AP to the corresponding benzoquinone monoamine with a ~1,000-fold rate enhancement relative to the background reaction [186].

The key mutations required for function, highlighted through the DFtet and DF1 constructs, were also transferred into a single-chain protein [187]. A 114-residue protein, DFsc, was computationally designed and bacterially expressed. It is made up of four helices connected by three loops (Figure 13), and promotes a wide range of chemical transformations. It is noteworthy that first-, second-, and third-shell modifications in DFsc scaffold alter the protein reactivity [188]. It was possible to reprogram the catalytic activity from the oxidation of hydroquinones to the *N*-hydroxylation of arylamines. Firstly, the first coordination sphere was altered to match that found in arylamine *N*-oxygenase (AurF), which involved the insertion of a third His residue ligand and the mutation of a clashing Tyr (I100H, Y18L). Secondly, a full set of second and third-sphere interactions was installed by mutating two more core residues to hydrogen-bond donating residues (L81H, I37N). The resulting 3His-G2DFsc and 3His-G4DFsc mutants catalyzed the selective arylamine *N*-hydroxylation, mimicking AurF [188]. Noteworthy, the zinc-containing protein 3His-G2DFsc was capable of stabilizing several reactive semiquinone radical species, such as 3,5-di-*tert*-butyl-semiquinone radical anion, $SQ^{\cdot-}$, a one-electron oxidized intermediate in the redox triad between DTBC and the corresponding quinone, Q ($H_2Q/SQ^{\cdot-}/Q$) [8,54,189]. This is a hallmark for protein *de novo* design, as it is a very general mechanism of protein function to stabilize a very reactive species in the protein interior, ready to be further processed or exploited.

The reported examples demonstrate that a diverse range of functionalities can be successfully engineered into these simplified scaffolds. Further work from our laboratories was aimed at increasing the evolutional complexity of DFs, introducing an allosteric regulation on the oxidase activity of the diiron center [190]. To this endeavor, a novel multi-domain architecture (MDA) strategy was developed to couple the DF domain with a small molecule binding domain. In particular PS1, a protein capable of binding a synthetic Zn-porphyrin (ZnP), was chosen as the second domain in order to examine how the binding of ZnP cofactor allosterically modulated the catalytic activity of the diiron-binding domain [191]. The first model, DFP1 (Due Ferri Porphyrin), was designed for maximal thermodynamic stability. The spectroscopic and structural characterization confirmed that the design strategy was successful in preserving the original structural and binding properties of both DF and PS1 proteins. Next, a new interhelical loop and a substrate-binding cleft leading to the diiron center were introduced into DFP1. The resulting protein, DFP3, not only bound the two cofactors but also allowed the allosteric communication between the domains to control the catalysis. The diiron form of the ZnP-bound protein showed significant phenol oxidase activity that was modulated by ZnP binding. Indeed, the binding of ZnP into PS1 domain markedly decreased K_m and k_{cat} values in the phenol oxidation at DF domain [190].

These studies paved the way for the design of artificial multi-domain proteins and established the feasibility of designing allosterically communicating sites, entirely from scratch.

Recently, Makhlynets and coworkers modified the DFsc dinuclear active site into a single metal-binding site, by mutating a bridging Glu residue to His (Uno Ferro single chain, UFsc) [192,193]. Following the DF redesign [8,54], Ala-to-Gly mutations were introduced to widen the substrate-access channel, and the resulting molecule was named 4G-UFsc. Both UFsc and 4G-UFsc were able to bind different metal ions such as Ni(II), Co(II), Mn(II) and Zn(II) in a 1:1 stoichiometry, displaying the highest affinity for zinc. Similar to the zinc-containing 3His-G2DFsc [189], both UFsc and 4G-UFsc stabilized $SQ^{\cdot-}$ produced by oxidation of DTBC to the corresponding quinone. It is noteworthy, for all proteins, that radical formation is irrespective of the nature of metal ion, with a single metal ion being sufficient for radical stabilization [192].

In a subsequent work, the same authors, by systematic mutagenesis, confirmed the role of the first and outer coordination spheres on modulating metal binding affinity [193]. All the results obtained with the UFsc family of proteins demonstrate that the robust and easy-to-modify DF scaffold affords competent catalysts and represents a versatile tool for mechanistic model studies.

In many cases, similar metal sites can display functional diversity depending on the specific environment created by the surrounding protein matrix. For example, Allen and coworkers designed five DF homodimeric analogs and tested them against catalase activity [194]. Contrarily to UFsc, the four-helix scaffold was altered to host up to three dinuclear sites by convenient mutation of core residues to metal-binding residues at the top and bottom of the bundle. Interestingly, 'P0' (one site), 'P2' and 'P4' (two sites) showed higher helical content with respect to 'P1' and 'P3' (three sites), compatible with the idea that the insertion of metal-binding hydrophilic residues comes at the cost of destabilizing the overall fold. Nevertheless, their dinuclear manganese cofactor, as found in natural Mn-catalases, was able to catalyze hydrogen peroxide dismutation. Both H_2O_2 consumption and O_2 formation were depending on enzyme concentration, the 'P1' and 'P3' variants, with three Mn_2-clusters, exhibiting higher activity. This last finding perfectly fits with the activity/stability tradeoff, as previously observed with DF and MID1sc proteins, in which higher activity could only be reached at the expense of higher structural flexibility.

Multi-nuclear sites have also been incorporated into peptide-based models with the aim of elucidating the key features determining the activity of natural metal clusters, and eventually to include these model peptides in engineered redox enzymes. Dutton and coworkers, in a pioneering work, achieved the incorporation of an iron carbonyl thiolate mimic of the [Fe-Fe]-hydrogenase active site into a *de novo* artificial peptide, creating the first peptide-based hydrogenase maquette (SynHid1) [195]. A 36-peptide was synthesized by solid-phase peptide synthesis, bearing a simple AAKAA penta-repeat. The third pentad was then mutated to host the CxxC binding motif, which provided the coordinating thiolates to the diiron hexacarbonyl metal cluster. Such a simple helical scaffold was not showing significant activity but undoubtedly represented the starting point for the following designed peptides.

Later on, Ghirlanda and coworkers inserted a diiron hexacarbonyl site into a α-helical peptide, via a NPAA (bearing a propanedithiol moiety) [196], thus mimicking the [FeFe]-hydrogenase active site. Starting from alanine-rich model peptides [197,198], they inserted an NPAA containing a 1,3-dithiol moiety to covalently anchor the diiron site in the peptide scaffold. The resulting molecule catalyzed photo-induced hydrogen production in water, at pH = 4.5, in the presence of a photosensitizer ($Ru(bpy)_3$) and a sacrificial electron donor (ascorbate), with high efficiency [196].

Hayashi and coworkers also succeeded in the design of a functional mimic of [FeFe]-hydrogenase active site [199]. They selected an 18-residue peptide containing the CxxCH motif of cytochrome c_{556} as peptide scaffold that is able to bind a diiron carbonyl cluster via two cysteines. Additionally, this peptide contained a histidine residue, which binds a photoactive Ru(bpy)(tpy) complex (bpy=2,2′-bipyridine, tpy=2,2′:6′,2″-terpyridine), acting as a photosensitizer for electron production. The modified peptide with the two metal centers was found to perform photocatalysis for hydrogen evolution in the presence of ascorbate as a sacrificial donor.

6. Summary

The case studies discussed in this chapter clearly demonstrate that the field of peptide design has spectacularly progressed in the past two decades. Either consisting of small sequences or complex supramolecular assemblies, peptides have been demonstrated to be proper candidates to host and tune the activity of a variety of metal-binding sites. By designing defined peptide sequences, it is possible to finely shape the metal-ion environment thanks to a subtle control over the first and second coordination sphere ligands, granted by amino acid residues. In some cases, this control goes beyond Nature's abilities, as peptide-based artificial metalloenzymes can be designed to catalyze also abiotic transformations. From other examples, it emerges that the structure–function relationship concept has been totally altered, as catalytic metal sites have been implanted into peptide scaffolds with structures completely different and unrelated to natural metalloenzymes.

This research field has strongly improved thanks to the development of different design strategies, computational methods, advances in molecular biology and high-throughput screening, whose combination appears very productive. Undoubtedly, peptide and protein designers have a formidable toolbox to develop any kind of functional peptide-based artificial metalloenzymes.

References

1. Crichton, R. R. (2019) *Biological Inorganic Chemistry: A New Introduction to Molecular Structure and Function*, 3rd edn. London, United Kingdom: Academic Press.
2. Maglio, O., Nastri, F. and Lombardi, A. (2012) Ionic interactions in natural and synthetic macromolecules. In *Structural and Functional Aspects of Metal Binding Sites in Natural and Designed Metalloproteins*, Ciferri, A. and Perico, A. eds., Chapter 11, pp. 361–450. Hoboken, NJ: John Wiley & Sons, Inc.
3. Valasatava, Y., Rosato, A., Furnham, N., Thornton, J. M. and Andreini, C. (2018) To what extent do structural changes in catalytic metal sites affect enzyme function? *J. Inorg. Biochem.* 179, pp. 40–53.
4. Valdez, C. E., Smith, Q. A., Nechay, M. R. and Alexandrova, A. N. (2014) Mysteries of metals in metalloenzymes. *Acc. Chem. Res.* 47, pp. 3110–3117.
5. Nastri, F., D'Alonzo, D., Leone, L., Zambrano, G., Pavone, V. and Lombardi, A. (2019) Engineering metalloprotein functions in designed and native scaffolds. *Trends Biochem. Sci.* 44, pp. 1022–1040.
6. Chino, M., Leone, L., Zambrano, G., Pirro, F., D'Alonzo, D., Firpo, V., Aref, D., Lista, L., Maglio, O., Nastri, F. and Lombardi, A. (2018) Oxidation catalysis by iron and manganese porphyrins within enzyme-like cages. *Biopolymers* 109, pp. e23107.
7. Nastri, F., Chino, M., Maglio, O., Bhagi-Damodaran, A., Lu, Y. and Lombardi, A. (2016) Design and engineering of artificial oxygen-activating metalloenzymes. *Chem. Soc. Rev.* 45, pp. 5020–5054.
8. Lombardi, A., Pirro, F., Maglio, O., Chino, M. and DeGrado, W. F. (2019) *de Novo* Design of four-helix bundle metalloproteins: One Scaffold, Diverse Reactivities. *Acc. Chem. Res.* 52, pp. 1148–1159.
9. Yu, F., Cangelosi, V. M., Zastrow, M. L., Tegoni, M., Plegaria, J. S., Tebo, A. G., Mocny, C. S., Ruckthong, L., Qayyum, H. and Pecoraro, V. L. (2014) Protein Design: Toward functional metalloenzymes. *Chem. Rev.* 114, pp. 3495–3578.
10. Zastrow, M. L. and Pecoraro, V. L. (2013) Designing Functional Metalloproteins: From Structural to Catalytic Metal Sites. *Coord. Chem. Rev.* 257, pp. 2565–2588.
11. Mocny, C. S. and Pecoraro, V. L. (2015) *de Novo* Protein Design as a Methodology for Synthetic Bioinorganic Chemistry. *Acc. Chem. Res.* 48, pp. 2388–2396.

12. Grayson, K. J. and Anderson, J. R. (2018) The ascent of man (made oxidoreductases). *Curr. Opin. Struct. Biol.* 51, pp. 149–155.
13. Bhagi-Damodaran, A., Hosseinzadeh, P., Mirts, E., Reed, J., Petrik, I. D., and Lu, Y. (2016) Design of heteronuclear metalloenzymes. In Pecoraro, V. L. *Methods in Enzymology*, vol. 580, pp. 501–537. Cambridge, MA: Academic Press.
14. Petrik, I. D., Liu, J., and Lu, Y. (2014) Metalloenzyme Design and Engineering Through Strategic Modifications of Native Protein Scaffolds. *Curr. Opin. Chem. Biol.* 19, pp. 67–75.
15. Lin, Y.-W. (2017) Rational design of metalloenzymes: From Single to Multiple Active Sites. *Coord. Chem. Rev.* 336, pp. 1–27.
16. Lewis, J. C. (2013) Artificial metalloenzymes and metallopeptide catalysts for organic synthesis. *ACS Catal.* 3, pp. 2954–2975.
17. Jeschek, M., Reuter, R., Heinisch, T., Trindler, C., Klehr, J., Panke, S. and Ward, T. R. (2016) Directed evolution of artificial metalloenzymes for *In Vivo* metathesis. *Nature.* 537, pp. 661–665.
18. Hyster, T. K. and Ward, T. R. (2016) Genetic optimization of Metalloenzymes: enhancing enzymes for non-natural reactions. *Angew. Chem. Int. Ed.* 55, pp. 7344–7357.
19. Jeschek, M., Panke, S. and Ward, T. R. (2018) Artificial metalloenzymes on the verge of new-to-nature metabolism. *Trends Biotechnol.* 36, pp. 60–72.
20. Schwizer, F., Okamoto, Y., Heinisch, T., Gu, Y., Pellizzoni, M. M. Lebrun, V., Reuter, R., Köhler, V., Lewis, J. C. and Ward, T. R. (2018) Artificial metalloenzymes: Reaction Scope and Optimization Strategies. *Chem. Rev.* 118, pp. 142–231.
21. Oohora, K., Onoda, A. and Hayashi, T. (2019) Hemoproteins reconstituted with artificial metal complexes as biohybrid catalysts. *Acc. Chem. Res.* 52, pp. 945–954.
22. Kleespies, S. T. Oloo, W. N. Mukherjee, A. and Que, L. (2015) C–H bond cleavage by bioinspired nonheme oxoiron(IV) Complexes, Including Hydroxylation of n-Butane. *Inorg. Chem.* 54, pp. 5053–5064.
23. Puri, M. and Que, L. (2015) Toward the synthesis of more reactive S = 2 non-heme oxoiron(IV) complexes. *Acc. Chem. Res.* 48, pp. 2443–2452.
24. Itoh, S. (2015) Developing mononuclear copper–active-oxygen complexes relevant to reactive intermediates of biological oxidation reactions. *Acc. Chem. Res.* 48, pp. 2066–2074.
25. Che, C.-M. and Huang, J.-S. (2009) Metalloporphyrin-based oxidation systems: From Biomimetic Reactions to Application in Organic Synthesis. *Chem. Commun.* pp. 3996–4015.
26. Costas, M. (2011) Selective C–H oxidation catalyzed by metalloporphyrins. *Coord. Chem. Rev.* 255, pp. 2912–2932.
27. Serrano-Plana, J., Garcia-Bosch, I., Company, A. and Costas, M. (2015) Structural and reactivity models for copper oxygenases: Cooperative Effects and Novel Reactivities. *Acc. Chem. Res.* 48, pp. 2397–2406.

28. Friedle, S., Reisner, E. and Lippard, S. J. (2010) Current challenges of modeling diiron enzyme active sites for dioxygen activation by biomimetic Synthetic Complexes. *Chem. Soc. Rev*. 39, pp. 2768–2779.
29. Hematian, S., Garcia-Bosch, I. and Karlin, K. D. (2015) Synthetic heme/copper assemblies: Toward an Understanding of Cytochrome c Oxidase Interactions with Dioxygen and Nitrogen Oxides. *Acc. Chem. Res*. 48, pp. 2462–2474.
30. Rolff, M., Schottenheim, J., Decker, H. and Tuczek, F. (2011) Copper–O2 reactivity of tyrosinase models towards external monophenolic substrates: Molecular Mechanism and Comparison with the Enzyme. *Chem. Soc. Rev*. 40, pp. 4077–4098.
31. Dalle, K. E. and Meyer, F. (2015) Modelling binuclear metallobiosites: insights from pyrazole-supported biomimetic and bioinspired complexes. *Eur. J. Inorg. Chem*. 2015, pp. 3391–3405.
32. Abdolahzadeh, S., Boer, J. W. de. and Browne, W. R. (2020) Redox-state dependent ligand exchange in manganese-based oxidation catalysis. *Eur. J. Inorg. Chem*. 2015, pp. 3432–3456.
33. Behrendt, R., White, P. and Offer, J. (2016) Advances in fmoc solid-phase peptide synthesis. *J. Pept. Sci*. 22, pp. 4–27.
34. Jad, Y. E., Kumar, A., El-Faham, A., de la Torre, B. G. and Albericio, F. (2019) Green transformation of solid-phase peptide synthesis. ACS Sustain. *Chem. Eng*. 7, pp. 3671–3683.
35. Gordon, C. P. (2018) The Renascence of continuous-flow peptide synthesis — An Abridged Account of Solid and Solution-Based Approaches. *Org. Biomol. Chem*. 16, pp. 180–196.
36. Góngora-Benítez, M., Tulla-Puche, J. and Albericio, F. (2013) Handles for fmoc solid-phase synthesis of protected peptides. *ACS Comb. Sci*. 15, pp. 217–228.
37. Rosano, G. L. and Ceccarelli, E. A. (2014) Recombinant protein expression in *escherichia coli*: Advances and Challenges. *Front. Microbiol*. 5.
38. Rodríguez, V., Asenjo, J. A. and Andrews, B. A. (2014) Design and implementation of a high yield production system for recombinant expression of peptides. *Microb. Cell Factories*. 13, pp. 65.
39. Liu, C. C. and Schultz, P. G. (2010) Adding new chemistries to the genetic code. *Annu. Rev. Biochem*. 79, pp. 413–444.
40. Baker, E. G., Bartlett, G. J., Porter Goff, K. L. and Woolfson, D. N. (2017) Miniprotein design: Past, Present, and Prospects. *Acc. Chem. Res*. 50, pp. 2085–2092.
41. Kuhlman, B. and Bradley, P. (2019) Advances in protein structure prediction and design. *Nat. Rev. Mol. Cell Biol*. 20, pp. 681–697.
42. Pan, X. and Kortemme, T. (2021) Recent advances in *de Novo* protein design: principles, Methods, and Applications. *J. Biol. Chem*. 296, pp. 100558.
43. Polizzi, N. F. and DeGrado, W. F. (2020) A Defined structural unit enables *de Novo* design of small-molecule–binding proteins. *Science* 369, pp. 1227–1233.

44. Wood, C. W., Bruning, M., Ibarra, A. Á., Bartlett, G. J., Thomson, A. R., Sessions, R. B., Brady, R. L. and Woolfson, D. N. (2014) CCBuilder: An interactive web-based tool for building, designing and assessing coiled-coil protein assemblies. *Bioinformatics* 30, pp. 3029–3035.
45. Gonzalez, G., Hannigan, B. and DeGrado, W. F. (2014) A Real-Time all-atom structural search engine for proteins. *PLoS Comput. Biol.* 10, pp. e1003750.
46. Zhou, J., Panaitiu, A. E. and Grigoryan, G. (2020) A General-purpose protein design framework based on mining sequence–structure relationships in known protein structures. *Proc. Natl. Acad. Sci.* 117, pp. 1059–1068.
47. Churchfield, L. A. and Tezcan, F. A. (2019) Design and Construction of Functional Supramolecular Metalloprotein Assemblies. *Acc. Chem. Res.* 52, pp. 345–355.
48. Alford, R. F., Leaver-Fay, A., Jeliazkov, J. R., O'Meara, M. J., DiMaio, F. P., Park, H., Shapovalov, M. V., Renfrew, P. D., Mulligan, V. K., Kappel, K., Labonte, J. W., Pacella, M. S., Bonneau, R., Bradley, P., Dunbrack, R. L., Das, R., Baker, D., Kuhlman, B., Kortemme, T. and Gray, J. J. (2017) The Rosetta all-atom energy function for macromolecular modeling and design. *J. Chem. Theory Comput.* 13, pp. 3031–3048.
49. Bhardwaj, G., Mulligan, V. K., Bahl, C. D., Gilmore, J. M., Harvey, P. J., Cheneval, O., Buchko, G. W., Pulavarti, S. V. S. R. K., Kaas, Q., Eletsky, A., Huang, P.-S., Johnsen, W. A., Greisen, P. J., Rocklin, G. J., Song, Y., Linsky, T. W., Watkins, A., Rettie, S. A., Xu, X., Carter, L. P., Bonneau, R., Olson, J. M., Coutsias, E., Correnti, C. E., Szyperski, T., Craik, D. J. and Baker, D. (2016) Accurate *de Novo* design of hyperstable constrained peptides. *Nature* 538, pp. 329–335.
50. Pan, X., Thompson, M. C., Zhang, Y., Liu, L., Fraser, J. S., Kelly, M. J. S. and Kortemme, T. (2020) Expanding the space of protein geometries by computational design of *de Novo* fold families. *Science* 369, pp. 1132–1136.
51. Moser, C. C., Sheehan, M. M., Ennist, N. M., Kodali, G., Bialas, C., Englander, M. T., Discher, B. M. and Dutton, P. L. (2016) *de Novo* Construction of redox active proteins. In Pecoraro, V. L. *Methods in Enzymology*, vol. 580, pp. 365–388. Cambridge, MA: Academic Press.
52. Lombardi, A., Nastri, F. and Pavone, V. (2001) Peptide-based heme–protein models. *Chem. Rev.* 101, pp. 3165–3190.
53. Leone, L., Chino, M., Nastri, F., Maglio, O., Pavone, V. and Lombardi, A. (2020) Mimochrome, a metalloporphyrin-Based Catalytic Swiss Knife†. *Biotechnol. Appl. Biochem.* 67, pp. 495–515.
54. Chino, M., Maglio, O., Nastri, F., Pavone, V., DeGrado, W. F. and Lombardi, A. (2015) Artificial diiron enzymes with a *De Novo* designed four-helix bundle structure. *Eur. J. Inorg. Chem.* 2015, pp. 3371–3390.

55. Manohar, M., Mooney, A. M., North, J. A., Nakkula, R. J., Picking, J. W., Edon, A., Fishel, R., Poirier, M. G. and Ottesen, J. J. (2009) Acetylation of histone H3 at the nucleosome dyad alters DNA-Histone binding. *J. Biol. Chem.* 284, pp. 23312–23321.
56. Hejjaoui, M., Butterfield, S., Fauvet, B., Vercruysse, F., Cui, J., Dikiy, I., Prudent, M., Olschewski, D., Zhang, Y., Eliezer, D. and Lashuel, H. A. (2012) Elucidating the role of C-terminal post-translational modifications using protein semisynthesis strategies: α-synuclein phosphorylation at tyrosine 125. *J. Am. Chem. Soc.* 134, pp. 5196–5210.
57. He, S., Bauman, D., Davis, J. S., Loyola, A., Nishioka, K., Gronlund, J. L., Reinberg, D., Meng, F., Kelleher, N. and McCafferty, D. G. (2003) Facile synthesis of site-specifically acetylated and methylated histone proteins: Reagents for Evaluation of the Histone Code Hypothesis. *Proc. Natl. Acad. Sci.* 100, pp. 12033–12038.
58. Unverzagt, C. and Kajihara, Y. (2013) Chemical assembly of *N*-glycoproteins: A refined toolbox to address a ubiquitous posttranslational modification. *Chem. Soc. Rev.* 42, pp. 4408–4420.
59. Piontek, C., Silva, D. V., Heinlein, C., Pöhner, C., Mezzato, S., Ring, P., Martin, A., Schmid, F. X. and Unverzagt, C. (2009) Semisynthesis of a homogeneous glycoprotein enzyme: ribonuclease C: Part 2. *Angew. Chem. Int. Ed.* 48, pp. 1941–1945.
60. Smolskaya, S. and Andreev, Y. A. (2019) Site-specific incorporation of unnatural amino acids into escherichia coli recombinant protein: Methodology Development and Recent Achievement. *Biomolecules* 9, p. 255.
61. Spicer, C. D. and Davis, B. G. (2014) Selective chemical protein modification. *Nat. Commun.* 5, p. 4740.
62. Erak, M., Bellmann-Sickert, K., Els-Heindl, S. and Beck-Sickinger, A. G. (2018) Peptide chemistry toolbox — transforming natural peptides into peptide therapeutics. *Bioorg. Med. Chem.* 26, pp. 2759–2765.
63. Tugyi, R., Uray, K., Iván, D., Fellinger, E., Perkins, A. and Hudecz, F. (2005) Partial D-amino acid substitution: Improved Enzymatic Stability and Preserved Ab Recognition of a MUC2 Epitope Peptide. *Proc. Natl. Acad. Sci.* 102, pp. 413–418.
64. Seebach, D., Beck, A. K. and Bierbaum, D. J. (2004) The world of β- and γ-peptides comprised of homologated proteinogenic amino acids and other components. *Chem. Biodivers.* 1, pp. 1111–1239.
65. Karle, I. L. and Balaram, P. (1990) Structural characteristics of alpha-hHelical peptide molecules containing Aib residues. *Biochemistry* 29, pp. 6747–6756.
66. Marshall, G. R., Hodgkin, E. E., Langs, D. A., Smith, G. D., Zabrocki, J. and Leplawy, M. T. (1990) Factors governing helical preference of peptides

containing multiple alpha, Alpha-Dialkyl Amino Acids. *Proc. Natl. Acad. Sci.* 87, pp. 487–491.

67. Di Costanzo, L., Dutta, S. and Burley, S. K. (2018) Amino Acid Modifications for Conformationally Constraining Naturally Occurring and Engineered Peptide Backbones: Insights from the Protein Data Bank. *Biopolymers* 109, p. e23230.
68. Drienovská, I., Rioz-Martínez, A., Draksharapu, A. and Roelfes, G. (2014) Novel artificial metalloenzymes by *In Vivo* incorporation of metal-binding unnatural amino acids. *Chem. Sci.* 6, pp. 770–776.
69. Mills, J. H., Khare, S. D., Bolduc, J. M., Forouhar, F., Mulligan, V. K., Lew, S., Seetharaman, J., Tong, L., Stoddard, B. L. and Baker, D. (2013) Computational design of an unnatural amino acid dependent metalloprotein with atomic level accuracy. *J. Am. Chem. Soc.* 135, pp. 13393–13399.
70. Clark, K. M., Tian, S., Donk, W. A. van der. and Lu, Y. (2016) Probing the role of the backbone carbonyl interaction with the cua center in azurin by replacing the peptide bond with an ester linkage. *Chem. Commun.* 53, pp. 224–227.
71. Caserta, G., Chino, M., Firpo, V., Zambrano, G., Leone, L., D'Alonzo, D., Nastri, F., Maglio, O., Pavone, V. and Lombardi, A. (2018) Enhancement of peroxidase activity in artificial mimochrome vi catalysts through rational design. *ChemBioChem.* 19, pp. 1823–1826.
72. Chino, M., Leone, L., Maglio, O., D'Alonzo, D., Pirro, F., Pavone, V., Nastri, F. and Lombardi, A. (2017) A *de Novo* Heterodimeric due ferri protein minimizes the release of reactive intermediates in dioxygen-dependent oxidation. *Angew. Chem. Int. Ed.* 56, pp. 15580–15583.
73. Koebke, K. J. and Pecoraro, V. L. (2019) Noncoded amino acids in *de novo* metalloprotein design: Controlling Coordination Number and Catalysis. *Acc. Chem. Res.* 52, pp. 1160–1167.
74. DeGrado, W. F., Summa, C. M., Pavone, V., Nastri, F. and Lombardi, A. (1999) *de Novo* Design and structural characterization of proteins and metalloproteins. *Annu. Rev. Biochem.* 68, pp. 779–819.
75. Koga, N., Tatsumi-Koga, R., Liu, G., Xiao, R., Acton, T. B., Montelione, G. T. and Baker, D. (2012) Principles for designing ideal protein structures. *Nature* 491, pp. 222–227.
76. Groß, A., Hashimoto, C., Sticht, H. and Eichler, J. (2016) Synthetic peptides as protein mimics. *Front. Bioeng. Biotechnol.* 3, 211. doi:10.3389/fbioe.2015.00211.
77. Lombardi, A., Marasco, D., Maglio, O., Di Costanzo, L., Nastri, F. and Pavone, V. (2000) Miniaturized metalloproteins: application to iron–sulfur proteins. *Proc. Natl. Acad. Sci.* 97, pp. 11922–11927.
78. Xing, G. and DeRose, V. J. (2001) Designing metal–peptide models for protein structure and function. *Curr. Opin. Chem. Biol.* 5, pp. 196–200.

79. Leone, L., D'Alonzo, D., Balland, V., Zambrano, G., Chino, M., Nastri, F., Maglio, O., Pavone, V. and Lombardi, A. (2018) Mn-Mimochrome VI*a: An artificial metalloenzyme with peroxygenase activity. *Front. Chem.* 6.
80. Firpo, V., Le, J. M., Pavone, V., Lombardi, A. and Bren, K. L. (2018) Hydrogen evolution from water catalyzed by cobalt-mimochrome VI*a, a synthetic mini-protein. *Chem. Sci.* 9, pp. 8582–8589.
81. Le, J. M., Alachouzos, G., Chino, M., Frontier, A. J., Lombardi, A. and Bren, K. L. (2020) Tuning mechanism through buffer dependence of hydrogen evolution catalyzed by a cobalt mini-enzyme. *Biochemistry* 59, pp. 1289–1297.
82. Roy, A., Sommer, D. J., Schmitz, R. A., Brown, C. L., Gust, D., Astashkin, A. and Ghirlanda, G. (2014) A *de Novo* Designed 2[4Fe-4S] ferredoxin mimic mediates electron transfer. *J. Am. Chem. Soc.* 136, pp. 17343–17349.
83. Smith, B. A. and Hecht, M. H. (2011) Novel proteins: from fold to function. *Curr. Opin. Chem. Biol.* 15, pp. 421–426.
84. Zhang, S.-Q., Chino, M., Liu, L., Tang, Y., Hu, X., DeGrado, W. F. and Lombardi, A. (2018) *de Novo* Design of tetranuclear transition metal clusters stabilized by hydrogen-bonded networks in helical bundles. *J. Am. Chem. Soc.* 140, pp. 1294–1304.
85. Koebke, K. J., Yu, F., Salerno, E., Van Stappen, C., Tebo, A. G., Penner-Hahn, J. E. and Pecoraro, V. L. (2018) Modifying the steric properties in the second coordination sphere of designed peptides leads to enhancement of nitrite reductase activity. *Angew. Chem. Int. Ed.* 57, pp. 3954–3957.
86. Chino, M., Zhang, S.-Q., Pirro, F., Leone, L., Maglio, O., Lombardi, A. and DeGrado, W. F. (2018) Spectroscopic and metal binding properties of a *de novo* metalloprotein binding a tetrazinc cluster. *Biopolymers* 109, pp. e23339.
87. Lin, Y.-W. (2019) Rational design of artificial metalloproteins and metalloenzymes with metal clusters. *Molecules*. 24, pp. 2743.
88. Koebke, K. J., Alfaro, V. S., Pinter, T. B. J., Deb, A., Lehnert, N., Tard, C., Penner-Hahn, J. E. and Pecoraro, V. L. (2020) Traversing the red–green–blue color spectrum in rationally designed cupredoxins. *J. Am. Chem. Soc.* 142, pp. 15282–15294.
89. Mathieu, E., Tolbert, A. E., Koebke, K. J., Tard, C., Iranzo, O., Penner-Hahn, J. E., Policar, C. and Pecoraro, V. (2020) Rational *de Novo* design of a cu metalloenzyme for superoxide dismutation. *Chem. – Eur. J.* 26, pp. 249–258.
90. Yin, L., Yuan, H., Liu, C., He, B., Gao, S.-Q., Wen, G.-B., Tan, X. and Lin, Y.-W. (2018) A rationally designed myoglobin exhibits a catalytic dehalogenation efficiency more than 1000-fold that of a native dehaloperoxidase. *ACS Catal.* 8, pp. 9619–9624.
91. Mirts, E. N., Petrik, I. D., Hosseinzadeh, P., Nilges, M. J. and Lu, Y. (2018) A designed heme-[4fe-4s] metalloenzyme catalyzes sulfite reduction like the native enzyme. *Science*. 361, pp. 1098–1101.

92. Liang, A. D., Serrano-Plana, J., Peterson, R. L. and Ward, T. R. (2019) Artificial metalloenzymes based on the biotin-streptavidin technology: Enzymatic Cascades and Directed Evolution. *Acc. Chem. Res.* 52, pp. 585–595.
93. Arnold, F. H. (2018) Directed evolution: bringing new chemistry to life. *Angew. Chem. Int. Ed.* 57, pp. 4143–4148.
94. Umezawa, N., Matsumoto, N., Iwama, S., Kato, N. and Higuchi, T. (2010) Facile synthesis of peptide–porphyrin conjugates: Towards Artificial Catalase. *Bioorg. Med. Chem.* 18, pp. 6340–6350.
95. Marques, H. M. (2007) Insights into porphyrin chemistry provided by the microperoxidases, The Haempeptides Derived From Cytochrome C. *Dalton Trans.* pp. 4371–4385.
96. Nicolis, S., Casella, L., Roncone, R., Dallacosta, C. and Monzani, E. (2007) Heme-peptide complexes as peroxidase models. *Comptes. Rendus. Chim.* 10, pp. 380–391.
97. Casella, L., De Gioia, L., Frontoso Silvestri, G., Monzani, E., Redaelli, C., Roncone, R. and Santagostini, L. (2000) Covalently modified microperoxidases as heme-peptide models for peroxidases. *J. Inorg. Biochem.* 79, pp. 31–40.
98. Dallacosta, C., Casella, L. and Monzani, E. (2004) Modified microperoxidases exhibit different reactivity towards phenolic substrates. *Chem Bio Chem.* 5, pp. 1692–1699.
99. Perutz, M. F., Hasnain, S. S., Duke, P. J., Sessler, J. L. and Hahn, J. E. (1982) Stereochemistry of iron in deoxyhaemoglobin. *Nature.* 295, pp. 535–538.
100. Nastri, F., Lombardi, A., Morelli, G., Maglio, O., D'Auria, G., Pedone, C. and Pavone, V. (1997) Hemoprotein models based on a covalent helix–heme–helix sandwich: 1. Design, Synthesis, and Characterization. *Chem. – Eur. J.* 3, pp. 340–349.
101. Lombardi, A., Nastri, F., Marasco, D., Maglio, O., Sanctis, G. D., Sinibaldi, F., Santucci, R., Coletta, M. and Pavone, V. (2003) Design of a new mimochrome with unique topology. *Chem. – Eur. J.* 9, pp. 5643–5654.
102. Di Costanzo, L., Geremia, S., Randaccio, L., Nastri, F., Maglio, O., Lombardi, A. and Pavone, V. (2004) Miniaturized heme proteins: crystal structure of Co(III)-mimochrome IV. *J. Biol. Inorg. Chem.* 9, pp. 1017–1027.
103. Vicari, C., Saraiva, I. H., Maglio, O., Nastri, F., Pavone, V., Louro, R. O. and Lombardi, A. (2014) Artificial heme-proteins: determination of axial ligand orientations through paramagnetic NMR shifts. *Chem. Commun.* 50, pp. 3852–3855.
104. Maglio, O., Chino, M., Vicari, C., Pavone, V., Louro, R. O. and Lombardi, A. (2021) Histidine orientation in artificial peroxidase regioisomers as determined by paramagnetic NMR shifts. *Chem. Commun.* 57, pp. 990–993.
105. Nastri, F., Lista, L., Ringhieri, P., Vitale, R., Faiella, M., Andreozzi, C., Travascio, P., Maglio, O., Lombardi, A. and Pavone, V. (2011) A

heme-peptide metalloenzyme mimetic with natural peroxidase-like activity. *Chem. - Eur. J.* 17, pp. 4444–4453.

106. Vitale, R., Lista, L., Cerrone, C., Caserta, G., Chino, M., Maglio, O., Nastri, F., Pavone, V. and Lombardi, A. (2015) Artificial heme-enzyme with enhanced catalytic activity: evolution, functional screening and structural characterization. *Org. Biomol. Chem.* 13, pp. 4858–4868.
107. Zambrano, G., Nastri, F., Pavone, V., Lombardi, A. and Chino, M. (2020) Use of an artificial miniaturized enzyme in hydrogen peroxide detection by chemiluminescence. *Sensors* 20, pp. 3793.
108. Leone, L., D'Alonzo, D., Maglio, O., Pavone, V., Nastri, F. and Lombardi, A. (2021) Highly selective indole oxidation catalyzed by a Mn-containing artificial mini-enzyme. *ACS Catal.* pp. 9407–9417.
109. Ranieri, A., Monari, S., Sola, M., Borsari, M., Battistuzzi, G., Ringhieri, P., Nastri, F., Pavone, V. and Lombardi, A. (2010) Redox and electrocatalytic properties of mimochrome VI, a synthetic heme peptide adsorbed on gold. *Langmuir* 26, pp. 17831–17835.
110. Zambrano, G., Ruggiero, E., Malafronte, A., Chino, M., Maglio, O., Pavone, V., Nastri, F. and Lombardi, A. (2018) Artificial heme enzymes for the construction of gold-based biomaterials. *Int. J. Mol. Sci.* 19, pp. 2896.
111. Vitale, R., Lista, L., Lau-Truong, S., Tucker, R. T., Brett, M. J., Limoges, B., Pavone, V., Lombardi, A. and Balland, V. (2014) Spectroelectrochemistry of FeIII- and CoIII-mimochrome VI Artificial enzymes immobilized on mesoporous ITO electrodes. *Chem. Commun.* 50, pp. 1894–1896.
112. Zambrano, G., Chino, M., Renzi, E., Girolamo, R. D., Maglio, O., Pavone, V., Lombardi, A. and Nastri, F. (2020) Clickable artificial heme-peroxidases for the development of functional nanomaterials. *Biotechnol. Appl. Biochem.* 67, pp. 549–562.
113. Venanzi, M., Cianfanelli, S. and Palleschi, A. (2014) Mimicking hemoproteins: a new synthetic metalloenzyme based on a Fe(III)-mesoporphyrin functionalized by two helical decapeptides: A Peptide Catalyst Mimicking Hemoproteins. *J. Pept. Sci.* 20, pp. 36–45.
114. Faiella, M., Maglio, O., Nastri, F., Lombardi, A., Lista, L., Hagen, W. R. and Pavone, V. (2012) *de Novo* Design, synthesis and characterisation of MP3, A new catalytic four-helix bundle hemeprotein. *Chem. – Eur. J.* 18, pp. 15960–15971.
115. Rodriguez-Lopez, J. N., Smith, A. T. and Thorneley, R. N. F. (1996) Role of arginine 38 in horseradish peroxidase: A Critical Residue for Substrate Binding and Catalysis. *J. Biol. Chem.* 271, pp. 4023–4030.
116. Koder, R. L., Anderson, J. L. R., Solomon, L. A., Reddy, K. S., Moser, C. C. and Dutton, P. L. (2009) Design and engineering of an O_2 transport protein. *Nature* 458, pp. 305–309.

117. Farid, T. A., Kodali, G., Solomon, L. A., Lichtenstein, B. R., Sheehan, M. M., Fry, B. A., Bialas, C., Ennist, N. M., Siedlecki, J. A., Zhao, Z., Stetz, M. A., Valentine, K. G., Anderson, J. L. R., Wand, A. J., Discher, B. M., Moser, C. C. and Dutton, P. L. (2013) Elementary Tetrahelical protein design for diverse oxidoreductase functions. *Nat. Chem. Biol.* 9, pp. 826–833.
118. Anderson, J. L. R., Armstrong, C. T., Kodali, G., Lichtenstein, B. R., Watkins, D. W., Mancini, J. A., Boyle, A. L., Farid, T. A., Crump, M. P., Moser, C. C. and Dutton, P. L. (2013) Constructing a man-made c-type cytochrome maquette *In Vivo*: Electron Transfer, Oxygen Transport and Conversion to a Photoactive Light Harvesting Maquette. *Chem. Sci.* 5, pp. 507–514.
119. Watkins, D. W., Jenkins, J. M. X., Grayson, K. J., Wood, N., Steventon, J. W., Le Vay, K. K., Goodwin, M. I., Mullen, A. S., Bailey, H. J., Crump, M. P., MacMillan, F., Mulholland, A. J., Cameron, G., Sessions, R. B., Mann, S. and Anderson, J. L. R. (2017) Construction and *in vivo* assembly of a catalytically proficient and hyperthermostable *de Novo* enzyme. *Nat. Commun.* 8, pp. 1–9.
120. Stenner, R., Steventon, J. W., Seddon, A. and Anderson, J. L. R. (2020) A *de Novo* peroxidase is also a promiscuous yet stereoselective carbene transferase. *Proc. Natl. Acad. Sci.* 117, pp. 1419–1428.
121. Moffet, D. A., Certain, L. K., Smith, A. J., Kessel, A. J., Beckwith, K. A. and Hecht, M. H. (2000) Peroxidase activity in heme proteins derived from a designed combinatorial library. *J. Am. Chem. Soc.* 122, pp. 7612–7613.
122. Patel, S. C., Bradley, L. H., Jinadasa, S. P. and Hecht, M. H. (2009) Cofactor binding and enzymatic activity in an unevolved superfamily of *de Novo* Designed 4-Helix Bundle Proteins. *Protein Sci.* 18, pp. 1388–1400.
123. Das, A. and Hecht, M. H. (2007) Peroxidase activity of *de Novo* heme proteins immobilized on electrodes. *J. Inorg. Biochem.* 101, pp. 1820–1826.
124. Patel, S. C. and Hecht, M. H. (2012) Directed evolution of the peroxidase activity of a *de Novo*-designed protein. *Protein Eng. Des. Sel.* 25, pp. 445–452.
125. Rufo, C. M., Moroz, Y. S., Moroz, O. V., Stöhr, J., Smith, T. A., Hu, X., DeGrado, W. F. and Korendovych, I. V. (2014) Short peptides self-assemble to produce catalytic amyloids. *Nat. Chem.* 6, pp. 303–309.
126. Richardson, J. S. and Richardson, D. C. (2002) Natural beta-sheet proteins use negative design to avoid edge-to-edge aggregation. *Proc. Natl. Acad. Sci. USA* 99, pp. 2754–2759.
127. Ouberai, M., Dolphin, G. T., Dumy, P. and Garcia, J. (2011) Amyloidogenesis highlighted by designed peptides forming supramolecular self-assemblies. *Chem. Sci.* 2, pp. 1293–1300.
128. Hughes, R. M. and Waters, M. L. (2006) Model systems for β-hairpins and β-sheets. *Curr. Opin. Struct. Biol.* 16, pp. 514–524.

129. Jiménez, M. A. (2014) Design of monomeric water-soluble β-hairpin and β-sheet peptides. In *Protein Design: Methods and Applications*, Köhler, V. ed., pp. 15–52. New York, NY: Springer.
130. Mahajan, M. and Bhattacharjya, S. (2013) β-Hairpin peptides: Heme Binding, Catalysis, and Structure in Detergent Micelles. *Angew. Chem. Int. Ed.* 52, pp. 6430–6434.
131. D'Souza, A., Torres, J. and Bhattacharjya, S. (2018) Expanding heme-protein folding space using designed multi-heme β-sheet mini-proteins. *Commun. Chem.* 1, pp. 78.
132. D'Souza, A., Mahajan, M. and Bhattacharjya, S. (2016) Designed multi-stranded heme binding β-sheet peptides in membrane. *Chem. Sci.* 7, pp. 2563–2571.
133. D'Souza, A., Wu, X., Yeow, E. K. L. and Bhattacharjya, S. (2017) Designed heme-cage β-sheet miniproteins. *Angew. Chem. Int. Ed.* 56, pp. 5904–5908.
134. D'Souza, A. and Bhattacharjya, S. (2021) *de Novo*-designed β-sheet heme proteins. *Biochemistry* 60, pp. 431–439.
135. Cordova, J. M., Noack, P. L., Hilcove, S. A., Lear, J. D. and Ghirlanda, G. (2007) Design of a functional membrane protein by engineering a heme-binding site in glycophorin A. *J. Am. Chem. Soc.* 129, pp. 512–518.
136. Cui, H., Webber, M. J. and Stupp, S. I. (2010) Self-Assembly of peptide amphiphiles: From Molecules to Nanostructures to Biomaterials. *Pept. Sci.* 94, pp. 1–18.
137. Solomon, L. A., Kronenberg, J. B. and Fry, H. C. (2017) Control of heme coordination and catalytic activity by conformational changes in peptide–amphiphile assemblies. *J. Am. Chem. Soc.* 139, pp. 8497–8507.
138. Zozulia, O. and Korendovych, I. V. (2020) Semi-rationally designed short peptides self-assemble and bind hemin to promote cyclopropanation. *Angew. Chem. Int. Ed.* 59, pp. 8108–8112.
139. Plegaria, J. S. and Pecoraro, V. L. (2015) Sculpting metal-binding environments in *de novo* designed three-helix bundles. *Isr. J. Chem.* 55, pp. 85–95.
140. Tebo, A. G. and Pecoraro, V. L. (2015) Artificial metalloenzymes derived from three-helix bundles. *Curr. Opin. Chem. Biol.* 25, pp. 65–70.
141. Pinter, T. B. J., Koebke, K. J. and Pecoraro, V. L. (2020) Catalysis and electron transfer in *de novo* designed helical scaffolds. *Angew. Chem. Int. Ed.* 59, pp. 7678–7699.
142. Dieckmann, G. R., McRorie, D. K., Lear, J. D., Sharp, K. A., DeGrado, W. F. and Pecoraro, V. L. (1998) The role of protonation and metal chelation preferences in defining the properties of mercury-binding coiled coils. *J. Mol. Biol.* 280, pp. 897–912.

143. Dieckmann, G. R., McRorie, D. K., Tierney, D. L., Utschig, L. M., Singer, C. P., O'Halloran, T. V., Penner-Hahn, J. E., DeGrado, W. F. and Pecoraro, V. L. (1997) *de Novo* Design of mercury-binding two- and three-helical bundles. *J. Am. Chem. Soc.* 119, pp. 6195–6196.
144. Lovejoy, B., Choe, S., Cascio, D., McRorie, D. K., DeGrado, W. F. and Eisenberg, D. (1993) Crystal structure of a synthetic triple-stranded alpha-helical bundle. *Science* 259, pp. 1288–1293.
145. O'Neil, K. T. and DeGrado, W. F. (1990) A thermodynamic scale for the helix-forming tendencies of the commonly occurring amino acids. *Science* 250, pp. 646–651.
146. Zastrow, M. L., Peacock, A. F. A., Stuckey, J. A. and Pecoraro, V. L. (2012) Hydrolytic catalysis and structural stabilization in a designed metalloprotein. *Nat. Chem.* 4, pp. 118–123.
147. Zastrow, M. L. and Pecoraro, V. L. (2014) Designing hydrolytic zinc metalloenzymes. *Biochemistry.* 53, pp. 957–978.
148. Tegoni, M., Yu, F., Bersellini, M., Penner-Hahn, J. E. and Pecoraro, V. L. (2012) Designing a functional type 2 copper center that has nitrite reductase activity within α-helical coiled coils. *Proc. Natl. Acad. Sci.* 109, pp. 21234–21239.
149. Koebke, K. J. and Pecoraro, V. L. (2018) Development of *de Novo* copper nitrite reductases: Where We are and Where We Need to Go. *ACS Catal.* 8, pp. 8046–8057.
150. Berwick, M. R., Lewis, D. J., Jones, A. W., Parslow, R. A., Dafforn, T. R., Cooper, H. J., Wilkie, J., Pikramenou, Z., Britton, M. M. and Peacock, A. F. A. (2014) *de Novo* Design of Ln(III) coiled coils for imaging applications. *J. Am. Chem. Soc.* 136, pp. 1166–1169.
151. Bryson, J. W., Desjarlais, J. R., Handel, T. M. and DeGrado, W. F. (1998) From coiled coils to small globular proteins: Design of a Native-Like Three-Helix Bundle. *Protein Sci.* 7, pp. 1404–1414.
152. Cangelosi, V. M., Deb, A., Penner-Hahn, J. E. and Pecoraro, V. L. (2014) A *de Novo* Designed metalloenzyme for the hydration of CO2. *Angew. Chem. Int. Ed.* 53, pp. 7900–7903.
153. Der, B. S., Edwards, D. R. and Kuhlman, B. (2012) Catalysis by a *de Novo* zinc-mediated protein interface: Implications for Natural Enzyme Evolution and Rational Enzyme Engineering. *Biochemistry* 51, pp. 3933–3940.
154. Studer, S., Hansen, D. A., Pianowski, Z. L., Mittl, P. R. E., Debon, A., Guffy, S. L., Der, B. S., Kuhlman, B. and Hilvert, D. (2018) Evolution of a highly active and enantiospecific metalloenzyme from short peptides. *Science* 362, pp. 1285–1288.
155. Basler, S., Studer, S., Zou, Y., Mori, T., Ota, Y., Camus, A., Bunzel, H. A., Helgeson, R. C., Houk, K. N., Jiménez-Osés, G. and Hilvert, D. (2021)

Efficient lewis acid catalysis of an abiological reaction in a *de novo* protein scaffold. *Nat. Chem.* 13, pp. 231–235.
156. Nomura, A. and Sugiura, Y. (2004) Hydrolytic Reaction by Zinc Finger Mutant Peptides: Successful redesign of structural zinc sites into catalytic zinc sites. *Inorg. Chem.* 43, pp. 1708–1713.
157. Dhanasekaran, M., Negi, S. and Sugiura, Y. (2006) Designer Zinc Finger Proteins: Tools for creating artificial DNA-binding functional proteins. *Acc. Chem. Res.* 39, pp. 45–52.
158. Patel, K., Srivastava, K. R. and Durani, S. (2010) Zinc-Finger Hydrolase: Computational selection of a linker and a sequence towards metal activation with a synthetic *αββ* protein. *Bioorg. Med. Chem.* 18, pp. 8270–8276.
159. Srivastava, K. R. and Durani, S. (2014) Design of a zinc-finger hydrolase with a synthetic *αββ* protein. *Plos One* 9, pp. e96234.
160. Carvalho, H. F., Branco, R. J. F., Leite, F. A. S., Matzapetakis, M., Roque, A. C. A. and Iranzo, O. (2019) Hydrolytic zinc metallopeptides using a computational multi-state design approach. *Catal. Sci. Technol.* 9, pp. 6723–6736.
161. Kiss, G., Çelebi-Ölçüm, N., Moretti, R., Baker, D. and Houk, K. N. (2013) Computational enzyme design. *Angew. Chem. Int. Ed.* 52, pp. 5700–5725.
162. Heinisch, T., Pellizzoni, M., Dürrenberger, M., Tinberg, C. E., Köhler, V., Klehr, J., Häussinger, D., Baker, D. and Ward, T. R. (2015) Improving the catalytic performance of an artificial metalloenzyme by computational design. *J. Am. Chem. Soc.* 137, pp. 10414–10419.
163. Khare, S. D., Kipnis, Y., Takeuchi, R., Ashani, Y., Goldsmith, M., Song, Y., Gallaher, J. L., Silman, I., Leader, H., Sussman, J. L., Stoddard, B. L., Tawfik, D. S. and Baker, D. (2012) Computational redesign of a mononuclear zinc metalloenzyme for organophosphate hydrolysis. *Nat. Chem. Biol.* 8, pp. 294–300.
164. Salgado, E. N., Radford, R. J. and Tezcan, F. A. (2010) Metal-directed protein self-assembly. *Acc. Chem. Res.* 43, pp. 661–672.
165. Radford, R. J., Brodin, J. D., Salgado, E. N. and Tezcan, F. A. (2011) Expanding the utility of proteins as platforms for coordination chemistry. *Coord. Chem. Rev.* 255, pp. 790–803.
166. Sontz, P. A., Song, W. J. and Tezcan, F. A. (2014) Interfacial metal coordination in engineered protein and peptide assemblies. *Curr. Opin. Chem. Biol.* 19, pp. 42–49.
167. Song, W. J. and Tezcan, F. A. (2014) A Designed supramolecular protein assembly with in vivo enzymatic activity. *Science* 346, pp. 1525–1528.
168. Song, W. J., Yu, J. and Tezcan, F. A. (2017) Importance of scaffold flexibility/rigidity in the design and directed evolution of artificial metallo-*β*-lactamases. *J. Am. Chem. Soc.* 139, pp. 16772–16779.

169. Churchfield, L. A., Alberstein, R. G., Williamson, L. M. and Tezcan, F. A. (2018) Determining the structural and energetic basis of allostery in a *de novo* designed metalloprotein assembly. *J. Am. Chem. Soc.* 140, pp. 10043–10053.
170. Rittle, J., Field, M. J., Green, M. T. and Tezcan, F. A. (2019) An efficient, step-economical strategy for the design of functional metalloproteins. *Nat. Chem.* 11, pp. 434–441.
171. Kakkis, A., Gagnon, D., Esselborn, J., Britt, R. D. and Tezcan, F. A. (2020) Metal-templated design of chemically switchable protein assemblies with high-affinity coordination sites. *Angew. Chem. Int. Ed.* 59, pp. 21940–21944.
172. Kamtekar, S. and Hecht, M. H. (1995) Protein motifs. 7. the four-helix bundle: what determines a fold? *FASEB J.* 9, pp. 1013–1022.
173. Peacock, A. F. (2016) Recent advances in designed coiled coils and helical bundles with inorganic prosthetic groups — from structural to functional applications. *Curr. Opin. Chem. Biol.* 31, pp. 160–165.
174. Lombardi, A., Summa, C. M., Geremia, S., Randaccio, L., Pavone, V. and DeGrado, W. F. (2000) Retrostructural analysis of metalloproteins: application to the design of a minimal model for diiron proteins. *Proc. Natl. Acad. Sci.* 97, pp. 6298–6305.
175. Maglio, O., Nastri, F., Pavone, V., Lombardi, A. and DeGrado, W. F. (2003) Preorganization of molecular binding sites in designed diiron proteins. *Proc. Natl. Acad. Sci. USA* 100, pp. 3772–3777.
176. Di Costanzo, L., Wade, H., Geremia, S., Randaccio, L., Pavone, V., DeGrado, W. F. and Lombardi, A. (2001) Toward the *de Novo* design of a catalytically active helix bundle: A Substrate-Accessible Carboxylate-Bridged Dinuclear Metal Center. *J. Am. Chem. Soc.* 123, pp. 12749–12757.
177. DeGrado, W. F., Di Costanzo, L., Geremia, S., Lombardi, A., Pavone, V. and Randaccio, L. (2003) Sliding helix and change of coordination geometry in a model di-mnii protein. *Angew. Chem. Int. Ed.* 42, pp. 417–420.
178. Lahr, S. J., Engel, D. E., Stayrook, S. E., Maglio, O., North, B., Geremia, S., Lombardi, A. and DeGrado, W. F. (2005) Analysis and design of turns in α-helical hairpins. *J. Mol. Biol.* 346, pp. 1441–1454.
179. Maglio, O., Nastri, F., Calhoun, J. R., Lahr, S., Wade, H., Pavone, V., DeGrado, W. F. and Lombardi, A. (2005) Artificial di-iron proteins: solution characterization of four helix bundles containing two distinct types of inter-helical loops. *J. Biol. Inorg. Chem.* 10, pp. 539–549.
180. Faiella, M., Andreozzi, C., de Rosales, R. T. M., Pavone, V., Maglio, O., Nastri, F., DeGrado, W. F. and Lombardi, A. (2009) An artificial di-iron oxo-protein with phenol oxidase activity. *Nat. Chem. Biol.* 5, pp. 882–884.
181. Torres Martin de Rosales, R., Faiella, M., Farquhar, E., Que, L., Andreozzi, C., Pavone, V., Maglio, O., Nastri, F. and Lombardi, A. (2010) Spectroscopic and

metal-binding properties of DF3: An Artificial Protein Able to Accommodate Different Metal Ions. *JBIC J. Biol. Inorg. Chem.* 15, pp. 717–728.

182. Kolb, H. C., Finn, M. G. and Sharpless, K. B. (2001) Click chemistry: Diverse chemical function from a few good reactions. *Angew. Chem. Int. Ed.* 40, pp. 2004–2021.
183. Chino, M., Leone, L., Maglio, O. and Lombardi, A. (2016) Designing covalently linked heterodimeric four-helix bundles. *Methods Enzymol.* 580, pp. 471–499.
184. Summa, C. M., Rosenblatt, M. M., Hong, J.-K., Lear, J. D. and DeGrado, W. F. (2002) Computational *de Novo* Design, and characterization of an A2B2 diiron protein. *J. Mol. Biol.* 321, pp. 923–938.
185. Marsh, E. N. G. and DeGrado, W. F. (2002) Noncovalent self-assembly of a heterotetrameric diiron protein. *Proc. Natl. Acad. Sci.* 99, pp. 5150–5154.
186. Kaplan, J. and DeGrado, W. F. (2004) *de Novo* Design of catalytic proteins. *Proc. Natl. Acad. Sci. USA* 101, pp. 11566–11570.
187. Calhoun, J. R., Kono, H., Lahr, S., Wang, W., DeGrado, W. F. and Saven, J. G. (2003) Computational design and characterization of a monomeric helical dinuclear metalloprotein. *J. Mol. Biol.* 334, pp. 1101–1115.
188. Reig, A. J., Pires, M. M., Snyder, R. A., Wu, Y., Jo, H., Kulp, D. W., Butch, S. E., Calhoun, J. R., Szyperski, T., Solomon, E. I. and DeGrado, W. F. (2012) Altering the O2-dependent reactivity of *de Novo* due ferri proteins. *Nat. Chem.* 4, pp. 900–906.
189. Ulas, G., Lemmin, T., Wu, Y., Gassner, G. T. and DeGrado, W. F. (2016) Designed metalloprotein stabilizes a semiquinone radical. *Nat. Chem.* 8, pp. 354–359.
190. Pirro, F., Schmidt, N., Lincoff, J., Widel, Z. X., Polizzi, N. F., Liu, L., Therien, M. J., Grabe, M., Chino, M., Lombardi, A. and DeGrado, W. F. (2020) Allosteric cooperation in a *de novo*-designed two-domain protein. *Proc. Natl. Acad. Sci.* 117, pp. 33246–33253.
191. Polizzi, N. F., Wu, Y., Lemmin, T., Maxwell, A. M., Zhang, S.-Q., Rawson, J., Beratan, D. N., Therien, M. J. and DeGrado, W. F. (2017) *de Novo* Design of a hyperstable non-natural protein-ligand complex with sub-Å accuracy. *Nat. Chem.* 9, pp. 1157–1164.
192. Yoon, J. H., Kulesha, A. V., Lengyel-Zhand, Z., Volkov, A. N., Rempillo, J. J., D'Souza, A., Costeas, C., Chester, C., Caselle, E. R. and Makhlynets, O. V. (2019) Uno ferro, a de novo designed protein, binds transition metals with high affinity and stabilizes semiquinone radical anion. *Chem. – Eur. J.* 25, pp. 15252–15256.
193. Kulesha, A., Yoon, J. H., Chester, C., D'Souza, A., Costeas, C. and Makhlynets, O. V. (2020) Contributions of primary coordination ligands and importance of outer sphere interactions in UFsc, A *de Novo* Designed Protein with High Affinity for Metal Ions. *J. Inorg. Biochem.* 212, pp. 111224.

194. Olson, T. L., Espiritu, E., Edwardraja, S., Canarie, E., Flores, M., Williams, J. C., Ghirlanda, G. and Allen, J. P. (2017) Biochemical and spectroscopic characterization of dinuclear mn-sites in artificial four-helix bundle proteins. *Biochim. Biophys. Acta BBA – Bioenerg.* 1858, pp. 945–954.
195. Jones, A. K., Lichtenstein, B. R., Dutta, A., Gordon, G. and Dutton, P. L. (2007) Synthetic hydrogenases: incorporation of an iron carbonyl thiolate into a designed peptide. *J. Am. Chem. Soc.* 129, pp. 14844–14845.
196. Roy, A., Madden, C. and Ghirlanda, G. (2012) Photo-Induced hydrogen production in a helical peptide incorporating a [FeFe] hydrogenase active site mimic. *Chem. Commun.* 48, pp. 9816–9818.
197. Chakrabartty, A., Kortemme, T. and Baldwin, R. L. (1994) Helix propensities of the amino acids measured in alanine-based peptides without helix-stabilizing side-chain interactions. *Protein Sci.* 3, pp. 843–852.
198. Marqusee, S., Robbins, V. H. and Baldwin, R. L. (1989) Unusually stable helix formation in short alanine-based peptides. *Proc. Natl. Acad. Sci. USA.* 86, pp. 5286–5290.
199. Sano, Y., Onoda, A. and Hayashi, T. (2012) Photocatalytic hydrogen evolution by a diiron hydrogenase model based on a peptide fragment of cytochrome c556 with an attached diiron carbonyl cluster and an attached ruthenium photosensitizer. *J. Inorg. Biochem.* 108, pp. 159–162.

https://doi.org/10.1142/9789811261664_0011

Chapter 11

Biohybrid Catalysts Harboring Synthetic Metal Complexes within β-Barrel Proteins

Akira Onoda[*, ‡], Shunsuke Kato[†], and Takashi Hayashi[†, §]

[*]*Faculty of Environmental Earth Science, Hokkaido University, Japan*
[†]*Department of Applied Chemistry, Graduate School of Engineering, Osaka University, Suita Japan*

[‡]*akira.onoda@ees.hokudai.ac.jp*
[§]*thayashi@chem.eng.osaka-u.ac.jp*

1. Introduction

Enzymes are elegant catalysts for living systems. They catalyze a wide range of reactions with high levels of selectivity and efficiency in a range of conditions in temperature, pH, pressure, and others. Advancements in protein engineering technology afford enzymes tailored for industrial production of chiral synthons and other applications [1]. Furthermore, directed evolution allows the improvement of properties or selectivities of enzymes. In contrast, achieving totally new activity in a given protein scaffold remains challenging [2–3].

Among the current strategies that allow proteins to have unnatural activity, the construction of artificial metalloenzymes is particularly promising [4–14]. This concept will lead to bridging the unique features of transition metal catalysis and biocatalysis. Artificial metalloenzymes are one of the biohybrid catalysts constructed by incorporating transition metal cofactor species into a protein scaffold. The rationale behind this concept is to combine the wide catalytic scope of transition metal complexes with the high activity and selectivity of the enzymes.

Sophisticated anchoring strategies have been demonstrated over the last decades for the conjugation of a non-native metal cofactor into a desired specific site within a protein matrix. These strategies involve dative, [15–22] supramolecular, [23–26] or covalent [27–34] approaches. Biohybrid catalysts comprising a synthetic transition metal complex and a protein scaffold have been shown to hold promise for the development of homogeneous catalysts with new chemical reactivity and selectivity to catalyze a variety of reactions such as hydrogenation, [35] Diels–Alder reaction, [26,36] sulfoxidation, [16,37,38] and benzannulation [39,40]. The reactivity and enantioselectivity in such reactions have been shown to be increased by optimization of the protein scaffolds generated by amino acid substitutions [5,41–56].

In this chapter, the authors review biohybrid catalysts harboring synthetic metal complexes within β-barrel protein scaffolds. The complexes were covalently linked between a maleimide moiety in the metal complexes and a cysteine residue, which locates in a hydrophobic cavity of the β-barrel protein. The authors have established a generalizable method enabling the directed evolution of the biohybrid catalysts with a covalently linked metal complex. The details on the methods and technology platforms for directed evolution of the biohybrid catalysts are also described.

2. CpRh-Linked Biohybrid Catalysts for Phenylacetylene Polymerization

Stereo-controlled C–C bond formation is a synthetically attractive target for a new class of biohybrid catalysts. The authors, therefore, prepared a biohybrid catalyst which promotes stereo-controlled polymerization within an engineered protein scaffold. *cis*-selective phenylacetylene polymerization has been shown to proceed by a variety of rhodium (Rh) complexes [57,58]. For example, it was reported that multiple Rh complexes immobilized within an internal surface of a spherical ferritin cage catalyze the polymerization of phenylacetylene [59,60]. To design and engineer a protein environment adjacent to the Rh complex, the authors developed biohybrid catalysts containing a single Rh active site in the rigid β-barrel structure of nitrobindin (Figure 1) [32]. This approach has proved that the protein environment adjacent to the Rh cofactor has a significant impact on stereo-controlled polymerization.

2.1. *Nitrobindin as a protein scaffold*

In the authors' group, biohybrid catalysts were developed using nitrobindin that has a robust β-barrel structure as a scaffold. Nitrobindin, a group of lipocalins and previously called nitrophorin, is found in *Arabidopsis thaliana*. This protein composed of 166-residues is involved in nitric oxide transport [61]. The protein forms a compact ten-stranded β-barrel that is structurally similar to the lipocalins and fatty acid binding proteins [62]. Such β-barrel structure is expected to provide a rigid platform to construct an artificial active site because proteins of this family retain their inherent barrel folding in the apo-form obtained by removal of the heme cofactor. The authors thus decided to utilize the hydrophobic cavity that accommodates the heme cofactor for incorporating a synthetic metal cofactor.

Native nitrobindin was engineered for use as a scaffold for biohybrid catalysts. First, nitrobindin contains a proximal histidine coordinating to heme iron. To facilitate removal of the heme cofactor and purification of

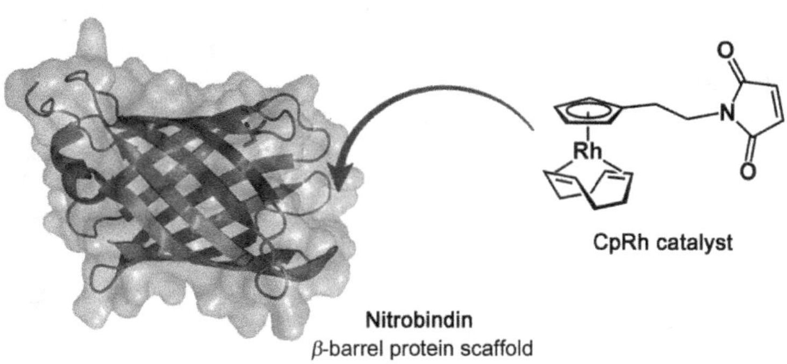

Fig. 1. Biohybrid catalyst with a covalently anchored Rh complex (CpRh) within a nitrobindin variant promotes *trans*-polyphenylacetylene synthesis. Reproduced with permission from Ref. [32]. Copyright 2012 The Royal Society of Chemistry.

the apo form of nitrobindin, His76 near the heme-binding site was replaced with Leu by site-directed mutagenesis. In addition, the two Met residues in the cavity were replaced with Leu because the thioether moiety might interact with a transition metal ion of the synthetic metal cofactor. In this chapter, heme-free engineered nitrobindin is abbreviated as NB. A strep-tag, His-tag or maltose binding tag was fused at the *N*-terminus to facilitate purification.

Furthermore, there is no Cys residue in native nitrobindin. Thus, one Cys residue was introduced into the hydrophobic cavity to covalently anchor a synthetic metal cofactor having a maleimide group for constructing and shaping the active site. The authors screened the positions for anchoring within the cavity, and then Gln96 was eventually identified as a suitable anchoring site for the synthetic metal cofactor.

2.2. *Cyclopentadienyl Rh complex*

An Rh complex with cyclopentadiene (Cp) and cyclooctadiene (cod) ligands was used as an artificial active site for an Rh-linked biohybrid catalyst to catalyze the polymerization of phenylacetylene. The Cp moiety was linked with a maleimide group which forms a covalent link with a Cys residue, as shown in Figure 2. The Cp and cod ligands bind to the Rh ion with η^5 and η^2 coordination modes, respectively (Figure 3(a)). The maleimide group of the cylopentadienyl Rh complex (CpRh) was confirmed to react selectively with the thiol group to form a covalent linkage. The 96th position, located at the entrance of the cavity, satisfies the utilization of the hydrophobic environment of the cavity together with the high efficiency in the conjugation of the Rh cofactor (Figure 3(b)). The molecular size of the complex was suitable for anchoring within the cavity (Figure 3(c)).

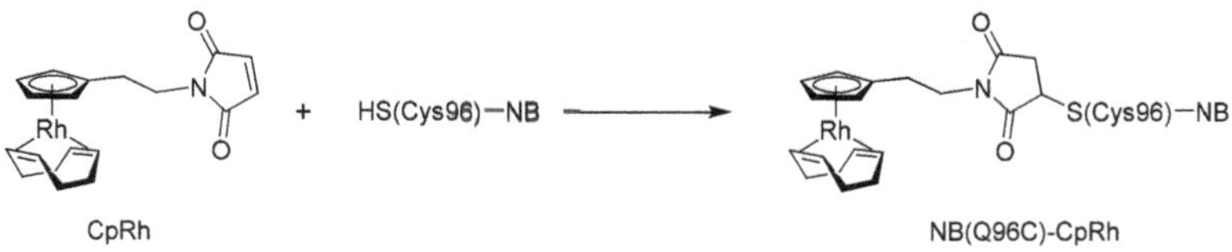

Fig. 2. Formation of a covalent linkage between the Cys residue and the maleimide moiety of the Rh complex.

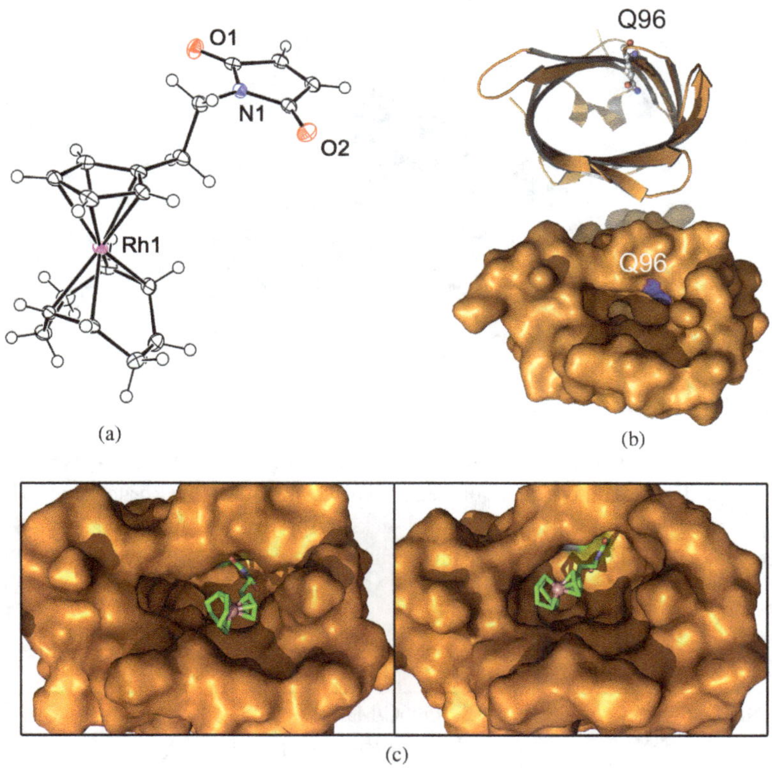

Fig. 3. (a) Crystal structure of CpRh (50% probability ellipsoids). (b) The position of the Q96 residue within the NB cavity. (c) Two possible MD structures of NB(Q96C)-CpRh catalyst. Reproduced with permission from Ref. [32]. Copyright 2012 The Royal Society of Chemistry.

2.3. *Cavity engineering*

To modulate size and shape of the cavity of the prototype biohybrid catalyst NB(Q96C)-CpRh, residues within a distance of 6 Å from the Rh center were engineered (Figure 4) [63]. The His76 and His158 residues were replaced with Ala and/or Leu to enlarge the cavity. In addition, Phe44, Leu75, His76, Lys127, Val128 or Leu148, were replaced with a Trp residue to tune the tightness of the cavity. NB variants that differed in size and shape of the cavity were used as a protein scaffold (Table 1). The structures of the cavities formed by NB's robust β-barrel scaffolds in all

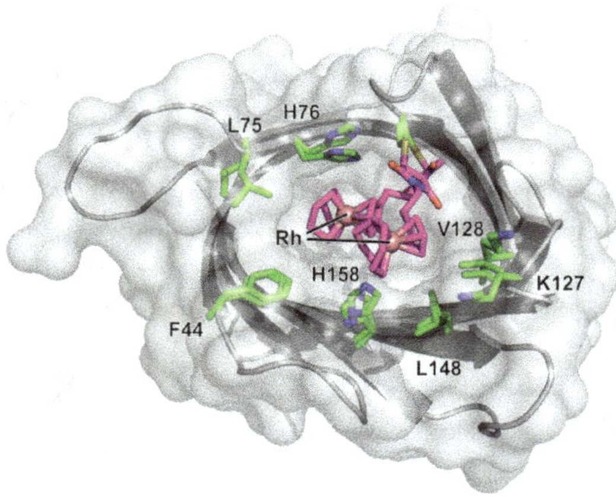

Fig. 4. The amino acid residues in the vicinity of the Rh complex within NB(Q96C)-CpRh. Two calculated stable conformations of the Rh complex are shown (the Rh atom and its ligand are represented by pink sphere and purple sticks, respectively). Met75 and Met148 were replaced by Leu in all variants. Used with permission from Ref. [63]. Copyright 2014 Wiley.

Table 1. List of NB variants.

NB variant	Mutations
NB(Q96C)	M75L/Q96C/M148L
NB1	M75L/H76A/Q96C/M148L/H158A
NB2	M75L/H76A/Q96C/M148L/H158L
NB3	M75L/H76L/Q96C/M148L/H158A
NB4	M75L/H76L/Q96C/M148L/H158L
NB5	F44W/M75L/H76L/Q96C/M148L/H158L
NB6	M75W/H76L/Q96C/M148L/H158L
NB7	M75L/H76W/Q96C/M148L/H158L
NB8	M75L/H76L/Q96C/K127W/M148L/H158L
NB9	M75L/H76L/Q96C/V128W/M148L/H158L
NB10	M75L/H76L/Q96C/M148W/H158L
NB4(L100E)	M75L/H76L/Q96C/L100E/M148L/H158L
NB4(S126E)	M75L/H76L/Q96C/S126E/M148L/H158L
NB4(V128E)	M75L/H76L/Q96C/V128E/M148L/H158L
NB4(T150E)	M75L/H76L/Q96C/M148L/T150E/H158L
NB4(T98E/L100E)	M75L/H76L/Q96C/T98E/L100E/M148L/H158L
NB4(L100E/A125E)	M75L/H76L/Q96C/L100E/A125E/M148L/H158L
NB4(L100E/V128E)	M75L/H76L/Q96C/L100E/V128E/M148L/H158L

variants are similar to that of the wild type as determined by the crystal structure analysis and molecular modeling (Figures 5 and 6) [62].

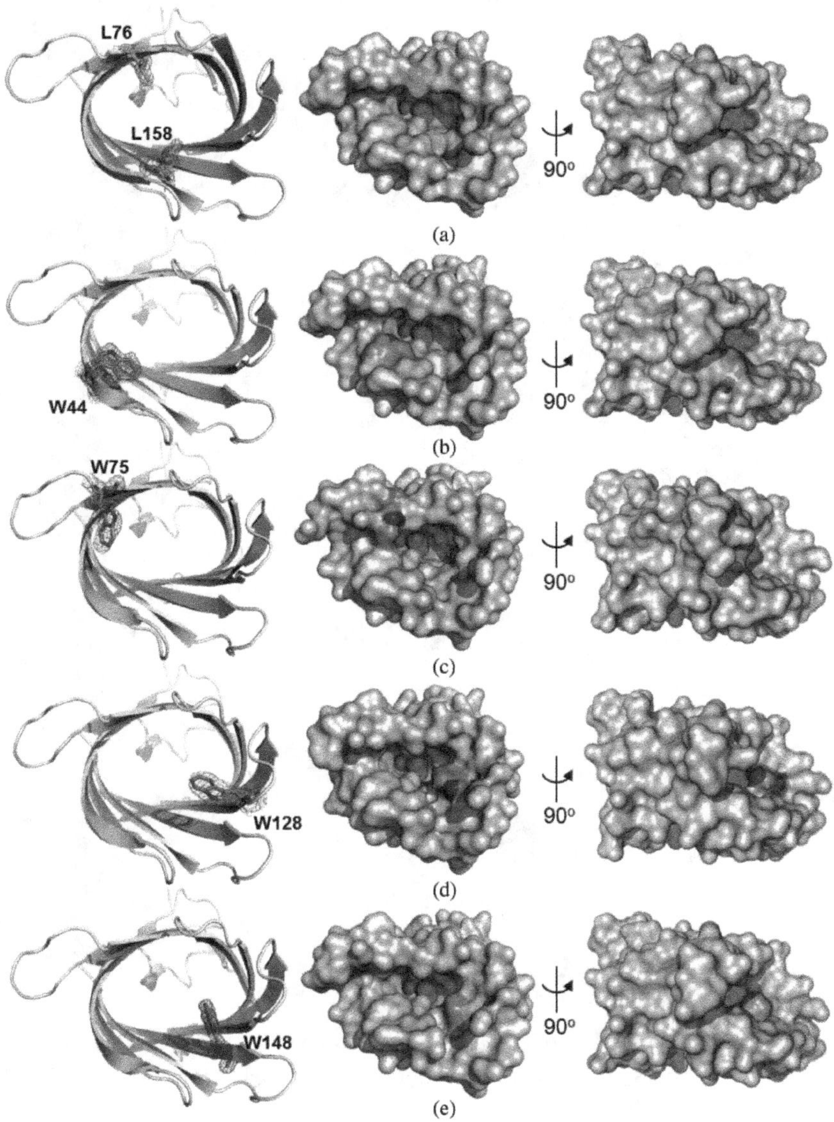

Fig. 5. Crystal structures of (a) NB4, (b) NB5, (c) NB6, (d) NB9, and (e) NB10. Leu and Trp residues are colored in green and orange, respectively. The β-barrel structures of the variants are superimposable with that of native NB (PDB: 2A13) with an RMSD value of less than 1.0 Å. Used with permission from Ref. [63]. Copyright 2014 Wiley.

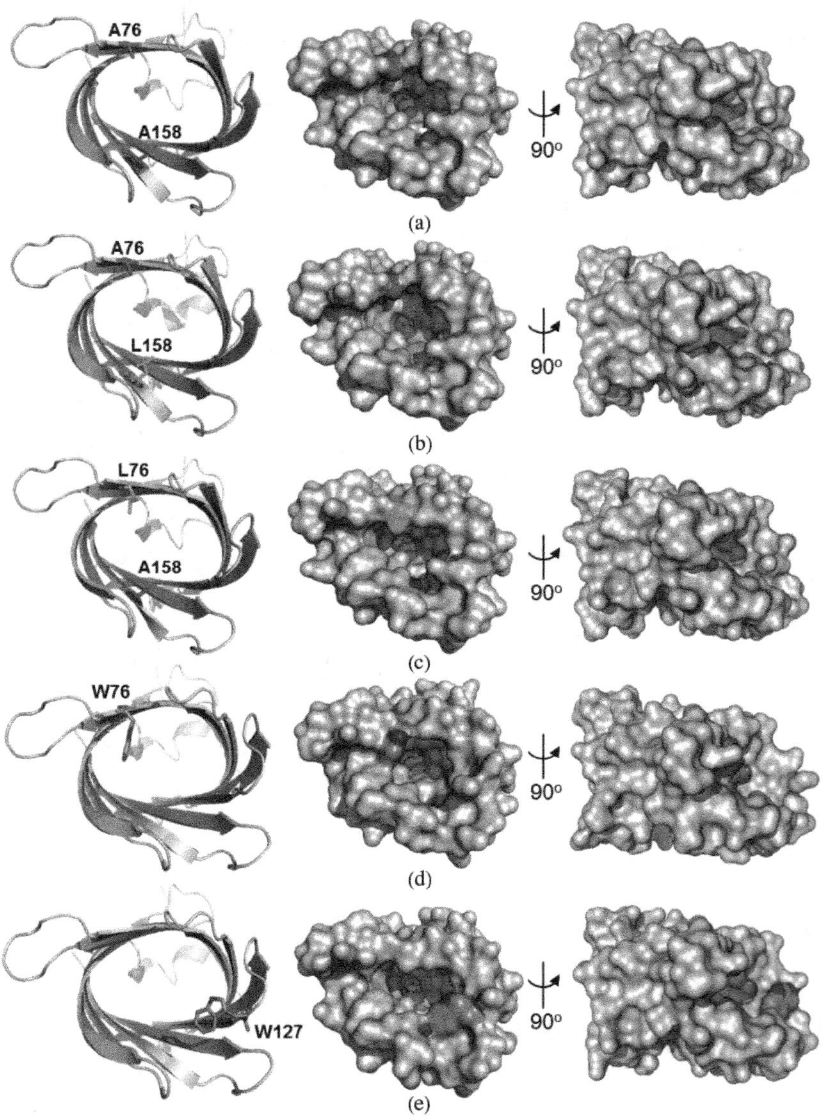

Fig. 6. Calculated structures of (a) NB1, (b) NB2, (c) NB3, (d) NB7, and (e) NB8. Ala, Leu, and Trp residues are colored in pink, green, and orange, respectively. Used with permission from Ref. [63]. Copyright 2014 Wiley.

2.4. *Preparation of CpRh-linked biohybrid catalysts*

NB1-CpRh — NB10-CpRh biohybrid catalysts (Table 1) were prepared by conjugating the Rh complex to each of the variant apo-proteins via the maleimide coupling to the Cys96 residue. The crystal structure of the biohybrid catalyst NB4-CpRh indicates that the Cp ligand is located in the hydrophobic surface consisting of L100, V128, I131, L148, L158 and L159 residues (Figure 7). The Rh center occupied by the labile cod ligand is thus oriented to favor the access of the monomer. In addition, the RMSD for the Cα atoms between NB4-CpRh and the apo-NB4 is 0.27 Å, therefore, the rigid *β*-barrel scaffold is retained in the Rh complex-linked NB as designed.

2.5. *Polymerization of phenylacetylene*

To get insights into the impact of the cavity engineering of CpRh-linked NBs, stereoselectivity in emulsion polymerizations of phenylacetylene was investigated (Table 2). A biohybrid catalyst, Mb(A125C)-CpRh, having the covalently-linked Rh complex on the surface of myoglobin produces polyphenylacetylene (PPA) with a high *cis* content (>91%) (Table 2, entry 1). In contrast, NB(Q96C)-CpRh harboring the Rh complex within the cavity of the NB(Q96C) yields PPA with a 54% *trans* content (Table 2, entry 2). The engineered biohybrid catalysts (NB1-CpRh, NB2-CpRh, and NB3-CpRh) have an enlarged cavity as a result of an Ala replacement. These catalysts produce PPA with moderate *trans* content, i.e., between 44% and 55%, indicating that the larger cavity does not enhance the *trans*-selectivity in PPA production (Table 2, entries 3–5). NB4-CpRh, in which two His residues are replaced with Leu residues, produces PPA with the highest *trans* content of 82% (Table 2, entry 6). The polymer produced by NB5-CpRh, with a cavity similar in size and shape to that of NB4-CpRh, produces PPA with a *trans* content of 77% (Table 2, entry 7). The biohybrid catalysts NB6-CpRh, NB7-CpRh, and NB8-CpRh, with small cavities, produce PPAs with lower *trans* content, i.e., between 39 and 28% (Table 2, entries 8–10). The bulky Trp residue adjacent to the Rh moiety could interface with the monomer access to the catalytic center, resulting in the reduction of the *trans* content. NB9-CpRh

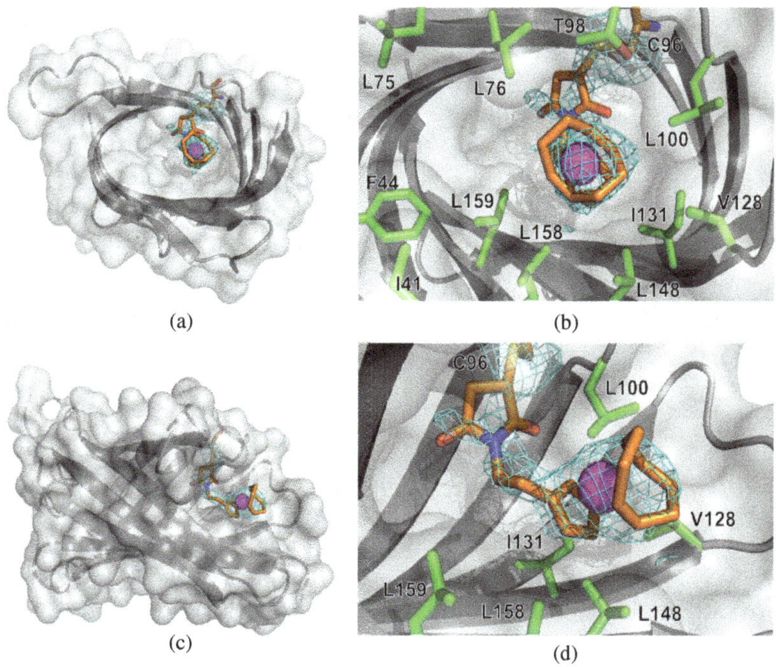

Fig. 7. Crystal structure of NB4-CpRh. (a) Front view, (b) enlarged front view around the Rh moiety, (c) side view, and (d) enlarged side view around the Rh moiety. The F_o–F_c omit map (light blue) is contoured at 3σ, covering the Rh complex and Cys96. (Rh in purple, carbon in orange, nitrogen in blue, oxygen in red, and the neighboring hydrophobic residues in green.) Reproduced with permission from Ref. [63]. Copyright 2014 Wiley.

and NB10-CpRh, with a crowded cavity, also produce PPA with lower *trans* content. (Table 2, entries 11 and 12) These data demonstrated that the cavity engineering of the CpRh-linked biohybrid catalysts contributes to high stereoselectivity in PPA synthesis.

2.6. *Computational structure*

Structural analysis was performed to understand how stereopreference is emerged within NB-CpRh biohybrid catalysts and how monomer access to the Rh center is controlled. Computational structures of NB1-CpRh, NB4-CpRh, and NB6-CpRh are superimposed in Figure 8. The total energy of the Rh complex and the surrounding 14 amino acid residues in the structures are plotted against the distance between the Rh ion and Cα of Leu75.

Table 2. Polymerization of phenylacetylene at 25°C with determined *trans*/*cis* ratios and molecular weight distributions.[a] Reproduced with permission from Ref. [63]. Copyright 2014 Wiley.

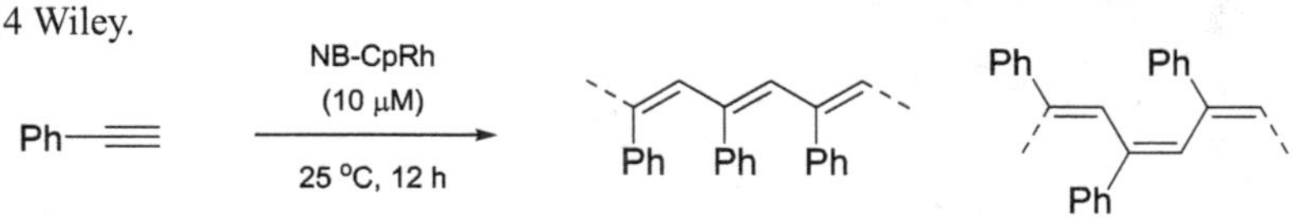

trans-PPA *cis*-PPA

Entry	Biohybrid cat.	*trans*:*cis*[b]	M_n[c]	M_w/M_n[c]
1	Mb(A125C)-CpRh	9:91	46,500	2.3
2	NB(Q96C)-CpRh	54:46	42,800	2.1
3	NB1-CpRh	44:56	36,500	2.6
4	NB2-CpRh	45:55	38,300	2.2
5	NB3-CpRh	55:45	36,800	2.2
6	NB4-CpRh	82:18	38,900	2.4
7	NB5-CpRh	77:23	38,300	2.3
8	NB6-CpRh	39:61	38,300	2.4
9	NB7-CpRh	34:66	31,100	2.5
10	NB8-CpRh	28:78	31,500	2.4
11	NB9-CpRh	40:60	34,600	2.1
12	NB10-CpRh	22:78	38,600	2.7

Notes: [a]The polymerization of phenylacetylene was performed in the presence of the biohybrid catalyst (10 μM) in buffer (10 mM Tris-HCl, pH 8.0) under emulsion conditions for 12 h at 25°C. [b]Determined by ^1H NMR. [c]The number average molecular weight (M_n) and the weight average molecular weight (M_w) were determined by gel permeation chromatography (GPC) in CHC_{13}.

The plots show the conformational distribution of the Rh complex within the cavity. NB1-CpRh exhibits two major conformations and the Rh active site is remarkably flexible (Figure 8(a)). Therefore, the decrease of *trans* selectivity in NB1-CpRh is explained by uncontrolled access of the monomer. The plots also suggest that the Rh complex has a defined orientation within the cavity of NB4, providing a confined environment for the polymerization (Figure 8(b)). In contrast, the NB6-CpRh produces PPA with lower *trans* content, although the Rh complex in NB6 shows a narrowly-distributed conformation. The access of the monomer to the Rh complex is disturbed in the tight cavity with the bulky Trp residue (Figure 8(c)).

The cavity of Rh complex-linked NB was engineered by site-directed mutagenesis, resulting in the identification of hot spot residues which modulate and significantly improve the *trans*/*cis*-stereoselectivity in PPA

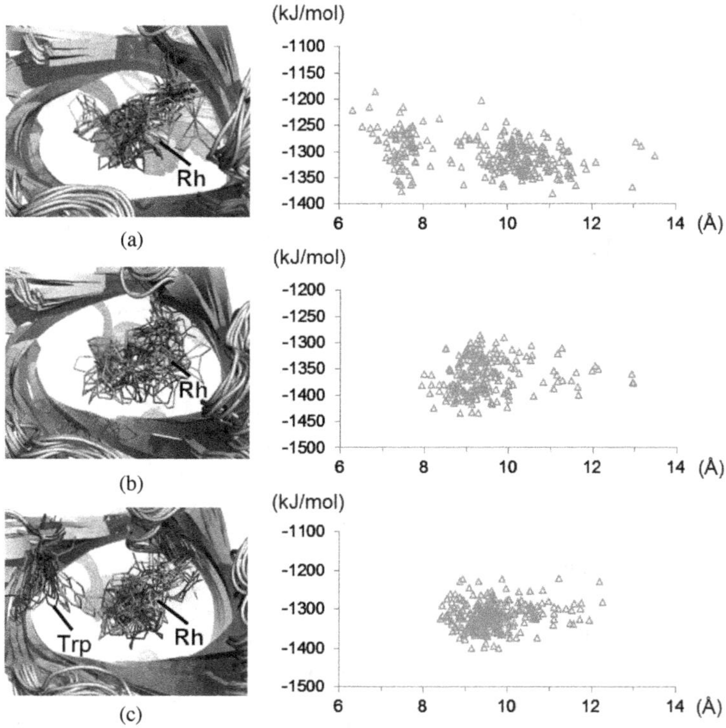

Fig. 8. The distribution of the Rh complex within the cavity of (a) NB1-CpRh, (b) NB4-CpRh and (c) NB6-CpRh during MD calculation at 298 K for 1500 ps. Selected 16 snapshot structures are shown in rainbow colors (left), and the total energy of the Rh complex and the surrounding 14 amino acid residues (positions 41, 44, 46, 75, 76, 96, 98, 100, 127, 128, 148, 150, 158, and 159) are plotted against the distance between the Rh ion and Cα of Leu75 (right). Total 240 minimized structures are plotted as green triangles. Reproduced with permission from Ref. [63]. Copyright 2014 Wiley.

[63]. As an extension of this biohybrid catalyst, polymerization of phenylacetylene was found to be also catalyzed by NB-CpRh displayed on the cell surface of *E. coli* [52].

3. Cp*Rh-Linked Biohybrid Catalysts

Encouraged by the successful development of the CpRh-linked biohybrid catalysts, the authors began the study on biohybrid catalysts using Cp*Rh(III) complexes, which catalyze a range of C(sp^2)–H bond functionalizations [64–67]. A biohybrid catalyst harboring the Cp*Rh(III) cofactor is expected to directly convert an inert C(sp^2)–H bond within a customizable protein environment. This was evidenced by the report demonstrating the asymmetric synthesis of dihydroisoquinolones catalyzed by a Cp*Rh(III) complex embedded within streptavidin [39–40].

To promote Cp*Rh(III)-catalyzed C(sp^2)–H bond functionalization in the protein environment, all the three coordination sites of the Cp*Rh(III) complex should be kept available for the reaction. The authors, therefore, developed a new Cp*Rh(III) cofactor with "latent" activity for being incorporated within the protein scaffold (Figure 9) [68]. First, the three coordination sites of the highly electrophilic Cp*Rh(III) complex are protected by two dithiophosphate ligands during the conjugation of the complex to the protein scaffold. The dithiophosphate ligands are then dissociated upon the addition of Ag^+ ion to activate the Cp*Rh(III)-linked biohybrid catalyst. This strategy enables covalent and specific conjugation of a highly reactive Cp*Rh(III) cofactor into a protein scaffold preventing nonspecific coordination of the nucleophiles such as cysteine and

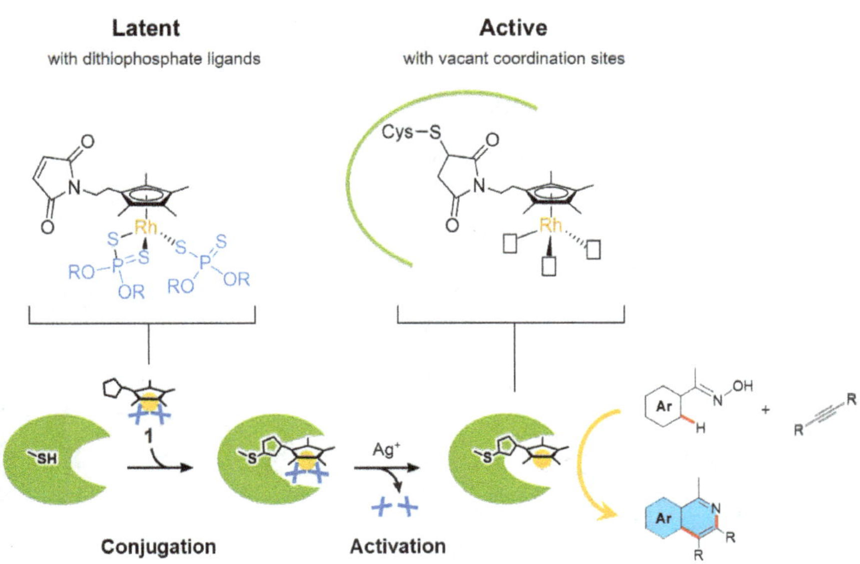

Fig. 9. Construction of the active Cp*Rh(III)-linked biohybrid catalyst for C(sp^2)–H bond functionalization using a Cp*Rh(III) cofactor with latent catalytic activity. Reproduced from Ref. [68].

histidine and deactivation of the catalyst. It was demonstrated that the biohybrid catalysts prepared using this method promote cycloaddition reaction of acetophenone oxime with diphenylacetylene.

3.1. *Cp*Rh(III) cofactor with latent catalytic activity*

Inert and catalytically inactive mononuclear Cp*Rh(III) complexes with sulfur-containing ligands **L1–L5** were tested as a Cp*Rh(III) cofactor with latent catalytic activity (Figure 10). Strong chelation of these ligands protects the coordination sites of the Cp*Rh(III) complex. Therefore, the nonspecific coordination of functional groups of amino acid residues is prevented. In addition, these ligands are capable of being dissociated upon the addition of Ag^+ ion. The sulfur atoms of the ligand preferentially coordinate to the Ag^+ ion by transmetalation, leading to the regeneration of an active Cp*Rh(III) complex with three available coordination sites.

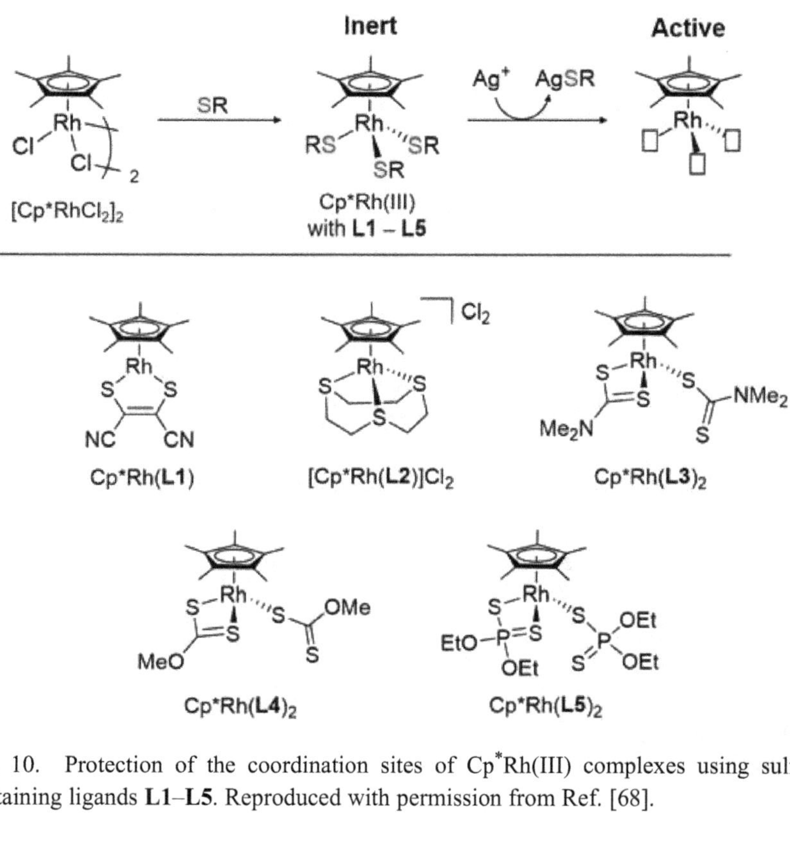

Fig. 10. Protection of the coordination sites of Cp*Rh(III) complexes using sulfur-containing ligands **L1–L5**. Reproduced with permission from Ref. [68].

In fact, the catalytic activity of Cp*Rh(III) complexes with ligand **L5** was recovered in the presence of Ag^+ ion (Table 3). Cycloaddition of 3′, 4′-ethylenedioxyacetophenone oxime (**1**) with diphenylacetylene (**2**) producing fluorescent isoquinoline **3** (λ_{em} = 453 nm) was used for facile and rapid evaluation of the catalytic activity of the Cp*Rh(III) complexes. The Cp*Rh(III) complexes with ligands **L1–L5** do not have catalytic activity in the absence of Ag^+ ion. The activity in the Cp*Rh complexes **L1–L4** (Table 3, entries 1–4) is recovered to some extent. In contrast, Cp*Rh(**L5**)$_2$ (Table 3, entry 5) gave **3** in 73% yield, which is in a similar yield range relative to [Cp*RhCl$_2$]$_2$ (Table 3, entry 6). The addition of sufficient amount of Ag^+ ion leads to full recover y of the catalytic activity of the Cp*Rh(III) complex with the protective ligands.

Cp*Rh(**L5**)$_2$ has two dithiophosphate ligands that coordinate in monodentate and in bidentate fashions. The Cp*Rh(III) complex with three coordination sites occupied with labile ligands such as solvent is

Table 3. Investigation of Cp*Rh(III) cofactors with latent catalytic activity.[a] Reproduced with permission from Ref. [68].

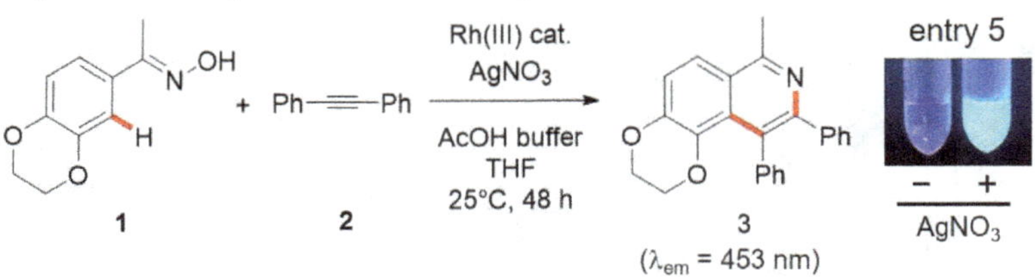

Entry	Catalyst	Yield (%)[b] 0 mM $AgNO_3$	10 mM $AgNO_3$
1	Cp*Rh(**L1**)	n.d.	5
2	[Cp*Rh(**L2**)]Cl$_2$	<1	6
3	Cp*Rh(**L3**)$_2$	n.d.	22
4	Cp*Rh(**L4**)$_2$	n.d.	51
5	Cp*Rh(**L5**)$_2$	n.d.	73
6	[Cp*RhCl$_2$]$_2$	68	67
7[c]	—	n.d.	n.d.

Note: [a]Reaction conditions: **1** (0.25 mM), **2** (5.0 mM), $AgNO_3$ (10 mM) and Cp*Rh(III) complex (25 μM, 10 mol%) in 400 μL AcOH buffer (100 mM AcOH, pH 4.0) and 100 μL THF, 48 h, 25°C. [b]Yields were calculated from the fluorescence intensity of isoquinoline product **3** at 453 nm. Cp*Rh(**L5**)$_2$ was found to exhibit promising catalytic activity in the presence of $AgNO_3$ (see the image of entry 5). [c]Without Cp*Rh(III) catalyst.

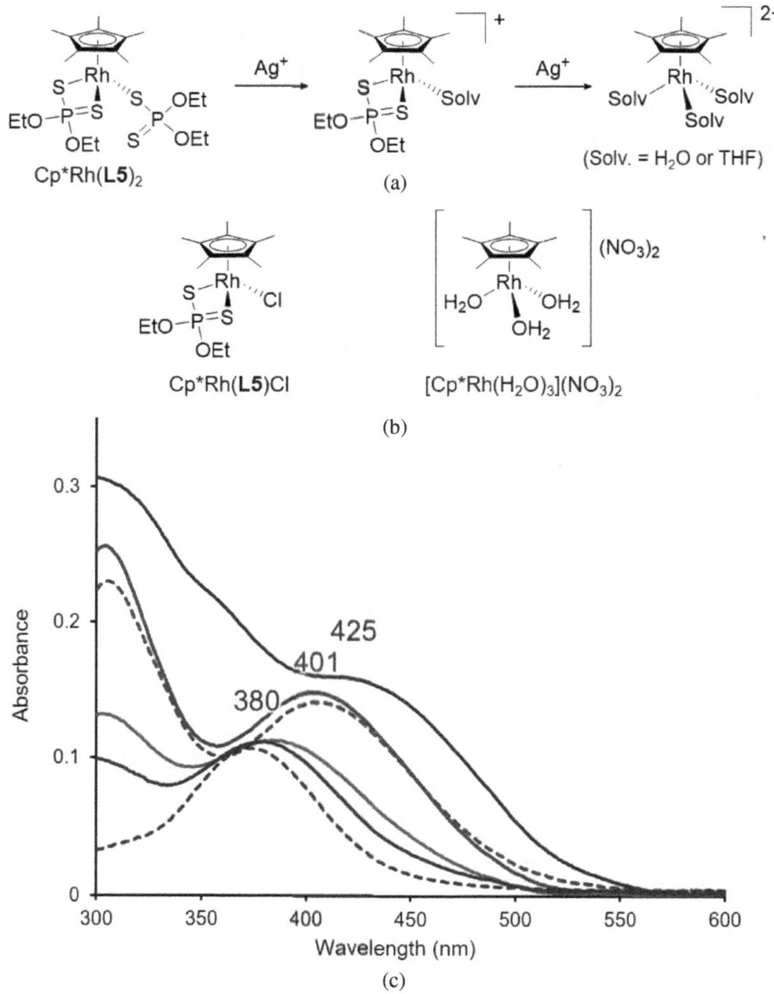

Fig. 11. (a) Plausible process for activation of Cp*Rh(**L5**)$_2$ (b) Chemical structures of Cp*Rh(**L5**)Cl and [Cp*Rh(H_2O)$_3$](NO_3)$_2$ (c) UV-vis spectral changes of Cp*Rh(**L5**)$_2$ (50 μM, 1.0 equiv) during the titration of Ag^+ ion; 0 equiv (black solid line), 1.0 equiv (red solid line), 4.0 equiv (green solid line), and 20 equiv (blue solid line) in H_2O/THF (1/1). UV-vis spectra of Cp*Rh(**L5**)Cl (red dotted line) and [Cp*Rh(H_2O)$_3$](NO_3)$_2$ (blue dotted lined) in H_2O/THF (1/1). Reproduced from Ref. [68].

generated upon the addition of Ag^+ ion through the dissociation of the two dithiophosphate ligands. This was confirmed using a titration experiment of Ag^+ ion using absorption and ESI-TOF MS analyzes (Figure 11).

3.2. *Construction of a Cp*Rh(III)-linked biohybrid catalyst*

A Rh(III)-dithiophosphate complex, Cp*Rh(**L5**)$_2$, containing a maleimide moiety, was linked with a Cys residue at position 96 of NB4. It was found that the dithiophosphate ligand **L5** completely suppresses the nonspecific binding of the Cp*Rh(III) complex on the protein. In contrast, NB4 is nonspecifically attached with three, four, and five molecules of Cp*Rh(III) when NB4 was mixed with [Cp*RhCl$_2$]$_2$. Therefore, the Cp*Rh(**L5**)$_2$ complex with the protecting dithiophosphate ligand enables specific conjugation between the maleimide moiety and the Cys96 residue without nonspecific interactions.

3.3. *Cycloaddition reaction catalyzed by Cp*Rh-linked biohybrid catalysts*

The catalytic activities of the biohybrid catalysts toward cycloaddition of **1** with **2** producing isoquinoline **3** and **4** are summarized in Table 4. The catalytic activity of NB4-Cp*Rh(**L5**)$_2$ (Table 4, entry 2) was recovered upon addition of Ag^+ ion in 15% yield. In the absence of Ag^+ ion, the product was not observed (Table 4, entry 1). However, NB-Cp*Rh(**L5**)$_2$ has lower catalytic activity relative to the Cp*Rh(**L5**)$_2$ complex (Table 4, entry 3). Therefore, the authors initiated the genetic engineering of the hydrophobic cavity of NB4 to improve the catalytic activity (Figure 12). Several NB4 variants with a Glu residue at different positions were tested on the basis of the known evidence that a carboxylate group contributes to acceleration of C(sp^2)–H bond functionalization [39]. The NB4(L100E) (Table 4, entry 4), NB4(S126E) (Table 4, entry 5), NB4(V128E) (Table 4, entry 6), and NB4(T150E) variants (Table 4, entry 7) were thus linked with Cp*Rh(**L5**)$_2$. It is noted that these variants show higher yields relative to NB4-Cp*Rh(**L5**)$_2$. Interestingly, NB4(L100E) afforded the products in 24% yield and therefore it was further engineered and tested (Table 4, entries 8–10). The NB4(L100E/A125E)-Cp*Rh(**L5**)$_2$ variant has the highest catalytic activity with 35% yield (Table 4, entry 8). This variant clearly shows higher activity in the concentration range of Ag^+ ion (0.25–1.0 mM) relative to original NB4-Cp*Rh(**L5**)$_2$. This indicates that the glutamate residues promote the access of Ag^+ ion into the hydrophobic cavity and the activation of the Cp*Rh(**L5**)$_2$ cofactor.

Table 4. Cycloaddition of **1** with **2** catalyzed by Cp*Rh(III)-incorporated biohybrid catalysts.[a] Reproduced from Ref. [68].

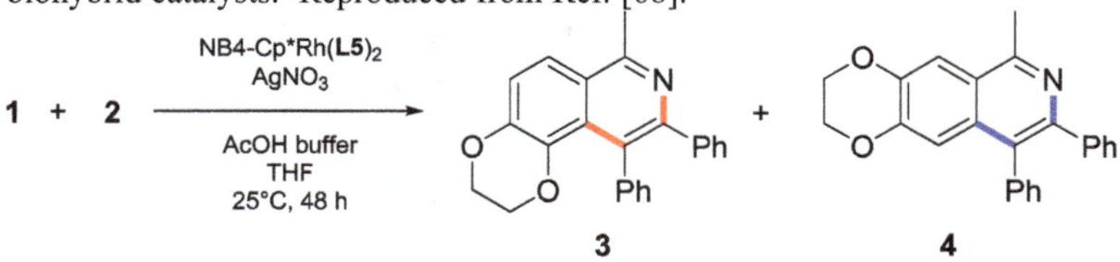

Entry	Rh catalyst	Yield (%)[b]	3/4
1[c]	NB4-CpRh(**L5**)$_2$	n.d.	—
2	NB4-Cp*Rh(**L5**)$_2$	15 ± 1	92/8
3	Cp*Rh(**L5**)$_2$	>95	89/11
4	NB4(L100E)-Cp*Rh(**L5**)$_2$	24 ± 1	91/9
5	NB4(S126E)-Cp*Rh(**L5**)$_2$	21 ± 1	91/9
6	NB4(V128E)-Cp*Rh(**L5**)$_2$	24 ± 1	90/10
7	NB4(T150E)-Cp*Rh(**L5**)$_2$	20 ± 1	91/9
8	NB4(T98E/L100E)-Cp*Rh(**L5**)$_2$	33 ± 1	90/10
9	NB4(L100E/A125E)-Cp*Rh(**L5**)$_2$	35 ± 1	89/11
10	NB4(L100E/V128E)-Cp*Rh(**L5**)$_2$	28 ± 1	91/9

Notes: [a]Reaction conditions: **1** (0.25 mM), **2** (5.0 mM), NB4-Cp*Rh(**L5**)$_2$ variants (25 μM, 10 mol%) and $AgNO_3$ (1.0 mM) in AcOH buffer (100 mM AcOH, 20% THF, pH 4.0), 48 h, 25°C. [b]Total yields of **3** and **4** were determined by GC-MS. [c]$AgNO_3$ (0 mM).

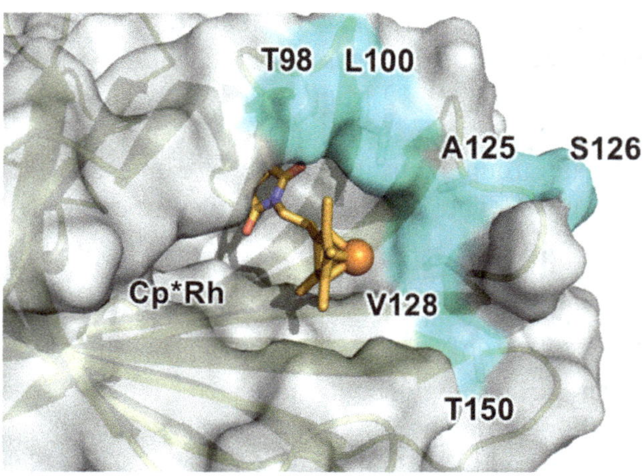

Fig. 12. MD structure of the biohybrid catalyst, NB4-Cp*Rh. The MD calculation was carried out based on the crystal structure of NB4 (PDB: 3WJB). Rh metal and the coordinating water molecules are shown in the sphere. The amino acid residues subjected to the mutation are highlighted in the cyan stick. Reproduced with permission from Ref. [68].

The authors developed a method for the construction of a biohybrid catalyst harboring a Cp*Rh(III) cofactor with “latent” activity. The coordination sites of the Cp*Rh(III) cofactor are protected using dithiophosphate ligands, thereby preventing nonspecific coordination of nucleophilic residues and allowing the selective conjugation of the Cp*Rh(III) cofactor to the Cys residue. The Cp*Rh(III)-linked biohybrid catalysts promote the cycloaddition of oxime with alkyne producing the isoquinoline product via $C(sp^2)$–H bond functionalization. This demonstrates that the reactive metal cofactor requiring multiple coordination sites can be accommodated into the protein scaffolds.

4. H_2-Evolving Diiron Complex-Linked Biohybrid Catalysts

Conjugating a protein scaffold with a metal catalyst for hydrogen evolution and oxidation has been studied for the purpose of organizing second and outer coordination spheres adjacent to the metal catalyst. In biological systems, hydrogenase catalyzes the reduction of protons and the capture of electrons from H_2 under mild conditions [69,70]. The active site of [FeFe]-H_2ase, an H-cluster, consists of an unusual bridging dithiolate ligand and diatomic ligands such as carbonyls and cyanides [71–73]. A variety of H-cluster model complexes containing a diiron cluster ($(\mu\text{-S})_2Fe_2(CO)_n$) have been synthesized [74–80]. These diiron model complexes have been demonstrated to function as hydrogen-evolving catalysts by cascading electrons from a visible light-driven photosensitizer [81–85]. Combining the $(\mu\text{-S})_2Fe_2(CO)_n$ model with biological scaffolds such as peptides and proteins has been studied to optimize the surrounding environment of the diiron core [19,86–88]. The authors demonstrated that an iron-carbonyl complex, $(\mu\text{-S})_2Fe_2(CO)_6$, covalently linked with the cavity of the NB scaffold promotes photocatalytic H_2 production [89].

4.1. *Construction of diiron complex-linked biohybrid catalyst*

An H_2-evolving diiron complex containing a dithiolate ligand with the maleimide group was linked onto the Cys96 residue of NB(Q96C). The diiron catalyst with the maleimide group was synthesized from a diiron hexacarbonyl complex, which includes a 2-carboxy-1,3-propanedithiol ligand (Figure 13(a)). The dithiolate ligand binds to two iron atoms in the typical

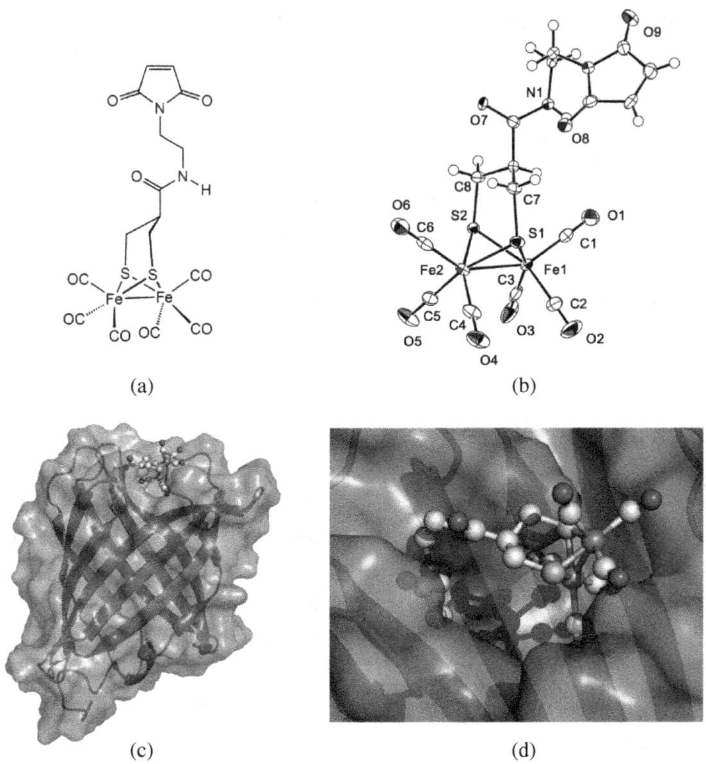

Fig. 13. (a) Chemical structure and (b) crystal structure of $(\mu\text{-S})_2Fe_2(CO)_6$ tethering a maleimide moiety (50% probability ellipsoids). (c) Side view and (d) zoomed view of the structure of NB(Q96C)-Fe_2 calculated by YASARA.[90] Iron in violet, sulfur in yellow, carbon in white, oxygen in red, and nitrogen in blue. Reproduced with permission from Ref. [89]. Copyright 2014 American Chemical Society.

coordination mode commonly found in the analogous $(\mu\text{-S})_2Fe_2(CO)_6$ complexes (Figure 13(b)). The molecular size was suitable for anchoring within the cavity as indicated by the X-ray crystal structure of the complex (Figures 13(c) and 13(d)).

The $(\mu\text{-S})_2Fe_2(CO)_6$ complexes (FeFe) with the maleimide group are specifically conjugated with NB(Q96C) to generate the biohybrid catalyst NB(Q96C)-FeFe. FT-IR measurement of NB(Q96C)-FeFe shows three characteristic bands assignable to the CO ligands at 2077, 2037, and 2005 cm^{-1}. The positions and the shapes of these bands are similar to those observed for reported (μ-S)$_2$Fe$_2$(CO)$_6$ complexes, indicating that the (μ-S)$_2$Fe$_2$ core with the six CO ligands is embedded within the protein cavity [75–76]. It is suggested that the CO ligands interact with the neighboring amino acid residues on the basis of the subtle spectral changes in the vicinity of 2,000 cm^{-1}.

4.2. *Photocatalytic H_2 production*

NB(Q96C)-FeFe photocatalytically produces H_2 in the presence of $[Ru(bpy)_3]^{2+}$ as a photosensitizer and excess ascorbate as a sacrificial reagent (Figure 14). The photocatalytic production of H_2 proceeds with a turnover number of ~130 per the hybrid catalyst after 6 h with a maximum turnover frequency of ~2.3 per minute. The result clearly indicates that the (μ-S)$_2$Fe$_2$(CO)$_6$ core within the NB protein retains photocatalytic H_2 evolution activity. The reactions within NB were, however, decelerated owing to decreased accessibility of the photosensitizer to the diiron active site [89].

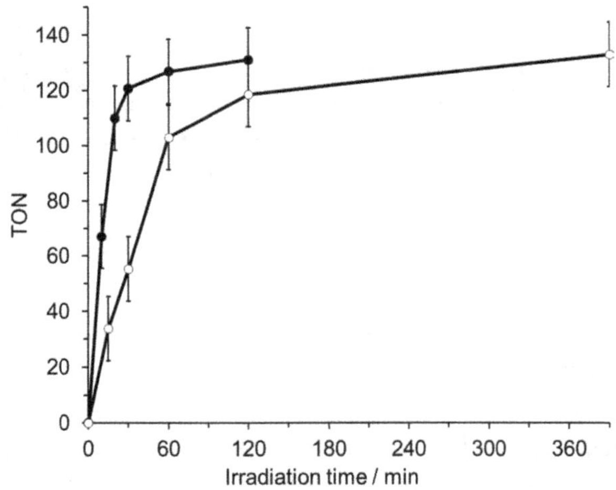

Fig. 14. Visible light-driven H_2 generation by NB(Q96C)-FeFe in 50 mM Tris/HCl (pH 4.0) (open circles) and the diiron complex (μ-S)$_2$Fe$_2$(CO)$_6$ in 50 mM Tris/HCl (pH 4.0) containing 4% (v/v) THF (filled circles) at 25°C. Reproduced with permission from Ref. [89]. Copyright 2014 American Chemical Society.

5. Biohybrid Catalysts Containing a Pyrene Molecule for Asymmetric Diels–Alder Reaction

Polycyclic aromatic groups such as pyrene have been reported to function as a binding and recognition moiety for a substrate via noncovalent interactions [91–94]. Under these grounds, the authors constructed a unique reaction cavity containing a pyrene moiety utilizing the rigid protein scaffold of NB. It was found that the pyrene-linked NB cavity promotes an asymmetric Diels–Alder (DA) reaction of ®-3-phenyl-yridinedin-2-yl) prop-2-en-1-one (**5**) with cyclopentadiene in the presence of Cu(II) ion (Figure 15) [95].

5.1. *Pyrene-linked biohybrid catalysts*

N-(1-pyrenyl)maleimide (Pyr) was conjugated to NB variants (NB1, NB2, NB4, NB5 and NB10) with different shapes of the hydrophobic cavity via the covalent link between Cys96 and the maleimide group (Figure 16(a)). The chiroptical properties of the pyrene moiety inside the cavity of the NB-Pyr variants indicate that two different orientations of the pyrene moiety are generated in the cavities of the NB variants. Since the access of Pyr depends on the feature of the cavity, the orientation of the pyrene group is selected during the coupling reaction as predicted by computational structures of NB4-Pyr (Figure 16(b)). This unique difference in the orientation of the pyrene moiety within the NB scaffold was utilized for the recognition of the substrate and selectivity of the product.

5.2. *Diels–Alder reaction*

To utilize the pyrene-linked cavity, a Cu(II)-catalyzed asymmetric DA reaction between **5** and cyclopentadiene was performed using the NB-Pyr variants as a reaction scaffold (Table 5). The DA reaction yields the *endo* and *exo* products as major and minor species, respectively (Figure 15(b)). The reaction in the absence of the pyrene-linked NB yields racemic cyclization products in 82% conversion with high *endo* selectivity. In contrast, the reactions proceed with higher *endo*-selectivity and enantioselectivity in the presence of NB-Pyr. The enantioselectivity is low in the case of NB1-Pyr (−6% *ee*) (Table 5, entry 2), NB6-Pyr (8% *ee*) (Table 5, entry 5), and NB10-Pyr (<5% *ee*) (Table 5, entry 6). NB2-Pyr exhibits a moderate

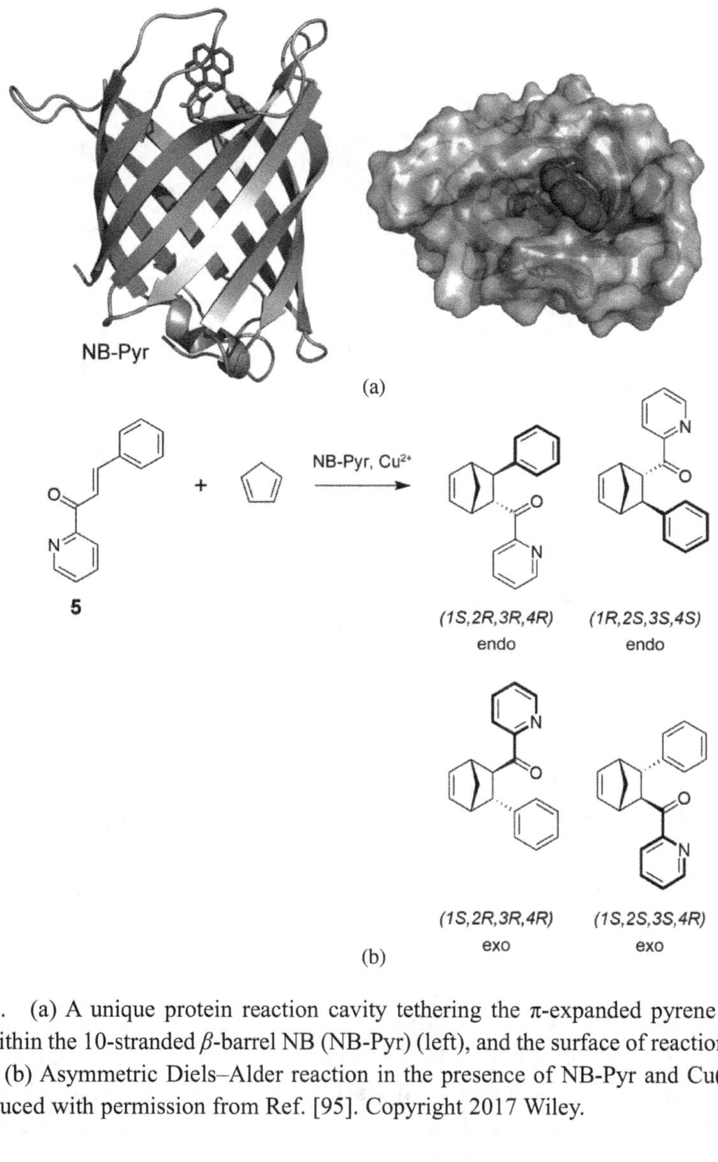

Fig. 15. (a) A unique protein reaction cavity tethering the π-expanded pyrene moiety (red) within the 10-stranded *β*-barrel NB (NB-Pyr) (left), and the surface of reaction cavity (right). (b) Asymmetric Diels–Alder reaction in the presence of NB-Pyr and Cu(II) ion. Reproduced with permission from Ref. [95]. Copyright 2017 Wiley.

ee value (34% *ee*) (Table 5, entry 3). Importantly, the NB4-Pyr conjugate shows the highest *endo*-selectivity (90% *diastereomeric excess (de)*) and the highest enantioselectivity (69% *ee*) (Table 5, entry 4). NB4 without the pyrene group produces low conversion (16%) and low

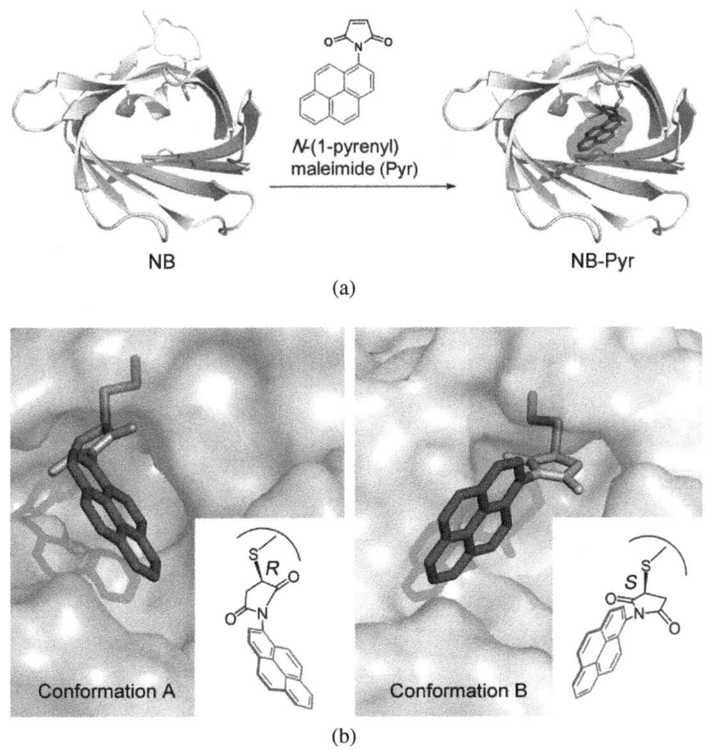

Fig. 16. (a) Preparation of NB-Pyr by covalent coupling between NB and Pyr. (b) The energy minimized structures of NB4-Pyr wi®(*R*)-configuration carbon (conformation A, left) and (*S*)-configuration carbon (conformation B, right) obtained by MD calculations using the YASARA software.[90] Reproduced with permission from Ref. [95]. Copyright 2017 Wiley.

enantioselectivity (−6% *ee*) (Table 5, entry 7). The yield (94%) and enantioselectivity (78% *ee*) clearly increase at a lower concentration of **5** (0.25 mM) under similar conditions (Table 5, entry 8). Therefore, the structure of the pyrene-linked protein cavity regulates the interaction with the substrate and the orientation between the two substrates during the DA reaction.

The effect of the pyrene moiety was investigated by replacing Pyr with other aromatic units such as *N*-benzylmaleimide (**6**), *N*-(1-naphthyl) maleimide (**7**), *N*-(2-pyrenyl)maleimide (**8**), and 1-(bromoacetyl)pyrene (**9**) (Figure 17). NB4-**6** with a benzyl moiety and NB4-**7** with a naphthyl

Table 5. Asymmetric Diels–Alder reaction in the presence of NB-Pyr and Cu(II) ion.[a]

Entry	NB conjugate	Conv. (%)	Endo:Exo	*ee* (%)[b]
1	—	82	92:8	<5
2	NB1-Pyr	45	93:7	−6
3	NB2-Pyr[c]	61	94:6	34
4	NB4-Pyr[c]	56	95:5	69
5	NB6-Pyr	40	92:8	8
6	NB10-Pyr	47	92:8	<5
7	NB4	16	89:11	−6
8	NB4-Pyr[d]	94	96:4	78
9	NB4-**6**	41	91:9	<5
10	NB4-**7**	57	93:7	15
11	NB4-**8**[e]	46	94:6	−10
12	NB4-**9**	54	92:8	−13

Notes: [a]Typical conditions: 1 mM **5**, 33 mM cyclopentadiene, 110 μM NB conjugates (11 mol%), and 100 μM $Cu(NO_3)_2$ (10 mol%) in 20 mM MOPS (pH 7.0) containing 150 mM NaCl for 3 days at 4°C. [b]Enantiomeric excess of *endo* isomers, positive *ee* means the preference of the product with the (1*R*,2*S*,3*S*,4*S*) configuration. [c]NB2-Pyr and NB4-Pyr are predicted to have conformation A. [d]0.25 mM **5**, 33 mM cyclopentadiene, 110 μM NB conjugates (44 mol%), and 100 µM $Cu(NO_3)_2$ (40 mol%). [e]Unpublished result.

group produce moderate conversion with low enantioselectivity (Table 5, entries 9 and 10). NB4-**8** tethering the pyrene group in a different position shows low enantioselectivity and opposite enantiopreference (Table 5, entry 11, unpublished result). NB4-**9** containing the pyrene group with the acetyl linker also shows low enantioselectivity and the opposite enantiopreference (Table 5, entry 12). The results indicate that the combination of **5** and the NB4 cavity is favorable for this reaction.

The recognition of **5** within NB-Pyr was predicted by docking simulation (Figure 16(b)). The docking simulation indicates that **5** is inserted into the cavity with its aryl group sandwiched between the pyrene group and the phenyl ring of the Phe44 residue in the protein cavity (Figure 18). The molecule of **5** exposes the *si* face of its double bond, which is preferentially attacked by cyclopentadiene to produce the *endo* product with (1*R*,2*S*,3*S*,4*S*) configuration. In contrast, the binding of **5** to the cavity having a different pyrene orientation is less favored because of the loss of interaction with the

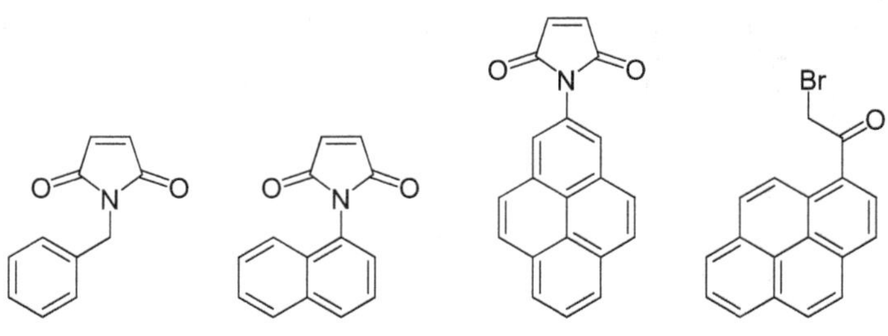

6 **7** **8** **9**

Fig. 17. Molecular structures of aromatic moieties linked to the cavity of NB4.

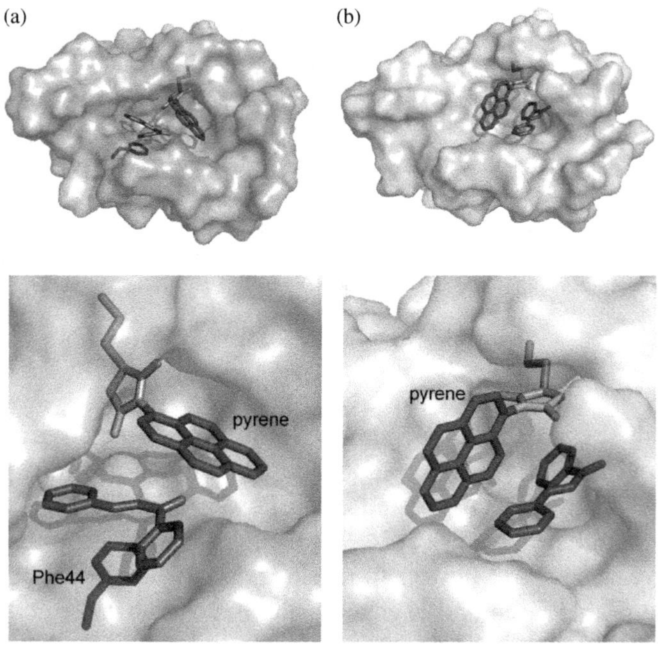

Fig. 18. The docking results of (a) conformation A and (b) conformation B estimated using the Glide program. The energy minimized structures were used as protein grids and azachalcone **5** was used as a ligand. The pyrene moiety (red), Phe44 residue (red), and **5** (in purple) are shown. Used with permission from Ref. [95]. Copyright 2017 Wiley.

pyrene and Phe44. The importance of the phenyl moiety was also supported by the DA reaction with substituted azachalcone derivatives **10–12** in the presence of NB4-Pyr (Figure 19). The DA reaction of the 4-methyl, 4-methoxy or 4-fluoro derivatives with cyclopentadiene has lower

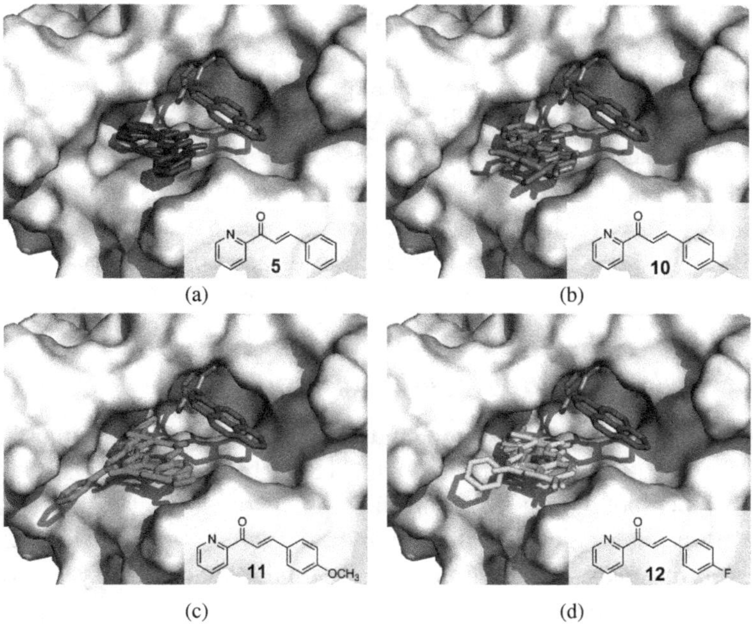

Fig. 19. Substrate scope of DA reaction. The docking results of (a) **5**, (b) **10**, (c) **11**, and (d) **12**. The energy minimized structures were used as protein grids and five docking structures are superimposed. Reproduced with permission from Ref. [95]. Copyright 2017 Wiley.

enantioselectivity albeit with lower yields. This indicates that the phenyl moiety of **5** substrate participate in an important interaction with the pyrene-linked cavity in NB4-Pyr. Interestingly, the docking structures of **5** showing high enantioselectivity indicate that substrate **5** is the best fit in the cavity supported by the pyrene. While **10, 11, 12** showing lower enantioselectivity has several different orientations within the cavity. This new strategy to utilize the protein scaffold linked with the pyrene moiety provides an attractive direction for the development of hybrid catalytic systems [95].

6. Directed Evolution of Cp*Rh-Linked Biohybrid Catalysts

Protein scaffolds offer infinite chemical diversity in the surrounding environment of the metal complexes by means of biotechnology. Directed evolution has been demonstrated as a powerful strategy for efficient discovery of the suitable combination of amino acid mutations in engineering the protein scaffold of biohybrid catalysts [3,45,96–101]. This approach explores the amino acid sequence space through an iterative cycle of random mutagenesis and library screening, leading to improvement in the performance of biohybrid catalysts. As described in this chapter, a biohybrid catalyst harboring a Cp*Rh(III) cofactor within the NB scaffold was developed (Figure 9) [68]. A directed evolution campaign of the Cp*Rh(III)-linked biohybrid catalyst was performed to further improve its activity toward the cycloaddition reaction of acetophenone oximes with alkynes producing a fluorescent isoquinoline product [102].

6.1. *HTS platform for biohybrid catalysts*

A reliable platform for high-throughput screening (HTS) is required for the directed evolution campaign. Although HTS for biohybrid catalysts is hampered by incorporating a synthetic metal cofactor, several excellent HTS platforms have been developed for biohybrid catalysts [43–47]. The screening platforms using periplasmic [48–50] and surface-displayed [51,52] protein scaffolds have been reported to increase the throughput of the directed evolution. The screening platform using a purified biohybrid catalyst will also be promising because a screening using cells or cell lysates may suffer from the deactivation of the metal cofactor [42,53–56]. In addition, the effect of background catalysis derived from an unconjugated metal cofactor can be ruled out. However, the screened library size in previous reports using conventional protein purification systems has been limited between a few dozen and a few hundred clones due to time- and cost-intensive feature.

The authors have developed an affinity purification system using a maltose-binding protein (MBP)-tag, enabling a reliable platform for HTS [103]. The use of the MBP-tag provides several advantages compared to the other standard purification tags. First, the MBP-tagged proteins can be purified in a facile one-step method using a custom-designed starch-agarose resin (Figure 20), which is easily prepared on a laboratory scale from inexpensive materials (Table 6) [102]. Second, the MBP-tag increases the solubility of a target protein, allowing the construction of a biohybrid catalyst library with high quality.

A newly established HTS platform for directed evolution of the Cp*Rh(III)-linked biohybrid catalyst using a 96-well format is shown in Figure 21. The target protein scaffold, NB4, is prepared as an MBP-tagged fusion protein, mbpNB4. Next, selected residues of the NB4 domain were

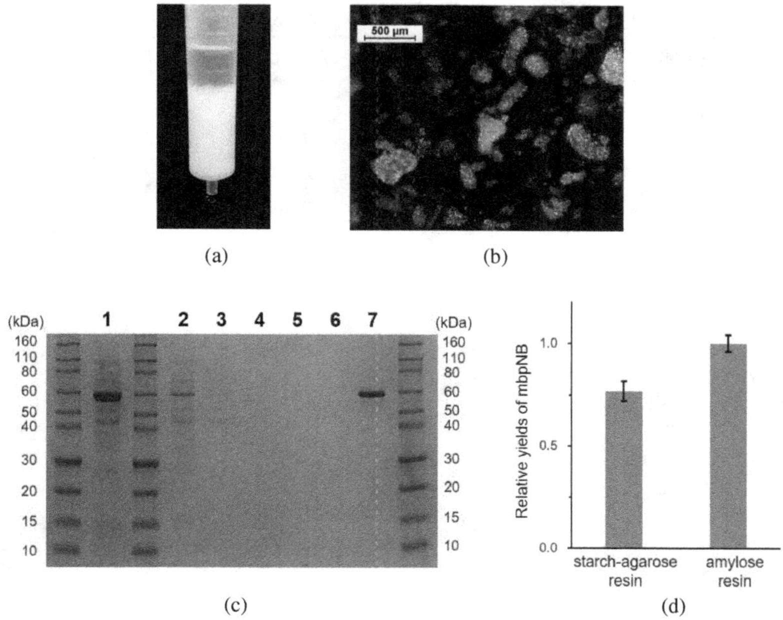

Fig. 20. (a) A photograph of starch-agarose resin. (b) An optical microscope image of starch-agarose. (c) SDS-PAGE analysis for the purification of mbpNB4 using starch-agarose resin. mbpNB4 is a fusion protein of NB4 with the MBP-tag (mbpNB4: 61 kDa). Lane 1: Crude cell lysate, lanes 2–6: Eluted fractions from the starch-agarose resin washed with an AcOH-MES buffer solution, and lane 7: First fraction eluted with AcOH-MES buffer containing 25 mM maltose. (d) Relative yields of mbpNB4 purified using the starch-agarose resin and commercially available amylose resin. Reproduced from with permission Ref. [102].

randomized via site-saturation mutagenesis (SSM). The library of mbpNB4 was expressed in *E. coli* cells. The cells harboring mbpNB4 variants were then lysed, and the mbpNB4 variants in the supernatant were directly subjected to conjugation with the Cp*Rh(III) complex tethering a maleimide group, which is protected by two *O,O'*-dicarboxyethoxyethyl dithiophosphate (**L6**) ligands. The reaction mixture was subjected to a 96-well filter plate packed with starch-agarose resin to purify the Cp*Rh(**L6**)$_2$-linked mbpNB4 (mbpNB4-Cp*Rh(**L6**)$_2$). Finally, mbpNB4-Cp*Rh(**L6**)$_2$ was eluted with a maltose solution to obtain a library of purified biohybrid catalysts. A removal of maltose is not required before screening because the maltose solution used in the elution step does not

Table 6. The costs for preparing 50 mL of starch-agarose resin[a] [102].

Chemicals	Price (JPY)	Amounts	Cost (JPY)
Agarose	86,500 (500 g)	1.6 g	277
Soluble starch	1,750 (500 g)	0.6 g	2.1
NaCl	2,000 (500 g)	0.36 g	1.4
Paraffin oil	7,040 (500 mL)	70 mL	9,856
Tween 80	2,700 (500 mL)	2.1 mL	11
			Total: 1,277

Note: [a]In the high-throughput screening for a biohybrid catalyst, c.a. 50 mL starch-agarose resin was packed into one 96-well filter plate (0.50 mL per each well).

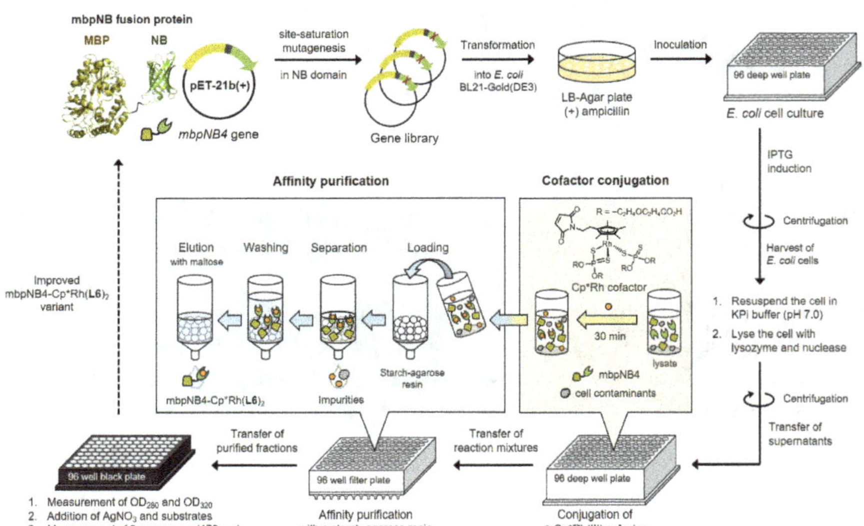

Fig. 21. Screening workflow for directed evolution of the Cp*Rh(III)-linked biohybrid catalyst. The four main steps of the HTS-platform include expression of mbpNB4 fusion protein, cofactor conjugation in a cell lysate, affinity purification using the starch-agarose resin, and evaluation in a 96-well format. Reproduced from with permission Ref. [102].

interfere with the catalysis of the Cp*Rh(III) cofactor. The mbpNB4-Cp*Rh(**L6**)$_2$ in the purified fraction was activated upon addition of Ag^+ ion, and subjected to screening through the cycloaddition reaction of 3′,4′-ethylenedioxyacetophenone oxime (**1**) with 1,4-dimethoxy-2-butyne (**13**)

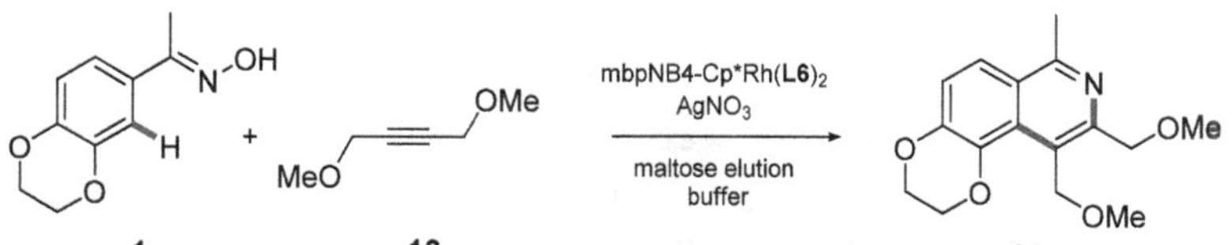

Fig. 22. Cycloaddition of acetophenone oxime **1** with alkyne **13**.

producing isoquinoline **14** (Figure 22). The activity of the mbpNB4-$Cp^*Rh(\mathbf{L6})_2$ variants was screened using a fluorescence microplate reader.

6.2. *Directed evolution of Cp*Rh-linked biohybrid catalysts*

The directed evolution of the Cp^*Rh(III)-linked biohybrid catalyst was performed using the developed HTS platform. Twenty-three NB4-positions (G36, Y38, T40, I41, F44, Y46, K68, S71, L75, L76, T98, L100, A125, K127, V128, K129, L148, T150, T151, T152, N153, L158, and L159) would function as the first, second, or outer coordination sphere of the Cp^*Rh(III) cofactor (Figure 23(a)). These prospective residues are located in the β-strands and loop regions forming the hydrophobic cavity (Figures 23(b) and 24). Therefore, these residues were randomized using SSM in the first round of the evolution. Three oligonucleotide primers including NHN, VNN and TGG codons that do not encode for a Cys residue were used for the randomization because the Cys substitution would provide an additional conjugation site for the cofactor (Table 7).

In the first round of directed evolution, more than 2,000 clones were screened. Ten Cp^*Rh(III)-linked mbpNB4 variants were identified as the first generation (Figure 25). In particular, two mbpNB4-$Cp^*Rh(\mathbf{L6})_2$ variants, T98H and N153I, have clearly higher activity relative to the parent mbpNB4-$Cp^*Rh(\mathbf{L6})_2$. However, the mbpNB4(N153I)-$Cp^*Rh(\mathbf{L6})_2$ variant, where Asn153 in NB4 was replaced with Ile, was obtained from the *E. coli* expression medium at a low concentration. Judging from the activity and expression level, mbpNB4(T98H)-$Cp^*Rh(\mathbf{L6})_2$ was finally selected for the next round of evolution.

Ten amino acid residues (G36, Y38, F44, Y46, S71, L100, A125, K127, K129, and N153) were selected for the SSM libraries and more than 1,000 clones were screened in the second round. Two promising variants, mbpNB4(T98H/L100K)-$Cp^*Rh(\mathbf{L6})_2$ and mbpNB4

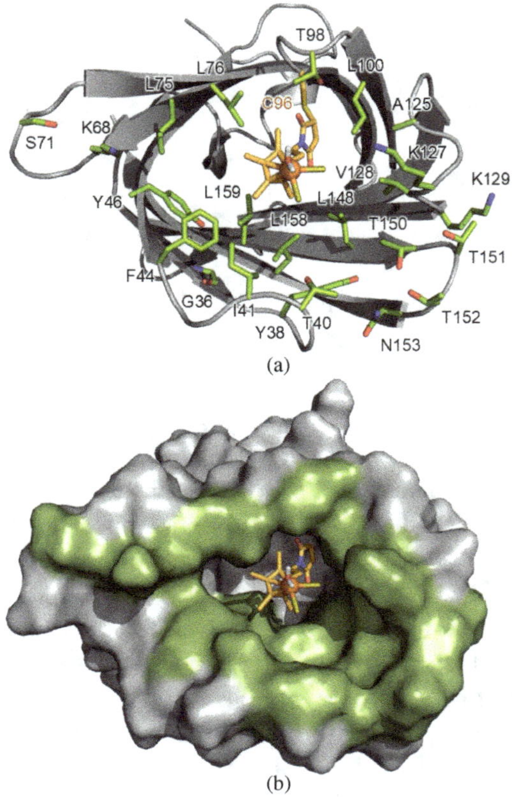

Fig. 23. MD structure of Cp*Rh(III)-linked NB4 with (a) cartoon and sticks and (b) modeled surfaces. The MD simulation was performed based on the crystal structure of NB4 (PDB: 3WJB). The dithiophosphate ligands of the Cp*Rh(III) cofactor were substituted with two chloride ions and one water molecule. The 23 residues subjected to SSM are highlighted in green. Reproduced with permission from Ref. [102].

(T98H/K127E)-Cp*Rh(**L6**)$_2$, were identified (Figure 26). A third round focusing on these two additional hot spot residues led to a discovery of the mbpNB4(T98H/L100K/K127E)-Cp*Rh(**L6**)$_2$ variant as the best performing biohybrid catalyst. These results indicate that two key substitutions, L100→K100 and K127→E127, enhance the activity in a cooperative manner. mbpNB4(T98H/L100K/K127E)-Cp*Rh(**L6**)$_2$ with the three substitutions has a 2.2-fold increase in catalytic activity. MD simulation suggests that Lys100 and Glu127 residues locate in the opposite side of the Rh metal center (Figure 27). Consequently, three mutations (T98→H98,

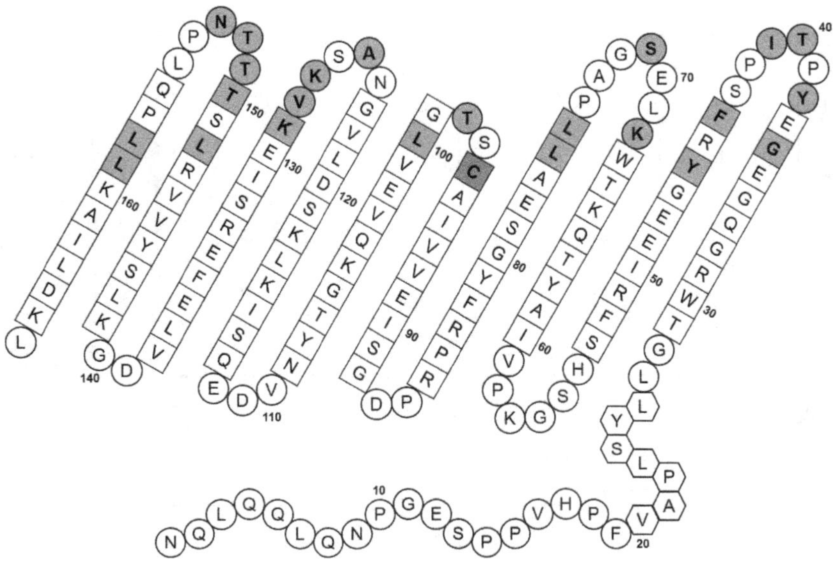

Fig. 24. A topology model of NB based on the crystal structure (PDB: 3WJB). Residues in the β-strands are shown in squares and residues in the α-helix structure are shown in hexagons. Cys96 residue is highlighted in red. The 23 positions subjected to site-saturation mutagenesis are highlighted in green [102].

Table 7. Degenerate codons and amino acids encoded [102].

Entry	**Codons**[a]	**Amino acids encoded**
1	NHN	A, N, D, Q, E, H, I, L, K, M, F, P, S, T, Y, V
2	VNN	A, R, N, D, Q, E, G, H, I, L, K, M, P, S, T, V
3	TGG	W

Notes: (N = A/C/G/T, H = A/C/T, V = A/C/G); [a]Three oligonucleotide primers containing NHN, VNN, and TGG codons were mixed in a ratio of 10:10:1 and used for site-saturation mutagenesis.

L100→K100 and K127→E127) in the NB4 cavity were determined as hot spots for improving the activity of the Cp*Rh(III) cofactor.

NB4(T98H/L100K/K127E)-Cp*Rh(**L5**)$_2$ without the MBP-tag provides product **14** with a 4.9-fold increase in activity relative to original NB4-Cp*Rh(**L5**)$_2$. In addition, NB4(T98H/L100K/K127E)-Cp*Rh(**L5**)$_2$ has the activity toward the cycloaddition of acetophenone oximes **1**, **15** and

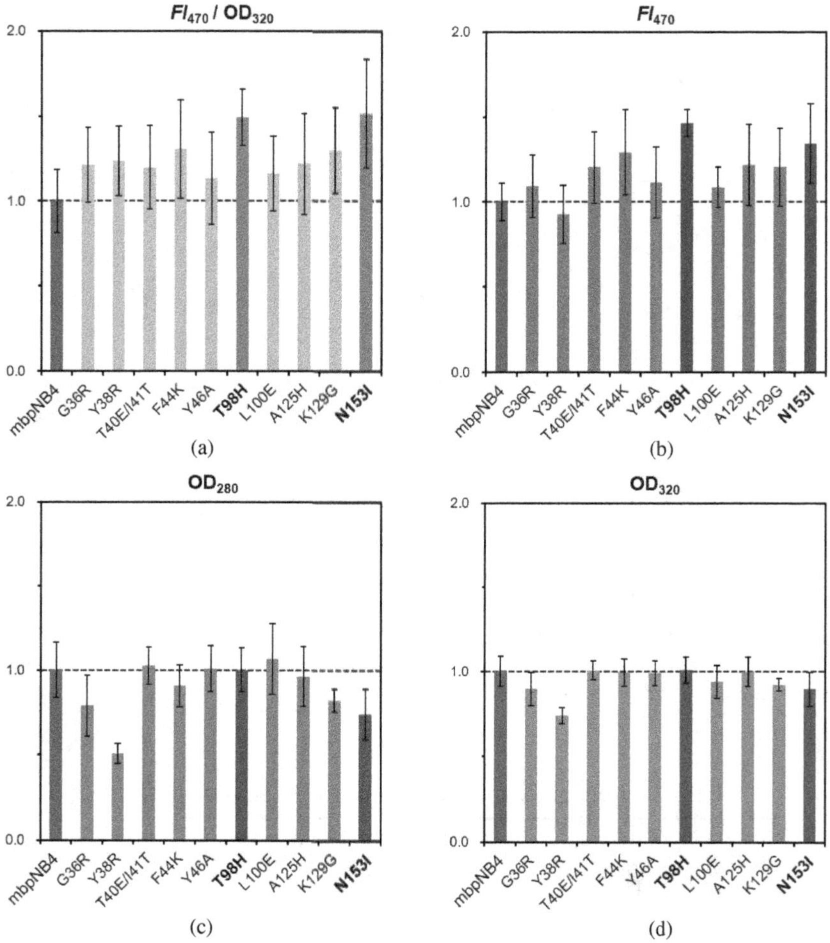

Fig. 25. mbpNB4-Cp*Rh(**L6**)$_2$ variants identified in the first round of directed evolution. (a) Relative catalytic activity of the mbpNB4-Cp*Rh(**L6**)$_2$ variants based on FI_{470}/OD$_{320}$. (b) Relative fluorescence intensity at 470 nm of reaction mixture (**1** + **13**). (c) Relative absorbance at 280 nm of the purified fraction containing each mbpNB4-Cp*Rh(**L6**)$_2$ variant. (d) Relative absorbance at 320 nm of the purified fraction containing each mbpNB4-Cp*Rh(**L6**)$_2$ variant. mbpNB4 and the mutations are shown in the bar graph. Reproduced with permission from Ref. [102].

16 with diphenylacetylene **2**. In the reaction of **1** with **2**, NB4(T98H/L100K/K127E)-Cp*Rh(**L5**)$_2$ provides **3** and **4** in 55% total yield with a 3, 4, fold increase in activity compared to NB4-Cp*Rh(**L5**)$_2$ (Figure 28).

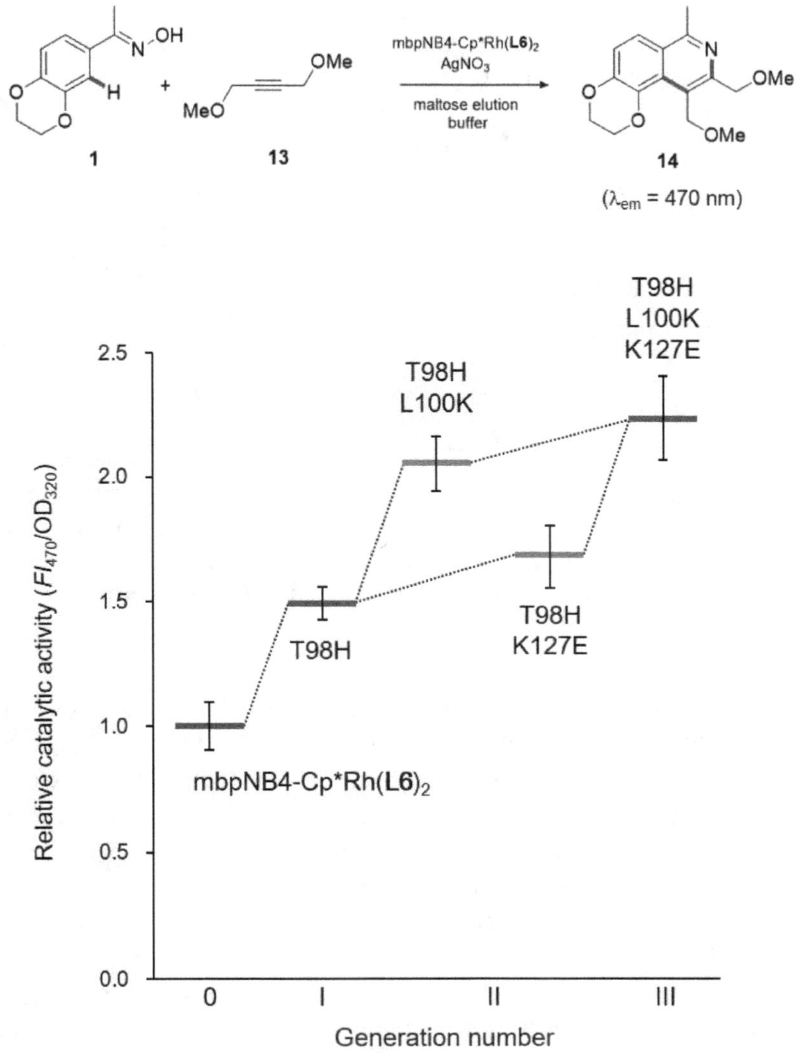

Fig. 26. Cycloaddition of oxime **1** with alkyne **13** catalyzed by evolved mbpNB4-Cp*Rh(**L6**)$_2$ variants. Reaction conditions: **1** (0.125 mM), **13** (2.0 mM) and $AgNO_3$ (1.0 mM) in a maltose elution buffer (25 mM maltose, 100 mM AcOH, 50 mM MES, 2% 1,4-dioxane, pH = 5.5) containing mbpNB4-Cp*Rh(**L6**)$_2$ variants (ca. 2 μM), 37°C for 72 h. Reproduced from with permission Ref. [102].

The catalysts also show higher activity toward the cycloaddition reactions with substrates **15** and **16** which differ in the ring size of catechol ether.

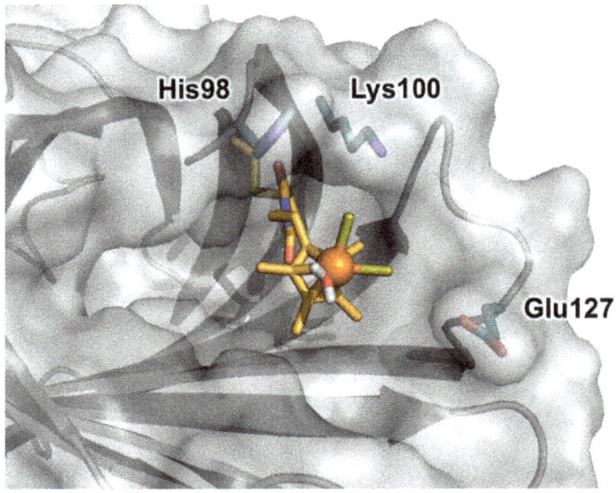

Fig. 27. An MD structure of Cp*Rh(III)-linked NB4(T98H/L100K/K127E). The MD calculation was carried out based on the crystal structure of NB4 (PDB: 3WJB). The two dithiophosphate ligands of the Cp*Rh(III) cofactor were substituted with two chloride ions and one water molecule. His98, Lys100 and Glu127 are highlighted as green sticks. [102].

The regioisomeric ratios of products did not change between NB4 (T98H/L100K/K127E)-Cp*Rh(**L5**)$_2$ and NB4-Cp*Rh(**L5**)$_2$ in all cases for the substrates **1**, **15**, and **16**. This result indicates that the His98 and Lys100 would interact with the cofactor and Glu127 would do with the Ag^+ ions during the exchange of the dithiophosphate ligands. These three residues are not apparently involved in substrate binding.

The reactivity of the Cp*Rh(III)-linked biohybrid catalysts toward the C(sp^2)–H bond functionalization was improved by directed evolution using newly developed HTS platforms, which includes affinity purification using an MBP-tag (Figure 29) [102]. Screening of more than 4,000 clones through three rounds of directed evolution led to the discovery of the promising Cp*Rh(III)-linked NB4(T98H/L100K/K127E) variant. This variant exhibits a clear increase relative to the original catalyst in terms of catalytic activity toward cycloaddition reactions of acetophenone oximes with alkynes. This HTS platform provides a versatile and powerful method for the directed evolution of biohybrid catalysts with a broad range of combination between metal cofactors and protein scaffolds.

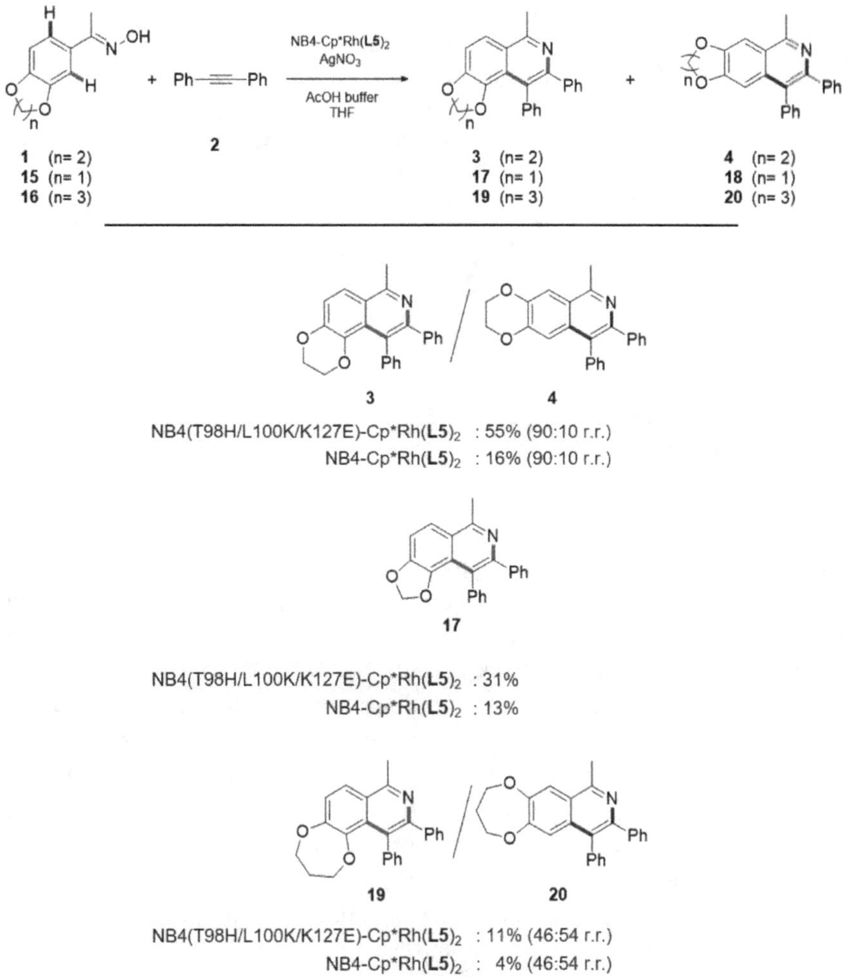

Fig. 28. Cycloaddition of **1**, **15** and **16** with diphenylacetylene **2** catalyzed by NB4-Cp*Rh(**L5**)$_2$ and NB4(T98H/L100K/K127E)-**1**. Reaction conditions: NB4-Cp*Rh(**L5**)$_2$ variant (20 μM), **1**, **15** and **16** (0.125 mM), **2** (2.0 mM) and $AgNO_3$ (1.0 mM) in AcOH buffer (100 mM AcOH, 20% THF, pH = 4.0), 25°C, 120 h. Total yields and regioisomeric ratio (r.r.) were determined by GC-MS. A trace amount of regioisomer **18** was generated (<1.0% yield). Reproduced with permission from Ref. [102].

7. Summary

In summary, biohybrid catalysts harboring various synthetic metal complexes within the β-barrel nitrobindin protein, which have been developed

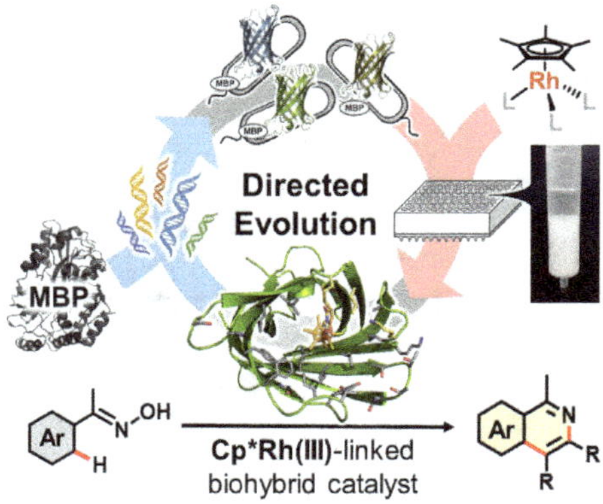

Fig. 29. Representative scheme of directed evolution for optimizing the Cp*Rh(III)-linked biohybrid catalysts. [102].

in the authors' groups, are described. The metal complexes were covalently linked to the Cys residue of the β-barrel protein via a maleimide moiety attached at the peripheral chain of the metal ligand. Nitrobindin has also been demonstrated to be a useful scaffold to accommodate other metal complexes in similar works that are not introduced in this chapter [104–106]. Furthermore, the use of transmembrane β-barrel protein such as FhuA is a promising direction for the whole cell catalysis and chemo-enzymatic cascade [33,107–110]. In addition, the authors have developed a method for directed evolution of the biohybrid catalysts with the covalently linked metal complex. This high-throughput screening platform using purified proteins provides a great opportunity to explore combinations of reactive synthetic metal complexes and protein scaffolds of interest, paving the way for discovery of a totally new activity and selectivity in biohybrid catalysts.

References

1. Wu, S., Snajdrova, R., Moore, J. C., Baldenius, K. and Bornscheuer, U. T. (2021) Biocatalysis: Enzymatic Synthesis for Industrial Applications. *Angew. Chem. Int. Ed.* 60, pp. 88–119.
2. Renata, H., Wang, Z. J. and Arnold, F. H. (2015) Expanding the Enzyme Universe: Accessing Non-natural Reactions by Mechanism-Guided Directed Evolution. *Angew. Chem. Int. Ed.* 54, pp. 3351–3367.

3. Chen, K. and Arnold, F. H. (2020) Engineering New Catalytic Activities in Enzymes. *Nat. Catal.* 3, pp. 203–213.
4. Thomas, C. M. and Ward, T. R. (2005) Artificial Metalloenzymes: Proteins as Hosts for Enantioselective Catalysis. *Chem. Soc. Rev.* 34, pp. 337–346.
5. Ward, T. R. (2011) Artificial Metalloenzymes Based on the Biotin-Avidin Technology: Enantioselective Catalysis and Beyond. *Acc. Chem. Res.* 44, pp. 47–57.
6. Reetz, M. T., Rentzsch, M., Pletsch, A., Maywald, M., Maiwald, P., Peyralans, J. J. P., Maichele, A., Fu, Y., Jiao, N., Hollmann, F., Mondiere, R. and Taglieber, A. (2007) Directed Evolution of Enantioselective Hybrid Catalysts: A Novel Concept in Asymmetric Catalysis. *Tetrahedron.* 63, pp. 6404–6414.
7. Reetz, M. T. (2019) Directed Evolution of Artificial Metalloenzymes: A Universal Means to Tune the Selectivity of Transition Metal Catalysts? *Acc. Chem. Res.* 52, pp. 336–344.
8. Schwizer, F., Okamoto, Y., Heinisch, T., Gu, Y., Pellizzoni, M. M., Lebrun, V., Reuter, R., Köhler, V., Lewis, J. C. and Ward, T. R. (2018) Artificial Metalloenzymes: Reaction Scope and Optimization Strategies. *Chem. Rev.* 118, pp. 142–231.
9. Lu, Y. (2006) Biosynthetic Inorganic Chemistry. *Angew. Chem. Int. Ed.* 45, pp. 5588–5601.
10. Yu, F., Cangelosi, V. M., Zastrow, M. L., Tegoni, M., Plegaria, J. S., Tebo, A. G., Mocny, C. S., Ruckthong, L., Qayyum, H. and Pecoraro, V. L. (2014) Protein Design: Toward Functional Metalloenzymes. *Chem. Rev.* 114, pp. 3495–3578.
11. Lewis, J. C. (2013) Artificial Metalloenzymes and Metallopeptide Catalysts for Organic Synthesis. *ACS Catal.* 3, pp. 2954–2975.
12. Roelfes, G. (2019) LmrR: A Privileged Scaffold for Artificial Metalloenzymes. *Acc. Chem. Res.* 52, pp. 545–556.
13. Deuss, P. J., den Heeten, R., Laan, W. and Kamer, P. C. J. (2011) Bioinspired Catalyst Design and Artificial Metalloenzymes. *Chem. Eur. J.* 17, pp. 4680–4698.
14. Ueno, T., Tabe, H. and Tanaka, Y. (2013) Artificial Metalloenzymes Constructed From Hierarchically-assembled Proteins. *Chem. Asian J.* 8, pp. 1646–1660.
15. Ohashi, M., Koshiyama, T., Ueno, T., Yanase, M., Fujii, H. and Watanabe, Y. (2003) Preparation of Artificial Metalloenzymes by Insertion of Chromium(III) Schiff Base Complexes into Apomyoglobin Mutants. *Angew. Chem. Int. Ed.* 42, pp. 1005–1008.
16. Mahammed, A. and Gross, Z. (2005) Albumin-Conjugated Corrole Metal Complexes: Extremely Simple Yet Very Efficient Biomimetic Oxidation Systems. *J. Am. Chem. Soc.* 127, pp. 2883–2887.

17. Jing, Q., Okrasa, K. and Kazlauskas, R. J. (2009) Stereoselective Hydrogenation of Olefins Using Rhodium-Substituted Carbonic Anhydrase — A New Reductase. *Chem. Eur. J.* 15, pp. 1370–1376.
18. Matsuo, T., Hayashi, A., Abe, M., Matsuda, T., Hisaeda, Y. and Hayashi, T. (2009) Meso-Unsubstituted Iron Corrole in Hemoproteins: Remarkable Differences in Effects on Peroxidase Activities between Myoglobin and Horseradish Peroxidase. *J. Am. Chem. Soc.* 131, pp. 15124–15125.
19. Sano, Y., Onoda, A. and Hayashi, T. (2011). A Hydrogenase Model System Based on the Sequence of Cytochrome *c*: Photochemical Hydrogen Evolution in Aqueous Media. *Chem. Commun.* 47, pp. 8229–8231.
20. Monnard, F. W., Nogueira, E. S., Heinisch, T., Schirmer, T. and Ward, T. R. (2013) Human Carbonic Anhydrase II as Host Protein for the Creation of Artificial Metalloenzymes: The Asymmetric Transfer Hydrogenation of Imines. *Chem. Sci.* 4, pp. 3269–3274.
21. Podtetenieff, J., Taglieber, A., Bill, E., Reijerse, E. J. and Reetz, M. T. (2010) An Artificial Metalloenzyme: Creation of a Designed Copper Binding Site in a Thermostable Protein. *Angew. Chem. Int. Ed.* 49, pp. 5151–5155.
22. Ball, Z. T. (2013) Designing Enzyme-like Catalysts: A Rhodium(II) Metallopeptide Case Study. *Acc. Chem. Res.* 46, pp. 560–570.
23. Wilson, M. E. and Whitesides, G. M. (1978) Conversion of a Protein to a Homogeneous Catalysts. *J. Am. Chem. Soc.* 100, pp. 306–307.
24. Collot, J., Gradinaru, J., Humbert, N., Skander, M., Zocchi, A. and Ward, T. R. (2003) Artificial Metalloenzymes for Enantioselective Catalysis Based on Biotin–Avidin. *J. Am. Chem. Soc.* 125, pp. 9030–9031.
25. Yamaguchi, H., Hirano, T., Kiminami, H., Taura, D. and Harada, A. (2006) Asymmetric Hydrogenation. *Org. Biomol. Chem.* 4, pp. 3571–3573.
26. Reetz, M. T. and Jiao, N. (2006) Copper–Phthalocyanine Conjugates of Serum Albumins as Enantioselective Catalysts in Diels–Alder Reactions. *Angew. Chem. Int. Ed.* 118, pp. 2476–2479.
27. Qi, D., Tann, C. M., Haring, D. and Distefano, M. D. (2001) Generation of New Enzymes via Covalent Modification of Existing Proteins. *Chem. Rev.* 101, pp. 3081–3111.
28. Reetz, M. T. (2002) Directed Evolution of Selective Enzymes and Hybrid Catalysts. *Tetrahedron.* 58, pp. 6595–6602.
29. Carey, J. R., Ma, S. K., Pfister, T. D., Garner, D. K., Kim, H. K., Abramite, J. A., Wang, Z., Guo, Z. and Lu, Y. (2004) A Site-Selective Dual Anchoring Strategy for Artificial Metalloprotein Design. *J. Am. Chem. Soc.* 126, pp. 10812–10813.
30. Haquette, P., Talbi, B., Barilleau, L., Madern, N., Fosse, C. and Salmain, M. (2011) Chemically Engineered Papain as Artificial Formate Dehydrogenase for NAD(P)H Regeneration. *Org. Biomol. Chem.* 9, pp. 5720–5727.

31. Matsuo, T., Imai, C., Yoshida, T., Saito, T., Hayashi, T. and Hirota, S. (2012) Creation of an Artificial Metalloprotein with a Hoveyda-Grubbs Catalyst Moiety Through the Intrinsic Inhibition Mechanism of α-Chymotrypsin. *Chem. Commun.* 48, pp. 1662–1664.
32. Onoda, A., Fukumoto, K., Arlt, M., Bocola, M., Schwaneberg, U. and Hayashi, T. (2012) A Rhodium Complex-Linked *β*-Barrel Protein as a Hybrid Biocatalyst for Phenylacetylene Polymerization. *Chem. Commun.* 48, pp. 9756–9758.
33. Philippart, F., Arlt, M., Gotzen, S., Tenne, S.-J., Bocola, M., Chen, H.-H., Zhu, L., Schwaneberg, U. and Okuda, J. (2013) A Hybrid Ring-Opening Metathesis Polymerization Catalyst Based on an Engineered Variant of the *β*-Barrel Protein FhuA. *Chem. Eur. J.* 19, pp. 13865–13871.
34. Bos, J., Garcia-Herraiz, A. and Roelfes, G. (2013) An Enantioselective Artificial Metallo-Hydratase. *Chem. Sci.* 4, pp. 3578–3582.
35. Zimbron, J. M., Heinisch, T., Schmid, M., Hamels, D., Nogueira, E. S., Schirmer, T., Ward, T. R., Zimbron, J. M., Heinisch, T., Schmid, M., Hamels, D., Nogueira, E. S., Schirmer, T. and Ward, T. R. (2013) A Dual Anchoring Strategy for the Localization and Activation of Artificial Metalloenzymes Based on the Biotin–Streptavidin Technology. *J. Am. Chem. Soc.* 135, pp. 5384–5388.
36. Bos, J., Fusetti, F., Driessen, A. J. M. and Roelfes, G. (2012) Enantioselective Artificial Metalloenzymes by Creation of a Novel Active Site at the Protein Dimer Interface. *Angew. Chem. Int. Ed.* 51, pp. 7472–7475.
37. Ueno, T., Koshiyama, T., Ohashi, M., Kondo, K., Kono, M., Suzuki, A., Yamane, T. and Watanabe, Y. (2005) Coordinated Design of Cofactor and Active Site Structures in Development of New Protein Catalysts. *J. Am. Chem. Soc.* 127, pp. 6556–6562.
38. Pordea, A., Creus, M., Panek, J., Duboc, C., Mathis, D. B., Novic, M. and Ward, T. R. (2008) Artificial Metalloenzyme for Enantioselective Sulfoxidation Based on Vanadyl-loaded Streptavidin. *J. Am. Chem. Soc.* 130, pp. 8085–8088.
39. Hyster, T. K., Knörr, L., Ward, T. R. and Rovis, T. (2012) Biotinylated Rh(III) Complexes in Engineered Streptavidin for Accelerated Asymmetric C–H Activation. *Science.* 338, pp. 500–503.
40. Hassan, I. S., Ta, A. N., Danneman, M. W., Semakul, N., Burns, M., Basch, C. H., Dippon, V. N., McNaughton, B. R. and Rovis, T. (2019) Asymmetric δ-Lactam Synthesis with a Monomeric Streptavidin Artificial Metalloenzyme. *J. Am. Chem. Soc.* 141, pp. 4815–4819.
41. Creus, M. and Ward, T. R. (2007) Designed Evolution of Artificial Metalloenzymes: Protein Catalysts Made to Order. *Org. Biomol. Chem.* 5, pp. 1835–1844.
42. Reetz, M. T., Peyralans, J. J. P., Maichele, A., Fu, Y. and Maywald, M. (2006) Directed Evolution of Hybrid Enzymes: Evolving Enantioselectivity of an

Achiral Rh-Complex Anchored to a Protein. *Chem. Commun.* pp. 4318–4320.

43. Yang, H., Swartz, A. M., Park, H. J., Srivastava, P., Ellis-Guardiola, K., Upp, D. M., Lee, G., Belsare, K., Gu, Y., Zhang, C., Moellering, R. E. and Lewis, J. C. (2018) Evolving Artificial Metalloenzymes via Random Mutagenesis. *Nat. Chem.* 10, pp. 318–324.
44. Hestericova, M., Heinisch, T., Alonso-Cotchico, L., Marechal, J. D., Vidossich, P. and Ward, T. R. (2018) Directed Evolution of an Artificial Imine Reductase. *Angew. Chem. Int. Ed.* 57, pp. 1863–1868.
45. Liang, A. D., Serrano-Plana, J., Peterson, R. L. and Ward, T. R. (2019) Artificial Metalloenzymes Based on the Biotin–Streptavidin Technology: Enzymatic Cascades and Directed Evolution. *Acc. Chem. Res.* 52, pp. 585–595.
46. Davis, H. J. and Ward, T. R. (2019) Artificial Metalloenzymes: Challenges and Opportunities. *ACS Cent. Sci.* 5, pp. 1120–1136.
47. Markel, U., Sauer, D. F., Schiffels, J., Okuda, J. and Schwaneberg, U. (2019) Towards the Evolution of Artificial Metalloenzymes–A Protein Engineer's Perspective. *Angew. Chem. Int. Ed.* 58, pp. 4454–4464.
48. Jeschek, M., Reuter, R., Heinisch, T., Trindler, C., Klehr, J., Panke, S. and Ward, T. R. (2016) Directed Evolution of Artificial Metalloenzymes for In Vivo Metathesis. *Nature* 537, pp. 661.
49. Zhao, J. M., Rebelein, J. G., Mallin, H., Trindler, C., Pellizzoni, M. M. and Ward, T. R. (2018) Genetic Engineering of an Artificial Metalloenzyme for Transfer Hydrogenation of a Self-Immolative Substrate in Escherichia Coil's Periplasm. *J. Am. Chem. Soc.* 140, pp. 13171–13175.
50. Zhao, J., Bachmann, D. G., Lenz, M., Gillingham, D. G. and Ward, T. R. (2018) An Artificial Metalloenzyme for Carbene Transfer Based on a Biotinylated Dirhodium Anchored within Streptavidin. *Cat. Sci. Technol.* 8, pp. 2294–2298.
51. Heinisch, T., Schwizer, F., Garabedian, B., Csibra, E., Jeschek, M., Vallapurackal, J., Pinheiro, V. B., Marliere, P., Panke, S. and Ward, T. R. (2018) *E. coli* Surface Display of Streptavidin for Directed Evolution of an Allylic Deallylase. *Chem. Sci.* 9, pp. 5383–5388.
52. Grimm, A. R., Sauer, D. F., Polen, T., Zhu, L., Hayashi, T., Okuda, J. and Schwaneberg, U. (2018) A Whole Cell *E. coli* Display Platform for Artificial Metalloenzymes: Poly(phenylacetylene) Production with a Rhodium–Nitrobindin Metalloprotein. *ACS Catal.* 8, pp. 2611–2614.
53. Creus, M., Pordea, A., Rossel, T., Sardo, A., Letondor, C., Ivanova, A., LeTrong, I., Stenkamp, R. E. and Ward, T. R. (2008) X-Ray Structure and Designed Evolution of an Artificial Transfer Hydrogenase. *Angew. Chem. Int. Ed.* 47, pp. 1400–1404.
54. Dydio, P., Key, H. M., Nazarenko, A., Rha, J. Y. E., Seyedkazemi, V., Clark, D. S. and Hartwig, J. F. (2016) An Artificial Metalloenzyme with the Kinetics of Native Enzymes. *Science* 354, pp. 102.

55. Key, H. M., Dydio, P., Clark, D. S. and Hartwig, J. F. (2016) Abiological Catalysis by Artificial Haem Proteins Containing Noble Metals in Place of Iron. *Nature* 534, pp. 534.
56. Mallin, H., Hestericova, M., Reuter, R. and Ward, T. R. (2016) Library Design and Screening Protocol for Artificial Metalloenzymes Based on the Biotin–Streptavidin Technology. *Nat. Protoc.* 11, pp. 835–852.
57. Tang, B. Z., Poon, W. H., Leung, S. M., Leung, W. H. and Peng, H. (1997) Synthesis of Stereoregular Poly(phenylacetylene)s by Organorhodium Complexes in Aqueous Media. *Macromolecules* 30, pp. 2209–2212.
58. Ikariya, T., Kishimoto, Y., Eckerle, P., Miyatake, T., Kainosho, M., Ono, A. and Noyori, R. (1999) Well-Controlled Polymerization of Phenylacetylenes with Organorhodium(I) Complexes: Mechanism and Structure of the Polyenes. *J. Am. Chem. Soc.* 121, pp. 12035–12044.
59. Abe, S., Hirata, K., Ueno, T., Morino, K., Shimizu, N., Yamamoto, M., Takata, M., Yashima, E. and Watanabe, Y. (2009) Polymerization of Phenylacetylene by Rhodium Complexes Within a Discrete Space of Apo-Ferritin. *J. Am. Chem. Soc.* 131, pp. 6958–6960.
60. Ke, Z., Abe, S., Ueno, T. and Morokuma, K. (2011) Rh-Catalyzed of Phenylacetylene: Theoretical Studies of the Reaction Mechanism, Regioselectivity, and Stereoregularity. *J. Am. Chem. Soc.* 133, pp. 7926–7941.
61. Amoia, A. M. and Montfort, W. R. (2007) Apo-Nitrophorin 4 at Atomic Resolution. *Protein Sci.* 16, pp. 2076–2081.
62. Bianchetti, C. M., Blouin, G. C., Bitto, E., Olson, J. S. and Phillips, G. N. (2010) The Structure and NO Binding Properties of the Nitrophorin-Like Heme-Binding Protein from *Arabidopsis thaliana* Gene Locus At1g79260.1. *Proteins* 78, pp. 917–931.
63. Fukumoto, K., Onoda, A., Mizohata, E., Bocola, M., Inoue, T., Schwaneberg, U. and Hayashi, T. (2014) A Rhodium Complex-Linked Hbrid Biocatalyst: Stereo-Controlled Phenylacetylene Polymerization Within an Engineered Protein Cavity. *ChemCatChem.* 6, pp. 1229–1235.
64. Song, G., Wang, F. and Li, X. (2012) C–C, C–O and C–N Bond Formation via Rhodium(III)-Catalyzed Oxidative C–H Activation. *Chem. Soc. Rev.* 41, pp. 3651–3678.
65. Song, G. and Li, X. (2015) Substrate Activation Strategies in Rhodium(III)-catalyzed Selective Functionalization of Arenes. *Acc. Chem. Res.* 48, pp. 1007–1020.
66. Chen, Z., Wang, B., Zhang, J., Yu, W., Liu, Z. and Zhang, Y. (2015) Transition Metal-Catalyzed C–H Bond Functionalizations by the Use of Diverse Directing Groups. *Org. Chem. Frontiers* 2, pp. 1107–1295.
67. Zhang, M., Zhang, Y., Jie, X., Zhao, H., Li, G. and Su, W. (2014) Recent Advances in Directed C-H Functionalizations Using Monodentate Nitrogen-Based Directing Groups. *Org. Chem. Frontiers* 1, pp. 843–895.

68. Kato, S., Onoda, A., Grimm, A. R., Tachikawa, K., Schwaneberg, U. and Hayashi, T. (2020) Incorporation of a Cp*Rh(III)-Dithiophosphate Cofactor with Latent Activity into a Protein Scaffold Generates a Biohybrid Catalyst Promoting C(sp^2)–H Bond Functionalization. *Inorg. Chem.* 59, pp. 14457–14463.
69. Cammack, R., Frey, M. and Robson, R., Eds. (2002) *Hydrogen as a Fuel: Learning from Nature*. CRC Press: London.
70. Armstrong, F. and Blundell, K., Eds. (2007) *Energy... Beyond Oil*. Oxford University Press: Oxford.
71. Peters, J. W. (1998) X-ray Crystal Structure of the Fe-Only Hydrogenase (Cpl) from Clostridium Pasteurianum to 1.8 Angstrom Resolution. *Science* 282, pp. 1853–1858.
72. Nicolet, Y., Piras, C., Legrand, P., Hatchikian, C. E. and Fontecilla-Camps, J. C. (1999) Desulfovibrio Desulfuricans Iron Hydrogenase: The Structure Shows Unusual Coordination to an Active Site Fe Binuclear Center. *Structure* 7, pp. 13–23.
73. Pandey, A. S., Harris, T. V., Giles, L. J., Peters, J. W. and Szilagyi, R. K. (2008) Dithiomethylether as a Ligand in the Hydrogenase H-Cluster. *J. Am. Chem. Soc.* 130, pp. 4533–4540.
74. Tard, C., Liu, X., Ibrahim, S. K., Bruschi, M., De Giola, L., Davies, S. C., Yang, X., Wang, L. S., Sawers, G. and Pickett, C. J. (2005) Synthesis of the H-Cluster Framework of Iron-Only Hydrogenase. *Nature* 433, pp. 610–613.
75. Jones, A. K., Lichtenstein, B. R., Dutta, A., Gordon, G. and Dutton, P. L. (2007) Synthetic Hydrogenases: Incorporation of an Iron Carbonyl Thiolate into a Designed Peptide. *J. Am. Chem. Soc.* 129, pp. 14844–14845.
76. Singleton, M. L., Reibenspies, J. H. and Darensbourg, M. Y. (2010) A Cyclodextrin Host/Guest Approach to a Hydrogenase Active Site Biomimetic Cavity. *J. Am. Chem. Soc.* 132, pp. 8870–8871.
77. Singleton, M. L., Crouthers, D. J., Duttweiler, R. P., Reibenspies, J. H. and Darensbourg, M. Y. (2011) Sulfonated Diiron Complexes as Water-Soluble Models of the [Fe–Fe]-Hydrogenase Enzyme Active Site. *Inorg. Chem.* 50, pp. 5015–5026.
78. Wang, N., Wang, M., Wang, Y., Zheng, D., Han, H., Ahlquist, M. S. G. and Sun, L. (2013) Catalytic Activation of H_2 under Mild Conditions by an [FeFe]-Hydrogenase Model via an Active μ-Hydride Species. *J. Am. Chem. Soc.* 135, pp. 13688–13691.
79. Hsieh, C.-H., Erdem, Ö. F., Harman, S. D., Singleton, M. L., Reijerse, E., Lubitz, W., Popescu, C. V., Reibenspies, J. H., Brothers, S. M., Hall, M. B. and Darensbourg, M. Y. (2012) Structural and Spectroscopic Features of Mixed Valent FeIIFeI Complexes and Factors Related to the Rotated

Configuration of Diiron Hydrogenase. *J. Am. Chem. Soc.* 134, pp. 13089–13102.

80. Camara, J. M. and Rauchfuss, T. B. (2012) Combining Acid–Base, Redox and Substrate Binding Functionalities to Give a Complete Model for the [FeFe]-Hydrogenase. *Nat. Chem.* 4, pp. 26–30.
81. Tard, C. and Pickett, C. J. (2009) Structural and Functional Analogues of the Active Sites of the [Fe]-, [NiFe]-, and [FeFe]-Hydrogenases. *Chem. Rev.* 109, pp. 2245–2274.
82. Sun, L., Åkermark, B. and Ott, S. (2005) Iron Hydrogenase Active Site Mimics in Supramolecular Systems Aiming for Light-Driven Hydrogen Production. *Coord. Chem. Rev.* 249, pp. 1653–1663.
83. Ott, S., Kritikos, M., Åkermark, B. and Sun, L. (2003) Synthesis and Structure of a Biomimetic Model of the Iron Hydrogenase Active Site Covalently Linked to a Ruthenium Photosensitizer. *Angew. Chem. Int. Ed.* 42, pp. 3285–3288.
84. Nann, T., Ibrahim, S. K., Woi, P. M., Xu, S., Ziegler, J. and Pickett, C. J. (2010) Water Splitting by Visible Light: A Nanophotocathode for Hydrogen Production. *Angew. Chem. Int. Ed.* 49, pp. 1574–1577.
85. Eckenhoff, W. T. and Eisenberg, R. (2012) Molecular Systems for Light Driven Hydrogen Production. *Dalton Trans.* 41, pp. 13004–13021.
86. Faiella, M., Roy, A., Sommer, D. and Ghirlanda, G. (2013) *De novo* Design of Functional Proteins: Toward Artificial Hydrogenases. *Pept. Sci.* 100, pp. 558–571.
87. Roy, A., Madden, C. and Ghirlanda, G. (2012) Photo-Induced Hydrogen Production in a Helical Peptide Incorporating a [FeFe]-Hydrogenase Active Site Mimic. *Chem. Commun.* 48, pp. 9816–9818.
88. Sano, Y., Onoda, A. and Hayashi, T. (2012) Photocatalytic Hydrogen Evolution by a Diiron Hydrogenase Model Based on a Peptide Fragment of Cytochrome c_{556} with an Attached Diiron Carbonyl Cluster and an Attached Ruthenium Photosensitizer. *J. Inorg. Biochem.* 108, pp. 159–162.
89. Onoda, A., Kihara, Y., Fukumoto, K., Sano, Y. and Hayashi, T. (2014) Photoinduced Hydrogen Evolution Catalyzed by a Synthetic Diiron Dithiolate Complex Embedded Within a Protein Matrix. *ACS Catal.* 4, pp. 2645–2648.
90. Krieger, E., Darden, T., Nabuurs, S., Finkelstein, A. and Vriend, G. (2004) Making Optimal Use of Empirical Energy Functions: Force-Field Parameterization in Crystal Space. *Proteins: Struct. Funct. Bioinf.* 57, pp. 678–683.
91. Knowles, R. R. and Jacobsen, E. N. (2010) Attractive Noncovalent Interactions in Asymmetric Catalysis: Links Between Enzymes and Small Molecule Catalysts. *Proc. Natl. Acad. Sci. USA* 107, pp. 20678–20685.

92. Kennedy, C. R., Lin, S. and Jacobsen, E. N. (2016) The Cation–π Interaction in Small-molecule Catalysis. *Angew. Chem. Int. Ed.* 55, pp. 12596–12624.
93. Cotelle, Y., Lebrun, V., Sakai, N., Ward, T. R. and Matile, S. (2016) Anion-π Enzymes. *ACS Central Sci.* 2, pp. 388–393.
94. Zhao, Y., Benz, S., Sakai, N. and Matile, S. (2015) Selective Acceleration of Disfavored Enolate Addition Reactions by Anion-π Interactions. *Chem. Sci.* 6, pp. 6219–6223.
95. Himiyama, T., Taniguchi, N., Kato, S., Onoda, A. and Hayashi, T. (2017) A Pyrene-linked Cavity within a β-Barrel Protein Promotes an Asymmetric Diels–Alder Reaction. *Angew. Chem. Int. Ed.* 56, pp. 13618–13622.
96. Reetz, M. T. (2004) Controlling the Enantioselectivity of Enzymes by Directed Evolution: Practical and Theoretical Ramifications. *Proc. Natl. Acad. Sci. USA* 101, pp. 5716–5722.
97. Prier, C. K. and Arnold, F. H. (2015) Chemomimetic Biocatalysis: Exploiting the Synthetic Potential of Cofactor-Dependent Enzymes to Create New Catalysts. *J. Am. Chem. Soc.* 137, pp. 13992–14006.
98. Leveson-Gower, R. B., Mayer, C. and Roelfes, G. (2019) The Importance of Catalytic Promiscuity for Enzyme Design and Evolution. *Nat. Rev. Chem.* 3, pp. 687–705.
99. Zeymer, C. and Hilvert, D. (2018) Directed Evolution of Protein Catalysts. *Annu. Rev. Biochem.* 87, pp. 131–157.
100. Romero, P. A. and Arnold, F. H. (2009) Exploring Protein Fitness Landscapes by Directed Evolution. *Nat. Rev. Mol. Cell. Biol.* 10, pp. 866–876.
101. Markel, U., Essani, K. D., Besirlioglu, V., Schiffels, J., Streit, W. R. and Schwaneberg, U. (2020) Advances in Ultrahigh-Throughput Screening for Directed Enzyme Evolution. *Chem. Soc. Rev.* 49, pp. 233–262.
102. Kato, S., Onoda, A., Taniguchi, N., Schwaneberg, U. and Hayashi, T. (2021) Directed Evolution of a $Cp^{*}Rh^{III}$-linked Biohybrid Catalyst Based on a Screening Platform with Affinity Purification. *Chem Bio Chem.* 22, pp. 679–685.
103. Ferenci, T. and Klotz, U. (1978) Affinity Chromatographic Isolation of the Periplasmic Maltose Binding Protein of *Escherichia coli*. *FEBS Lett.* 94, pp. 213–217.
104. Himiyama, T., Sauer, D. F., Onoda, A., Spaniol, T. P., Okuda, J. and Hayashi, T. (2016) Construction of a Hybrid Biocatalyst Containing a Covalently-Linked Terpyridine Metal Complex Within a Cavity of Aponitrobindin. *J. Inorg. Biochem.* 158, pp. 55–61.
105. Sauer, D. F., Himiyama, T., Tachikawa, K., Fukumoto, K., Onoda, A., Mizohata, E., Inoue, T., Bocola, M., Schwaneberg, U., Hayashi, T. and Okuda, J. (2015) A Highly Active Biohybrid Catalyst for Olefin Metathesis

in Water: Impact of a Hydrophobic Cavity in a β-Barrel Protein. *ACS Catal.* 5, pp. 7519–7522.

106. Grimm, A. R., Sauer, D. F., Davari, M. D., Zhu, L., Bocola, M., Kato, S., Onoda, A., Hayashi, T., Okuda, J. and Schwaneberg, U. (2018) Cavity Size Engineering of a β-Barrel Protein Generates Efficient Biohybrid Catalysts for Olefin Metathesis. *ACS Catal.* pp. 3358–3364.
107. Sauer, D. F., Bocola, M., Broglia, C., Arlt, M., Zhu, L.-L., Brocker, M., Schwaneberg, U. and Okuda, J. (2015) Hybrid Ruthenium ROMP Catalysts Based on an Engineered Variant of β-Barrel Protein FhuA ΔCVFtev: Effect of Spacer Length. *Chem. Asian J.* 10, pp. 177–182.
108. Osseili, H., Sauer, D. F., Beckerle, K., Arlt, M., Himiyama, T., Polen, T., Onoda, A., Schwaneberg, U., Hayashi, T. and Okuda, J. (2016) Artificial Diels-Alderase Based on the Transmembrane Protein FhuA. *Beilstein J. Org. Chem.* 12, pp. 1314–1321.
109. Thiel, A., Sauer, D. F., Mertens, M. A. S., Polen, T., Chen, H. H., Schwaneberg, U. and Okuda, J. (2018) Cyclotrimerization of Phenylacetylene Catalyzed by a Cobalt Half-Sandwich Complex Embedded in an Engineered Variant of Transmembrane Protein FhuA. *Org. Biomol. Chem.* 16, pp. 5452–5456.
110. Mertens, M. A. S., Sauer, D. F., Markel, U., Schiffels, J., Okuda, J. and Schwaneberg, U. (2019) Chemoenzymatic Cascade for Stilbene Production from Cinnamic Acid Catalyzed by Ferulic Acid Decarboxylase and an Artificial Metathease. *Cat. Sci. Technol.* 9, pp. 5572–5576.

https://doi.org/10.1142/9789811261664_0012

Chapter 12

Chemistry for a Better Life: Elaborating Artificial Metalloenzymes for Eco-compatible Chemical Synthesis Procedures and Therapeutic Applications

Frédéric Avenier, Wadih Ghattas, Rémy Ricoux, and Jean-Pierre Mahy*

Institut de Chimie Moléculaire et des Matériaux d'Orsay (ICMMO), Laboratoire de Chimie Bioorganique et Bioinorganique, Université Paris-sud, Université Paris-Saclay, France

**jean-pierre.mahy@u-psud.fr*

1. Introduction

Considering current economic and ecological contexts, the questions of setting up clean and eco-efficient processes as well as saving our energy resources appear to be of fundamental importance. We need to develop reactions that would address the problem of the selective transformation of chemicals under mild conditions. This urges industries to develop "green chemistry" procedures that not only include catalytic processes to limit waste, but also to use harmless solvents, the ideal of which would be water, with low temperatures and pressures to limit energy consumption. Enzymes, and in particular metalloenzymes, are biocatalysts that already fulfill such conditions. Because their properties are complementary to those of chemical catalysts, it is conceivable to design catalysts that would combine the robustness and wide range of reactions of chemical catalysts with the ability of enzymes to work under mild conditions in aqueous medium and with high selectivity. This can be realized by associating metal complexes with proteins to afford new artificial metalloenzymes that would be able to catalyze selective reactions under eco-compatible conditions. The properties of the obtained proteins-stability, efficiency and selectivity- can be both optimized by chemical engineering of the metal ligand and biochemical engineering of the protein, using, in particular, the recently discovered directed evolution techniques. This chapter not only focuses on artificial metalloenzymes that typically catalyze abiotic reactions, including olefin metathesis, polymerization of phenylacetylene, allylic deallylations, nitrene and carbene transfer reactions and Diels–Alder reactions, but also on their production in living cells and presents their potential as new tools both for synthetic applications under eco-compatible conditions and also for various analytical and therapeutic applications.

2. Olefin Metathesis

Olefin metathesis can be defined as an olefin rearrangement process catalyzed by an organometallic catalyst, most of the time involving Mo, W or Ru metal ions. These reactions are classified into three categories: (i) cross-metathesis, (ii) ring-closing metathesis, and (iii) ring-opening metathesis polymerization. All these reactions are nowadays commonly used for organic synthesis thanks to the work of Chauvin, Schrock and Grubbs, who were awarded the Nobel Prize of Chemistry for the discovery and development of these reactions [1–3]. The mechanism suggested by Chauvin involves the formation of Schrock-type carbenes or alkylidenes, catalyzed by organometallic complexes which are now commercially available for some of them (Figure 1).

Original catalysts were largely considered being sensitive towards air and moisture, but the incorporation of chelating styrene and *N*-heterocyclic carbene ligands led to more stable compounds commonly named as Grubbs–Hoveyda-type catalysts [4] which can even be used in fully aqueous solution [5]. Such properties have propelled olefin metathesis as a promising strategy for biorthogonal applications since no comparable natural biological reaction is known to date. Interestingly, olefin

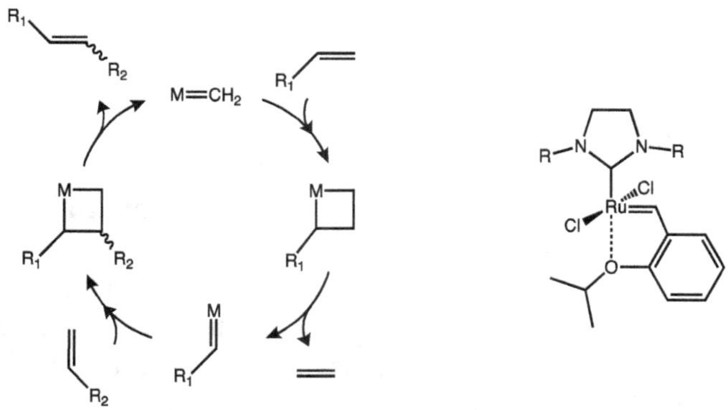

Fig. 1. (left) Catalytic mechanism for ring-closing metathesis suggested by Chauvin and (right) general structure for Grubbs–Hoveyda-type catalysts.

metathesis reactions have already been used to perform post-translational protein modifications. For example, the Davies group has shown that a protein bearing an allyl sulfide formed at a cysteine position allows to graft various olefin molecules at the surface of the protein via cross-metathesis reaction catalyzed by Hoveyda–Grubbs second generation catalysts in aqueous medium [6]. Another group managed to graft a ruthenium catalyst at the surface of a protein to catalyze ring-openingcross-metathesis metathesis polymerization at the surface of the protein in order to get protein modified with PEG chain at their surface [7]. These examples clearly illustrate the potential of olefin metathesis for specific applications based on biorthogonal chemistry in biological media. This could include implementation of olefin metathesis into natural metabolic pathways or new strategies for specific drug delivery.

The main problem for such applications is the potential deactivation of the catalyst when entering the living cell medium that is quite different from simple *in vitro* aqueous media. Living cells are indeed complex entities containing very large amounts of potential inhibitors for unprotected ruthenium catalysts. One way to protect ruthenium catalysts for *in vivo* applications is their incorporation into a protein scaffold. This not only protects the catalysts from the living cell environment but also helps their solubilization in aqueous media. A few examples of artificial metalloprotein bearing a ruthenium complex and catalyzing olefin metathesis in the aqueous medium have been published in the last 20 years.

2.1. *Artificial metalloenzymes for* in vitro *and* in vivo *olefin metathesis*

The first examples of such artificial metalloenzymes for *in vitro* use were published in 2011 by the groups of Ward and Hilvert. In one case, a Grubbs–Hoveyda-type catalyst was grafted to a cysteine-containing variant of a small heat shock protein from Methanocaldococcus jannaschii via an electrophilic bromoacetamid group. The resulting artificial metalloenzyme was able to catalyze a benchmark ring-closing metathesis reaction up to 25 turnovers in the acidic aqueous medium within 12 hours at 42°C [8]. In the other case, the same ring-closing metathesis reaction was catalyzed by a biotinylated Hoveyda–Grubbs catalyst specifically inserted within (strep)avidin proteins giving conversions values up to 95% at pH 4 [9]. Another strategy involved an Hoveyda–Grubbs catalyst equipped with *L*-phenylalanine chloromethylketone which was incorporated into α-chymotrypsin through the intrinsic inhibition mechanism of the protein. This clearly inhibited the natural enzyme activity and allowed ring-closing metathesis to operate in water with up to 20 turnovers at 37°C [10] The group of Okuda also incorporated a Hoveyda–wild-typeGrubbs catalyst via covalent binding into a protein. In this case, the ruthenium catalyst bearing a maleimide or a bromo acetyl bromide group was specifically reacted with the single accessible cysteine of an engineered variant of the β-barrel protein FhuA. The resulting metalloenzymes catalyzed ring-opening metathesis polymerization with good conversion (up to 77%, 955 TON) [11]. It was also demonstrated that the spacer length between the cysteine and the ruthenium complex could improve the activity and increase the *cis* content of the double bond in the synthesized polymer [12]. Finally, the Gebbink group synthesized a ruthenium complex functionalized with a phosphonate ester that can be used as a suicide inhibitor of serine hydroxylase enzymes such as the lipase cutinase. This covalent binding of the catalyst at the active site of the enzyme generated new artificial metalloproteins active in the ring-closing metathesis of the benchmark substrtate (*N,N*-diallyl-*p*-toluenesulfonamide) and the cross-metathesis of allylbenzene in good yields [13].

All these interesting examples of artificial metalloenzyme with good olefin metathesis activity in the aqueous medium clearly demonstrate the high potential of olefin metathesis for biorthogonal applications in living cells. However, catalyzing reactions in bacteria, eukaryote cells or plant cells is an even tougher challenge due to the presence of multiple potential inhibitors such as glutathione which has clearly been identified as a major inhibitor for precious metal catalysts in the aqueous medium [14]. With this problem in mind, Wards and coworkers have developed an interesting strategy based on the *in cellulo* production of streptavidin and its exportation to the periplasm of the bacteria thanks to its fusion with the OmpA signal peptide. Once in this compartment, the streptavidin is easily accessible to exogeneous molecules such as a synthetic biotinylated Hoveyda–Grubbs ruthenium complex to form the artificial metalloenzyme directly in the bacteria periplasm. The choice of periplasm as a catalytic compartment was not only to make accessible the protein to ruthenium complex and substrates, but also to take advantage of the fact that this compartment is less concentrated in glutathione than the cytoplasm. Once assembled in the periplasm, the artificial "metathase" can perform ring-closing metathesis. This was clearly demonstrated *in vivo* by the transformation of a non-fluorescent substrate **1** into the fluorescent umbelliferone **2** via a biorthogonal ring-closing metathesis reaction at the periplasm location (Figure 2).

The scope of the reaction was then extended to the water-soluble benchmark **3**, giving relatively poor yields in **4** when the wild-type streptavidin was produced and used in *Escherichia coli (E. coli)*. Interestingly,

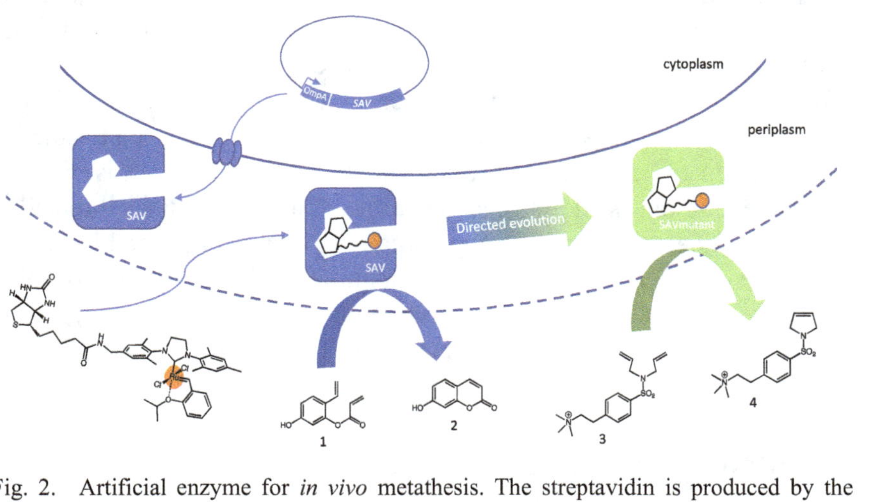

Fig. 2. Artificial enzyme for *in vivo* metathesis. The streptavidin is produced by the bacteria and exported to the periplasm where it incorporates a biotinylated ruthenium complex to form the artificial metalloenzyme [15].

the authors took advantage of this low activity in order to engineer *in cellulo* a better catalyst via successive rounds of directed evolution of the artificial metalloenzyme and managed to get a 5-fold improvement with a quintuple mutant for the cell-specific activity (Figure 2) [15].

This work clearly demonstrates the possibility to apply the streptavidin-biotin technology to the development of artificial metalloenzyme in order to catalyze olefin metathesis in living cells, a reaction that is not present among natural enzymes activities. This system was even improved within the living cell by directed evolution, opening a wide range of applications in the fields of biotechnology and medicine by setting new bio-orthogonal tools.

In terms of application, a new kind of biosensor sensitive to ethylene was recently engineered based on the incorporation of a second-generation Hoveyda–Grubbs catalyst grafted with a fluorescent 7-diethylamino-coumarin (DEAC) and a DABCYL quencher into the hydrophobic pocket of a human serum albumin protein. In such edifice, the DABCYL quencher suppresses DEAC fluorescence. However, in the presence of ethylene gas, the ruthenium complex catalyzes a cross-metathesis reaction, releasing the DABCYL quencher in solution and thus allowing the DEAC to fluoresce (Figure 3(a)). Such a system is highly original and could allow the easy detection of ethylene in different samples including living plants or fruits [16]. For example, thin slices of kiwifruit were incubated with the artificial metalloenzyme and the production of ethylene was followed by fluorescence imaging. These experiments clearly showed a significant increase of fluorescence in the outer pericarp of ripened fruits (Figure 3(b)). In this case, although the macroscopic analysis does not demonstrate the activity within living cells, it clearly shows that the artificial metalloenzyme is active within the tissues of a living organism.

Such strategy may be used for diagnostic applications as it is the case for ethylene in this work, but the versatility of albumin artificial metallo-enzymes may also allow other applications in living cells, notably thanks to the development of glycosylated albumin artificial metalloenzymes, which are efficiently protecting the ruthenium catalyst from the high concentration in glutathione present in cells [17].

3. Polymerization of Phenylacetylene

The formation of stereo-controlled C–C bonds is a synthetically attractive target because it results in the formation of sought-for compounds [18].

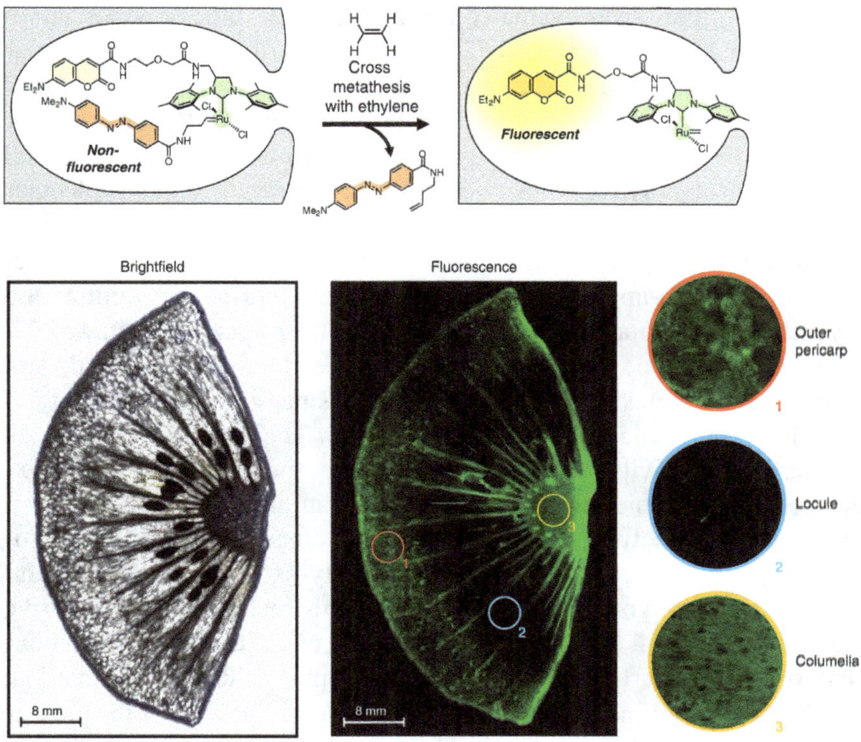

Fig. 3. General mechanism for the ethylene detection by the albumin artificial metalloenzyme (a) and fluorescence imaging of a kiwifruit slice incubated with the albumin artificial metalloenzyme [16].

Therefore, several research teams have explored the use of hybrid biocatalysts to explore the possibility of controlling the synthesis of polymers by relying on interactions provided by a protein scaffold. The hydrophobic environment of binding cavity of the protein could not only favor the polymerization reaction, but also orchestrate the position of the substrates, hence influencing the size and the polydispersity of the polymer.

3.1. *Artificial metalloenzymes for* in vitro *and* in vivo *polymerization of phenylacetylene*

In 2009, Watanabe *et al.* encapsulated a rhodium catalyst $[Rh(nbd)Cl]_2$ (nbd = norbornadiene) **5** in the interior cavity of apo-ferritin. The obtained biohybrid was evaluated for the catalysis of the polymerization of phenylacetylene (Figure 4). The stereoregularity and the molecular weight of the polymer resulting from the catalysis by the biohybrid Rh(nbd) — apo-ferritin were examined by SEC and NMR analyzes. The results showed that Rh(nbd) — apo-ferritin provided a *cis*-transoidal main chain of polyphenylacetylene with a number average molecular weight (Mn) of 13.1×10^3 (Mw/Mn = 2.6) while catalysis by **5** provided an Mn of 63.7×10^3 (Mw/Mn = 21.4) (Figure 4) [19]. The crystal structure of Rh(nbd)-apo-ferritin was solved at 1.80 Å resolution and revealed that the total number of rhodium atoms *per* apo-ferritin was 72. However, it was concluded that most of the rhodium sites could not serve as active sites for the polymerization since only a few chains of polyphenylacetylene are formed in the cavity. The extent of Rh(nbd) — apo-ferritin reactivity with phenylacetylene derivatives bearing carboxylic acid, phosphonic acid groups was also examined. No polymerization of these phenylacetylene derivatives was obtained. This lack of polymerization could be explained by the difficulty of anionic monomers to penetrate the biohybrid cavity due to the repulsion between the negative monomer loads and the anionic inner surface of the channel, which consists of three aspartic acids and three glutamic acids of the spherical apo-ferritin [19]. Finally, in 2012, the catalytic mechanism of the polymerization of phenylacetylene catalyzed by rhodium inside apo-ferritin was studied by QM/MM [20]. The study proposed a mechanism for the catalysis of polymerization by the rhodium-containing sites. It also demonstrated the central role of hydrophobic amino acid residues in promoting polymer elongation and resulted in identifying the most efficient sites. The same year, the Hayashi group used the covalent bond strategy to obtain a hybrid catalyst capable of polymerizing phenylacetylene. The authors thus linked covalently via a maleimide bond a rhodium complex inside the cavity of a variant of aponitrobindin, NB (Q96C). The catalytic activity was examined and showed that Rh-NB (Q96C) promoted the polymerization of phenylacetylene resulting in a polymer with 53% *trans* content, while the Rh catalyst without the protein matrix gave almost exclusively polyphenylacetylene with a *cis* content greater than 93% [21]. Thanks to the crystal structure of the protein and to molecular modeling K. Fukumoto *et al.* were able to re-engineer the cavity of nitrobindin resulting in a biohybrid with improved stereoselectivity as the polymerization of phenylacetylene reached a *trans* content of 82% [22].

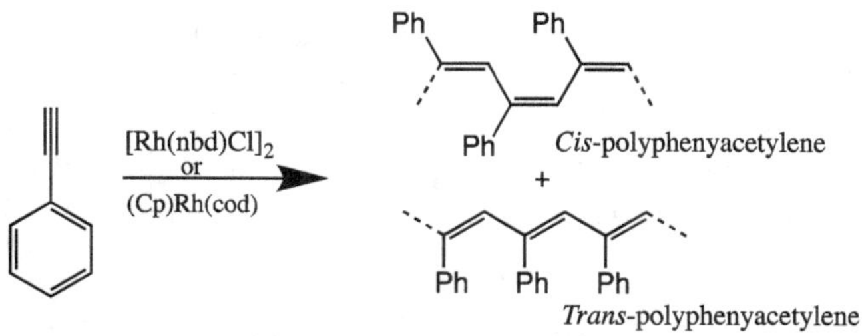

Fig. 4. Catalysis of the polymerization of phenylacetylene by rhodium complexes.

Recently, Grimm *et al.* transposed this type of reaction on whole cell catalytic systems [23]. The authors thus constructed a variant of NB fused with an autotransporter of esterase (EstA) which resulted in displaying the host protein NB on the outer membrane of *E. coli*. After the covalent anchoring of (maleimide-Cp)Rh(cod) **6** (Cp = cyclopentadiene, cod = cyclopentadiene) to NB4 nitrobindin at the surface of the bacterial cells, the catalytic performances of the generated biohybrind bugs were evaluated. This cellular system provided the polyphenylacetylene with 80% of *trans* content and with a TON per cell as high as 39×10^6.

4. Allylic Deallylase

The bioorthogonal catalysis of the uncaging of amines from the allyl carbamate-protecting group by organometallic ruthenium complexes has been shown to function under biologically relevant conditions and even inside living cells.

The catalysis of the deprotection of *N*-(allyloxycarbonyl)aminocoumarin in water/DMO (200/1) in the presence of glutathione (10 equiv.) led to the formation of fluorescent aminocoumarin and allowed the kinetic follow-up of the reaction. Several organometallic ruthenium complexes were assayed at 1% mol loading and [(Cp)(Me_2NQ)(ally)Ru]PF_6 **7** (Cp = η^5-cyclopentadieny, Me_2NQ = 4-(*N,N*-dimethylamino)-2-quinolinecarboxyl) showed the highest TON of 270 and the highest stability for at least 24 h [24]. Catalysis using complex **7** was subsequently assayed inside cells. HeLa cells were incubated with bis[*N*-(allyloxycarbonyl)]rhodamine 110 then washed with buffer (PBS) and exposed to complex **7**. Rhodamine 110 was uncaged as the fluorescence increase in the cytoplasm reached 130-fold in 10 min indicating that the complex was up-taken by the cells and that it remained active. Similarly, HeLa cells were incubated with prodrug *N*-(allyloxycarbonyl)doxorubicin, after washing, the addition of complex **7** led to cell death indicating that the uncaging of cytotoxic doxorubicin was successful (Figure 5) [24].

4.1. *Artificial Allylic deallylases for* in vitro *and* in vivo *catalysis*

Thereafter, complex **7** was covalently bound to biotin and incubated with streptavidin to form an artificial allylic deallylase. The binding to biotin resulted in a reduced activity as TON reached only 7. However, the activity was restored inside the four binding pockets of streptavidin as the catalysis using the biohybrid reached a TON of 26 *per* pocket. Two methods were used to enable the artificial enzyme to cross the cellular membrane and preform artificial enzymatic bioorthogonal catalysis *in cellulo*. In the first method, cell-penetrating benzopentasulfides (B5S) were bound to biotin and the four streptavidin binding pockets of the artificial enzyme

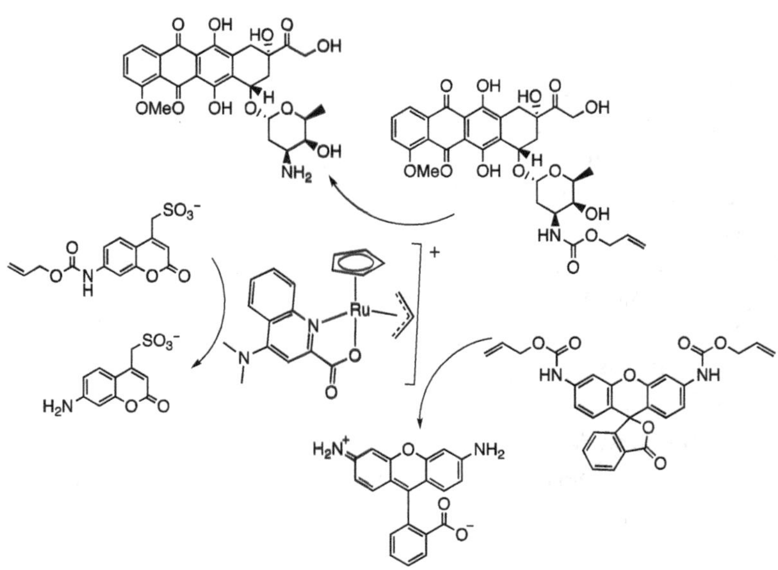

Fig. 5. Catalysis of the uncaging of coumarin, rhodamine and doxorubicin by the allylic deallylases by ruthenium complex **7**.

were shared between biotin bound complex **7** and biotin bound B5S. Such artificial enzymes could accumulate in the cytoplasm of HeLa Kyoto cells, wherein they catalyzed the uncaging of rhodamine 110. In the second method, cell-penetrating B5S were covalently bound to streptavidin leaving four binding pockets available for the binding of biotin bound complex **7**. Indeed, the artificial enzyme also accumulated in the cytoplasm and could be fully exploited as its four binding pockets were available for catalysis (Figure 6(a)) [25]. Bacterial cells were also used as a platform for biorthogonal catalysis by artificial enzymes. Directed evolution was used to further improve the activity of the artificial allylic deallylase and streptavidin was expressed exposed at the surface of *E. coli* to facilitate the selection process (Figure 6(b)). This was achieved by the expression of streptavidin fused to the *C*-terminus of a part of the outer membrane protein OmpA (residues 46–159) that was also fused to truncated *E. coli* lipoprotein Lpp (residues 1–9). The activity of the mutants i.e., uncaging of aminocoumarin, was measured in 98 well plates and the most efficient mutants were identified as double mutants S112Y– K121S and S112M–K121A yielded about 20-fold increased activity vs. the wild-type artificial enzyme after normalization with respect to expression levels. The activity of the purified mutants proved that they are indeed more active than the wild-type artificial enzyme but with only a 6-fold increased activity *in vitro*. The crystal structure of the double mutant S112M–K121A revealed the role of the mutated residues. Indeed, the M112 residue stabilized the binding of the complex by a methionine-aromatic interaction with the quinoline ligand. Additionally, both M112 and A121 residues participated in the formation of a pocket that harbored the ligand [26]. In addition to bacterial cells and human cells, algae cells were also exploited to display the artificial allylic deallylase. Here, the followed strategy consisted firstly in the directed evolution of streptavidin *in vitro* to improve the allylic deallylase activity of the artificial enzyme in the uncaging of aminocoumarin. From 34 single mutants, streptavidin S112M and streptavidin K121R were shown to form the most active artificial enzymes. The combination of these mutations in streptavidin S112M-K121R was not successful in further increasing the TON. Surprisingly when the mutation of the fourth-best single mutant i.e., streptavidin S112Y was combined with K121R, the obtained streptavidin S112Y-K121R provided the most active artificial allylic deallylase with 7-fold increased activity vs. wild-type streptavidin-based artificial enzyme. Secondly, biotine was bound to *N*-hydroxysuccinimide and incubated with *Chlamydomonas reinhardtii*

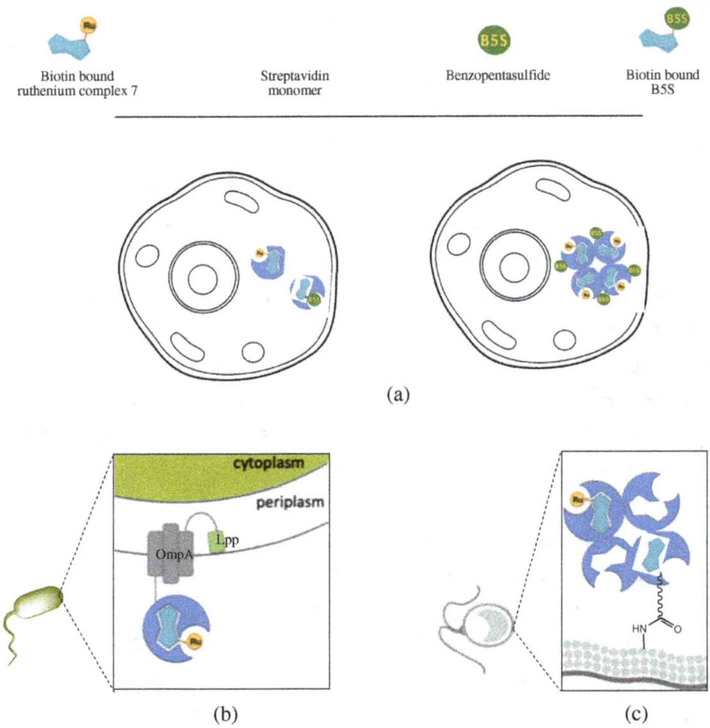

Fig. 6. (a) Hela cells containing an artificial allylic deallylase formed either by sharing the four binding pockets of streptavidin between complex 7 and cell-penetrating B5S (left) or binding the four binding pockets of B5S-modified streptavidin by complex 7 (right). (b) *E. coli* cells displaying an artificial allylic deallylase at the surface of the outer membrane. (c) Artificial allylic deallylase displayed at the surface of *C. reinhardtii*.

cells (Figure 6(c)). *N*-hydroxysuccinimide esters reacted with available amines and thiols at the cell surface and thus resulted in algae cells that displayed biotin at their cellular surface. These cells were incubated with either wild-type streptavidin or streptavidin S112Y K121R, which could then bind one of the displayed biotins in one of their four binding pockets. The remaining three binging pockets were then used to bind the ruthenium complex. The so-formed artificial allylic deallylases displayed at the surface of algae cells were used for catalysis. The displayed artificial enzyme derived from the double mutant streptavidin showed 6-fold increase of activity when compared with the one derived from the wild-type protein and which is similar to the results obtained *in vitro* [27].

5. Artificial Metalloenzymes for the *in vitro* and *in vivo* Catalysis of C–N and C–C Bond Formation

The formation of C–N and C–C bond stands among the most important processes that gives access to useful intermediates in organic synthesis such as, respectively, amines and aziridines, and cyclopropanes and carbocycles. There is thus a crucial need for developing catalysts that would perform such reactions under ecocompatible conditions, that is, under atmospheric pressure at room temperature and in non-polluting solvents, the ideal of which would be water.

Among these reactions, nitrene and carbene transfer reactions catalyzed by transition metal complexes (Cu, Fe, Mn, Rh....) have long been developed, but they take place in organic solvents (CH_2Cl_2, CH_3CN...) and often use harmful reagents such as respectively tosylimidoiodobenzene, tosylazide or chloroamines, or diazoacetate derivatives (Figure 7)

These reactions can be classified as a biological reactions, although a specific cytochrome P450 enzyme (Bez E) was recently reported by a Japanese group to be able to catalyze the intramolecular transfer of natural nitrene into a C=C bond leading to an aziridine intermediate in the biosynthesis of benzastatin (Figure 8) [28].

There have thus recently been significant efforts dedicated to the development of biocatalysts capable of catalyzing nitrene and carbene transfer reactions in water under eminently eco-compatible conditions.

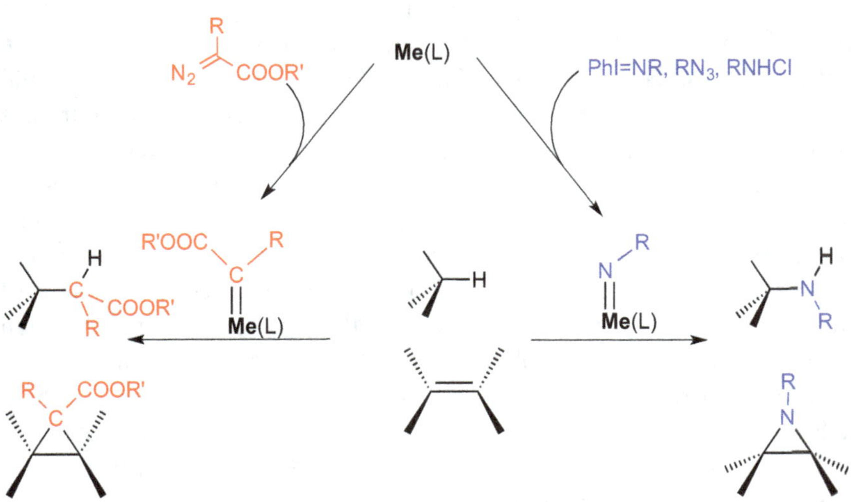

Fig. 7. Cabene and nitrene transfer reactions catalyzed by metal complexes.

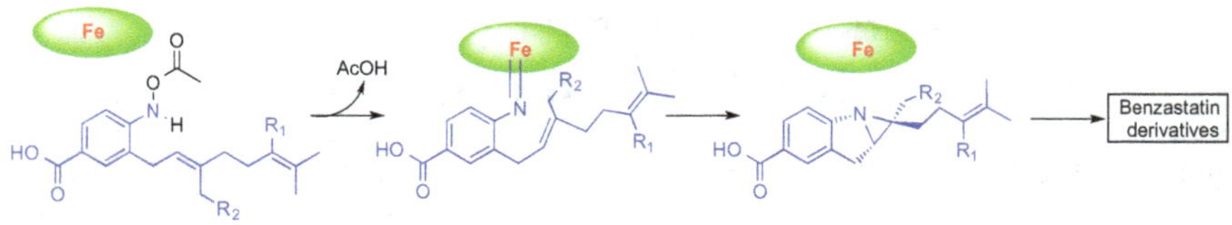

Fig. 8. Nitrene transfer reaction catalyzed "*in vivo*" by a cytochrome P450 (Bez E).

Artificial hemoproteins have first been constructed by supramolecular anchoring of synthetic metalloporphyrins into proteins, which led to promising preliminary results in the catalysis of oxene and carbene transfer reactions. However, in these biocatalysts, the protein pocket has not been specifically designed for the metalloporphyrin host, and presents a rather low affinity for it with K_ds in the micromolar range. This causes an equilibrium between bound and unbound metalloporphyrin as well as a competition with the non-specific binding at the surface of the protein that are both deleterious for the selectivity of the catalyzed reaction.

People have thus thought about using the already existing hemoproteins such as myoglobin and cytochromes P450 to redesign their active site in order to produce new artificial hemoproteins with new catalytic activities, in particular to make them able to perform abiological reactions. This has been made possible with the development of new tools in molecular biology and biochemistry, in particular with directed evolution that was the subject of the 2018 Nobel Prize attributed to Frances Arnold [29]. This has allowed imparting hemoproteins such as cytochromes P450s and myoglobin with new carbene and nitrene transfer activities, providing promising tools for the catalysis of reactions such as cyclopropanation reactions, C–H bond functionalization as well as nitrene transfer reactions, with high efficiencies as described in the following paragraphs (**Scheme 1**). In addition, in all the cases, after a few rounds of mutagenesis, mutants that were able to catalyze those reactions with high enantioselectivity could be obtained. Finally, several groups showed that these new artificial metalloenzymes could also be used, even in whole cells, for the preparative scale-production of compounds with excellent enantioselectivity, opening new ways for the industrial synthesis of compounds of pharmaceutical interest.

5.1. *Engineered hemoproteins catalyzing nitrene transfer reactions*

This reactivity was initiated with iron porphyrins by Breslow and Gellman [30,31] and Mansuy's group [32] in the early 1980s. Breslow, Dawson *et al.* [33] also showed in 1985 that aliphatic amination could be catalyzed *in vitro* by a cytochrome P450.

These enzymatic nitrene transfer studies were taken up 25 years later by several groups. First, Fasan and coworkers used cytochrome $P450_{BM3}$ and variants to catalyze intramolecular C–H amination of a series of trisubstituted sulfonyl azides **8a-c** that led to the desired benzosultam product **9a-c**[34] as well as to the cyclization of carbonazidates **11** that allowed the synthesis of oxazolidinones **12** (Figure 9) [35].

Those reactions took place under anaerobic conditions, and required the presence of NADPH as a reductant, which consequently also led to the reduction of the sulfonyl azides into sulfonamides that occurred in competition with the intramolecular amination. Whereas $P450_{BM3}$ showed a modest activity, engineered variants of $P450_{BM3}$, containing from 2 to 6 mutations, appeared to be more efficient catalysts for the intramolecular

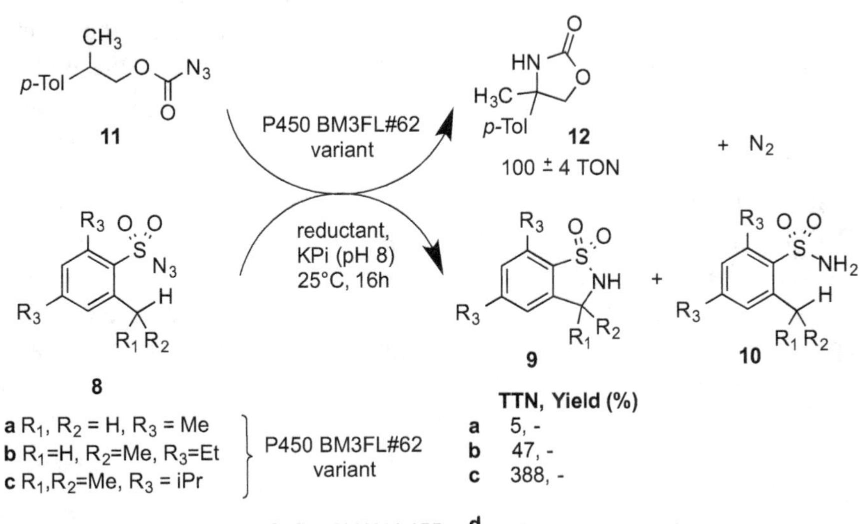

Fig. 9. Intramolecular nitrene transfer reactions catalyzed by cytochrome P450 BM3 and 119 variants selected after directed evolution.

C-H amination reactions. The best of them, the FL#62 variant, that contained five mutations with respect to WT $P450_{BM3}$, had the best C-H amination activity leading not only to up to 20-times higher TTN for the formation of benzosultams **9a-c**, but also leading to 20 turnovers in oxazolidinone **12**.

The mechanism involved the formation of an iron(IV)-nitrene intermediate that could lead either to the benzosultam or oxazolidone product after nitrene insertion into the C–H bond, or to the corresponding sulfonamide after protonation of the nitrogen atom mediated by a highly conserved threonine T268 in the active site of $P450_{BM3}$. Mutation of this threonine by alanine led to T268A mutants of all the variants that showed a clear enhancement of the C–H amination by a factor 2 to 6 with respect to the sulfonamide formation [34] The conversion of sulfonyl azides (**8d**,**e**) into sultams (**9d**,**e**) was also investigated by Hartwig and coworkers. They built up new hemoproteins by replacing the heme iron of a P450 derived from a thermophilic organism, CYP119 by iridium to obtain Ir(Me)-CYP119-WT hemoproteins that were found to be the most active and the most chemoselective ones for the intramolecular C–H amination [36]. Using protein engineering, they selected a CYP119 variant, Ir(Me)-CYP119-Max-L155G, that contained five mutations in its active site, which led to product **9e** with a 98% yield, but with a modest 63:37 enantiomeric ratio(er). The enantioselectivity of this reaction could be improved by creating a library of CYP119 variants containing mutations at a subset of eight different positions within the active site of the enzyme. The activity of the CYP119 mutants containing Ir(Me)-PPIX cofactors was evaluated directly in cell lysates, The products from C–H amination were formed in up to 98% yield and ~300 TON and, in all cases, the chemoselectivity for C–H bond amination was greater than 20:1. In one case, the enantiomeric excess even reached a 95:5 er.

The intermolecular nitrene transfer reactions were investigated by Arnold and coworkers. They were the first to show that new hemoproteins engineered from Cyt P450s, cytochromes P411, that contained a serine axial ligand to the heme iron in place of the wild-type cysteine ligand were able to catalyze, in the presence of NADPH as reductant, the intermolecular transfer of nitrene moieties into benzylic C–H bonds under anaerobic conditions (Figure 10) [37]. After directed evolution, on the protein, the best mutant obtained, $P411_{CHA,}$ was found capable of catalyzing the benzylic tosylamidation of 4-ethylanisole (**13a**) by tosyl azide

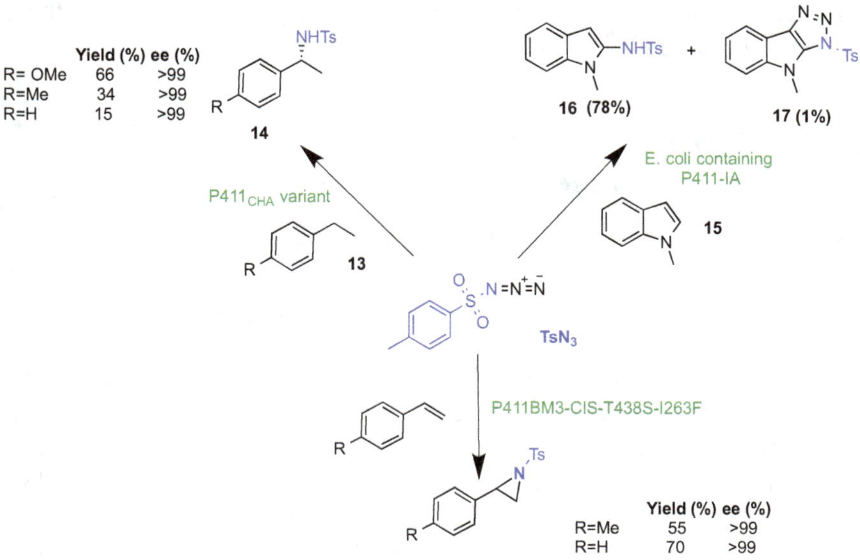

Fig. 10. Intermolecular nitrene transfer reactions catalyzed by cytochrome P411 variants selected after directed evolution.

(TsN_3) to form the benzylic *N*-tosylamide (**14a**), with up to 1,300 turnovers, a 66% yield and a very good enantioselectivity (99% ee) even on preparative scale or in whole *E. coli* cells.

Further investigations by Arnold and coworkers led them to select other cytochromes P450 variants in whole *E. coli* cells that were found able to catalyze the tosylamidation of indoles, such as 1-methylindole **15,** to form the C-2 tosylamide **16** (Figure 10) [38]. Two undesired side reactions were observed: formation of sulfonamide **17** and also the formation of triazole **17** resulting from a cycloaddition between the tosylazide and indole **15**. Directed evolution involving mutagenesis of both the heme and reductase domains allowed to obtain P411 variants that favored the tosylamidation reaction over those two unwanted reactions. The best variant obtained, P411-IA, provided the desired indole amidation products with up to 8400 turnovers and a 90% yield, with a chemoselectivity of 110:12:1 in favor of nitrene transfer over reduction or triazole formation. Finally, of all the enzymes tested, a variant of P411BM3-CIS-T438S having a single active-site substitution, I263F, was the most active to catalyze the aziridination of a series of styrene derivatives, being more productive with the less electron-rich 4-methylstyrene and styrene substrates with up to 600 TON, a 70% yield and a 99% ee (Figure 10) [39].

5.2. *Artificial metalloenzymes and engineered hemoproteins catalyzing carbene transfer reactions*

Two artificial metalloenzymes were shown to be able to catalyze carbene transfer reactions. The first one was an artificial hemoprotein that was prepared by Roelfes and coworkers by incorporation of heme into a homodimeric protein with a wide hydrophobic cavity, Lactoccocal multidrug resistance Regulator (LmrR) [40–42]. Using different LmrR mutants led to the cyclopropanation of styrene derivatives by ethyldiazoacetate **18** (EDA) (Figure 11), the benchmark reaction for cyclopropanation catalysis, with a good activity and a moderate enantioselectivity (Table 1) [43].

The second one, which was reported by Ward and coworkers, was obtained by incorporation of a biotinylated dirhodium complex that was

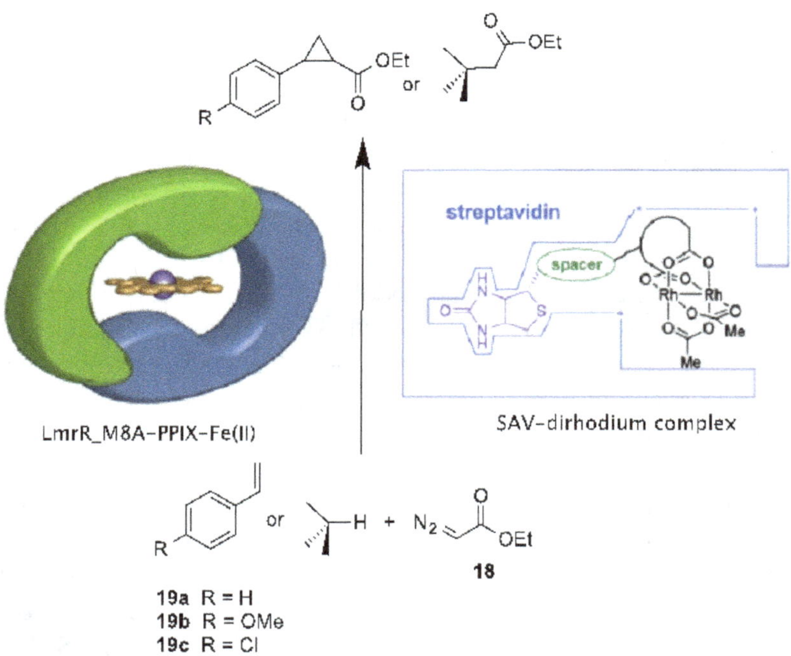

Fig. 11. Carbene transfer reactions catalyzed by an artificial hemoprotein or by a biotinylated dirhodium complex embedded within engineered streptavidin variants.

Table 1. Results obtained for the cyclopropanation of styrene 1 and derivatives by EDA catalyzed by artificial hemoproteins.

Group	Protein	Mutant	Metal complex	Subs.	Yield	TON	ee (%)
Roelfes	LmrR	LmrR_ M8A	heme	19a	39	391	38
				19b	36	359	44
				19c	35	351	25
Ward	Sav	Sav WT	Rh_2complex	19a		54	−66 *trans*
Brustad	$P450_{BM3}$	T268A	heme	19a	68	339	−97 *trans*
		WIVS-FM* T268A C400G	Ir(Me)DPIX	19a	48	240	0
		T268A	heme	19a	57	284	−97 *trans*
		WIVS-FM* T268A	FeDPIX	19a	44	221	−46 *trans*
Fasan	myoglobin	H64V, V68A	heme	19a	99	>500	99.9
		H64V, V68A		19c	4	180	99.8
		H64V, V68A + cells		19c	80	365	99.8
Arnold	$P450_{BM3}$	T268A	heme	19a	65	323	−96 trans

embedded within engineered streptavidin variants, following the so-called "Trojan Horse" strategy. Using ethyldiazoacetate **18** (EDA) as a transfer agent, the resulting biohybrids were found to be able to catalyze the carbene insertion into the double of styrene leading to the corresponding cyclopropane with up to 80 TON and a 1.5/1 *trans*/*cis* ratio. The insertion of the carbene moiety of trifluoro-ethylphenyldiazoacetate into allylic C–H bonds of cyclohexadiene was also catalyzed with up to 60 TON but no enantioselectivity could be observed. Chemical- and genetic optimization allowed to modulate the catalytic activity of the artificial metalloenzymes which could even be expressed in the periplasm of *E. coli* cells. The best *in vivo* artificial enzyme was then obtained by assembling a rhodium complex with the streptavidin K121C mutant expressed in the periplasm of *E. coli*. It was shown to be active for the cyclopropanation of styrene with up to 20 turnovers [44].

The directed evolution of $P450_{BM3}$ has been employed by several groups, among which is that of Frances Arnold who was the first to be able to enhance the activity and the selectivity of cytochrome $P450_{BM3}$ for the catalysis of cyclopropanation reactions. The best mutant obtained, $P450_{BM3}$-T268A, catalyzed the cyclopropanation of styrene **19a** by EDA **18** (Figure 11) with 65% yield and 96% ee (Table 1) [45].

Later, artificial hemoproteins were produced by Brustad and coworkers who used orthogonal expression techniques to introduce mutations in the heme pocket to allow the direct "*in cellulo*" incorporation into the apoprotein of metal complexes of Deuteroporphyrin IX as cofactors instead of the heme. Incorporation of Fe(Me)-Deuteroporphyrin IX and Ir(Me)-Deuteroporphyrin IX in the WIVS-FM*T268A variant, derived cyt. $P450_{BM3,}$ led to artificial hemoproteins that catalyzed the cyclopropanation of styrene **19a** by EDA **18** with good efficiencies and selectivities (Table 1) [46, 47].

Directed evolution of myoglobin (Mb) was also used by Fasan and coworkers to produce artificial hemoproteins that were found to be able to catalyze cyclopropanation reactions. The H64V-V68A double mutant catalyzed the benchmark reaction with excellent yield (99%) and enantioselectivity (ee = 99,9%) [48, 49] (Table 1). It is noteworthy that this mutant was also found to be able to catalyze the C–H functionalization of indoles by **18**, with an excellent conversion of 85% and a TON of 106 leading to a single product [50]. It is noteworthy that this reaction could even be performed in whole cells, with a conversion of 99% and a TON of 82.

Very recently, Hayashi and coworkers found out that myoglobin reconstituted (rMb) with iron(II)-porphycene (FePc) was able to catalyze the cyclopropanation of styrene **19a** by EDA **18**, and was 26-fold more efficient than native myoglobin (nMb) [51, 52]. UV-visible studies allowed to show the involvement of an iron(IV)-metallocarbene as the active species in this cyclopropanation reaction.

Substituting the native Fe ion not only by Co, Cu or Mn, but also by noble metals including Ru, Rh, Pd, Ag and Ir, into the metalloporphyrin IX (M-PIX) cofactor allowed Hartwig and coworkers to generate new hemoproteins that catalyzed the intramolecular carbene insertion of a diazoester into a C–H bond to form a dihydrobenzofuran product as well as the enantio- and diastereoselective cyclopropanation of unactivated olefins. Among the eight studied engineered myoglobins, Ir(Me)-PIX-Mb appeared to be the best catalyst for these reactions [53]. Hartwig and coworkers then turned again to their mutants of CYP119, in which they substituted the heme iron by an iridium methyl unit and found that the Ir(Me)-CYP119-C317G mutant was able to catalyze the intramolecular carbene insertion in C-H bonds of 2-alkyl-benzenesulfonylazides [54, 55] leading to a 14% enantiomeric excess and a TOF of 0.13 min^{-1}. Further directed evolution, focusing on amino acids close to the active site, allowed to select, after four rounds of evolution, four mutants, CYP119-Max: C317G, T213G, L69V, V254L, that were able to catalyze the reaction with 94% ee and a TOF of 43 min^{-1}.

Finally, Arnold and coworkers demonstrated that one of their engineered cytochrome P450s, the P411-PFA variant was able to catalyze the insertion of fluoroalkyl carbene intermediates into α-amino $C(sp^3)$–H bonds, performing this reaction on a wide range of substrates with enantiomeric excesses up to 99% and up to 4070 TTN [56]. The reaction could even be performed on a preparative scale with a yield of 64% (116 mg) and 98% ee for the reaction of *N*-phenylpyrrolidine with 2,2,2-trifluoro-1-diazoethane. This strategy thus provided a very powerful method for the synthesis of chiral organofluorine molecules, which is otherwise not possible with small-molecule catalysts.

5.3. *Artificial enzymes catalyzing the Diels–Alder reaction*

The Diels–Alder cycloaddition is a cornerstone in organic synthesis [57], but it very often takes place in organic solvents and requires the use of polluting catalysts. It can be classified as a [4+2] cycloaddition that starts from 1,3-diene and alkene (dienophile) and yields a substituted cyclohexene system forming two carbon–carbon bonds and up to four new stereogenic centers in one step (Figure 12). In principle, the Diels–Alder reaction proceeds in a concerted manner through a cyclic transition state (Figure 12), thus the stereochemistry of substrate alkenes is completely retained and the reaction produces a limited number of diastereomers (Four at the most) in an excellent yield.

Natural enzymes that catalyze these reactions are rare, even if a few of them have recently been reported in the literature [58–62]. In those enzymes, the catalysis is mainly due to a template effect, in which molecular interactions between the active site amino acid side chains and the substrates substituents help the relative positioning of the diene with respect to the dienophile to lead to the corresponding stabilized conformation of the transition state (Figure 12(a)).

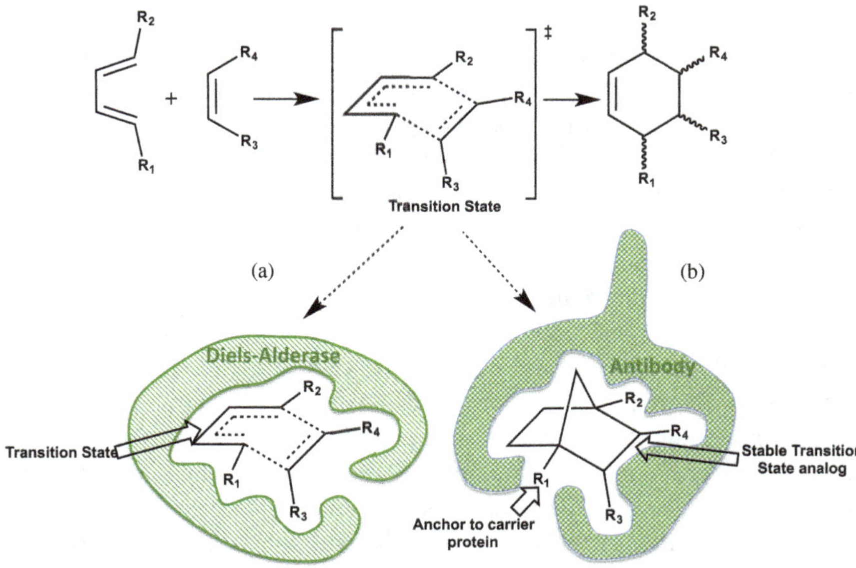

Fig. 12. Mechanism of the Diels–Alder reaction and, (a) stabilization of the transition state by natural Diels–Alderases, (b) generation of antibodies, raised against a stable transition state analog, that possess a Diels–Alderase activity.

The two reasons mentioned above have very often incited scientists to prepare artificial biocatalysts that could function under ecofriendly conditions. Inspired by the suggested template effect described above, several groups produced antibodies that were raised against a stable transition state analog (Figure 12(b)), so that these antibodies could also bind and stabilize the transition state and thus catalyze the Diels–Alder reactions. Using this strategy, catalytic antibodies that catalyzed Diels–Alder cycloadditions with rate enhancements k_{cat}/k_{uncat} up to 10^3 [63–65] and even, in one case, a catalytic antibody was found to catalyze the disfavored *exo* Diels–Alder transformation yielding a single regioisomer in high enantiomeric excess [66].

More recently, Siegel and coworkers described the *de novo* computational design and experimental characterization of enzymes catalyzing a bimolecular Diels–Alder reaction with high stereoselectivity and substrate specificity [67]. They started with a computational model of the transition state, which sets the geometrical arrangement of the two substrates in the enzyme active site, and placed hydrogen-donating and accepting amino acid side chains near the dienophile and diene, respectively, to lower the energy barrier to reaction. Quantum-mechanical simulations led them to generate an ensemble of ~10^{19} so-called theozymes, which varied the two assisting amino acid side chains and their orientation relative to the model of the transition state. Using an adequate algorithm, they compared their theozyme conformers with a library of 207 known protein scaffolds to identify approximately 10^6 theozymes that fit into one or more of the scaffolds. They further selected 84 candidates with apparent optimized active site geometry that they synthesized by protein expression. Two of the produced proteins showed k_{cat}/k_{uncat} rate enhancements that were comparable with those already observed for catalytic antibodies, and also excellent stereoselectivity and for multiple reaction cycles.

5.4. *Artificial metalloenzymes enzymes catalyzing the Diels–Alder reaction*

Though it was suspected for some time that Mg(II)-macrophomate synthase could be a metallo-Diels–Alderase, it has been demonstrated later that in fact it catalyzed a Michael addition followed by an aldol addition [68–70]. There is thus no known natural metalloenzyme that catalyzes the DA reaction to date.

As a consequence, many teams in the world have been tackling the elaboration of new artificial metalloenzymes that would catalyze the Diels–Alder reaction under ecofriendly conditions. It has been shown that Cu^{II} was the most efficient water-compatible transition metal for the lewis acid catalysis of this cycloaddition [71–73] and therefore most artificial metallo-Diels–Alderases have been prepared by incorporating Cu^{II} complexes into biomacromolecules covalently or non-covalently, thereby generating a single artificial metalloenzyme which can then be optimized by molecular biological methods (Table 2).

The first simple strategy that was used was the supramolecular insertion of metal cofactors into proteins using either the "host–guest strategy" or the "Trojan-horse strategy". Reetz and coworkers first inserted Cu^{II}-phtalocyanine into a variety of serum albumins including the bovine (BSA) and human ones [74, 75], whereas Roelfes *et al*. incorporated into DNA Cu^{II} complexes of aromatic nitrogen bi- and ter-pyridine ligands that intercalated between base pairs [76]. In an original approach, Palomo *et al.* generated a heterogeneous artificial Diels–Alderase by assembling Cu^{II}-phenanthroline-lipase at the surface of sepabeads [77]. Finally, following the "Trojan horse" strategy, a Cu^{II}-1,10-phenanthroline coupled to a testosterone anchor, was inserted into the neo-carzinostatin variant NCS-3.24, thanks to its affinity for the testosterone moiety [78].

The covalent anchoring strategy was the most frequently employed and involved most of the time the reaction of a cysteine residue of the protein with a reactive maleimide or bromoacetamide function carried by the ligand. (η^6-arene)-Ru^{II} complexes were then inserted into papain by Salmain *et al.* [79], whereas Di Méo *et al.* anchored Cu^{II}-phenanthroline and terpyridine complexes into F119C and Y26C mutants of dimeric (A3) [80] and single-chain (A3_A3') [81] synthetic alpha-repeat proteins. Cu^{II}-pyrenyl and -terpyridine complexes were anchored, respectively, into Nitrobindin [82] and ferric hydroxamate uptake protein component A (Fhu A) [82] by Hayashi's group. Deuss *et al.* also introduced Cu^{II}-phenanthroline and -dipicolylamine complexes in two unique cysteine-containing sterol carrier protein type 2 like domain (SCP-2L) mutants to perform Diels–Alder reactions between azachalcone and cyclopentadiene [83]. Finally, to perform the same reaction, the Cu^{II}-1,10-phenanthroline complex was introduced into the mutant M89C of the lactococcal multidrug resistance regulator (LmrR) by Roelfes and coworkers [84].

All of the prepared artificial metalloenzymes catalyzed the Diels–Alder cycloaddition involving the benchmark substrates 2-azachalcon (**1a**) and cyclopentadiene (**2**) which provides up to four product isomers (**3**) (Figure 13). The mechanism of the reaction has been described to proceed by the bidentate coordination of dienophile **1a** on Cu^{II} via the nitrogen and the oxygen of its amino and carbonyl groups, respectively.

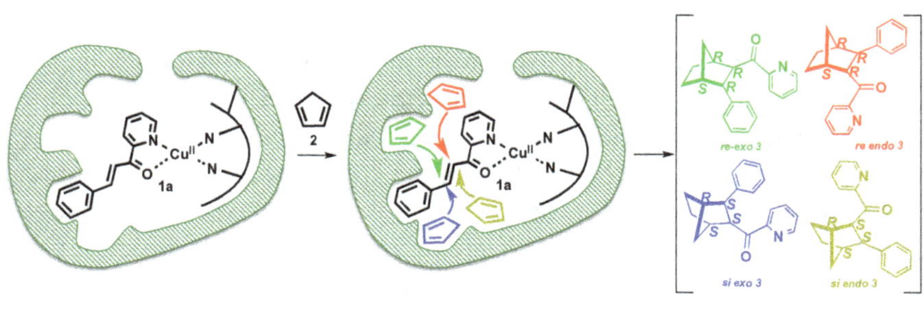

Fig. 13. Diels–Alder reaction catalyzed by artificial metalloenzymes: bidentate coordination of dienophile 1a to copper(II), approach of cyclopentadiene 2 controlled by the active site amino acids and the four stereosimers formed.

The reactivity of **1a** is thus increased thanks to the Lewis acidity of Cu^{II} that makes it more electron-deficient and more prone to react with diene **2**. Interactions of the active site amino acids with the cyclopentadiene allow the control of its approach relatively to **1a**, which determines the relative ratio of the four isomers obtained (Figure 13).

The main results obtained are summarized in Table 2. Yields ranging between 11% and 98% could be obtained with the various biohybrids, whereas the *endo* isomer was always the major isomers obtained with *endo/exo* ratios ranging from 66/34 to 96/4. The obtained enantiomeric excesses also greatly varied as a function of the biocatalyst with values between 0% and 100%. Overall, the most efficient of these biocatalysts were the heterogeneous Cu^{II}-Phen-SB-Lys-GTL*/196 catalyst [77] and the one prepared by the covalent anchoring of a 1,10-Cu^{II}-phenanthroline complex into the mutant M89C of LmrR [84] that both provided 3a in respectively 98% and 93% yield and 97% ee with an *endo/exo* ratio of 95:5.

Two other original strategies have recently been used to generate very efficient and selective Diels–Alderases. The first one, developed by Reetz team, relies on the concept of directed evolution of hybrid catalysts that was proposed some time ago. In the quest to construct an appropriate experimental platform for asymmetric Diels–Alder reactions amenable to this Darwinian approach to catalysis, they developed a strategy based on the design of a Cu(II)-specific binding site in a thermostable protein host (tHisF). The introduction of a His-His-Asp coordinating triade for the Cu^{II} ion into tHisF led to interesting results in the catalysis of Diels–Alder reaction with a 73% yield, a 93/7 *endo/exo* ratio and a 46% ee [75, 85] This sets the stage for genetic fine-tuning using the methods of directed evolution.

The second original strategy relies on the substitution of the native metal ion of metalloenzyme by another metal ion to induce a new — possibly abiological — catalytic activity. This was recently applied by Ghattas *et al.* to a monocupine enzyme 1-aminocyclopropane carboxylic acid oxidase, in which the Fe^{II} ion was coordinated by a His-His-Asp triade. Substitution of the Fe^{II} by a Cu^{II} ion afforded the most efficient artificial Diels–Alderase ever reported, that provided the (*1S,2R,3R,4R*) product isomer (Figure 13) with a quantitative yield and >99% ee [86]. This unprecedented performance was rationalized by molecular modeling as only one docking pose of 2-azachalcone was possible in the active site of the enzyme and this was the one that leads to the (*1S,2R,3R,4R*) product isomer.

Table 2. Results obtained for the cyclopropanation of styrene 1 and derivatives by EDA catalyzed by artificial hemoproteins.

Protein[a]	Cu(II) ligand[b]	Yield (%)	Endo/Exo	ee (%)	Reference
Supramolecular Anchoring					
SB-Lys-GTL*/196	Phen	98	95/5	97	[77]
BSA,	Phtalocyanin	78	96/4	85–98	[74,75]
HSA		89	91/9		
DNA	Dmbpy	>80	>95/5	48–100	[76]
Supramolecular anchoring: Trojan Horse strategy					
NCS-3.24	Phen-testosterone	84	84/16	0	[78]
Covalent anchoring					
Papain	(η^6-arene)[c]	90	nd	0	[79]
NB	Pyrenyl	22	90/10	nd	[82]
Fhu A	Terpy	15	66/34	nd	[82]
V83C-SCP-2L	Phen	19.6	88/12	25	[83]
	Dipicolylamine	86.8	94/6	4	
F119C- Y26C-A3,	Phen.	11	86/14	62	[80]
F119C-Y26C A3-A3'	Phen	15	93/7	52	[81]
	Terpy	38	92/8	5	
M89C-LmrR	Phen	93	95/5	97	[84]
Protein engineering: introduction of a coordination site for Cu(II)					
THisF	His,His,Asp	73	93/7	46	[75, 85]
Metal substitution: Fe(II) by Cu(II)					
ACC Oxidase	His,His,Asp	100	99/1	95	[86]

Notes: [a]LmrR, *Lactococcal* multidrug resistance regulator; SB-Lys-GTL*/196, Sepabeads Lys196 mutant of *Geobacillus thermocatenulatus* lipase; HSA, human serum albumin; A3, αRep A3 protein; SCP-2L, sterol carrier protein type 2-like domain; NCS, neocarzinostatin; NB, nitrobindin; FhuA, ferric hydroxamate uptake protein component A, [b]Phen: phenanthroline, Terpy: terpyridine, Dmbpy: 4,4′-dimethyl-2,2′-bipyridine, [c]metal cation: Ru(II)

Finally, Ghattas *et al.* prepared and characterized artificial metalloenzymes based on the A_{2A} adenosine receptor embedded in the cytoplasmic membranes of living human cells. For this, they used the "Trojan Horse" strategy to assemble the metalloenzyme by inserting in the wild-type receptor conjugates of strong antagonists covalently bound to copper(II) catalysts (Figure 14).

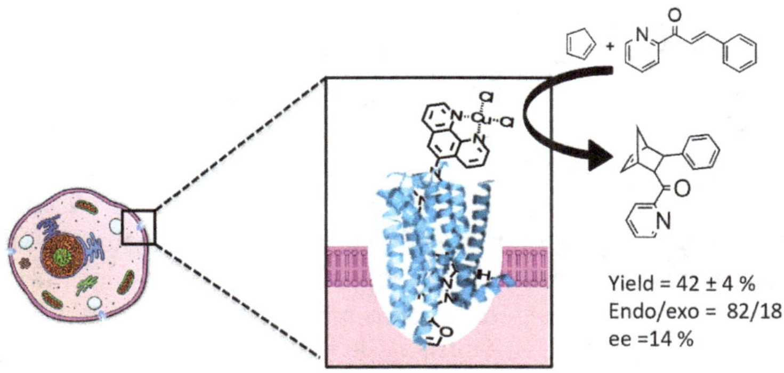

Fig. 14. Insertion of a Cu^{II}-phenanthroline-A_2A agonist conjugate in the A_2A adenosine receptor, using the "Trojan Horse" strategy Diels–Alder reaction catalyzed by an artificial metalloenzyme assembled at the surface of a leaving HEK cell.

The resulting cells enantioselectively catalyzed the abiotic Diels–Alder cycloaddition reaction of cyclopentadiene and azachalcone with a 42% yield, an 82/18 *endo*/ratio and a 14% yield [87].

The prospects of this strategy lie in the organ-confined *in vivo* preparation of receptor-based artificial metalloenzymes for the catalysis of reactions exogenous to the human metabolism. These could be used for the targeted synthesis of either drugs or deficient metabolites and for the activation of prodrugs, leading to therapeutic tools with unforeseen applications.

6. Conclusion

As shown in this chapter, in the last 10 years, there has been a burst in the production of artificial metalloenzymes that catalyze under eco-compatible conditions abiotic reactions, including olefin metathesis, polymerization of phenylacetylene, allylic deallylations, nitrene and carbene transfer reactions and Diels–Alder reactions. In the last few years, increasing efforts have been devoted to the production of such artificial metalloenzymes in living cells with the objective of producing new tools that would present important applications in various socio-economic domains.

Most of these systems will first find applications in synthetic chemistry for the production of valuable chemical intermediates. Several groups thus showed that new artificial metalloenzymes that are able to catalyze C–N and C–C bond formation constitute tools of choice in organic synthesis, even in whole cells, for the preparative scale-production of compounds with an excellent enantioselectivity, opening new ways for the industrial synthesis of compounds of pharmaceutical interest.

In this context, using directed evolution techniques, Arnold and coworkers selected cytochromes P450 variants that were found capable of catalyzing in whole *E. coli* cells the tosylamidation of indoles [38]. They also selected other engineered cytochrome P450s, the P411-PFA variants, that were able to catalyze very efficiently the enantioselective insertion of fluoroalkyl carbene intermediates into α-amino C(sp^3)–H bonds [56]. This reaction could even be performed on a preparative scale, which thus provided a very powerful method for the synthesis of chiral organofluorine molecules, which is otherwise not possible with small-molecule catalysts.

In the field of polymer chemistry, an artificial metallopolymerase, prepared by covalent anchoring of a Rhodium complex to a Q96C nitrobindin mutant, could be expressed as a fusion protein with an autotranspoter of esterase on the outer membrane of the bacterial *E. coli* cells. It promoted the stereoselective polymerization of phenylacetylene, leading to the formation of precious compounds having useful properties such as electrical conductivity, light emission and liquid crystallinity [23].

The streptavidin-biotin technology has proven to be a tool of choice for the expression or assembling in the periplasm of *E. coli* cells and HeLa cells of artificial enzymes that could catalyze various kinds of reactions and whose catalytic activity could be both chemically and genetically optimized.

An *in vivo* efficient artificial enzyme for the cyclopropanation of styrene was then obtained by assembling a rhodium-biotin conjugate with the streptavidin K121C mutant expressed in the periplasm of *E. coli* [44]. Using a similar strategy, an artificial metalloenzyme that catalyzed olefin metathesis was produced in living *E. coli* cells, by assembling in their periplasm synthetic biotinylated Hoveyda–Grubbs ruthenium complexes with streptavidin and mutants [15]. This opened a wide range of applications in the fields of biotechnology and medicine by setting new bioorthogonal tools. It also led to the conception of a new kind of bio-sensor sensitive to ethylene that could be engineered based on the incorporation of a second-generation Hoveyda–Grubbs catalyst grafted with a fluorescent 7-diethylaminocoumarin and a DABCYL quencher into the hydrophobic pocket of a human serum albumin. This biosensor was active in living fruit tissues for the detection of ethylene [16].

This technique was also used to prepare artificial metalloenzymes that were found able to catalyze Diels–Alder reactions at the surface of leaving human cells. The metalloenzyme was assembled by inserting in the wild-notable type A_{2A} adenosine receptor embedded in the cytoplasmic membrane of these cells conjugates of strong antagonists covalently bound to copper(II) catalysts [87]. This opens a new way for the *in vivo* targeted synthesis of either drugs or deficient metabolites and for the activation of prodrugs, leading to therapeutic tools with unforeseen applications.

The bioorthogonal catalysis of the uncaging of amines from the allyl carbamate protecting group by organometallic ruthenium complexes was also shown to function under biologically relevant conditions and even inside living cells, giving access to new tools for future applications in therapy and imaging. Ru complexes were shown to be able to perform the uncaging of the drug doxorubicin from the prodrug *N*-(allyloxycarbonyl) doxorubicin directly into the leaving HeLa cells [24]. The same complex was covalently bound to biotin and incubated with streptavidin to form an artificial allylic deallylase that could be assembled in the periplasm of *E. coli* and HeLa cells in order to perform artificial enzymatic bioorthogonal catalysis *in cellulo* [25–27]. Covalent attachment of the biotinylated ruthenium complex at the surface of algae cells followed by addition of streptavidin allowed to form artificial allylic deallylases that could be used for catalysis.

Overall, the production of new artificial metalloenzyme that catalyze *in vivo* abiological reactions, also called biorthogonal reactions, offers new promising tools that will be of prime importance for future applications in several socio-economical areas of interest: green chemistry, through bioconversion processes for synthesis of high added value molecules; technology by the production of polymers of interest for electrical conductivity and light emission; environment by the elaboration of gas biosensors and finally health, by setting new therapeutic and imaging tools thanks to the *in vivo* catalysis of drug synthesis or the activation of pro-drugs or probes.

No doubt that in the current context of sustainable growth, and with regard to the numerous potential applications it offers, exponentially increasing efforts will be devoted to the new field of research that constitutes the *in vivo* production of artificial metalloenzymes.

References

1. Chauvin, Y. (2006) Olefin Metathesis: The Early Days (Nobel Lecture). *Angew. Chem. Int. Ed.* 45, pp. 3740–3747.
2. Schrock, R. R. (2006) Multiple Metal–Carbon Bonds for Catalytic Metathesis Reactions (Nobel Lecture). *Angew. Chem. Int. Ed.* 45, pp. 3748–3759.
3. Grubbs, R. H. (2006) Olefin-Metathesis Catalysts for the Preparation of Molecules and Materials (Nobel Lecture). *Angew. Chem. Int. Ed.* 45, pp. 3760–3765.
4. Garber, S. B., Kingsbury, J. S., Gray, B. L. and Hoveyda, A. H. (2000) Efficient and Recyclable Monomeric and Dendritic Ru-based Metathesis Catalysts. *J. Am. Chem. Soc.* 122, pp. 8168–8179.
5. Burtscher, D. and Grela, K. (2009) Aqueous Olefin Metathesis. *Angew. Chem. Int. Ed.* 48, pp. 442–454.
6. Lin, Y. A., Chalker, J. M., Floyd, N., Bernardes, G. J. L. and Davis, B. G. (2008) Allyl Sulfides Are Privileged Substrates in Aqueous Cross-Metathesis: Application to Site-Selective Protein Modification. *J. Am. Chem. Soc.* 130, pp. 9642–9643.
7. Isarov, S. A. and Pokorski, J. K. (2015) Protein ROMP: Aqueous Graft-from Ring-Opening Metathesis Polymerization. *ACS Macro Lett.* 4, pp. 969–973.
8. Mayer, C., Gillingham, D. G., Ward, T. R. and Hilvert, D. (2011) An Artificial Metalloenzyme for Olefin Metathesis. *Chem. Commun.* 47, pp. 12068–12070.
9. Lo, C., Ringenberg, M. R., Gnandt, D., Wilson, Y. and Ward, T. R. (2011) Artificial Metalloenzymes for Olefin Metathesis Based on the Biotin-(strept)avidin Technology. *Chem. Commun.* 47, pp. 12065–12067.
10. Matsuo, T., Imai, C., Yoshida, T., Saito, T., Hayashi, T. and Hirota, S. (2012) Creation of an Artificial Metalloprotein with a Hoveyda–Grubbs Catalyst Moiety Through the Intrinsic Inhibition Mechanism of α-Chymotrypsin. *Chem. Commun.* 48, pp. 1662–1664.
11. Philippart, F., Arlt, M., Gotzen, S., Tenne, S.-J., Bocola, M., Chen, H.-H., Zhu, L., Schwaneberg, U. and Okuda, J. (2013) A Hybrid Ring-Opening Metathesis Polymerization Catalyst Based on an Engineered Variant of the β-Barrel Protein FhuA. *Chem. Eur. J.* 19, pp. 13865–13871.
12. Sauer, D. F., Bocola, M., Broglia, C., Arlt, M., Zhu, L.-L., Brocker, M., Schwaneberg, U. and Okuda, J. (2015) Hybrid Ruthenium ROMP Catalysts Based on an Engineered Variant of β-Barrel Protein FhuA ΔCVF^{tev}: Effect of Spacer Length. *Chem. Asian J.* 10, pp. 177–182.
13. Basauri-Molina, M., Verhoeven, D. G. A., van Schaik, A. J., Kleijn, H. and Klein Gebbink, R. J. M. (2015) Ring-Closing and Cross-Metathesis with Artificial Metalloenzymes Created by Covalent Active Site-Directed Hybridization of a Lipase. *Chem. Eur. J.* 21, pp. 15676–15685.

14. Wilson, Y. M., Dürrenberger, M., Nogueira, E. S. and Ward, T. R. (2014) Neutralizing the Detrimental Effect of Glutathione on Precious Metal Catalysts. *J. Am. Chem. Soc.* 136, pp. 8928–8932.
15. Jeschek, M., Reuter, R., Heinisch, T., Trindler, C., Klehr, J., Panke, S. and Ward, T. R. (2016) Directed Evolution of Artificial Metalloenzymes for *in vivo* Metathesis. *Nature* 537, pp. 661–665.
16. Vong, K., Eda, S., Kadota, Y., Nasibullin, I., Wakatake, T., Yokoshima, S., Shirasu, K., and Tanaka, K. (2019) An Artificial Metalloenzyme Biosensor can Detect Ethylene Gas in Fruits and Arabidopsis Leaves. *Nat Commun.* 10, pp. 5746.
17. Eda, S., Nasibullin, I., Vong, K., Kudo, N., Yoshida, M., Kurbangalieva, A., and Tanaka, K. (2019) Biocompatibility and Therapeutic Potential of Glycosylated Albumin Artificial Metalloenzymes. *Nat Catal.* 2, pp. 780–792.
18. Liu, J., Lam, J. W. Y. and Tang, B. Z. (2009) Acetylenic Polymers: Syntheses, Structures, and Functions. *Chem. Rev.* 109, pp. 5799–5867.
19. Abe, S., Hirata, K., Ueno, T., Morino, K., Shimizu, N., Yamamoto, M., Takata, M., Yashima, E. and Watanabe, Y. (2009) Polymerization of Phenylacetylene by Rhodium Complexes within a Discrete Space of apo-Ferritin. *J. Am. Chem. Soc.* 131, pp. 6958–6960.
20. Ke, Z., Abe, S., Ueno, T. and Morokuma, K. (2012) Catalytic Mechanism in Artificial Metalloenzyme: QM/MM Study of Phenylacetylene Polymerization by Rhodium Complex Encapsulated in *apo*-Ferritin. *J. Am. Chem. Soc*, 134, pp. 15418–15429.
21. Onoda, A., Fukumoto, K., Arlt, M., Bocola, M., Schwaneberg, U. and Hayashi, T. (2012) A Rhodium Complex-Linked β-Barrel Protein as a Hybrid Biocatalyst for Phenylacetylene Polymerization. *Chem. Commun.* 48, pp. 9756–9758.
22. Fukumoto, K., Onoda, A., Mizohata, E., Bocola, M., Inoue, T., Schwaneberg, U. and Hayashi, T. (2014) Rhodium-Complex-Linked Hybrid Biocatalyst: Stereo-Controlled Phenylacetylene Polymerization within an Engineered Protein Cavity. *ChemCatChem.* 6, pp. 1229–1235.
23. Grimm, A. R., Sauer, D. F., Polen, T., Zhu, L., Hayashi, T., Okuda, J. and Schwaneberg, U. (2018) A Whole Cell *E. coli* Display Platform for Artificial Metalloenzymes: Poly(phenylacetylene) Production with a Rhodium–Nitrobindin Metalloprotein. *ACS Catal.* 8, pp. 2611–2614.
24. Völker, T., Dempwolff, F., Graumann, P. L. and Meggers, E. (2014) Progress towards Bio-orthogonal Catalysis with Organometallic Compounds. *Angew. Chem. Int. Ed.* 53, pp. 10536–10540.
25. Cheng, Y., Zong, L., López-Andarias, J., Bartolami, E., Okamoto, Y., Ward, T. R., Sakai, N. and Matile, S. (2019) Cell-Penetrating Dynamic-Covalent Benzopolysulfane Networks. *Angew. Chem. Int. Ed.* 58, pp. 9522–9526.

26. Heinisch, T., Schwizer, F., Garabedian, B., Csibra, E., Jeschek, M., Vallapurackal, J., Pinheiro, V. B., Marlière, P., Panke, S. and Ward, T. R. (2018) *E. coli* Surface Display of Streptavidin for Directed Evolution of an Allylic Deallylase. *Chem. Sci.* 9, pp. 5383–5388.
27. Szponarski, M., Schwizer, F., Ward, T. R. and Gademann, K. (2018) On-Cell Catalysis by Surface Engineering of Live Cells with an Artificial Metalloenzyme. *Commun. Chem.* 1, 84.
28. Tsutsumi, H., Katsuyama, Y., Izumikawa, M., Takagi, M., Fujie, M., Satoh, N., Shin-ya, K. and Ohnishi, Y. (2018) Unprecedented Cyclization Catalyzed by a Cytochrome P450 in Benzastatin Biosynthesis. *J. Am. Chem. Soc.* 140, pp. 6631–6639.
29. Arnold, F. H. (2018) Directed Evolution: Bringing New Chemistry to Life. *Angew. Chem. Int. Ed.* 57, pp. 4143–4148.
30. Breslow, R. and Gellman, S. H. (1982) Tosylamidation of Cyclohexane by a Cytochrome P-450 Model. *J. Chem. Soc. Chem. Commun.* pp. 1400–1401.
31. Breslow, R. and Gellman, S. H. (1983) Intramolecular Nitrene Carbon-Hydrogen Insertions Mediated by Transition-Metal Complexes as Nitrogen Analogs of Cytochrome P-450 Reactions. *J. Am. Chem. Soc.* 105, pp. 6728–6729.
32. Mansuy, D., Mahy, J.-P., Dureault, A., Bedi, G. and Battioni, P. (1984) Iron- and Manganese-Porphyrin Catalysed Aziridination of Alkenes by Tosyl- and Acyl-Iminoiodobenzene. *J. Chem. Soc. Chem. Commun.* pp. 1161–1163.
33. Svastits, E. W., Dawson, J. H., Breslow, R. and Gellman, S. H. (1985) Functionalized Nitrogen Atom Transfer Catalyzed by Cytochrome P-450. *J. Am. Chem. Soc.* 107, pp. 6427–6428.
34. Singh, R., Bordeaux, M. and Fasan, R. (2014) P450-Catalyzed Intramolecular sp^3 C–H Amination with Arylsulfonyl Azide Substrates. *ACS Catal.* 4, pp. 546–552.
35. Singh, R., Kolev, J. N., Sutera, P. A. and Fasan, R. (2015) Enzymatic C(sp^3)-H Amination: P450-Catalyzed Conversion of Carbonazidates into Oxazolidinones. *ACS Catal.* 5, pp. 1685–1691.
36. Dydio, P., Key, H. M., Hayashi, H., Clark, D. S. and Hartwig, J. F. (2017) Chemoselective, Enzymatic C–H Bond Amination Catalyzed by a Cytochrome P450 Containing an Ir(Me)-PIX Cofactor. *J. Am. Chem. Soc.* 139, pp. 1750–1753.
37. Prier, C. K., Zhang, R. K., Buller, A. R., Brinkmann-Chen, S. and Arnold, F. H. (2017) Enantioselective, Intermolecular Benzylic C–H Amination Catalysed by an Engineered Iron-Haem Enzyme. *Nature Chem.* 9, pp. 629–634.
38. Brandenberg, O. F., Miller, D. C., Markel, U., Ouald Chaib, A. and Arnold, F. H. (2019) Engineering Chemoselectivity in Hemoprotein-Catalyzed Indole Amidation. *ACS Catal.* 9, pp. 8271–8275.

39. Farwell, C. C., Zhang, R. K., McIntosh, J. A., Hyster, T. K. and Arnold, F. H. (2015) Enantioselective Enzyme-Catalyzed Aziridination Enabled by Active-Site Evolution of a Cytochrome P450. *ACS Cent. Sci.* 1, pp. 89–93.
40. Roelfes, G. (2019) LmrR: A Privileged Scaffold for Artificial Metalloenzymes. *Acc. Chem. Res.* 52, pp. 545–556.
41. Bos, J., Browne, W. R., Driessen, A. J. M. and Roelfes, G. (2015) Supramolecular Assembly of Artificial Metalloenzymes Based on the Dimeric Protein LmrR as Promiscuous Scaffold. *J. Am. Chem. Soc.* 137, pp. 9796–9799.
42. Chordia, S., Narasimhan, S., Lucini Paioni, A., Baldus, M. and Roelfes, G. (2021) *In Vivo* Assembly of Artificial Metalloenzymes and Application in Whole-Cell Biocatalysis. *Angew. Chem. Int. Ed.* 60, pp. 5913–5920.
43. Villarino, L., Splan, K. E., Reddem, E., Alonso-Cotchico, L., Gutiérrez de Souza, C., Lledós, A., Maréchal, J.-D., Thunnissen, A.-M. W. H. and Roelfes, G. (2018) An Artificial Heme Enzyme for Cyclopropanation Reactions. *Angew. Chem. Int. Ed.* 57, pp. 7785–7789.
44. Zhao, J., Bachmann, D. G., Lenz, M., Gillingham, D. G. and Ward, T. R. (2018) An Artificial Metalloenzyme for Carbene Transfer Based on a Biotinylated Dirhodium Anchored within Streptavidin. *Catal. Sci. Technol.* 8, pp. 2294–2298.
45. Coelho, P. S., Brustad, E. M., Kannan, A. and Arnold, F. H. (2013) Olefin Cyclopropanation via Carbene Transfer Catalyzed by Engineered Cytochrome P450 Enzymes. *Science* 339, pp. 307–310.
46. Reynolds, E. W., McHenry, M. W., Cannac, F., Gober, J. G., Snow, C. D. and Brustad, E. M. (2016) An Evolved Orthogonal Enzyme/Cofactor Pair. *J. Am. Chem. Soc.* 138, pp. 12451–12458.
47. Reynolds, E. W., Schwochert, T. D., McHenry, M. W., Watters, J. W. and Brustad, E. M. (2017) Orthogonal Expression of an Artificial Metalloenzyme for Abiotic Catalysis. *Chem Bio Chem.* 18, pp. 2380–2384.
48. Tinoco, A., Wei, Y., Bacik, J.-P., Carminati, D. M., Moore, E. J., Ando, N., Zhang, Y. and Fasan, R. (2019) Origin of High Stereocontrol in Olefin Cyclopropanation Catalyzed by an Engineered Carbene Transferase. *ACS Catal.* 9, pp. 1514–1524.
49. Tinoco, A., Steck, V., Tyagi, V. and Fasan, R. (2017) Highly Diastereo- and Enantioselective Synthesis of Trifluoromethyl-Substituted Cyclopropanes via Myoglobin-Catalyzed Transfer of Trifluoromethylcarbene. *J. Am. Chem. Soc.* 139, pp. 5293–5296.
50. Vargas, D. A., Tinoco, A., Tyagi, V. and Fasan, R. (2018) Myoglobin-Catalyzed C−H Functionalization of Unprotected Indoles. *Angew. Chem. Int. Ed.* 57, pp. 9911–9915.
51. Oohora, K., Meichin, H., Zhao, L., Wolf, M. W., Nakayama, A., Hasegawa, J., Lehnert, N. and Hayashi, T. (2017) Catalytic Cyclopropanation by Myoglobin

Reconstituted with Iron Porphycene: Acceleration of Catalysis due to Rapid Formation of the Carbene Species. *J. Am. Chem. Soc.* 139, pp. 17265–17268.
52. Oohora, K., Onoda, A. and Hayashi, T. (2019) Hemoproteins Reconstituted with Artificial Metal Complexes as Biohybrid Catalysts. *Acc. Chem. Res.* 52, pp. 945–954.
53. Key, H. M., Dydio, P., Clark, D. S. and Hartwig, J. F. (2016) Abiological Catalysis by Artificial Haem Proteins Containing Noble Metals in Place of Iron. *Nature* 534, pp. 534–537.
54. Dydio, P., Key, H. M., Nazarenko, A., Rha, J. Y.-E., Seyedkazemi, V., Clark, D. S. and Hartwig, J. F. (2016) An Artificial Metalloenzyme with the Kinetics of Native Enzymes. *Science* 354, pp. 102–106.
55. Natoli, S. N., Hartwig and J. F. (2019) Noble−Metal Substitution in Hemoproteins: An Emerging Strategy for a biological Catalysis. *Acc. Chem. Res.* 52, pp. 326–335.
56. Zhang, J., Huang, X., Zhang, R. K. and Arnold, F. H. (2019) Enantiodivergent α-Amino C–H Fluoroalkylation Catalyzed by Engineered Cytochrome P450s. *J. Am. Chem. Soc.* 141, pp. 9798–9802.
57. Funel, J.-A. and Abele, S. (2013) Industrial Applications of the Diels–Alder Reaction. *Angew. Chem. Int. Ed.* 52, pp. 3822–3863.
58. Oikawa, H. (2016) Nature's Strategy for Catalyzing Diels–Alder Reaction. *Cell Chem. Biol.* 23, pp. 429–430.
59. Kim, H. J., Ruszczycky, M. W., Choi, S., Liu, Y. and Liu, H. (2011) Enzyme-Catalysed [4+2] Cycloaddition is a Key Step in the Biosynthesis of Spinosyn A. *Nature*. 473, pp. 109–112.
60. Byrne, M. J., Lees, N. R., Han, L.-C., van der Kamp, M. W., Mulholland, A. J., Stach, J. E. M., Willis, C. L. and Race, P. R. (2016) The Catalytic Mechanism of a Natural Diels–Alderase Revealed in Molecular Detail. *J. Am. Chem. Soc.* 138, pp. 6095–6098.
61. Li, L., Yu, P., Tang, M.-C., Zou, Y., Gao, S.-S., Hung, Y.-S., Zhao, M., Watanabe, K., Houk, K. N. and Tang, Y. (2016) Biochemical Characterization of a Eukaryotic Decalin-Forming Diels–Alderase. *J. Am. Chem. Soc.* 138, pp. 15837–15840.
62. Tan, D., Jamieson, C. S., Ohashi, M., Tang, M.-C., Houk, K. N. and Tang, Y. (2019) Genome-Mined Diels–Alderase Catalyzes Formation of the *cis*-Octahydrodecalins of Varicidin A and B. *J. Am. Chem. Soc.* 141, pp. 769–773.
63. Hilvert, D., Hill, K. W., Nared, K. D. and Auditor, M. T. M. (1989) Antibody Catalysis of the Diels–Alder Reaction. *J. Am. Chem. Soc.* 111, pp. 9261–9262.
64. Braisted, A. C. and Schultz, P. G. (1990) An Antibody-Catalyzed Bimolecular Diels–Alder Reaction. *J. Am. Chem. Soc.* 112, pp. 7430–7431.

65. Gouverneur, V., Houk, K., de Pascual-Teresa, B., Beno, B., Janda, K. and Lerner, R. (1993) Control of the Exo and Endo Pathways of the Diels–Alder Reaction by Antibody Catalysis. *Science* 262, pp. 204–208.
66. Heine, A. (1998) An Antibody exo Diels–Alderase Inhibitor Complex at 1.95 Angstrom Resolution. *Science* 279, pp. 1934–1940.
67. Siegel, J. B., Zanghellini, A., Lovick, H. M., Kiss, G., Lambert, A. R., St. Clair, J. L., Gallaher, J. L., Hilvert, D., Gelb, M. H., Stoddard, B. L., Houk, K. N., Michael, F. E., Baker, D. (2010) Computational Design of an Enzyme Catalyst for a Stereoselective Bimolecular Diels–Alder Reaction. *Science* 329, pp. 309–313.
68. Klas, K., Tsukamoto, S., Sherman, D. H. and Williams, R. M. (2015) Natural Diels–Alderases: Elusive and Irresistable. *J. Org. Chem.* 80, pp. 11672–11685.
69. Ose, T., Watanabe, K., Mie, T., Honma, M., Watanabe, H., Yao, M., Oikawa, H. and Tanaka, I. (2003) Insight into a Natural Diels–Alder Reaction from the Structure of Macrophomate Synthase. *Nature* 422, pp. 185–189.
70. Guimarães, C. R. W., Udier-Blagović, M. and Jorgensen, W. L. (2005) Macrophomate Synthase: QM/MM Simulations Address the Diels–Alder versus Michael–Aldol Reaction Mechanism. *J. Am. Chem. Soc.* 127, pp. 3577–3588.
71. Otto, S., Bertoncin, F. and Engberts, J. B. F. N. (1996) Lewis Acid Catalysis of a Diels–Alder Reaction in Water. *J. Am. Chem. Soc.* 118, pp. 7702–7707.
72. Otto, S. and Engberts, J. B. F. N. (1999) A Systematic Study of Ligand Effects on a Lewis-Acid-Catalyzed Diels–Alder Reaction in Water. Water-Enhanced Enantioselectivity. *J. Am. Chem. Soc.* 121, pp. 6798–6806.
73. Mubofu, E. B. and Engberts, J. B. F. N. (2004) Specific Acid Catalysis and Lewis Acid Catalysis of Diels–Alder Reactions in Aqueous Media. *J. Phys. Org. Chem.* 17, pp. 180–186.
74. Reetz, M. T. and Jiao, N. (2006) Copper–Phthalocyanine Conjugates of Serum Albumins as Enantioselective Catalysts in Diels–Alder Reactions. *Angew. Chem. Int. Ed.* 45, pp. 2416–2419.
75. Reetz, M. T. (2012) Artificial Metalloenzymes as Catalysts in Stereoselective Diels–Alder Reactions. *Chem Rec.* 12, pp. 391–406.
76. Roelfes, G., Boersma, A. J. and Feringa, B. L. (2006) Highly Enantioselective DNA-Based Catalysis. *Chem. Commun.* pp. 635–637.
77. Filice, M., Romero, O., Gutiérrez-Fernández, J., de las Rivas, B., Hermoso, J. A. and Palomo, J. M. (2015) Synthesis of a Heterogeneous Artificial Metallolipase with Chimeric Catalytic Activity. *Chem. Commun.* 51, pp. 9324–9327.
78. Ghattas, W., Cotchico-Alonso, L., Maréchal, J.-D., Urvoas, A., Rousseau, M., Mahy, J.-P. and Ricoux, R. (2016) Artificial Metalloenzymes with the

Neocarzinostatin Scaffold: Toward a Biocatalyst for the Diels–Alder Reaction. *ChemBioChem.* 17, pp. 433–440.

79. Talbi, B., Haquette, P., Martel, A., de Montigny, F., Fosse, C., Cordier, S., Roisnel, T., Jaouen, G. and Salmain, M. (2010) (η6-Arene) Rthenium(ii) Complexes and Metallo-Papain Hybrid as Lewis Acid Catalysts of Diels–Alder Reaction in Water. *Dalton Trans.* 39, pp. 5605.
80. Di Meo, T., Ghattas, W., Herrero, C., Velours, C., Minard, P., Mahy, J.-P., Ricoux, R. and Urvoas, A. (2017) αRep A3: A Versatile Artificial Scaffold for Metalloenzyme Design. *Chem. Eur. J.* 23, pp. 10156–10166.
81. Di Meo, T., Kariyawasam, K., Ghattas, W., Valerio-Lepiniec, M., Sciortino, G., Maréchal, J.-D., Minard, P., Mahy, J.-P., Urvoas, A. and Ricoux, R. (2019) Functionalized Artificial Bidomain Proteins Based on an α-Solenoid Protein Repeat Scaffold: A New Class of Artificial Diels–Alderases. *ACS Omega* 4, pp. 4437–4447.
82. Himiyama, T., Taniguchi, N., Kato, S., Onoda, A. and Hayashi, T. (2017) A Pyrene-Linked Cavity within a β-Barrel Protein Promotes an Asymmetric Diels–Alder Reaction. *Angew. Chem. Int. Ed.* 56, pp. 13618–13622.
83. Deuss, P. J., Popa, G., Slawin, A. M. Z., Laan, W. and Kamer, P. C. J. (2013) Artificial Copper Enzymes for Asymmetric Diels–Alder Reactions. *ChemCatChem.* 5, pp. 1184–1191.
84. Bos, J., Fusetti, F., Driessen, A. J. M. and Roelfes, G. (2012) Enantioselective Artificial Metalloenzymes by Creation of a Novel Active Site at the Protein Dimer Interface. *Angew. Chem. Int. Ed.* 51, pp. 7472–7475.
85. Podtetenieff, J., Taglieber, A., Bill, E., Reijerse, E. J. and Reetz, M. T. (2010) An Artificial Metalloenzyme: Creation of a Designed Copper Binding Site in a Thermostable Protein. *Angew. Chem. Int. Ed.* 49, pp. 5151–5155.
86. Ghattas, W., Dubosclard, V., Tachon, S., Beaumet, M., Guillot, R., Réglier, M., Simaan, A. J. and Mahy, J.-P. (2019) Cu^{II}-Containing 1-Aminocyclopropane Carboxylic Acid Oxidase is an Efficient Stereospecific Diels–Alderase. *Angew. Chem. Int. Ed.* 58, pp. 14605–14609.
87. Ghattas, W., Dubosclard, V., Wick, A., Bendelac, A., Guillot, R., Ricoux, R. and Mahy, J.-P. (2018) Receptor-Based Artificial Metalloenzymes on Living Human Cells. *J. Am. Chem. Soc.* 140, pp. 8756–8762.

https://doi.org/10.1142/9789811261664_bmatter

Index

www.ingramcontent.com/pod-product-compliance
Lightning Source LLC
LaVergne TN
LVHW010326220926
848484LV00004BB/845
* 9 7 8 9 8 1 1 2 6 1 6 5 7 *